Medical Group Management Association

Cost Survey

2004 REPORT BASED ON 2003 DATA

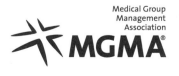

Medical Group
Management
Association

MGMA®

www.mgma.com

2004 MGMA Survey Advisory Committee Members

Fred Simmons, Jr., CPA, *Chair*
Chief Executive Officer
Clearwater Cardiovascular and
Interventional Consultants
Clearwater, FL

David Taylor, CMPE
Director of Operations
Cox Health Systems
Springfield, MO

Glen Lawson, MHA, CMPE
Administrator
Rehlen, Bartlow and Goodman MDs, Inc.
Santa Ana, CA

Bruce A. Johnson, JD, MPA
Principal
MGMA Health Care Consulting Group
Medical Group Management Association
Erie, CO

Board Liaison
Michael L. Nochomovitz, MD
President & Chief Medical Officer
University Primary & Specialty Care Practices
University Hospitals Health System
Cleveland, OH

Julie Lineberger, FACMPE
Administrator
Orthopedic Surgery Center of Idaho
Solutions Group
Boise, ID

Jane Dodds, MPH, FACMPE
Administrator
Orthopedic Associates of Rochester
Rochester, NY

Jeffrey Mossoff, CMPE
Executive Vice President
University Clinical Associates
University of Mississippi
Jackson, MS

David Gortner, MD
Section Head, Internal Medicine
Virginia Mason Medical Center
Seattle, WA

Academic Practice Committee Chair
Herb Stanley
Interim Executive Director
University Physicians
University of Missouri Columbia
Columbia, MO

The *Cost Survey: 2004 Report Based on 2003 Data* was compiled by the Medical Group Management Association (MGMA) Survey Operations Department. The Survey Operations Department staff members responsible for this and other MGMA surveys are:

Ruth Gaulke, MAPW, Survey Analyst III
Allison Gault, Data Specialist
Suman Elizabeth Graeber, MHA, Survey Manager
Danielle C. Guillen, Data Specialist
Rusalyn A. Herington, MBA, Production Manager
Fran L. Iannucci, MS, Survey Analyst II
Heather C. Jones, Department Coordinator

Mariann Lowery, Production Coordinator
Lori L. McNeilley, Survey Analyst II
Mark W. Peterson, MS, Survey Analyst I
Daniel P. Stech, MBA, CMPE, Director
Emma Vazirabadi, Survey Analyst I
Brooke L. Whitten, Survey Analyst II
Jay Y. Whitten, Data Specialist

Desktop Publishing by
Vivian Heggie, Heggie Enterprises, Inc.

For further information or questions, please contact Suman Elizabeth Graeber, MHA, Survey Manager or Lori L. McNeilley, Survey Analyst II, toll-free 877.ASK.MGMA (275.6462), ext. 1895.

ISSN #1064-4571
ISBN #1-56829-063-2

September 2004

Dear Colleague:

Thank you for using the Medical Group Management Association (MGMA) **Cost Survey: 2004 Report Based on 2003 Data.** The MGMA survey reports are the leading financial benchmark references of the medical group management profession.

If you have this report because your practice participated in the survey, we appreciate your contributions to the data. A major benefit of participating in the surveys is a complimentary copy of the report. You can also take pride in knowing that you have helped build the most comprehensive database of medical group practice information available.

If you are involved in the management of a practice that did not submit data, I strongly encourage you to take part in next yearís survey. Greater participation makes the survey report even more credible and valuable to you, your practice and your colleagues. The survey process is not difficult and MGMA Survey Operations Department staff is available to provide assistance.

The report is organized to allow you to easily compare your practiceís performance and key data to those of your peers. The executive summary and appendices include important information that will help you understand the data and make more meaningful comparisons. I am sure you will agree that the survey data are an important tool in managing, evaluating and assisting a medical practice.

We are always looking for ways to improve our surveys and the survey process. The MGMA Survey Advisory Committee and staff welcome any suggestions you may have that advance our efforts.

Again, thanks for helping to make MGMA survey reports the ìgold standardî in our profession.

Sincerely,

Frederic R. Simmons Jr. CPA
Chair, 2004 MGMA Survey Advisory Committee

Table of Contents

Executive Summary

Demographic Tables and Graphs

Multispecialty Practices

Primary Care Single Specialty Practices by Ownership

Single Specialty Practices, Not Hospital or IDS Owned

Appendices

Important Notice and Disclaimer

The information contained in the *Cost Survey: 2004 Report Based on 2003 Data* is presented solely for the purpose of informing readers of ranges of medical practice charges, revenue, expenses, earnings and staffing, reported by Medical Group Management Association member organizations. These data may not be used for the purpose of limiting competition, restraining trade, or reducing or stabilizing salary or benefit levels. Such improper use is prohibited by federal and state antitrust laws and will violate the antitrust compliance program established and enforced by the MGMA Board of Directors.

MGMA publications are intended to provide current and accurate information, and are designed to assist readers in becoming more familiar with the subject matter covered. MGMA published the *Cost Survey: 2004 Report Based on 2003 Data* for a general audience as well as for MGMA members. Such publications are distributed with the understanding that MGMA does not render any legal, accounting, or professional advice that may be construed as specifically applicable to individual situations. No representations or warranties are made concerning the application of legal or other principles discussed in MGMA publications to any specific factual situation, nor is any prediction made concerning how any particular judge, government official, or other person will interpret or apply such principles. Specific factual situations should be discussed with professional advisors.

Executive Summary

Introduction

Purpose: The Medical Group Management Association (MGMA) *Cost Survey: 2004 Report Based on 2003 Data* is a comprehensive financial census of the MGMA membership designed to assist medical practice administrators in measuring and improving their organization's performance. Information is presented on revenue, staffing, operating costs and other critical performance metrics for practices reporting at least three full-time equivalent (FTE) physicians. Ongoing assessment of these areas can provide the framework for the continuous quality improvement (CQI) process that can help practices become more efficient and reduce costs.

Effective management of cost and quality is essential in the ever-changing and increasingly competitive business of health care. This report is a practical tool that can be used to evaluate efficiency and, in conjunction with other MGMA products, assist practices in maximizing quality and managing costs.

Description: The first MGMA *Cost Survey* was conducted in 1947. For 57 years, the annual *Cost Survey* has provided MGMA members and others with a comparison tool to assist in improving the management of their practices. The *Cost Survey Report* summarizes the financial performance and productivity of responding medical practices. A comprehensive fiscal picture of medical group practice is presented in the report.

Significant metrics contained in the report are: staffing ratios, medical revenue, staff salary costs, total operating costs, revenue after operating costs, provider cost and net practice income/loss. Accounts receivable, payer mix, collection percentages, financial ratios and balance sheet information are also included in the report.

Analyzing productivity is important in assessing the performance of a practice. The *Cost Survey* has productivity measures of Resource-Based Relative Value Scale (RBRVS) units, RBRVS physician work units, patients and procedures.

Data are reported for 20 different types of single-specialty practices and for multispecialty practices. Multispecialty information is reported for all practices, for practices owned by a hospital, practices not owned by a hospital, for primary care only practices, and by geographic section, group size and level of capitation revenue. "All Multispecialty" practice information does not include multispecialty practices with specialty care only.

MGMA Survey Products: In addition to the *Cost Survey,* the MGMA Survey Operations Department conducts other annual surveys of MGMA member practices.

The *Physician Compensation and Production Survey* reports individual physician and nonphysician provider compensation data. This survey report also has productivity data including collections, professional gross charges, ambulatory encounters, hospital encounters, surgical/anesthesia cases, total RBRVS units and physician work RVUs. Ratios of compensation to gross charges and compensation per physician work RVU are calculated.

Another compensation survey conducted by MGMA is the *Management Compensation Survey.* The report includes compensation, bonus and retirement benefit amounts for physician executives and for various upper and middle level manager positions.

MGMA also conducts a parallel survey in the academic sector. The *Academic Practice Compensation and Production Survey for Faculty & Management* provides compensation and productivity levels for medical school physician faculty. Clinical science department and practice plan managerial compensation and benefit information is also reported.

The MGMA *Cost Survey Report* and *Physician Compensation and Production Survey Report* are available in both printed format and as an interactive CD, which includes more comprehensive statistics and additional data not found in the printed report.

A *Cost Survey* respondent ranking report, comparing the respondent's data against the survey medians, is computed and distributed only to respondents to enable them to easily identify measures that might warrant further review and improvement.

Also, surveys have been conducted of selected clinical specialties and special interest groups within MGMA. Cost survey reports will be available for anesthesia practices, cardiovascular/thoracic surgery and cardiology practices, orthopedic practices, pediatric practices, urology practices and for practices within integrated delivery systems.

Additional reports are available for ambulatory surgery centers and management services organizations.

Better Performing Practices: The *Cost Survey* database is the basis for selecting medical groups that meet or exceed standards of financial success. An in-depth analysis of "better performing" medical group practices is presented in a companion publication, the *Performance and Practices of Successful Medical Groups.*

Survey Advisory Committee: The MGMA Survey Advisory Committee provided guidance on the format and content of this report as well as the related questionnaire and guide to ensure that the survey addresses current and relevant practice management areas. The committee members are listed on page two.

Survey Methodology

Changes to the Instrument and Report: Only minor modifications were made to the survey questionnaire and report in response to suggestions by survey users and the Survey Advisory Committee.

The report itself is similar to last year's report.

Data Collection: Survey questionnaires were mailed in early April 2004 to MGMA member and nonmember organizations. While predominantly medical group practices, the MGMA membership includes many other types of organizations involved in physician practice management. Printed questionnaires were mailed to selected organizations that were, or were presumed to be, affiliated with medical practices. Available on the MGMA Web site were a downloadable electronic version of the questionnaire and a printable version.

Participation Burden: Under the direction of the Survey Advisory Committee, a short form version of the *Cost Survey Questionnaire* was distributed to a random sample of practices, in order to ease the participation burden and increase responses from single specialty practices. Including only 48 key variables, the short form version was also mailed to practices in the specialties of anesthesiology, hematology/oncology, pediatrics and urology. The data captured through the traditional, comprehensive *Questionnaire* and the short form versions were combined and are included within the tables in this report.

Data Editing: A critical aspect of the survey process is the editing phase. Editing is the process of identifying reported errors, mathematical miscalculations, inconsistencies and extreme values for follow-up and resolution. Questionnaires were classified as valid cases, ineligible, or incomplete cases. By default, all cases were valid initially. Practices that identified themselves as an academic practice, or a freestanding ambulatory surgery center were reclassified as ineligible. Practices having fewer than three full-time equivalent (FTE) physicians were also considered ineligible, as has historically been the case. However, an exception was made this year for the first time to include practices with fewer than three FTE if they were

hospital/IDS owned single-specialty practices in allergy/immunology and surgical: neurological.

Questionnaires were classified as incomplete if any of the following key information was not reported:

- Fiscal year
- Practice type
- Single-specialty practice type for single-specialty practices
- Freestanding ambulatory surgery center
- Medical school faculty practice plan
- Majority owner
- Total medical revenue
- Total support staff FTE and cost
- Total general operating cost
- Total operating cost
- Total medical revenue after operating cost
- Total physician FTE and cost
- Organization name
- State

Guidelines were developed to structure the editing process. The MGMA Survey Operations Department *Cost Survey* team examined all questionnaires. Extreme data were analyzed on a practice, variable by variable, and on a case by case basis. These outliers were also examined by multispecialty and single-specialty type. For accounts receivable aging, balance sheet and payer mix, all data in each section were suppressed if any of the questions in the section were not answered.

Response Rate: In January 2004, 11,054 organizations were identified in the MGMA constituent database. A goal of this survey was to obtain as many responses as possible from medical practices. The frame selection had two objectives: 1) to solicit increased participation, and 2) to focus resources intended to generate response primarily from eligible organizations. Eligible organizations are those organizations defined by MGMA as "medical practices" having three or more FTE physicians, or noted exceptions described previously. Other organizations that own or manage medical practices such as hospitals, management services organizations and integrated delivery systems may participate in the survey on behalf of their respective medical practices. Additional non-member organizations were mailed a questionnaire due to MGMA's collaboration with the American Urological Association (AUA) (additional 743 organizations) and the American Academy of Pediatrics (AAP) (additional 828 organizations).

Ultimately 12,614 organizations received questionnaires, some of which may not have been eligible to respond to the *Cost Survey*. Examples of these organizations that were not qualified to respond include medical service and supply vendors and pharmaceutical companies. If an organization had no identifying information in the database, it was excluded from the survey frame to promote a more known and homogenous sample.

Of the survey questionnaires mailed to member and nonmember individuals associated with one of the previously mentioned organizations, 195 were determined to be undeliverable.

Ultimately, the number of questionnaires actually distributed to organizations identified in the MGMA database was 12,419. Respondents returned 1,608 questionnaires, including 874 surveys in electronic format and 734 paper surveys. Of these returned questionnaires, 366 questionnaires were determined to be ineligible or incomplete and were not included in the tables within this report.

In total, data from 1,242 responses were included in this report. The response rate for this survey was 12.9 percent. Hospitals, integrated health systems, management services organizations and other entities that provide or assist in the provision of physician services comprised 223 responses.

This survey continues to capture an increasing number of organizations not formally affiliated with MGMA through membership.

Limitations of the Data: It is recommended to use caution in interpreting the data in this report. The report is based on a voluntary response by primarily MGMA member practices and data may not be representative of all providers in medical practices. Additionally, note that the respondents vary from year to year. Therefore, conclusions about longitudinal trends or year-to-year fluctuations in summary statistics may not be appropriate.

Other sources of potential bias exist. Since the survey is designed primarily for traditional medical practices, organizations that have diverged from this model may find the questionnaire design difficult for reporting their financial information. The user of this report should also be mindful of the number of respondents (listed as "counts") reported within the tables.

Other findings were discovered in connection with measures of certain specialties where widely varying data were reported among the observed practices between 2002 and 2003 data. While significant resources were dedicated to validating the data, some questions remain regarding observed shifts in the data. Report users are urged to exercise caution when basing decisions on these data.

Confidentiality: The MGMA and MGMA Center for Research Policy on Data Confidentiality states: "All data submitted to MGMA and the MGMA Center for Research will be kept confidential. All submitted data and related materials that identify a specific organization or individual will be safeguarded and will not be published or voluntarily released within the public domain without written permission."

Only summary statistics will be published. A summary statistic will be reported only if there are sufficient responses to be statistically reliable and if the anonymity of those submitting data is protected.

In compliance with the MGMA policy, an asterisk (*) denotes data that have been suppressed to ensure confidentiality.

When counts are low, 10 to 15 responses, it is important to understand that the information reported may not be reflective of the industry. For example, "Radiology" displays a maximum of 12 responses per value in the 15.* tables. Although extensive editing was conducted for this specialty, the participants portrayed here may not reflect all Radiology practices, and exhibit some variations from prior years.

Data Computations

Calculations: Most of the data presented in the report are calculated variables. Calculations were performed to create financial measures such as return on equity, to convert data into percentages or ratios, to calculate totals such as total cost, or to normalize the data to accommodate differences in the size of responding practices. The calculations used in the report appear in Appendix C: Calculations and Formulas on page 266.

Data Normalization: The survey respondents included in the report were practices ranging from three physicians (see exceptions under data editing section) to several hundred. Since performance data are directly related to the size of the practice, it was necessary to normalize the data to neutralize the impact of group size. For example, reporting median revenue is not very helpful when differences can be attributed to size and not performance. Reporting revenue *per FTE physician* provides a more meaning-ful measure. The calculations for data normalization appear in Appendix C: Calculations and Formulas on page 266. The variables used as denominators to normalize data in the *Cost Survey Report* are:

Per FTE physician

As a percent of total medical revenue

Per FTE provider
Per square foot
Per total RVU
Per work RVU
Per patient

How to Use This Report

It is important to understand how the information is collected and defined in the survey. Appendices E and F reproduce the *Cost Survey: 2004 Questionnaire Based on 2003 Data* and the *Cost Survey: 2004 Guide to the Questionnaire Based on 2003 Data*. These Appendices are a very important reference for the user since they provide detailed definitions and formulas for the questions on the questionnaire.

Report Organization: Data results begin on page 27. There are 16 data sections in the report. Multispecialty practice data are reported in the first eight, followed by three sections of primary care specialties: family practice, internal medicine and pediatrics, displayed with not hospital-owned and all owner values. The final five sections of data represent 17 not hospital-owned single specialties. The section number is the first number that appears in the table number (before the decimal point).

Each data section contains multiple tables. The table number appears after the decimal point (i.e., Table 4.5b means section 4, table 5b). The first three tables present staffing, accounts receivable, collection percentages, financial ratios and payer mix data. Tables *.4a through *.4f present staffing breakouts, charges and revenue, operating cost, provider cost, net income and balance sheet information — all normalized by FTE physician. Tables *.5a through *.5e present similar information as a percent of total medical revenue. Data are also reported per FTE provider (Tables *.6a through *.6b); per square foot (Tables *.7a through *.7b); per total RVU (Tables *.8a through *.8b); per physician work RVU (Tables *.9a through *.9b); and per patient (Tables *.10a through *.10b). Tables *.11a through *.11h present procedural and charge data. Page headers and sidebars assist in table location.

Statistical Interpretation: The median is reported in all tables. The term "median" can be used synonymously with 50th percentile rank. In addition to the median, some tables include the 10th, 25th, 75th, and 90th percentiles along with the mean and standard deviation, so the reader can better understand the distribution of the data. The reader is strongly encouraged to use the median as the measure of central tendency, as the median is not subject to the distortion that may occur in the mean

when extremely high or low values are in the data set.

When interpreting the meaning of percentile ranks, the reader must exercise judgment as to the desirability of high or low ranking. In considering the value "Total medical revenue after operating cost" displayed in Table 2.5c, the astute user of this report will realize that a practice ranking in the 90th percentile has been more profitable in the year 2003 than practices ranking in the 10th percentile. While, in contrast, observing "Total operating cost" in Table 2.5b shows identical percentile rankings, but the meaning of a high ranking here is less desirable to the medical practice. Practices typically strive for cost containment and those ranking in the 10th percentile would have achieved more desirable levels of performance than those ranking in the 90th percentile.

The reader must also exercise caution in evaluating the meaning of median values in specific tables. An example of this is the accounts receivable aging data in Table 1.2. A reader may believe the medians for the aging categories should sum to 100%. By their nature, however, the sum of the medians probably will not equal 100%. This is because the practice that is at the median for 31 to 60 days in AR may not be the same practice that is at the median for 61 to 90 days in AR. The means, however, when summed, will equal 100% if two conditions exist; the respondents reported data for all categories and each individual response adds to 100%. The survey methodology ensures that the first condition is met, but not the second. Although the data editing staff attempts to edit all responses, not all arithmetic errors are resolved, particularly those with errors less than 10%. The prioritization of data editing activities directs editing resources to those responses with the highest percentage of arithmetic errors. Therefore, means will not necessarily add to 100%. The same situation occurs with the support staff FTE breakouts not equaling total FTE support staff in Table 1.4a, as well as all situations where the components of sums are reported in the tables.

Another example of questionable use of the medians concerns using medians to calculate ratios or other financial indicators. Dividing median net fee-for-service (FFS) revenue by median gross FFS charges will not necessarily equal the median gross FFS collection percent in Table 1.2. Once again, this is because the practice that is at the median for net FFS revenue is probably different from the practice that is at the median for gross FFS charges, both of which are probably different form the practice that is the median for gross FFS collection percent. The gross FFS collection percentage is most appropriately calculated individually for each respondent prior to the median being generated.

Key Findings: The key to success for medical practices is providing quality care in an efficient manner. The *Cost Survey Report* can be used as a management tool to gauge a practice's efficiency and performance. The survey includes historical data in several important areas:

Cost structure: Graph 1 on page 17 depicts the breakdown of total cost. This breakdown includes three cost categories: support staff, operating and provider. There are multiple breakouts of operating cost. For the purpose of this graph, only the main breakouts of building and occupancy, medical/surgical supply, information systems, ancillary service and other general operating cost are shown. Physician cost is the largest expense, followed by support staff cost.

Collection percentages: The billing (charges) and collection (revenue) functions are critical components of practice management. Graph 2 on page 17 shows that since the 1980s, the gross FFS collection percent has steadily declined, and that trend continued into 2003. This is not surprising given medical practices' experience away from managed care and towards FFS reimbursements. This is a shift from the past few years where the growth of managed care and the downward pressure on reimbursement were factors driving down the collection percentages.

The adjusted FFS collection percent reflects collections after adjustment to the billed charge (contractual adjustments, Medicare/Medicaid charge restrictions, etc.), indicating the efficacy of billing and collection functions. This percentage has exhibited very small fluctuations over the past 10 years.

Changes in revenue and expenses: Graph 3 on page 18 depicts the 15-year trend for total medical revenue, total operating cost and total medical revenue after operating cost for multispecialty practices. Since 1989, total medical revenue per FTE physician has increased 66.4%, from $352,334 to $586,381. Total operating cost per FTE physician, however, increased 84.3%, from $189,462 to $349,090. The result has been an increase in revenue after operating cost from $152,903 to $232,052, a 14-year increase of 51.8%.

Changes in Operating Cost as a Percent of Total Medical Revenue: Graph 4 on page 18 depicts the change in practice "overhead" in the 15-year period for multispecialty, family practice, orthopedic surgery and cardiology practices. This ratio is a calculation of total operating cost divided by total medical revenue and provides the reader with an understanding of the relationship between cost and revenue.

Feedback: If you have questions concerning the survey results or comments on how this report, the survey questionnaire or the guide can be improved, please contact the MGMA Survey Operations Department toll-free, 877.ASK-MGMA (275.6462), ext. 895, or e-mail surveys@mgma.com. Purchasing information for the MGMA survey reports appears on the inside back cover of this report.

List of Data Tables

The layout of this report includes 16 sections grouped by – multispecialty practices, primary care single-specialty practices by ownership and single-specialty practices, not hospital or IDS owned. Each section contains category breakouts consisting of 14 pages of tables. The following list provides the title for each table. The asterisks indicate a section number from 1 through 16.

NOTES:

THIS PAGE INTENTIONALLY LEFT BLANK

Demographic Tables and Graphs

Table A: Multispecialty (Primary and Specialty Care), Multispecialty (Primary Care Only) and Selected Single Specialties
Median Values for Key Practice Indicators per 10,000 Encounters

	Multispecialty with primary and specialty care	Multispecialty with primary care only	Internal Medicine*	Family Practice*	Pediatrics*
Total gross charges	$177	$116	$119	$116	$115.00
Medical revenue after operating cost	$47	$32	$34	$35	$31.00
Total cost	$115	$79	$90	$84	$88.00
Total general operating cost	$32.98	$22.00	$25.00	$23.00	$24.00
Total support staff FTE	9.88	7.20	9	8	*
Total support staff cost	$34.87	$23.10	$35	$27	*
Physician work RVUs	1	0.80	1.00	0.89	*
Total RVUs	2	2	1.40	1.86	*
Square feet	0.38	0.28	0.33	0.35	0.28
Encounters per patient	3	3	4	3	*

* Data includes hospital/IDS owned single specialty groups.

Table A: Multispecialty (Primary and Specialty Care), Multispecialty (Primary Care Only) and Selected Single Specialties
Median Values for Key Practice Indicators per 10,000 Encounters (continued)

	Cardiology*	Gastroenterology*	OB/GYN*	Ophthalmology*	Surgery: General*
Total gross charges	$444.00	$392.00	$235.00	$229.00	$360.00
Medical revenue after operating cost	$103.00	$112.00	$68.00	$69.00	$109.00
Total cost	$195.00	$179.00	$150.00	$137.00	$184.00
Total general operating cost	$46.00	$31.00	$36.00	$36.00	$37.00
Total support staff FTE	11	13	10	14	11
Total support staff cost	$48.00	$42.00	$39.00	$42.00	$43.00
Physician work RVUs	1.88	2.52	1.95	2.4	2.36
Total RVUs	4	4.3	4.12	4.53	5.03
Square feet	0.34	0.42	0.39	0.44	0.43
Encounters per patient	3	2	2	2	2.28

* Data includes hospital/IDS owned single specialty groups.

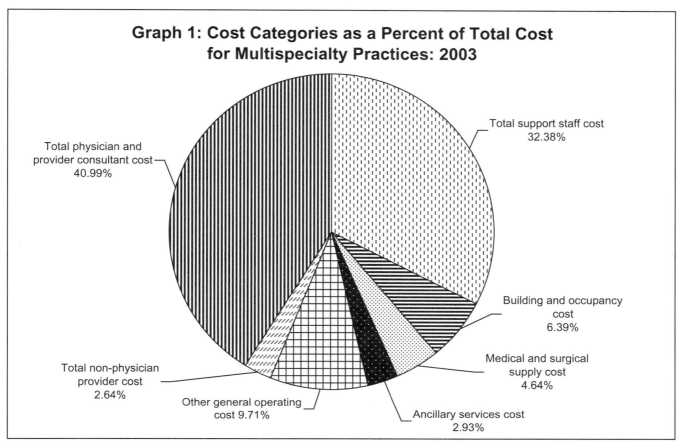

Graph 1: Cost Categories as a Percent of Total Cost for Multispecialty Practices: 2003

Total support staff cost
32.38%

Total physician and provider consultant cost
40.99%

Building and occupancy cost
6.39%

Medical and surgical supply cost
4.64%

Total non-physician provider cost
2.64%

Other general operating cost 9.71%

Ancillary services cost
2.93%

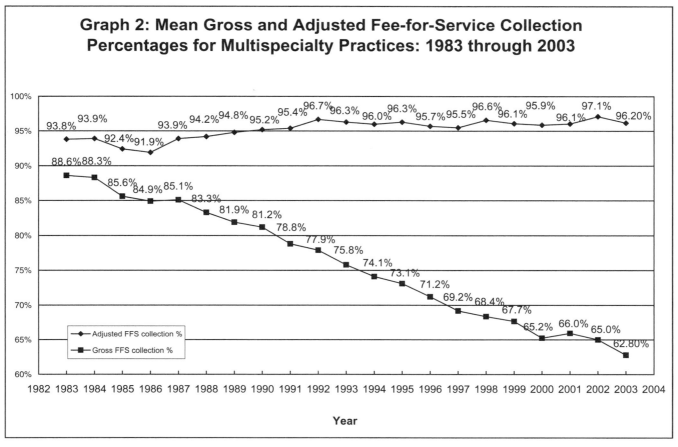

Graph 2: Mean Gross and Adjusted Fee-for-Service Collection Percentages for Multispecialty Practices: 1983 through 2003

Adjusted FFS collection %: 93.8%, 93.9%, 92.4%, 91.9%, 93.9%, 94.2%, 94.8%, 95.2%, 95.4%, 96.7%, 96.3%, 96.0%, 96.3%, 95.7%, 95.5%, 96.6%, 96.1%, 95.9%, 96.1%, 97.1%, 96.20%

Gross FFS collection %: 88.6%, 88.3%, 85.6%, 84.9%, 85.1%, 83.3%, 81.9%, 81.2%, 78.8%, 77.9%, 75.8%, 74.1%, 73.1%, 71.2%, 69.2%, 68.4%, 67.7%, 65.2%, 66.0%, 65.0%, 62.80%

Year

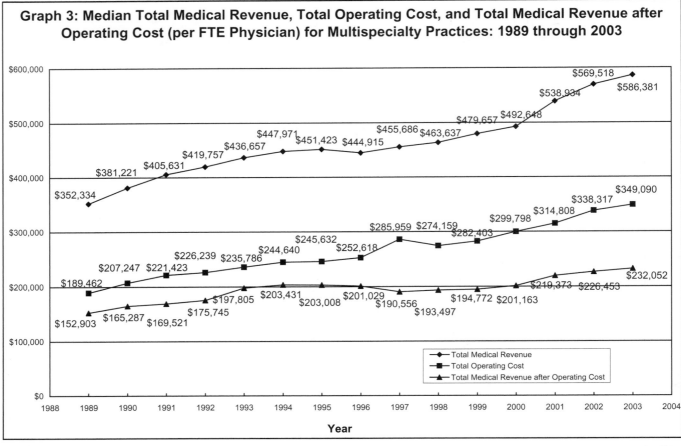

Graph 3: Median Total Medical Revenue, Total Operating Cost, and Total Medical Revenue after Operating Cost (per FTE Physician) for Multispecialty Practices: 1989 through 2003

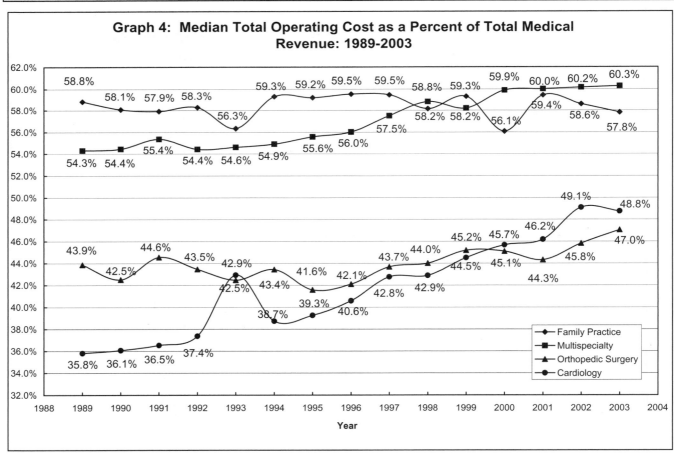

Graph 4: Median Total Operating Cost as a Percent of Total Medical Revenue: 1989-2003

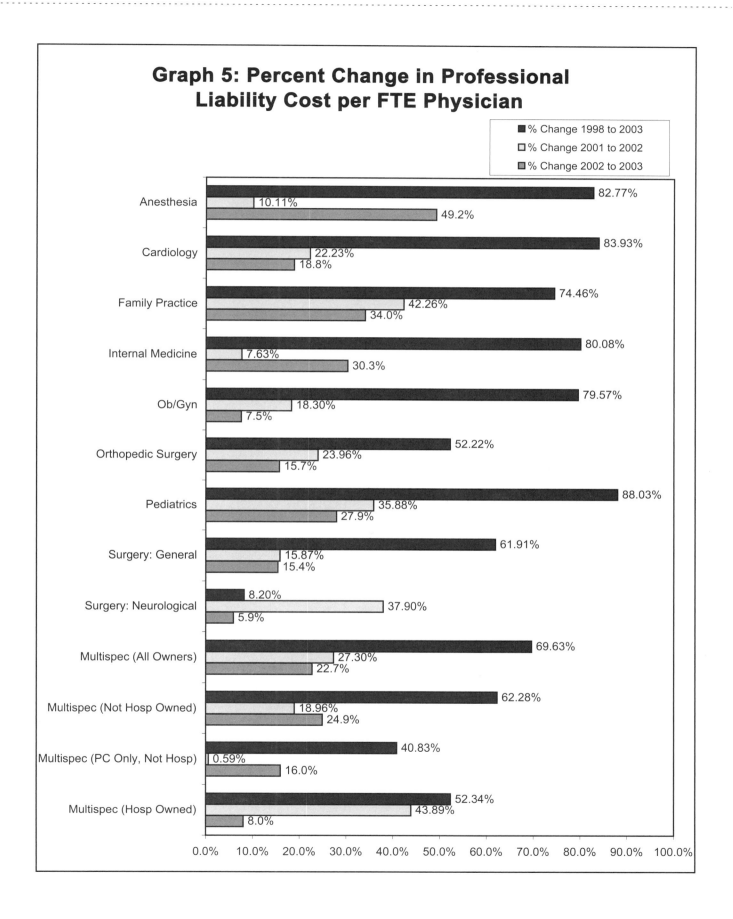

Graph 5: Percent Change in Professional Liability Cost per FTE Physician

Legend:
- ■ % Change 1998 to 2003
- □ % Change 2001 to 2002
- ▨ % Change 2002 to 2003

Category	% Change 1998 to 2003	% Change 2001 to 2002	% Change 2002 to 2003
Anesthesia	82.77%	10.11%	49.2%
Cardiology	83.93%	22.23%	18.8%
Family Practice	74.46%	42.26%	34.0%
Internal Medicine	80.08%	7.63%	30.3%
Ob/Gyn	79.57%	18.30%	7.5%
Orthopedic Surgery	52.22%	23.96%	15.7%
Pediatrics	88.03%	35.88%	27.9%
Surgery: General	61.91%	15.87%	15.4%
Surgery: Neurological	8.20%	37.90%	5.9%
Multispec (All Owners)	69.63%	27.30%	22.7%
Multispec (Not Hosp Owned)	62.28%	18.96%	24.9%
Multispec (PC Only, Not Hosp)	40.83%	0.59%	16.0%
Multispec (Hosp Owned)	52.34%	43.89%	8.0%

0.0% 10.0% 20.0% 30.0% 40.0% 50.0% 60.0% 70.0% 80.0% 90.0% 100.0%

Medical Practice Demographics

1. Responses Received*

	Count
Questionnaires received	1,608
Ineligible/incomplete cases	366
Eligible/complete cases	1,242

2. Geographic Section

	Count	Percent
Eastern section	328	26.41%
Midwest section	302	24.32%
Southern section	348	28.02%
Western section	264	21.26%
Total	1,242	100.00%

3. Demographic Classification

	Count	Percent
Non-metropolitan (under 50,000)	192	21.60%
Metropolitan (50,001 to 250,000)	275	30.93%
Metropolitan (250,001 to 1,000,000)	270	30.37%
Metropolitan (over 1,000,000)	152	17.10%
Total	889	100.00%

4. State

	Count	Percent
Alaska	1	.08%
Alabama	18	1.45%
Arkansas	18	1.45%
Arizona	14	1.13%
California	48	3.86%
Colorado	44	3.54%
Connecticut	15	1.21%
District of Columbia	2	.16%
Delaware	5	.40%
Florida	47	3.78%
Georgia	46	3.70%
Hawaii	2	.16%
Iowa	26	2.09%
Idaho	7	.56%
Illinois	34	2.74%
Indiana	36	2.90%
Kansas	24	1.93%
Kentucky	14	1.13%
Louisiana	16	1.29%
Massachusetts	15	1.21%
Maryland	17	1.37%
Maine	15	1.21%
Michigan	49	3.95%
Minnesota	38	3.06%
Missouri	22	1.77%
Mississippi	6	.48%
Montana	13	1.05%
Nebraska	17	1.37%
New Hampshire	8	.64%
New Jersey	21	1.69%
New Mexico	1	.08%
Nevada	7	.56%
New York	40	3.22%
North Carolina	106	8.53%
North Dakota	4	.32%
Ohio	60	4.83%
Oklahoma	5	.40%
Oregon	51	4.11%
Pennsylvania	42	3.38%
Rhode Island	3	.24%
South Carolina	20	1.61%
South Dakota	8	.64%
Tennessee	45	3.62%
Texas	67	5.39%
Utah	13	1.05%
Virginia	37	2.98%
Washington	59	4.75%
Wisconsin	30	2.42%
West Virginia	2	.16%
Wyoming	4	.32%
Total	1,242	100.00%

Medical Practice Demographics (continued)

5. Legal Organization

	Count	Percent
Business corporation	227	18.31%
Limited liability company	100	8.06%
Not-for-profit corporation/foundation	156	12.58%
Partnership	56	4.52%
Professional corporation/association	672	54.19%
Sole proprietorship	1	.08%
Other	28	2.26%
Total	1,240	100.00%

6. Organization Ownership

	Count	Percent
Government	3	.24%
IDS or hospital	197	15.86%
Insurance company or HMO	1	.08%
MSO or PPMC	6	.48%
Physicians	1,019	82.05%
Other	16	1.29%
Total	1,242	100.00%

7. Group Type

	Count	Percent
Single specialty	918	73.91%
Multispecialty with primary and spec care	233	18.76%
Multispecialty with primary care only	66	5.31%
Multispecialty with specialty care only	25	2.01%
Total	1,242	100.00%

8. Single-specialty Group Type

	Count	Percent
Allergy/Immunology	11	1.20%
Anesthesiology	62	6.75%
Anesthesiology: Pain Management	32	3.49%
Cardiology	88	9.59%
Dermatology	3	.33%
Dermatology: MOHS Surgery	1	.11%
Emergency Medicine	5	.54%
Family Practice	102	11.11%
Gastroenterology	37	4.03%
Hematology/Oncology	32	3.49%
Internal Medicine	31	3.38%
Neonatal Medicine	2	.22%
Nephrology	8	.87%
Neurology	16	1.74%
Ob/Gyn	57	6.21%
Ob/Gyn: Gynecological Oncology	2	.22%
Ob/Gyn: Maternal & Fetal Medicine	1	.11%
Ophthalmology	22	2.40%
Ophthalmology: Retina	2	.22%
Orthopedics (Nonsurgical)	9	.98%
Orthopedic Surgery	100	10.89%
Otorhinolaryngology	15	1.63%
Pathology	8	.87%
Pediatrics	89	9.69%
Pediatric Cardiology	1	.11%
Physiatry	1	.11%
Pulmonary Medicine	10	1.09%
Radiation Oncology	1	.11%
Radiology	12	1.31%
Rheumatology	4	.44%
Surg: Cardiovascular	14	1.53%
Surg: Colon and Rectal	2	.22%
Surgery: General	23	2.51%
Surg: Neurological	10	1.09%
Surg: Oral	11	1.20%
Surg: Pediatric	3	.33%
Surg: Plastic & Reconstruction	2	.22%
Surg: Thoracic	1	.11%
Surg: Vascular	3	.33%
Urology	84	9.15%
Other Single Specialty	1	.11%
Total	918	100.00%

Medical Practice Demographics (continued)

9. MSO or PPMC Provided Services

	Count	Percent
Yes	88	9.81%
No	809	90.19%
Total	897	100.00%

10. Square Footage of All Facilities

	Count	Percent
6,000 sq ft or less	193	16.86%
6,001 to 12,000 sq ft	298	26.03%
12,001 to 28,000 sq ft	321	28.03%
28,001 sq ft or more	333	29.08%
Total	1,145	100.00%

11. Number of Branch Clinics

	Count	Percent
1 to 2 branches	224	38.29%
3 to 4 branches	125	21.37%
5 to 6 branches	64	10.94%
7 branches or more	172	29.40%
Total	585	100.00%

12. Practice Derived Revenue from Capitation Contracts

	Count	Percent
Yes	185	20.67%
No	710	79.33%
Total	895	100.00%

13. Practice Maintained IBNR Liability Account for Capitated Patients

	Count	Percent
Yes	39	21.55%
No	142	78.45%
Total	181	100.00%

14. Net Capitation Revenue Percent of Total Medical Revenue

	Count	Percent
No capitation	720	81.73%
10% or less	88	9.99%
11% to 50%	65	7.38%
51% to 100%	8	.91%
Total	881	100.00%

15. Tax Reporting Accounting Method

	Count	Percent
Cash	655	73.10%
Accrual	241	26.90%
Total	896	100.00%

16. Internal Management Accounting Method

	Count	Percent
Cash or modified cash	613	67.96%
Accrual	289	32.04%
Total	902	100.00%

17. Re-age Accounts Receivable

	Count	Percent
Yes	404	34.15%
No	779	65.85%
Total	1,183	100.00%

18. FTE Physicians

	Count	Percent
10 FTE or less	705	56.76%
11 to 25 FTE	312	25.12%
26 to 50 FTE	112	9.02%
51 to 75 FTE	50	4.03%
76 to 150 FTE	43	3.46%
151 FTE or more	20	1.61%
Total	1,242	100.00%

19. FTE Nonphysician Providers

	Count	Percent
1 FTE or less	185	21.59%
2 to 3 FTE	255	29.75%
4 to 6 FTE	178	20.77%
7 FTE or more	239	27.89%
Total	857	100.00%

20. FTE Providers

	Count	Percent
10 FTE or less	309	36.06%
11 to 25 FTE	270	31.51%
26 to 50 FTE	137	15.99%
51 to 75 FTE	58	6.77%
76 to 150 FTE	52	6.07%
151 FTE or more	31	3.62%
Total	857	100.00%

Medical Practice Demographics (continued)

21. Nonphysician Providers per FTE Physician

	Count	Percent
No nonphysician providers	627	73.16%
1 FTE or less	198	23.10%
2 FTE	20	2.33%
3 to 4 FTE	11	1.28%
5 to 8 FTE	1	.12%
Total	857	100.00%

22. FTE Support Staff

	Count	Percent
15 FTE or less	234	18.84%
16 to 30 FTE	327	26.33%
31 to 75 FTE	330	26.57%
76 FTE or more	351	28.26%
Total	1,242	100.00%

23. Net Income with Financial Support

	Count	Percent
Loss	29	42.03%
Zero	2	2.90%
Profit	38	55.07%
Total	69	100.00%

24. Net Income without Financial Support

	Count	Percent
Loss	371	33.88%
Zero	22	2.01%
Profit	702	64.11%
Total	1,095	100.00%

25. Net Income Excluding Financial Support (All Practices)

	Count	Percent
Loss	433	37.20%
Zero	22	1.89%
Profit	709	60.91%
Total	1,164	100.00%

26. Hours to Complete Survey Questionnaire

	Count	Percent
2 hours or less	139	13.80%
3 to 4 hours	256	25.42%
5 to 8 hours	267	26.51%
9 hours or more	345	34.26%
Total	1,007	100.00%

THIS PAGE INTENTIONALLY LEFT BLANK

Multispecialty Practices

Multispecialty Practices

Multispecialty — All Practices

Table 1.1: Staffing and Practice Data

	Count	Mean	Std. Dev.	10th %tile	25th %tile	Median	75th %tile	90th %tile
Total provider FTE	264	65.37	79.47	9.66	17.70	39.24	80.30	158.74
Total physician FTE	299	51.08	70.35	6.30	12.00	27.00	64.82	116.00
Total nonphysician provider FTE	264	12.15	18.48	1.55	2.50	6.00	14.74	33.05
Total support staff FTE	299	255.10	323.12	29.10	56.50	139.62	305.70	633.20
Number of branch clinics	225	10	13	1	3	6	12	21
Square footage of all facilities	277	106,987	154,365	12,900	22,383	50,735	129,356	263,405

Table 1.2: Accounts Receivable Data, Collection Percentages and Financial Ratios

	Count	Mean	Std. Dev.	10th %tile	25th %tile	Median	75th %tile	90th %tile
Total AR/physician	275	$125,962	$64,280	$56,739	$78,144	$113,677	$167,140	$208,650
Total AR/provider	245	$104,927	$53,612	$50,153	$64,509	$96,197	$132,738	$171,497
0-30 days in AR	276	50.38%	14.09%	31.36%	41.75%	51.99%	59.91%	68.22%
31-60 days in AR	276	15.44%	5.01%	9.69%	11.91%	15.07%	18.00%	22.04%
61-90 days in AR	276	8.41%	2.86%	5.33%	6.36%	8.18%	10.06%	11.82%
91-120 days in AR	276	5.75%	2.40%	3.28%	4.10%	5.48%	6.73%	8.46%
120+ days in AR	276	20.02%	11.81%	7.80%	12.22%	17.52%	25.91%	35.89%
Re-aged: 0-30 days in AR	110	52.97%	12.77%	34.48%	43.81%	53.26%	62.39%	71.52%
Re-aged: 31-60 days in AR	110	15.15%	5.30%	9.48%	11.63%	14.47%	17.65%	22.14%
Re-aged: 61-90 days in AR	110	8.08%	2.93%	5.34%	5.85%	7.55%	9.78%	12.06%
Re-aged: 91-120 days in AR	110	5.56%	2.47%	3.21%	3.98%	5.11%	6.55%	8.45%
Re-aged: 120+ days in AR	110	18.24%	9.60%	6.51%	11.81%	16.91%	22.85%	31.21%
Not re-aged: 0-30 days in AR	154	48.33%	14.19%	29.10%	39.14%	49.99%	58.20%	64.31%
Not re-aged: 31-60 days in AR	154	15.57%	4.88%	9.73%	11.96%	15.54%	18.41%	21.93%
Not re-aged: 61-90 days in AR	154	8.67%	2.83%	5.43%	6.88%	8.37%	10.38%	11.91%
Not re-aged: 91-120 days in AR	154	5.96%	2.37%	3.42%	4.35%	5.89%	7.06%	8.60%
Not re-aged: 120+ days in AR	154	21.47%	12.59%	8.46%	12.73%	18.56%	28.37%	37.65%
Months gross FFS charges in AR	247	1.72	.58	1.14	1.34	1.61	1.97	2.40
Days gross FFS charges in AR	247	52.37	17.67	34.63	40.68	49.11	59.93	73.02
Gross FFS collection %	267	62.81%	10.97%	49.56%	55.42%	63.35%	69.86%	75.45%
Adjusted FFS collection %	258	96.23%	9.73%	92.63%	95.74%	97.39%	98.66%	99.55%
Gross FFS + cap collection %	105	65.99%	16.17%	50.58%	56.62%	64.71%	72.25%	81.24%
Net cap rev % of gross cap chrg	87	78.27%	29.88%	40.59%	62.77%	76.89%	94.95%	113.61%
Current ratio	155	4.31	10.28	.64	1.08	1.66	2.82	7.00
Tot asset turnover ratio	155	6.25	6.33	1.55	2.51	4.08	6.67	14.70
Debt to equity ratio	155	4.04	7.26	.23	.85	1.77	3.97	8.10
Debt ratio	155	59.79%	24.87%	18.38%	45.82%	63.92%	79.87%	89.01%
Return on total assets	146	9.99%	44.03%	-19.44%	-2.31%	2.82%	13.80%	49.70%
Return on equity	146	31.05%	188.52%	-68.65%	-8.03%	8.57%	34.22%	141.22%

Table 1.3: Breakout of Total Gross Charges by Type of Payer

	Count	Mean	Std. Dev.	10th %tile	25th %tile	Median	75th %tile	90th %tile
Medicare: fee-for-service	274	25.44%	13.71%	7.42%	15.15%	25.26%	34.56%	42.05%
Medicare: managed care FFS	274	1.24%	3.98%	.00%	.00%	.00%	.00%	3.78%
Medicare: capitation	274	.97%	3.37%	.00%	.00%	.00%	.00%	1.45%
Medicaid: fee-for-service	274	6.60%	6.96%	.00%	1.78%	4.59%	9.00%	15.00%
Medicaid: managed care FFS	274	1.84%	6.45%	.00%	.00%	.00%	.26%	5.19%
Medicaid: capitation	274	.65%	2.34%	.00%	.00%	.00%	.00%	1.30%
Commercial: fee-for-service	274	36.42%	21.98%	3.10%	19.75%	39.12%	52.28%	63.60%
Commercial: managed care FFS	274	13.93%	21.27%	.00%	.00%	.00%	22.43%	48.90%
Commercial: capitation	274	4.59%	12.35%	.00%	.00%	.00%	2.00%	15.00%
Workers' compensation	274	1.49%	2.95%	.00%	.07%	1.00%	1.72%	3.01%
Charity care and prof courtesy	274	.51%	1.32%	.00%	.00%	.00%	.50%	1.47%
Self-pay	274	5.52%	5.52%	1.00%	2.00%	3.89%	7.00%	12.18%
Other federal government payers	274	.81%	4.07%	.00%	.00%	.00%	.29%	1.30%

Multispecialty — All Practices
(per FTE Physician)

Table 1.4a: Staffing, RVUs, Patients, Procedures and Square Footage

	Count	Mean	Std. Dev.	10th %tile	25th %tile	Median	75th %tile	90th %tile
Total provider FTE/physician	**264**	**1.26**	**.21**	**1.08**	**1.12**	**1.21**	**1.33**	**1.51**
Prim care phy/physician	261	.69	.25	.36	.48	.70	.94	1.00
Nonsurg phy/physician	178	.26	.17	.06	.14	.22	.38	.46
Surg spec phy/physician	172	.22	.15	.06	.11	.21	.29	.39
Total NPP FTE/physician	264	.26	.21	.08	.12	.21	.33	.51
Total support staff FTE/phy	**299**	**5.12**	**1.60**	**3.38**	**4.07**	**4.95**	**5.92**	**7.04**
Total empl support staff FTE	272	5.11	1.57	3.42	4.00	4.94	5.89	7.04
General administrative	260	.31	.19	.12	.18	.27	.38	.54
Patient accounting	247	.72	.36	.30	.48	.67	.92	1.24
General accounting	207	.09	.06	.04	.05	.08	.11	.15
Managed care administrative	116	.14	.16	.01	.03	.08	.17	.38
Information technology	166	.10	.08	.02	.05	.08	.14	.21
Housekeeping, maint, security	155	.12	.14	.02	.04	.07	.18	.27
Medical receptionists	252	.98	.42	.46	.73	.94	1.24	1.55
Med secretaries,transcribers	194	.28	.26	.04	.11	.22	.36	.59
Medical records	223	.41	.23	.14	.25	.39	.54	.70
Other admin support	143	.22	.52	.03	.05	.09	.20	.44
***Total administrative supp staff**	**146**	**3.05**	**1.02**	**2.00**	**2.41**	**3.00**	**3.55**	**4.16**
Registered Nurses	230	.49	.39	.09	.18	.39	.73	.96
Licensed Practical Nurses	225	.55	.45	.08	.20	.44	.86	1.13
Med assistants, nurse aides	240	.77	.49	.22	.41	.70	1.06	1.45
***Total clinical supp staff**	**232**	**1.64**	**.54**	**1.08**	**1.31**	**1.56**	**1.90**	**2.30**
Clinical laboratory	199	.34	.19	.10	.21	.32	.43	.56
Radiology and imaging	213	.27	.17	.08	.14	.24	.39	.50
Other medical support serv	150	.32	.41	.04	.10	.21	.41	.60
***Total ancillary supp staff**	**148**	**.86**	**.41**	**.33**	**.57**	**.87**	**1.12**	**1.44**
Tot contracted supp staff	97	.18	.26	.02	.04	.11	.24	.41
Tot RVU/physician	115	14,633	39,083	6,443	8,507	10,251	13,307	17,450
Physician work RVU/physician	122	5,390	1,675	3,997	4,596	5,280	5,982	6,704
Patients/physician	136	1,953	1,204	930	1,134	1,574	2,332	3,805
Tot procedures/physician	222	11,411	5,353	5,483	8,672	11,187	13,759	16,055
Square feet/physician	277	2,143	1,037	1,242	1,543	2,025	2,532	3,040

*See pages 260 and 261 for definition.

Table 1.4b: Charges and Revenue

	Count	Mean	Std. Dev.	10th %tile	25th %tile	Median	75th %tile	90th %tile
Net fee-for-service revenue	270	$545,006	$208,590	$292,888	$390,593	$536,134	$669,127	$821,633
Gross FFS charges	268	$892,241	$402,959	$452,117	$595,395	$844,830	$1,116,224	$1,405,219
Adjustments to FFS charges	254	$337,887	$223,541	$111,926	$190,067	$280,154	$438,844	$631,246
Adjusted FFS charges	258	$566,985	$224,507	$311,977	$401,137	$557,566	$695,954	$857,714
Bad debts due to FFS activity	244	$17,839	$16,128	$3,529	$7,097	$12,521	$23,699	$38,628
Net capitation revenue	106	$124,715	$207,897	$4,222	$14,980	$45,531	$147,865	$372,749
Gross capitation charges	87	$175,316	$300,176	$9,273	$30,270	$73,886	$199,034	$432,412
Capitation revenue	102	$202,022	$414,331	$4,464	$17,237	$50,876	$202,288	$610,207
Purch serv for cap patients	29	$258,490	$376,856	$4,584	$32,442	$113,531	$382,923	$701,462
Net other medical revenue	197	$24,848	$47,359	$917	$3,819	$12,294	$29,028	$51,070
Gross rev from other activity	189	$37,240	$62,403	$1,380	$5,557	$15,562	$36,207	$98,627
Other medical revenue	154	$20,042	$47,858	$743	$2,616	$8,744	$18,143	$36,380
Rev from sale of goods/services	109	$40,405	$63,352	$953	$3,979	$14,663	$53,539	$107,240
Cost of sales	66	$33,560	$47,494	$1,645	$3,806	$10,927	$40,597	$132,173
Total gross charges	**289**	**$916,900**	**$335,849**	**$497,853**	**$654,980**	**$892,829**	**$1,133,353**	**$1,372,638**
Total medical revenue	**299**	**$606,151**	**$217,739**	**$344,052**	**$458,238**	**$586,381**	**$746,763**	**$885,787**

Multispecialty — All Practices
(per FTE Physician)

Table 1.4c: Operating Cost

	Count	Mean	Std. Dev.	10th %tile	25th %tile	Median	75th %tile	90th %tile
Total support staff cost/phy	**299**	**$188,473**	**$65,328**	**$114,860**	**$142,181**	**$177,128**	**$226,263**	**$274,615**
Total empl supp staff cost/phy	276	$150,818	$51,168	$95,785	$111,542	$144,460	$176,095	$221,337
General administrative	261	$18,080	$11,843	$7,744	$10,619	$15,598	$22,677	$30,711
Patient accounting	250	$18,417	$8,754	$7,814	$13,168	$17,812	$23,226	$29,487
General accounting	209	$3,445	$2,541	$1,297	$2,018	$2,796	$3,971	$5,716
Managed care administrative	115	$4,841	$7,033	$618	$1,299	$2,572	$5,099	$12,611
Information technology	167	$4,301	$3,467	$1,050	$1,914	$3,426	$5,301	$8,504
Housekeeping, maint, security	156	$2,846	$2,739	$349	$860	$1,939	$3,955	$6,439
Medical receptionists	253	$21,789	$9,931	$9,801	$15,425	$20,796	$27,938	$34,179
Med secretaries,transcribers	196	$7,339	$6,259	$1,049	$2,978	$5,962	$9,923	$15,333
Medical records	224	$8,350	$4,927	$2,763	$4,695	$7,518	$10,897	$14,873
Other admin support	146	$5,880	$12,727	$675	$1,271	$2,608	$5,484	$11,150
***Total administrative supp staff**	**139**	**$85,082**	**$30,644**	**$52,524**	**$67,750**	**$82,284**	**$98,201**	**$120,473**
Registered Nurses	231	$19,704	$15,328	$3,404	$7,711	$15,732	$30,145	$39,343
Licensed Practical Nurses	222	$15,673	$12,371	$2,733	$5,962	$13,054	$23,448	$31,259
Med assistants, nurse aides	237	$19,241	$12,314	$5,222	$9,939	$17,216	$27,122	$35,561
***Total clinical supp staff**	**229**	**$48,263**	**$16,835**	**$30,561**	**$36,596**	**$45,316**	**$57,449**	**$70,459**
Clinical laboratory	199	$10,061	$5,892	$2,568	$5,939	$9,823	$13,226	$16,746
Radiology and imaging	215	$11,161	$16,198	$2,793	$5,064	$8,764	$14,517	$19,581
Other medical support serv	155	$12,125	$16,626	$1,230	$3,099	$7,147	$14,573	$23,708
***Total ancillary supp staff**	**172**	**$28,580**	**$17,980**	**$6,852**	**$15,966**	**$28,138**	**$37,854**	**$49,482**
Total empl supp staff benefits	290	$37,621	$15,829	$19,093	$25,991	$35,897	$47,276	$60,275
Tot contracted supp staff	149	$5,315	$7,283	$290	$972	$2,438	$6,710	$13,877
Total general operating cost	**299**	**$181,399**	**$92,919**	**$90,471**	**$122,413**	**$168,111**	**$218,841**	**$271,374**
Information technology	271	$10,910	$7,110	$3,826	$5,599	$9,248	$13,632	$21,381
Medical and surgical supply	274	$39,947	$50,389	$8,946	$14,549	$27,669	$49,282	$82,434
Building and occupancy	274	$41,009	$17,204	$21,360	$28,766	$38,125	$50,635	$60,065
Furniture and equipment	239	$10,160	$12,054	$1,249	$3,243	$7,584	$13,159	$21,604
Admin supplies and services	271	$12,182	$7,760	$4,945	$6,941	$10,592	$15,291	$21,245
Prof liability insurance	289	$14,583	$9,706	$5,440	$8,013	$12,001	$18,431	$25,310
Other insurance premiums	231	$2,133	$3,108	$369	$645	$1,192	$2,547	$4,389
Outside professional fees	253	$6,320	$14,309	$697	$1,536	$3,380	$6,692	$12,344
Promotion and marketing	257	$2,829	$2,652	$373	$1,078	$2,111	$3,616	$6,328
Clinical laboratory	232	$15,085	$10,183	$1,409	$8,067	$14,002	$20,776	$28,749
Radiology and imaging	216	$10,905	$12,521	$739	$2,289	$5,558	$17,158	$28,949
Other ancillary services	118	$9,702	$19,900	$195	$869	$2,890	$10,826	$20,473
Billing purchased services	160	$5,367	$8,606	$197	$836	$1,937	$4,465	$20,022
Management fees paid to MSO	30	$22,863	$17,211	$1,240	$8,633	$22,325	$29,555	$53,875
Misc operating cost	268	$11,416	$12,185	$2,046	$4,169	$7,937	$14,359	$24,196
Cost allocated to prac from par	35	$16,573	$20,902	$1,131	$3,932	$11,879	$22,589	$39,153
Total operating cost	**299**	**$369,688**	**$141,139**	**$217,125**	**$281,700**	**$349,090**	**$446,094**	**$548,446**

*See pages 260 and 261 for definition.

Multispecialty — All Practices
(per FTE Physician)

Table 1.4d: Provider Cost

	Count	Mean	Std. Dev.	10th %tile	25th %tile	Median	75th %tile	90th %tile
Total med rev after oper cost	299	$238,074	$112,198	$105,629	$162,855	$232,052	$303,102	$373,944
Total provider cost/physician	299	$260,424	$80,313	$169,603	$202,539	$248,611	$302,930	$365,209
Total NPP cost/physician	270	$22,026	$18,201	$5,868	$9,383	$18,040	$28,077	$45,737
Nonphysician provider comp	254	$18,057	$14,974	$5,045	$7,558	$14,469	$22,713	$34,945
Nonphysician prov benefit cost	235	$4,082	$3,815	$800	$1,434	$3,104	$5,340	$8,854
Provider consultant cost	98	$12,192	$12,454	$1,370	$3,542	$7,628	$18,108	$28,238
Total physician cost/physician	299	$237,058	$76,496	$151,183	$182,866	$221,703	$280,578	$332,803
Total phy compensation	276	$206,924	$70,746	$133,289	$157,849	$192,217	$242,493	$302,701
Total phy benefit cost	273	$32,448	$13,652	$14,224	$23,646	$31,594	$42,225	$49,705

Table 1.4e: Net Income or Loss

	Count	Mean	Std. Dev.	10th %tile	25th %tile	Median	75th %tile	90th %tile
Total cost	299	$630,112	$194,051	$393,317	$493,336	$608,717	$753,696	$871,733
Net nonmedical revenue	243	$20,045	$60,442	-$3,797	$350	$4,148	$19,122	$63,103
Nonmedical revenue	214	$27,077	$231,221	$227	$836	$4,010	$12,192	$39,626
Fin support for oper costs	39	$68,812	$110,992	$1,493	$15,034	$50,000	$83,960	$158,059
Goodwill amortization	48	$4,596	$9,568	$15	$145	$940	$5,004	$13,288
Nonmedical cost	102	$33,777	$292,371	$9	$156	$1,345	$5,466	$17,215
Net inc, prac with fin sup	37	-$693	$110,359	-$68,414	-$27,638	$0	$6,946	$36,739
Net inc, prac w/o fin sup	246	-$5,368	$59,635	-$88,307	-$20,360	$784	$18,827	$46,290
Net inc, excl fin supp (all prac)	283	-$13,531	$65,676	-$103,826	-$39,663	-$1	$14,795	$44,107

Table 1.4f: Assets and Liabilities

	Count	Mean	Std. Dev.	10th %tile	25th %tile	Median	75th %tile	90th %tile
Total assets	160	$208,174	$198,208	$49,820	$75,629	$150,427	$253,696	$484,668
Current assets	162	$105,048	$83,682	$10,747	$32,268	$94,803	$156,146	$216,020
Noncurrent assets	162	$100,749	$153,295	$9,325	$22,482	$47,107	$117,927	$283,861
Total liabilities	162	$117,426	$123,326	$15,652	$35,150	$77,124	$157,185	$301,210
Current liabilities	162	$60,053	$56,424	$5,587	$18,032	$47,636	$87,362	$136,562
Noncurrent liabilities	162	$57,373	$86,573	$0	$1,542	$20,130	$66,884	$202,759
Working capital	162	$44,995	$60,430	-$15,782	$2,650	$27,345	$76,513	$127,644
Total net worth	162	$88,371	$132,668	$5,656	$16,657	$52,986	$111,091	$188,223

Multispecialty — All Practices
(as a % of Total Medical Revenue)

Table 1.5a: Charges and Revenue

	Count	Mean	Std. Dev.	10th %tile	25th %tile	Median	75th %tile	90th %tile
Net fee-for-service revenue	270	90.02%	17.86%	68.22%	89.74%	97.53%	99.81%	100.00%
Net capitation revenue	106	18.06%	21.01%	.72%	2.81%	9.48%	24.27%	46.52%
Net other medical revenue	197	3.95%	6.68%	.14%	.74%	1.87%	4.28%	9.11%
Total gross charges	**296**	**156.87%**	**31.28%**	**123.18%**	**137.61%**	**153.68%**	**171.12%**	**193.05%**

Table 1.5b: Operating Cost

	Count	Mean	Std. Dev.	10th %tile	25th %tile	Median	75th %tile	90th %tile
Total support staff cost	**299**	**32.60%**	**11.97%**	**23.57%**	**26.69%**	**31.08%**	**35.44%**	**43.11%**
Total empl support staff cost	276	25.78%	9.38%	18.68%	21.00%	24.81%	27.94%	33.27%
General administrative	261	3.16%	2.53%	1.44%	1.76%	2.55%	3.61%	5.50%
Patient accounting	250	3.10%	1.64%	1.39%	2.07%	2.88%	3.74%	5.04%
General accounting	209	.60%	.59%	.19%	.31%	.43%	.69%	1.12%
Managed care administrative	115	.78%	1.35%	.10%	.20%	.36%	.82%	1.62%
Information technology	167	.62%	.48%	.18%	.31%	.54%	.80%	1.10%
Housekeeping, maint, security	156	.44%	.53%	.06%	.14%	.28%	.58%	.94%
Medical receptionists	253	4.05%	2.69%	1.42%	2.36%	3.32%	5.17%	7.75%
Med secretaries,transcribers	196	1.18%	1.06%	.19%	.47%	.95%	1.60%	2.33%
Medical records	224	1.40%	1.10%	.56%	.82%	1.20%	1.74%	2.43%
Other admin support	146	1.05%	2.49%	.09%	.19%	.39%	.89%	1.98%
*Total administrative supp staff	139	13.56%	7.32%	9.01%	10.35%	12.84%	14.93%	17.61%
Registered Nurses	231	3.39%	3.38%	.69%	1.32%	2.66%	4.34%	6.53%
Licensed Practical Nurses	222	2.70%	2.29%	.46%	1.10%	2.05%	3.87%	5.88%
Med assistants, nurse aides	237	3.54%	2.65%	.73%	1.68%	2.75%	4.97%	7.32%
*Total clinical supp staff	229	8.30%	3.63%	4.98%	6.14%	7.52%	9.52%	12.28%
Clinical laboratory	199	1.60%	1.25%	.51%	.97%	1.38%	2.00%	2.99%
Radiology and imaging	215	1.69%	3.28%	.51%	.86%	1.48%	2.00%	2.45%
Other medical support serv	155	1.74%	2.56%	.17%	.53%	1.07%	1.92%	3.76%
*Total ancillary supp staff	172	4.07%	2.15%	1.47%	2.72%	3.80%	5.14%	6.71%
Total empl supp staff benefits	290	6.47%	2.86%	3.72%	4.82%	6.13%	7.39%	9.31%
Tot contracted supp staff	149	.91%	1.55%	.05%	.14%	.39%	1.20%	2.29%
Total general operating cost	**299**	**29.85%**	**8.71%**	**21.47%**	**24.69%**	**28.87%**	**33.39%**	**38.17%**
Information technology	271	1.83%	1.17%	.78%	1.04%	1.54%	2.27%	3.52%
Medical and surgical supply	274	5.95%	4.36%	1.89%	3.06%	4.68%	7.33%	11.47%
Building and occupancy	274	7.08%	2.99%	3.91%	5.14%	6.71%	8.27%	10.36%
Furniture and equipment	239	1.56%	1.38%	.30%	.57%	1.26%	2.10%	3.25%
Admin supplies and services	272	2.07%	1.30%	.94%	1.25%	1.77%	2.46%	3.80%
Prof liability insurance	289	2.57%	1.78%	.94%	1.39%	2.07%	3.25%	4.91%
Other insurance premiums	229	.33%	.49%	.07%	.11%	.21%	.40%	.65%
Outside professional fees	253	.93%	1.31%	.14%	.25%	.53%	1.06%	1.97%
Promotion and marketing	257	.45%	.40%	.07%	.21%	.35%	.59%	.92%
Clinical laboratory	232	2.42%	1.89%	.31%	1.12%	2.21%	3.29%	4.79%
Radiology and imaging	219	1.52%	1.55%	.12%	.36%	.90%	2.29%	3.91%
Other ancillary services	118	1.30%	2.16%	.05%	.14%	.51%	1.44%	3.61%
Billing purchased services	160	1.14%	2.11%	.03%	.14%	.32%	.71%	4.91%
Management fees paid to MSO	32	4.77%	4.95%	.16%	1.23%	3.19%	6.44%	12.16%
Misc operating cost	268	1.88%	1.80%	.39%	.74%	1.38%	2.42%	3.72%
Cost allocated to prac from par	35	3.60%	4.64%	.30%	.82%	2.41%	5.44%	8.76%
Total operating cost	**299**	**62.30%**	**15.79%**	**49.69%**	**55.22%**	**60.30%**	**66.05%**	**74.81%**

*See pages 260 and 261 for definition.

Multispecialty — All Practices
(as a % of Total Medical Revenue)

Table 1.5c: Provider Cost

	Count	Mean	Std. Dev.	10th %tile	25th %tile	Median	75th %tile	90th %tile
Total med rev after oper cost	299	38.34%	12.81%	25.66%	34.00%	39.83%	44.83%	50.32%
Total provider cost	299	45.03%	11.65%	33.57%	38.70%	43.25%	49.45%	60.46%
Total NPP cost	270	3.76%	3.48%	.92%	1.71%	2.88%	4.69%	7.03%
Nonphysician provider comp	254	3.06%	2.81%	.81%	1.38%	2.37%	3.79%	5.47%
Nonphysician prov benefit cost	235	.68%	.70%	.15%	.27%	.50%	.86%	1.40%
Provider consultant cost	98	1.70%	1.62%	.22%	.51%	1.22%	2.59%	3.58%
Total physician cost	299	41.14%	11.31%	29.83%	34.09%	39.78%	45.97%	56.34%
Total phy compensation	276	35.42%	9.98%	25.31%	28.79%	34.21%	39.55%	48.38%
Total phy benefit cost	273	5.70%	2.72%	2.41%	4.21%	5.52%	6.93%	8.56%

Table 1.5d: Net Income or Loss

	Count	Mean	Std. Dev.	10th %tile	25th %tile	Median	75th %tile	90th %tile
Total cost	299	107.33%	20.90%	94.24%	98.55%	100.79%	110.36%	127.05%
Net nonmedical revenue	243	4.85%	17.10%	-.70%	.06%	.60%	3.56%	12.02%
Nonmedical revenue	214	5.96%	56.85%	.04%	.16%	.56%	2.00%	6.44%
Fin support for oper costs	39	18.70%	33.59%	.24%	2.57%	9.11%	20.87%	36.77%
Goodwill amortization	48	.75%	1.14%	.00%	.02%	.12%	1.22%	2.57%
Nonmedical cost	102	7.83%	71.87%	.00%	.03%	.23%	.88%	2.42%
Net inc, prac with fin sup	37	-1.17%	34.94%	-18.55%	-6.67%	.00%	1.31%	6.29%
Net inc, prac w/o fin sup	246	-2.23%	12.51%	-18.48%	-3.33%	.09%	2.77%	6.91%
Net inc, excl fin supp (all prac)	283	-4.47%	15.28%	-23.72%	-7.88%	.00%	2.35%	6.27%

Table 1.5e: Assets and Liabilities

	Count	Mean	Std. Dev.	10th %tile	25th %tile	Median	75th %tile	90th %tile
Total assets	162	31.70%	31.38%	6.52%	14.07%	24.12%	39.76%	63.70%
Current assets	162	15.97%	12.18%	1.78%	5.82%	15.63%	23.41%	29.78%
Noncurrent assets	162	15.73%	24.28%	1.45%	3.82%	7.49%	17.03%	40.77%
Total liabilities	162	17.94%	18.29%	2.62%	5.56%	12.62%	23.57%	44.16%
Current liabilities	162	8.86%	7.02%	.85%	3.21%	7.68%	13.01%	16.88%
Noncurrent liabilities	162	9.08%	14.16%	.00%	.22%	3.45%	11.06%	28.39%
Working capital	162	7.11%	9.70%	-2.63%	.29%	4.21%	11.55%	20.50%
Total net worth	162	13.76%	21.19%	1.09%	2.75%	8.48%	17.11%	28.97%

Multispecialty — All Practices
(per FTE Provider)

Table 1.6a: Staffing, RVUs, Patients, Procedures and Square Footage

	Count	Mean	Std. Dev.	10th %tile	25th %tile	Median	75th %tile	90th %tile
Total physician FTE/provider	**264**	**.81**	**.11**	**.66**	**.75**	**.83**	**.89**	**.93**
Prim care phy/provider	233	.55	.21	.28	.37	.54	.73	.87
Nonsurg phy/provider	164	.22	.15	.05	.11	.20	.31	.41
Surg spec phy/provider	158	.17	.11	.05	.09	.17	.24	.29
Total NPP FTE/provider	264	.19	.11	.07	.11	.17	.25	.34
Total support staff FTE/prov	**264**	**4.18**	**1.08**	**3.01**	**3.47**	**4.09**	**4.83**	**5.53**
Total empl supp staff FTE/prov	243	4.17	1.05	2.98	3.44	4.08	4.82	5.57
General administrative	235	.25	.15	.11	.14	.23	.31	.46
Patient accounting	228	.59	.30	.27	.40	.55	.72	1.02
General accounting	194	.07	.04	.03	.04	.06	.09	.13
Managed care administrative	107	.11	.13	.01	.03	.06	.14	.29
Information technology	158	.08	.06	.02	.04	.07	.11	.17
Housekeeping, maint, security	147	.09	.09	.01	.03	.06	.15	.22
Medical receptionists	227	.79	.32	.37	.61	.78	.96	1.17
Med secretaries,transcribers	183	.23	.21	.03	.09	.18	.28	.44
Medical records	209	.33	.18	.12	.20	.31	.45	.57
Other admin support	136	.18	.42	.02	.04	.08	.16	.34
***Total administrative supp staff**	**138**	**2.42**	**.71**	**1.61**	**1.90**	**2.45**	**2.86**	**3.29**
Registered Nurses	210	.39	.30	.07	.14	.30	.58	.77
Licensed Practical Nurses	204	.44	.36	.07	.16	.35	.67	.89
Med assistants, nurse aides	217	.63	.39	.16	.31	.57	.91	1.19
***Total clinical supp staff**	**212**	**1.32**	**.38**	**.89**	**1.07**	**1.28**	**1.51**	**1.83**
Clinical laboratory	188	.27	.14	.09	.18	.26	.35	.44
Radiology and imaging	203	.22	.14	.07	.11	.20	.31	.41
Other medical support serv	142	.24	.26	.03	.08	.19	.32	.47
***Total ancillary supp staff**	**141**	**.69**	**.33**	**.26**	**.47**	**.69**	**.89**	**1.10**
Tot contracted supp staff	90	.13	.14	.01	.03	.08	.19	.34
Tot RVU/provider	100	9,121	3,656	5,583	7,057	8,282	10,648	13,343
Physician work RVU/provider	112	4,388	1,329	3,168	3,630	4,273	4,955	5,745
Patients/provider	125	1,633	1,036	730	947	1,348	1,999	2,922
Tot procedures/provider	197	9,321	3,316	5,151	7,402	9,380	10,941	13,374
Square feet/provider	246	1,735	652	1,040	1,305	1,659	2,030	2,457
Total support staff FTE/phy	**299**	**5.12**	**1.60**	**3.38**	**4.07**	**4.95**	**5.92**	**7.04**

*See pages 260 and 261 for definition.

Table 1.6b: Charges, Revenue and Cost

	Count	Mean	Std. Dev.	10th %tile	25th %tile	Median	75th %tile	90th %tile
Total gross charges	262	$791,259	$333,508	$440,602	$545,355	$742,311	$975,199	$1,213,307
Total medical revenue	264	$501,253	$176,601	$309,168	$382,374	$488,528	$588,998	$710,969
Net fee-for-service revenue	241	$452,510	$167,839	$250,160	$346,324	$435,153	$541,952	$663,707
Net capitation revenue	95	$102,388	$171,557	$3,632	$9,689	$42,179	$132,114	$276,795
Net other medical revenue	183	$17,423	$24,715	$785	$3,487	$10,078	$22,184	$34,064
Total support staff cost/prov	264	$153,975	$48,055	$101,129	$118,306	$147,628	$182,519	$217,454
Total general operating cost	264	$151,124	$78,457	$75,077	$103,981	$140,059	$178,174	$220,312
Total operating cost	264	$305,006	$114,370	$180,825	$230,348	$290,963	$361,167	$434,527
Total med rev after oper cost	264	$197,444	$90,181	$97,922	$143,949	$191,092	$244,461	$305,838
Total provider cost/provider	264	$213,758	$65,478	$133,441	$169,720	$206,515	$251,292	$301,089
Total NPP cost/provider	263	$15,976	$9,627	$5,402	$8,345	$14,811	$20,997	$28,748
Provider consultant cost	92	$10,019	$10,298	$1,228	$2,829	$5,903	$14,290	$22,215
Total physician cost/provider	264	$194,810	$66,655	$114,160	$149,156	$186,716	$230,646	$285,748
Total phy compensation	247	$169,966	$60,861	$101,455	$128,868	$163,172	$200,542	$251,056
Total phy benefit cost	244	$26,421	$11,379	$11,056	$18,129	$26,024	$34,453	$41,050
Total cost	264	$518,764	$157,646	$348,628	$407,323	$499,874	$603,343	$714,445
Net nonmedical revenue	220	$16,189	$51,785	-$3,880	$348	$3,109	$16,193	$49,798
Net inc, prac with fin sup	33	-$902	$100,473	-$63,748	-$24,919	$0	$6,988	$55,914
Net inc, prac w/o fin sup	217	-$3,159	$45,682	-$59,823	-$11,611	$1,040	$15,364	$33,632
Net inc, excl fin supp (all prac)	250	-$10,150	$52,735	-$84,572	-$29,069	$3	$13,697	$31,715
Total support staff FTE/phy	**299**	**5.12**	**1.60**	**3.38**	**4.07**	**4.95**	**5.92**	**7.04**

Multispecialty — All Practices
(per Square Foot)

Table 1.7a: Staffing, RVUs, Patients and Procedures

	Count	Mean	Std. Dev.	10th %tile	25th %tile	Median	75th %tile	90th %tile
Total prov FTE/10,000 sq ft	**246**	**6.71**	**4.56**	**4.07**	**4.93**	**6.03**	**7.66**	**9.62**
Total phy FTE/10,000 sq ft	277	5.60	3.70	3.29	3.95	4.94	6.48	8.05
Prim care phy/10,000 sq ft	242	3.68	2.06	1.45	2.03	3.33	4.89	6.53
Nonsurg phy/10,000 sq ft	165	1.42	1.25	.27	.65	1.11	1.84	2.73
Surg spec phy/10,000 sq ft	161	1.14	.86	.26	.51	.96	1.49	2.16
Total NPP FTE/10,000 sq ft	246	1.23	1.09	.38	.58	1.03	1.50	2.15
Total supp stf FTE/10,000 sq ft	**277**	**26.22**	**8.08**	**16.80**	**21.11**	**25.29**	**30.47**	**36.95**
Total empl supp stf/10,000 sq ft	253	25.83	7.79	16.58	20.99	25.21	29.59	35.75
General administrative	245	1.58	1.04	.57	.83	1.38	1.96	2.92
Patient accounting	233	3.65	2.27	1.46	2.40	3.26	4.45	6.10
General accounting	194	.44	.34	.17	.26	.37	.52	.78
Managed care administrative	110	.69	.77	.07	.15	.40	.95	1.77
Information technology	158	.50	.36	.11	.26	.41	.69	1.06
Housekeeping, maint, security	146	.50	.45	.09	.16	.32	.74	1.11
Medical receptionists	235	5.04	2.61	1.85	3.33	4.57	6.55	8.71
Med secretaries,transcribers	182	1.43	1.49	.20	.49	1.03	1.77	2.82
Medical records	210	2.04	1.15	.68	1.20	1.89	2.68	3.69
Other admin support	136	1.09	2.13	.12	.25	.45	1.09	2.04
*Total administrative supp staff	140	14.32	4.87	8.54	11.48	13.79	17.14	20.37
Registered Nurses	215	2.31	1.79	.48	.89	1.94	3.16	4.62
Licensed Practical Nurses	211	2.57	2.16	.59	.98	2.09	3.78	5.04
Med assistants, nurse aides	226	4.21	3.17	.87	1.83	3.24	5.62	8.84
*Total clinical supp staff	221	8.07	3.23	4.76	5.81	7.39	9.67	11.80
Clinical laboratory	189	1.60	1.02	.54	1.01	1.50	1.94	2.74
Radiology and imaging	199	1.31	.80	.41	.68	1.16	1.78	2.41
Other medical support serv	141	1.63	2.94	.17	.55	1.02	1.75	3.15
*Total ancillary supp staff	143	4.14	2.35	1.24	2.61	3.69	5.67	6.80
Tot contracted supp staff	96	.95	1.50	.07	.15	.53	1.02	2.03
Tot RVU/sq ft	109	7.55	14.88	2.99	4.30	5.71	7.56	9.54
Physician work RVU/sq ft	116	3.04	3.11	1.68	2.06	2.66	3.35	4.19
Patients/sq ft	127	1.08	.77	.40	.53	.88	1.37	2.04
Tot procedures/sq ft	209	5.86	2.92	3.11	4.13	5.46	6.88	9.37
Total support staff FTE/phy	**299**	**5.12**	**1.60**	**3.38**	**4.07**	**4.95**	**5.92**	**7.04**

*See pages 260 and 261 for definition.

Table 1.7b: Charges, Revenue and Cost

	Count	Mean	Std. Dev.	10th %tile	25th %tile	Median	75th %tile	90th %tile
Total gross charges	**275**	**$518.18**	**$510.77**	**$256.92**	**$346.23**	**$463.96**	**$587.59**	**$748.21**
Total medical revenue	**277**	**$324.22**	**$213.43**	**$180.30**	**$229.26**	**$304.60**	**$374.15**	**$440.61**
Net fee-for-service revenue	249	$281.03	$120.09	$145.61	$203.68	$268.64	$351.91	$412.76
Net capitation revenue	97	$63.67	$93.67	$2.75	$7.16	$26.28	$82.41	$178.09
Net other medical revenue	182	$11.38	$18.81	$.47	$1.62	$5.19	$12.74	$30.39
Total support staff cost/sq ft	**277**	**$97.56**	**$35.69**	**$56.64**	**$77.23**	**$92.91**	**$111.68**	**$144.47**
Total general operating cost	**277**	**$91.98**	**$44.46**	**$47.75**	**$67.13**	**$86.10**	**$110.65**	**$133.94**
Total operating cost	**277**	**$189.62**	**$71.61**	**$115.00**	**$144.92**	**$183.75**	**$220.06**	**$266.93**
Total med rev after oper cost	**277**	**$135.01**	**$175.96**	**$49.61**	**$84.25**	**$119.47**	**$161.29**	**$202.62**
Total provider cost/sq ft	**277**	**$143.81**	**$142.92**	**$76.99**	**$97.43**	**$129.84**	**$163.38**	**$200.41**
Total NPP cost/sq ft	251	$10.76	$11.06	$2.90	$4.94	$8.82	$13.82	$19.57
Provider consultant cost	94	$5.59	$5.87	$.85	$1.59	$3.70	$7.09	$13.88
Total physician cost/sq ft	277	$132.47	$135.53	$68.10	$89.03	$117.45	$149.06	$187.47
Total phy compensation	255	$108.00	$47.31	$57.72	$76.16	$102.69	$127.25	$162.92
Total phy benefit cost	253	$16.98	$8.86	$6.63	$10.78	$16.05	$21.16	$29.48
Total cost	**277**	**$333.42**	**$182.85**	**$203.97**	**$251.45**	**$320.05**	**$377.31**	**$453.23**
Net nonmedical revenue/sq ft	223	$10.15	$26.54	-$1.71	$.21	$1.79	$10.40	$30.64
Net inc, prac with fin sup	35	-$7.80	$52.11	-$44.01	-$18.34	-$2.30	$3.99	$11.01
Net inc, prac w/o fin sup	227	$.83	$43.55	-$35.85	-$7.10	$.61	$9.12	$22.47
Net inc, excl fin supp (all prac)	262	-$5.09	$46.42	-$51.44	-$19.62	$.00	$7.23	$19.57
Total support staff FTE/phy	**299**	**5.12**	**1.60**	**3.38**	**4.07**	**4.95**	**5.92**	**7.04**

Multispecialty — All Practices
(per Total RVU)

Table 1.8a: Staffing, Patients, Procedures and Square Footage

	Count	Mean	Std. Dev.	10th %tile	25th %tile	Median	75th %tile	90th %tile
Total prov FTE/10,000 tot RVU	**100**	**1.40**	**1.46**	**.75**	**.94**	**1.21**	**1.42**	**1.79**
Total phy FTE/10,000 tot RVU	115	1.18	1.14	.57	.75	.98	1.18	1.55
Prim care phy/10,000 tot RVU	104	.81	.82	.27	.43	.64	.89	1.34
Nonsurg phy/10,000 tot RVU	76	.33	.82	.07	.13	.21	.30	.54
Surg spec phy/10,000 tot RVU	67	.18	.12	.05	.09	.16	.25	.37
Total NPP FTE/10,000 tot RVU	100	.27	.35	.07	.13	.20	.32	.41
Total supp stf FTE/10,000 tot RVU	**115**	**5.58**	**5.59**	**2.98**	**3.68**	**4.53**	**5.67**	**7.26**
Tot empl supp stf/10,000 tot RVU	107	5.45	5.40	3.03	3.61	4.53	5.57	7.14
General administrative	103	.30	.26	.10	.17	.23	.37	.48
Patient accounting	99	.69	.81	.17	.40	.55	.81	1.24
General accounting	85	.10	.15	.02	.04	.07	.10	.19
Managed care administrative	53	.16	.28	.01	.04	.08	.17	.36
Information technology	68	.11	.15	.03	.04	.08	.14	.22
Housekeeping, maint, security	66	.13	.27	.01	.03	.06	.12	.23
Medical receptionists	98	1.11	1.05	.40	.61	.85	1.32	1.81
Med secretaries,transcribers	76	.29	.38	.03	.10	.18	.30	.77
Medical records	87	.44	.42	.13	.20	.34	.56	.84
Other admin support	61	.28	.66	.02	.04	.09	.19	.43
***Total administrative supp staff**	**60**	**3.41**	**4.02**	**1.70**	**1.97**	**2.67**	**3.30**	**5.63**
Registered Nurses	98	.53	.54	.10	.21	.40	.63	1.13
Licensed Practical Nurses	94	.47	.64	.05	.13	.25	.53	1.19
Med assistants, nurse aides	97	.88	.89	.22	.39	.69	1.13	1.63
***Total clinical supp staff**	**99**	**1.77**	**1.72**	**.75**	**1.05**	**1.36**	**2.02**	**2.68**
Clinical laboratory	84	.30	.25	.09	.18	.25	.37	.56
Radiology and imaging	84	.25	.20	.07	.13	.21	.33	.44
Other medical support serv	64	.50	1.42	.04	.08	.17	.36	.79
***Total ancillary supp staff**	**60**	**.99**	**1.27**	**.34**	**.46**	**.74**	**1.06**	**1.43**
Tot contracted supp staff	45	.32	.85	.01	.03	.08	.28	.72
Physician work RVU/tot RVU	95	.51	.15	.38	.44	.49	.52	.68
Patients/tot RVU	75	.23	.38	.07	.10	.14	.22	.39
Tot procedures/tot RVU	95	1.22	1.48	.58	.73	.93	1.23	1.85
Square feet/tot RVU	109	.22	.19	.10	.13	.18	.23	.33
Total support staff FTE/phy	**299**	**5.12**	**1.60**	**3.38**	**4.07**	**4.95**	**5.92**	**7.04**

*See pages 260 and 261 for definition.

Table 1.8b: Charges, Revenue and Cost

	Count	Mean	Std. Dev.	10th %tile	25th %tile	Median	75th %tile	90th %tile
Total gross charges	**114**	**$105.59**	**$118.11**	**$59.40**	**$69.21**	**$86.24**	**$105.43**	**$141.55**
Total medical revenue	**115**	**$66.83**	**$71.77**	**$39.47**	**$45.74**	**$52.54**	**$68.27**	**$90.64**
Net fee-for-service revenue	107	$56.85	$60.42	$31.86	$39.57	$46.67	$59.87	$74.96
Net capitation revenue	50	$13.22	$17.74	$.48	$1.94	$6.31	$17.43	$32.88
Net other medical revenue	84	$4.61	$13.56	$.09	$.61	$1.27	$3.08	$9.11
Total supp staff cost/tot RVU	**115**	**$21.42**	**$20.46**	**$11.31**	**$14.15**	**$16.59**	**$22.57**	**$31.80**
Total general operating cost	**115**	**$19.70**	**$25.07**	**$9.87**	**$12.03**	**$15.56**	**$19.77**	**$27.42**
Total operating cost	**115**	**$41.14**	**$44.87**	**$23.95**	**$25.91**	**$32.64**	**$41.19**	**$59.22**
Total med rev after oper cost	**115**	**$25.68**	**$30.58**	**$11.88**	**$16.91**	**$22.03**	**$26.78**	**$35.18**
Total provider cost/tot RVU	**115**	**$28.34**	**$25.85**	**$16.93**	**$20.57**	**$23.98**	**$29.77**	**$39.54**
Total NPP cost/tot RVU	102	$2.32	$2.90	$.49	$1.14	$1.81	$2.51	$3.86
Provider consultant cost	45	$1.29	$2.04	$.14	$.27	$.75	$1.60	$2.99
Total physician cost/tot RVU	115	$25.90	$22.52	$14.93	$17.65	$21.42	$28.08	$36.30
Total phy compensation	107	$21.56	$20.54	$12.36	$15.00	$18.47	$23.08	$29.10
Total phy benefit cost	107	$3.54	$2.78	$1.34	$2.20	$2.95	$4.32	$5.36
Total cost	**93**	**$70.22**	**$45.32**	**$45.20**	**$54.08**	**$62.58**	**$71.94**	**$103.20**
Net nonmedical revenue	92	$2.45	$4.77	-$.29	$.06	$.38	$2.98	$8.80
Net inc, prac with fin sup	21	-$2.43	$5.85	-$7.61	-$5.67	-$1.10	$.47	$2.18
Net inc, prac w/o fin sup	90	$.88	$9.49	-$6.35	-$1.07	$.06	$1.23	$5.01
Net inc, excl fin supp (all prac)	111	-$.99	$10.17	-$11.61	-$3.93	$.00	$.89	$3.36
Total support staff FTE/phy	**299**	**5.12**	**1.60**	**3.38**	**4.07**	**4.95**	**5.92**	**7.04**

Multispecialty — All Practices
(per Work RVU)

Table 1.9a: Staffing, Patients, Procedures and Square Footage

	Count	Mean	Std. Dev.	10th %tile	25th %tile	Median	75th %tile	90th %tile
Total prov FTE/10,000 work RVU	112	2.67	2.35	1.74	2.02	2.34	2.75	3.16
Tot phy FTE/10,000 work RVU	122	2.16	1.77	1.49	1.67	1.89	2.18	2.50
Prim care phy/10,000 work RVU	110	1.45	1.12	.58	.84	1.31	1.77	2.33
Nonsurg phy/10,000 work RVU	79	.48	.28	.13	.29	.45	.64	.84
Surg spec phy/10,000 work RVU	76	.36	.22	.10	.19	.35	.48	.64
Total NPP FTE/10,000 work RVU	112	.52	.59	.15	.26	.41	.63	.84
Total supp stf FTE/10,000 wrk RVU	122	10.59	9.29	6.22	7.93	9.39	11.36	13.69
Tot empl supp stf/10,000 work RVU	114	10.66	9.33	6.36	8.05	9.36	10.89	13.59
General administrative	110	.64	.49	.27	.38	.51	.80	1.12
Patient accounting	107	1.44	1.46	.45	.93	1.20	1.69	2.18
General accounting	91	.18	.23	.05	.08	.13	.20	.28
Managed care administrative	58	.29	.51	.03	.05	.15	.36	.58
Information technology	75	.23	.27	.05	.10	.18	.29	.40
Housekeeping, maint, security	74	.26	.48	.03	.08	.14	.33	.47
Medical receptionists	108	2.08	1.52	1.01	1.34	1.83	2.44	3.20
Med secretaries,transcribers	86	.53	.64	.08	.23	.38	.65	1.04
Medical records	99	.84	.72	.28	.44	.73	1.02	1.50
Other admin support	67	.48	1.21	.04	.08	.16	.37	.74
***Total administrative supp staff**	70	6.36	6.78	3.33	4.41	5.32	6.51	8.01
Registered Nurses	104	1.00	.89	.17	.41	.85	1.32	1.83
Licensed Practical Nurses	99	1.03	1.20	.12	.31	.64	1.41	2.36
Med assistants, nurse aides	104	1.66	1.57	.40	.73	1.30	2.10	3.33
***Total clinical supp staff**	103	3.40	2.86	1.82	2.30	2.97	3.90	4.78
Clinical laboratory	89	.60	.45	.15	.36	.56	.74	1.02
Radiology and imaging	93	.52	.34	.14	.26	.49	.70	.82
Other medical support serv	69	.69	1.27	.09	.14	.43	.76	1.23
***Total ancillary supp staff**	64	1.88	1.92	.75	1.06	1.66	2.15	2.76
Tot contracted supp staff	46	.38	.59	.02	.06	.17	.47	1.03
Tot RVU/work RVU	95	2.60	5.13	1.46	1.93	2.03	2.27	2.65
Patients/work RVU	73	.42	.69	.15	.21	.29	.44	.65
Tot procedures/work RVU	103	2.48	2.76	1.28	1.71	2.06	2.45	3.09
Square feet/work RVU	116	.43	.33	.24	.30	.38	.49	.59
Total support staff FTE/phy	299	5.12	1.60	3.38	4.07	4.95	5.92	7.04

*See pages 260 and 261 for definition.

Table 1.9b: Charges, Revenue and Cost

	Count	Mean	Std. Dev.	10th %tile	25th %tile	Median	75th %tile	90th %tile
Total gross charges	121	$201.91	$206.70	$118.31	$135.78	$179.93	$213.13	$263.85
Total medical revenue	122	$130.34	$125.07	$81.15	$92.93	$112.90	$137.75	$166.08
Net fee-for-service revenue	114	$112.45	$105.93	$66.39	$80.46	$98.23	$122.39	$147.37
Net capitation revenue	51	$27.78	$36.29	$1.17	$3.59	$12.12	$38.73	$75.32
Net other medical revenue	92	$8.51	$25.44	$.09	$.79	$2.35	$5.79	$17.30
Total supp staff cost/work RVU	122	$40.40	$33.52	$22.70	$28.36	$35.29	$46.19	$55.51
Total general operating cost	122	$39.16	$44.19	$19.88	$25.10	$33.68	$42.07	$55.33
Total operating cost	122	$79.62	$76.70	$48.30	$53.45	$69.96	$86.00	$104.71
Total med rev after oper cost	122	$50.72	$50.81	$25.52	$34.78	$46.09	$55.09	$63.59
Total provider cost/work RVU	122	$55.14	$44.26	$36.20	$42.19	$49.99	$58.17	$66.72
Total NPP cost/work RVU	114	$4.52	$5.19	$1.16	$2.11	$3.37	$5.49	$8.09
Provider consultant cost	49	$2.83	$3.94	$.27	$.73	$1.33	$4.05	$5.15
Total physician cost/work RVU	122	$50.03	$38.30	$32.54	$39.13	$45.70	$52.87	$60.87
Total phy compensation	113	$42.96	$36.06	$27.72	$32.76	$38.95	$44.01	$51.08
Total phy benefit cost	113	$6.76	$4.40	$2.69	$4.70	$6.07	$8.03	$9.51
Total cost	122	$134.76	$119.78	$86.97	$101.15	$118.17	$140.74	$168.30
Net nonmedical revenue	101	$5.80	$16.56	-$.52	$.21	$.99	$5.75	$17.11
Net inc, prac with fin sup	23	$1.34	$28.32	-$14.04	-$6.23	$.00	$1.13	$13.29
Net inc, prac w/o fin sup	94	-$.21	$15.47	-$12.87	-$4.22	$.17	$2.49	$7.43
Net inc, excl fin supp (all prac)	117	-$3.13	$16.95	-$21.55	-$8.87	-$.28	$1.95	$5.82
Total support staff FTE/phy	299	5.12	1.60	3.38	4.07	4.95	5.92	7.04

Multispecialty — All Practices
(per Patient)

Table 1.10a: Staffing, RVUs, Procedures and Square Footage

	Count	Mean	Std. Dev.	10th %tile	25th %tile	Median	75th %tile	90th %tile
Total prov FTE/10,000 patients	**125**	**8.65**	**8.90**	**3.42**	**5.00**	**7.42**	**10.56**	**13.69**
Total phy FTE/10,000 pat	137	7.08	7.49	2.59	4.25	6.34	8.80	10.75
Prim care phy/10,000 pat	132	4.36	2.18	1.68	2.85	3.96	5.52	7.61
Nonsurg phy/10,000 pat	90	2.19	3.15	.38	.84	1.51	2.74	4.23
Surg spec phy/10,000 pat	86	2.13	5.41	.21	.46	1.24	2.41	3.31
Total NPP FTE/10,000 pat	125	1.57	1.51	.33	.60	1.13	2.13	3.33
Total supp staff FTE/10,000 pat	**137**	**35.05**	**28.86**	**13.42**	**20.11**	**30.01**	**43.31**	**58.28**
Total empl supp staff/10,000 pat	137	34.68	28.74	13.42	19.39	29.98	43.25	58.27
General administrative	132	2.28	2.79	.58	.94	1.67	2.88	4.03
Patient accounting	125	4.99	5.06	1.44	2.17	3.94	6.39	9.17
General accounting	114	.60	.49	.16	.27	.52	.86	1.12
Managed care administrative	68	.92	1.22	.08	.19	.39	1.01	3.25
Information technology	91	.76	.77	.12	.25	.52	1.02	1.68
Housekeeping, maint, security	80	.74	.83	.06	.15	.47	1.12	2.00
Medical receptionists	130	6.54	4.75	1.84	3.51	5.92	8.70	11.42
Med secretaries,transcribers	104	1.80	2.07	.15	.60	1.13	2.49	3.98
Medical records	115	2.68	1.92	.85	1.21	2.15	4.13	5.59
Other admin support	77	1.33	4.41	.17	.27	.59	1.18	1.98
*****Total administrative supp staff**	**71**	**22.62**	**21.60**	**8.51**	**12.51**	**18.62**	**27.44**	**37.92**
Registered Nurses	121	3.55	5.57	.39	1.02	2.44	4.59	6.72
Licensed Practical Nurses	120	3.65	3.37	.48	1.15	2.13	5.66	8.24
Med assistants, nurse aides	124	4.51	3.14	1.24	2.28	3.97	6.21	9.00
*****Total clinical supp staff**	**112**	**10.95**	**8.33**	**4.05**	**6.93**	**9.91**	**13.68**	**17.70**
Clinical laboratory	108	2.10	1.57	.47	.90	1.52	3.19	4.18
Radiology and imaging	108	2.00	2.83	.33	.80	1.38	2.58	4.14
Other medical support serv	80	2.05	2.23	.15	.39	1.35	3.08	4.64
*****Total ancillary supp staff**	**72**	**6.61**	**6.03**	**1.51**	**2.66**	**5.04**	**8.75**	**12.77**
Tot contracted supp staff	53	.95	1.21	.07	.22	.53	1.15	2.41
Tot RVU/patient	75	7.80	4.80	2.54	4.54	6.93	10.34	14.42
Physician work RVU/patient	73	3.71	1.84	1.55	2.26	3.44	4.76	6.56
Tot procedures/patient	124	7.81	4.98	2.73	4.71	7.15	10.67	12.90
Square feet/patient	127	1.43	1.28	.49	.73	1.13	1.87	2.53
Total support staff FTE/phy	**299**	**5.12**	**1.60**	**3.38**	**4.07**	**4.95**	**5.92**	**7.04**

*See pages 260 and 261 for definition.

Table 1.10b: Charges, Revenue and Cost

	Count	Mean	Std. Dev.	10th %tile	25th %tile	Median	75th %tile	90th %tile
Total gross charges	**137**	**$713.98**	**$949.18**	**$253.77**	**$357.59**	**$508.11**	**$815.82**	**$1,277.87**
Total medical revenue	**137**	**$450.21**	**$565.73**	**$152.41**	**$233.50**	**$341.86**	**$555.20**	**$803.37**
Net fee-for-service revenue	135	$391.85	$544.36	$120.96	$199.77	$282.68	$456.99	$719.39
Net capitation revenue	62	$95.05	$145.81	$2.64	$10.40	$28.71	$128.55	$289.01
Net other medical revenue	104	$20.13	$36.70	$.67	$3.45	$9.46	$18.97	$42.63
Total support staff cost/patient	**137**	**$133.40**	**$133.91**	**$49.66**	**$69.72**	**$105.50**	**$162.96**	**$243.12**
Total general operating cost	**137**	**$129.85**	**$150.27**	**$43.61**	**$63.51**	**$101.69**	**$153.28**	**$247.94**
Total operating cost	**137**	**$262.50**	**$281.66**	**$90.00**	**$141.78**	**$205.19**	**$318.18**	**$448.83**
Total med rev after oper cost	**137**	**$187.71**	**$291.44**	**$48.46**	**$90.89**	**$138.08**	**$217.55**	**$320.88**
Total provider cost/patient	**137**	**$195.91**	**$289.08**	**$64.84**	**$97.80**	**$144.72**	**$230.92**	**$329.06**
Total NPP cost/patient	128	$12.79	$11.89	$2.85	$4.88	$8.52	$18.79	$28.31
Provider consultant cost	52	$7.20	$7.25	$.58	$1.71	$5.02	$10.37	$17.80
Total physician cost/patient	137	$181.24	$281.55	$54.89	$89.80	$139.16	$207.11	$311.97
Total phy compensation	136	$157.40	$250.02	$46.76	$77.01	$116.35	$175.79	$273.53
Total phy benefit cost	134	$23.72	$34.16	$5.82	$10.43	$18.84	$28.88	$41.09
Total cost	**137**	**$458.41**	**$564.73**	**$150.77**	**$238.31**	**$352.38**	**$558.09**	**$781.78**
Net nonmedical revenue	115	$10.28	$30.51	-$3.75	$.06	$1.63	$8.72	$32.28
Net inc, prac with fin sup	17	-$11.13	$38.79	-$60.14	-$14.57	$2.53	$3.83	$18.26
Net inc, prac w/o fin sup	114	$3.96	$44.25	-$33.04	-$3.50	$3.24	$13.05	$33.30
Net inc, excl fin supp (all prac)	131	-$3.09	$50.23	-$61.31	-$14.32	$1.71	$10.41	$32.16
Total support staff FTE/phy	**299**	**5.12**	**1.60**	**3.38**	**4.07**	**4.95**	**5.92**	**7.04**

Multispecialty — All Practices
(Procedure and Charge Data)

Table 1.11a: Activity Charges to Total Gross Charges Ratios

	Count	Mean	Std. Dev.	10th %tile	25th %tile	Median	75th %tile	90th %tile
Total proc gross charges	225	93.19%	7.32%	82.26%	90.23%	95.53%	98.36%	100.00%
Medical proc-inside practice	224	48.09%	19.21%	26.09%	34.00%	43.79%	62.51%	76.20%
Medical proc-outside practice	197	10.23%	8.22%	3.05%	5.70%	8.84%	13.13%	18.08%
Surg proc-inside practice	212	7.17%	6.08%	2.32%	3.92%	5.64%	8.36%	13.87%
Surg proc-outside practice	169	15.79%	11.42%	2.32%	7.08%	14.77%	21.36%	29.18%
Laboratory procedures	219	10.43%	7.11%	1.34%	4.96%	10.11%	14.09%	20.02%
Radiology procedures	206	7.83%	5.56%	1.10%	3.29%	6.58%	12.12%	15.34%
Tot nonproc gross charges	196	7.93%	7.72%	1.23%	2.53%	5.54%	10.83%	18.10%
Total support staff FTE/phy	299	5.12	1.60	3.38	4.07	4.95	5.92	7.04

Table 1.11b: Medical Procedure Data (inside the practice)

	Count	Mean	Std. Dev.	10th %tile	25th %tile	Median	75th %tile	90th %tile
Gross charges/procedure	218	$77.24	$26.47	$52.58	$63.08	$73.88	$85.29	$104.44
Total cost/procedure	195	$64.95	$21.17	$42.43	$50.68	$61.75	$75.45	$94.20
Operating cost/procedure	180	$40.19	$16.74	$24.52	$29.36	$37.26	$46.12	$62.66
Provider cost/procedure	198	$25.04	$7.68	$15.60	$19.64	$24.39	$29.85	$34.40
Procedures/patient	125	3.70	2.02	1.53	2.32	3.57	4.73	5.73
Gross charges/patient	126	$270.58	$161.98	$108.90	$159.11	$241.23	$335.64	$455.53
Procedures/physician	221	5,728	2,302	3,310	4,345	5,456	6,718	8,193
Gross charges/physician	224	$415,235	$149,499	$256,868	$325,546	$391,049	$485,997	$581,377
Procedures/provider	197	4,664	1,914	2,763	3,568	4,399	5,369	6,621
Gross charges/provider	201	$338,628	$128,850	$207,585	$263,297	$317,256	$393,575	$471,760
Gross charge to total cost ratio	195	1.22	.32	.87	1.05	1.19	1.39	1.55
Oper cost to total cost ratio	180	.61	.07	.53	.57	.61	.65	.70
Prov cost to total cost ratio	195	.39	.07	.30	.35	.40	.44	.48
Total support staff FTE/phy	299	5.12	1.60	3.38	4.07	4.95	5.92	7.04

Table 1.11c: Medical Procedure Data (outside the practice)

	Count	Mean	Std. Dev.	10th %tile	25th %tile	Median	75th %tile	90th %tile
Gross charges/procedure	192	$122.19	$46.17	$81.14	$98.37	$114.94	$140.82	$170.90
Total cost/procedure	171	$58.45	$29.08	$36.82	$44.44	$54.46	$68.27	$81.18
Operating cost/procedure	161	$23.13	$11.84	$13.51	$16.33	$20.96	$26.87	$33.59
Provider cost/procedure	174	$35.20	$19.20	$21.17	$26.54	$32.77	$41.06	$49.26
Procedures/patient	114	.64	.73	.10	.25	.45	.76	1.35
Gross charges/patient	115	$75.40	$94.69	$13.19	$28.14	$44.35	$87.94	$172.50
Procedures/physician	194	862	826	225	411	674	1,097	1,481
Gross charges/physician	197	$99,805	$100,302	$28,761	$49,477	$80,105	$108,898	$177,275
Procedures/provider	176	688	579	185	338	538	881	1,245
Gross charges/provider	181	$82,601	$74,326	$25,650	$41,528	$63,324	$94,698	$151,141
Gross charge to total cost ratio	171	2.20	.55	1.58	1.85	2.14	2.48	2.78
Oper cost to total cost ratio	161	.39	.08	.29	.34	.39	.44	.48
Prov cost to total cost ratio	171	.61	.08	.52	.56	.61	.66	.70
Total support staff FTE/phy	299	5.12	1.60	3.38	4.07	4.95	5.92	7.04

Multispecialty — All Practices
(Procedure and Charge Data)

Table 1.11d: Surgery/Anesthesia Procedure Data (inside the practice)

	Count	Mean	Std. Dev.	10th %tile	25th %tile	Median	75th %tile	90th %tile
Gross charges/procedure	208	$137.31	$147.53	$30.69	$57.54	$97.54	$168.46	$260.26
Total cost/procedure	186	$118.51	$113.16	$27.16	$50.40	$82.80	$144.94	$253.21
Operating cost/procedure	172	$74.83	$72.68	$17.09	$32.84	$52.13	$92.25	$167.07
Provider cost/procedure	188	$45.60	$44.76	$9.64	$18.27	$32.90	$57.04	$87.85
Procedures/patient	118	.56	.54	.06	.16	.37	.87	1.41
Gross charges/patient	119	$54.00	$109.02	$8.13	$15.45	$31.40	$57.70	$112.02
Procedures/physician	209	761	646	136	275	554	1,165	1,568
Gross charges/physician	212	$70,194	$67,243	$15,145	$28,211	$50,972	$83,341	$147,782
Procedures/provider	187	648	546	130	239	480	959	1,325
Gross charges/provider	190	$61,206	$60,279	$14,614	$24,886	$43,198	$71,393	$132,668
Gross charge to total cost ratio	186	1.22	.32	.87	1.05	1.19	1.37	1.53
Oper cost to total cost ratio	172	.61	.07	.53	.57	.61	.65	.70
Prov cost to total cost ratio	186	.39	.07	.30	.35	.40	.44	.48
Total support staff FTE/phy	299	5.12	1.60	3.38	4.07	4.95	5.92	7.04

Table 1.11e: Surgery/Anesthesia Procedure Data (outside the practice)

	Count	Mean	Std. Dev.	10th %tile	25th %tile	Median	75th %tile	90th %tile
Gross charges/procedure	165	$818.69	$465.51	$199.58	$450.87	$816.26	$1,089.72	$1,404.74
Total cost/procedure	151	$398.48	$244.23	$94.17	$228.94	$374.45	$519.31	$698.58
Operating cost/procedure	142	$153.74	$105.51	$35.54	$83.03	$138.14	$196.97	$278.57
Provider cost/procedure	152	$244.35	$148.22	$52.92	$137.39	$234.12	$326.04	$427.84
Procedures/patient	95	.28	.48	.01	.06	.12	.27	.61
Gross charges/patient	93	$119.72	$105.85	$12.43	$37.31	$83.27	$207.61	$275.71
Procedures/physician	168	330	551	21	81	193	303	779
Gross charges/physician	169	$172,464	$176,209	$16,140	$58,311	$144,789	$249,241	$322,068
Procedures/provider	153	273	428	17	60	156	267	637
Gross charges/provider	155	$139,792	$133,047	$12,175	$42,679	$119,069	$197,092	$257,803
Gross charge to total cost ratio	151	2.21	.57	1.59	1.87	2.13	2.47	2.83
Oper cost to total cost ratio	142	.39	.08	.29	.34	.39	.44	.48
Prov cost to total cost ratio	151	.61	.08	.53	.56	.61	.66	.71
Total support staff FTE/phy	299	5.12	1.60	3.38	4.07	4.95	5.92	7.04

Multispecialty — All Practices
(Procedure and Charge Data)

Table 1.11f: Clinical Laboratory/Pathology Procedure Data

	Count	Mean	Std. Dev.	10th %tile	25th %tile	Median	75th %tile	90th %tile
Gross charges/procedure	213	$33.42	$49.44	$14.88	$19.79	$29.06	$37.03	$46.08
Total cost/procedure	191	$26.47	$45.26	$12.21	$17.39	$22.25	$27.75	$35.69
Operating cost/procedure	177	$15.12	$6.19	$7.80	$11.16	$14.33	$18.38	$22.58
Provider cost/procedure	195	$9.74	$15.59	$4.16	$5.96	$7.94	$10.12	$13.02
Procedures/patient	122	2.35	1.82	.29	.85	2.19	3.28	5.13
Gross charges/patient	124	$69.78	$59.40	$5.68	$23.39	$51.21	$103.61	$166.02
Procedures/physician	215	3,367	2,345	477	1,569	3,300	4,604	6,318
Gross charges/physician	219	$103,081	$76,479	$8,267	$45,136	$96,168	$148,067	$194,925
Procedures/provider	192	2,822	1,688	512	1,554	2,826	3,712	5,120
Gross charges/provider	196	$89,097	$60,353	$10,862	$50,865	$82,831	$124,778	$162,929
Gross charge to total cost ratio	192	1.30	.34	.92	1.10	1.28	1.45	1.70
Oper cost to total cost ratio	177	.64	.09	.53	.58	.65	.69	.73
Prov cost to total cost ratio	192	.37	.09	.27	.31	.36	.42	.49
Total support staff FTE/phy	299	5.12	1.60	3.38	4.07	4.95	5.92	7.04

Table 1.11g: Diagnostic Radiology and Imaging Procedure Data

	Count	Mean	Std. Dev.	10th %tile	25th %tile	Median	75th %tile	90th %tile
Gross charges/procedure	202	$158.75	$120.76	$64.24	$82.02	$133.60	$198.48	$282.02
Total cost/procedure	181	$130.91	$104.48	$58.81	$75.64	$101.41	$158.89	$231.73
Operating cost/procedure	172	$85.08	$68.67	$35.94	$46.84	$71.97	$104.32	$148.49
Provider cost/procedure	185	$45.69	$37.56	$18.27	$24.36	$36.57	$58.11	$81.94
Procedures/patient	117	.48	.89	.04	.12	.30	.61	.82
Gross charges/patient	116	$84.64	$202.69	$5.68	$16.31	$35.73	$108.79	$171.62
Procedures/physician	205	574	426	50	244	555	766	1,100
Gross charges/physician	206	$90,828	$87,520	$6,232	$26,821	$64,044	$132,686	$210,200
Procedures/provider	187	477	346	53	228	470	620	858
Gross charges/provider	188	$78,029	$74,505	$7,400	$22,057	$52,767	$114,912	$182,480
Gross charge to total cost ratio	182	1.25	.34	.92	1.05	1.24	1.42	1.66
Oper cost to total cost ratio	173	.65	.10	.51	.59	.65	.71	.75
Prov cost to total cost ratio	182	.35	.10	.25	.29	.35	.41	.49
Total support staff FTE/phy	299	5.12	1.60	3.38	4.07	4.95	5.92	7.04

Table 1.11h: Nonprocedural Gross Charge Data

	Count	Mean	Std. Dev.	10th %tile	25th %tile	Median	75th %tile	90th %tile
Gross charges/patient	111	$78.72	$160.56	$3.90	$12.52	$32.34	$90.25	$191.95
Nonproc gross charges/physician	196	$89,674	$109,647	$7,761	$21,856	$49,720	$113,900	$200,486
Gross charges/provider	178	$79,953	$97,058	$7,300	$20,013	$42,441	$112,605	$190,674
Total support staff FTE/phy	299	5.12	1.60	3.38	4.07	4.95	5.92	7.04

Multispecialty — Not Hospital or IDS Owned

Table 2.1: Staffing and Practice Data

	Count	Mean	Std. Dev.	10th %tile	25th %tile	Median	75th %tile	90th %tile
Total provider FTE	192	**61.61**	**76.73**	**9.53**	**15.77**	**34.79**	**75.38**	**156.84**
Total physician FTE	213	49.24	70.93	6.38	11.88	26.00	61.46	112.45
Total nonphysician provider FTE	192	12.21	19.47	1.48	2.50	5.57	14.74	33.97
Total support staff FTE	213	**261.03**	**337.62**	**31.76**	**56.70**	**140.00**	**313.60**	**641.48**
Number of branch clinics	158	8	8	1	2	5	9	18
Square footage of all facilities	199	105,636	161,664	13,000	22,390	49,500	120,000	263,351

Table 2.2: Accounts Receivable Data, Collection Percentages and Financial Ratios

	Count	Mean	Std. Dev.	10th %tile	25th %tile	Median	75th %tile	90th %tile
Total AR/physician	197	**$135,359**	**$64,947**	**$62,489**	**$86,798**	**$127,291**	**$178,104**	**$215,213**
Total AR/provider	180	**$111,403**	**$54,471**	**$55,929**	**$72,314**	**$102,466**	**$139,708**	**$177,973**
0-30 days in AR	198	50.29%	14.52%	30.76%	41.48%	51.67%	60.13%	69.43%
31-60 days in AR	198	15.23%	5.22%	9.22%	11.13%	14.81%	18.03%	22.68%
61-90 days in AR	198	8.18%	2.89%	4.98%	6.14%	7.82%	9.86%	11.59%
91-120 days in AR	198	5.61%	2.52%	3.07%	3.87%	5.33%	6.64%	8.48%
120+ days in AR	198	20.70%	12.22%	8.14%	12.98%	18.22%	26.47%	35.74%
Re-aged: 0-30 days in AR	78	53.62%	12.38%	36.22%	45.18%	53.57%	63.25%	70.17%
Re-aged: 31-60 days in AR	78	14.74%	5.04%	9.16%	10.46%	13.79%	17.65%	22.34%
Re-aged: 61-90 days in AR	78	7.81%	2.64%	4.83%	5.81%	7.12%	9.17%	11.58%
Re-aged: 91-120 days in AR	78	5.42%	2.51%	3.03%	3.83%	4.87%	6.29%	8.10%
Re-aged: 120+ days in AR	78	18.40%	9.37%	7.40%	12.36%	16.94%	22.85%	30.87%
Not re-aged: 0-30 days in AR	112	47.89%	14.64%	27.15%	38.83%	49.07%	58.27%	65.88%
Not re-aged: 31-60 days in AR	112	15.52%	5.39%	9.18%	11.22%	15.37%	18.76%	23.22%
Not re-aged: 61-90 days in AR	112	8.49%	3.06%	5.01%	6.68%	8.05%	9.98%	11.98%
Not re-aged: 91-120 days in AR	112	5.80%	2.56%	3.11%	3.91%	5.46%	7.00%	8.75%
Not re-aged: 120+ days in AR	112	22.31%	13.04%	8.98%	14.47%	18.97%	28.41%	37.41%
Months gross FFS charges in AR	173	1.71	.51	1.16	1.35	1.63	1.96	2.33
Days gross FFS charges in AR	173	52.07	15.45	35.20	41.12	49.70	59.71	70.74
Gross FFS collection %	186	62.65%	11.31%	49.80%	55.23%	62.54%	69.76%	75.73%
Adjusted FFS collection %	178	96.20%	11.51%	92.63%	95.88%	97.67%	98.89%	99.85%
Gross FFS + cap collection %	71	65.04%	13.42%	50.89%	56.29%	64.69%	72.97%	81.05%
Net cap rev % of gross cap chrg	60	79.14%	29.97%	42.69%	64.27%	77.01%	94.37%	115.52%
Current ratio	126	4.82	11.33	.57	1.05	1.64	2.96	8.73
Tot asset turnover ratio	126	6.80	6.76	1.57	2.78	4.37	7.40	17.74
Debt to equity ratio	126	4.07	7.31	.25	.83	1.79	4.65	8.08
Debt ratio	126	60.58%	24.57%	20.22%	45.22%	64.20%	82.29%	88.98%
Return on total assets	116	16.58%	45.31%	-6.92%	-.67%	3.52%	18.37%	65.27%
Return on equity	116	58.49%	175.99%	-20.20%	-2.04%	10.97%	54.10%	182.43%

Table 2.3: Breakout of Total Gross Charges by Type of Payer

	Count	Mean	Std. Dev.	10th %tile	25th %tile	Median	75th %tile	90th %tile
Medicare: fee-for-service	195	25.88%	14.48%	6.95%	14.40%	26.00%	35.28%	44.24%
Medicare: managed care FFS	195	1.32%	3.64%	.00%	.00%	.00%	.00%	4.01%
Medicare: capitation	195	1.16%	3.76%	.00%	.00%	.00%	.00%	2.80%
Medicaid: fee-for-service	195	6.07%	6.82%	.00%	1.00%	4.00%	8.40%	14.24%
Medicaid: managed care FFS	195	1.60%	5.22%	.00%	.00%	.00%	.06%	5.00%
Medicaid: capitation	195	.67%	2.30%	.00%	.00%	.00%	.00%	1.69%
Commercial: fee-for-service	195	37.56%	21.67%	5.30%	20.85%	39.30%	53.00%	65.03%
Commercial: managed care FFS	195	12.78%	20.24%	.00%	.00%	.00%	21.00%	43.02%
Commercial: capitation	195	4.45%	11.78%	.00%	.00%	.00%	2.00%	15.40%
Workers' compensation	195	1.63%	3.28%	.00%	.13%	1.00%	1.80%	3.42%
Charity care and prof courtesy	195	.51%	1.44%	.00%	.00%	.00%	.50%	1.50%
Self-pay	195	5.50%	5.28%	1.00%	2.00%	3.87%	7.51%	12.64%
Other federal government payers	195	.86%	4.47%	.00%	.00%	.00%	.40%	1.57%

Multispecialty — Not Hospital or IDS Owned
(per FTE Physician)

Table 2.4a: Staffing, RVUs, Patients, Procedures and Square Footage

	Count	Mean	Std. Dev.	10th %tile	25th %tile	Median	75th %tile	90th %tile
Total provider FTE/physician	**192**	**1.27**	**.22**	**1.08**	**1.12**	**1.22**	**1.35**	**1.52**
Prim care phy/physician	187	.65	.25	.35	.42	.64	.90	1.00
Nonsurg phy/physician	132	.28	.18	.06	.15	.26	.39	.52
Surg spec phy/physician	130	.23	.15	.07	.12	.22	.29	.39
Total NPP FTE/physician	192	.27	.22	.08	.12	.22	.35	.52
Total support staff FTE/phy	**213**	**5.39**	**1.60**	**3.64**	**4.41**	**5.31**	**6.20**	**7.21**
Total empl support staff FTE	190	5.39	1.57	3.70	4.38	5.32	6.15	7.21
General administrative	185	.32	.19	.13	.19	.27	.38	.54
Patient accounting	184	.77	.35	.38	.53	.71	.94	1.28
General accounting	157	.09	.07	.04	.06	.08	.11	.15
Managed care administrative	89	.14	.14	.03	.04	.10	.18	.39
Information technology	125	.12	.08	.03	.06	.10	.15	.22
Housekeeping, maint, security	122	.13	.15	.02	.04	.07	.19	.31
Medical receptionists	182	.96	.42	.41	.72	.92	1.20	1.49
Med secretaries,transcribers	151	.29	.26	.05	.12	.23	.36	.59
Medical records	169	.43	.23	.16	.28	.40	.55	.70
Other admin support	109	.16	.17	.03	.05	.09	.17	.45
*Total administrative supp staff	**114**	**3.21**	**1.05**	**2.09**	**2.56**	**3.12**	**3.82**	**4.22**
Registered Nurses	166	.50	.39	.09	.22	.41	.74	.97
Licensed Practical Nurses	160	.56	.48	.08	.20	.43	.90	1.13
Med assistants, nurse aides	171	.79	.49	.22	.43	.72	1.05	1.45
*Total clinical supp staff	**171**	**1.67**	**.57**	**1.12**	**1.36**	**1.58**	**1.94**	**2.34**
Clinical laboratory	157	.36	.19	.16	.25	.35	.44	.58
Radiology and imaging	161	.31	.17	.11	.18	.29	.41	.53
Other medical support serv	115	.31	.26	.05	.12	.26	.44	.61
*Total ancillary supp staff	**123**	**.91**	**.41**	**.36**	**.61**	**.93**	**1.20**	**1.49**
Tot contracted supp staff	81	.19	.27	.01	.03	.11	.25	.44
Tot RVU/physician	81	17,014	46,415	6,400	9,036	11,316	14,375	19,387
Physician work RVU/physician	82	5,609	1,931	3,797	4,689	5,570	6,154	7,684
Patients/physician	103	2,056	1,316	965	1,148	1,569	2,494	4,048
Tot procedures/physician	159	12,542	5,649	7,382	9,837	12,141	14,472	16,502
Square feet/physician	199	2,170	1,126	1,148	1,539	2,038	2,532	3,005

*See pages 260 and 261 for definition.

Table 2.4b: Charges and Revenue

	Count	Mean	Std. Dev.	10th %tile	25th %tile	Median	75th %tile	90th %tile
Net fee-for-service revenue	189	$596,700	$209,957	$340,125	$470,723	$592,212	$742,459	$857,387
Gross FFS charges	187	$981,103	$422,302	$522,663	$693,994	$922,776	$1,196,790	$1,498,074
Adjustments to FFS charges	174	$378,885	$241,368	$138,502	$220,551	$326,711	$491,938	$684,238
Adjusted FFS charges	178	$623,469	$230,016	$340,907	$487,323	$609,252	$763,960	$886,326
Bad debts due to FFS activity	166	$18,677	$17,053	$3,145	$6,825	$13,567	$25,933	$40,390
Net capitation revenue	72	$128,485	$169,948	$4,379	$17,728	$54,019	$197,340	$396,474
Gross capitation charges	60	$208,942	$349,902	$10,873	$33,539	$88,130	$220,924	$570,621
Capitation revenue	70	$190,602	$271,788	$5,059	$20,806	$64,068	$263,103	$631,683
Purch serv for cap patients	23	$178,668	$205,506	$8,730	$38,498	$91,199	$258,790	$588,848
Net other medical revenue	139	$29,220	$54,474	$1,158	$5,929	$14,396	$31,200	$57,909
Gross rev from other activity	136	$43,628	$70,034	$1,805	$7,204	$18,276	$40,659	$116,204
Other medical revenue	110	$23,211	$55,872	$957	$3,099	$8,561	$18,143	$37,738
Rev from sale of goods/services	82	$45,931	$69,237	$1,138	$6,108	$17,207	$56,238	$125,566
Cost of sales	52	$36,102	$49,776	$1,822	$3,764	$13,602	$43,503	$132,517
Total gross charges	**203**	**$992,741**	**$337,503**	**$569,752**	**$734,131**	**$965,521**	**$1,216,186**	**$1,480,361**
Total medical revenue	**213**	**$651,733**	**$199,479**	**$400,125**	**$515,182**	**$633,096**	**$772,072**	**$907,235**

Multispecialty — Not Hospital or IDS Owned
(per FTE Physician)

Table 2.4c: Operating Cost

	Count	Mean	Std. Dev.	10th %tile	25th %tile	Median	75th %tile	90th %tile
Total support staff cost/phy	213	$196,771	$66,621	$124,948	$152,374	$187,639	$230,486	$291,066
Total empl supp staff cost/phy	194	$158,293	$51,998	$98,680	$121,931	$152,448	$186,254	$226,453
General administrative	186	$18,816	$12,599	$8,199	$11,003	$16,006	$23,146	$31,133
Patient accounting	186	$19,516	$8,236	$10,488	$13,917	$18,526	$23,702	$29,766
General accounting	159	$3,551	$2,583	$1,509	$2,083	$2,833	$4,210	$5,716
Managed care administrative	88	$4,791	$5,845	$842	$1,490	$2,665	$5,443	$12,613
Information technology	127	$4,786	$3,423	$1,296	$2,557	$4,008	$6,173	$9,179
Housekeeping, maint, security	124	$3,056	$2,837	$544	$1,061	$2,046	$4,364	$7,018
Medical receptionists	182	$21,005	$9,684	$8,727	$14,448	$20,044	$26,319	$33,625
Med secretaries,transcribers	151	$7,537	$6,233	$1,390	$3,306	$6,282	$9,733	$15,261
Medical records	170	$8,601	$5,007	$2,882	$5,287	$7,732	$10,915	$14,461
Other admin support	110	$3,944	$4,633	$753	$1,271	$2,313	$4,997	$9,084
*****Total administrative supp staff**	110	$89,476	$31,763	$56,419	$69,902	$85,289	$102,071	$135,129
Registered Nurses	166	$20,253	$15,484	$3,631	$8,280	$16,832	$30,736	$39,821
Licensed Practical Nurses	157	$15,880	$13,122	$2,752	$5,904	$12,811	$23,863	$31,699
Med assistants, nurse aides	168	$19,755	$12,317	$5,322	$10,414	$17,834	$27,252	$35,431
*****Total clinical supp staff**	166	$48,721	$17,284	$30,854	$37,055	$45,637	$58,831	$70,461
Clinical laboratory	157	$10,904	$5,703	$4,260	$7,343	$10,653	$13,746	$17,745
Radiology and imaging	162	$11,262	$6,510	$3,816	$6,005	$10,257	$15,204	$19,930
Other medical support serv	119	$12,282	$14,901	$1,516	$4,100	$8,451	$14,573	$23,942
*****Total ancillary supp staff**	139	$31,015	$18,417	$10,741	$18,352	$29,427	$39,189	$52,797
Total empl supp staff benefits	208	$38,739	$16,042	$20,110	$26,302	$36,702	$49,246	$61,453
Tot contracted supp staff	114	$5,278	$7,683	$292	$987	$2,398	$6,470	$13,647
Total general operating cost	213	$193,325	$79,173	$102,446	$135,509	$179,697	$244,222	$301,382
Information technology	192	$12,074	$7,443	$4,862	$6,848	$10,158	$15,558	$23,000
Medical and surgical supply	192	$41,191	$35,813	$9,586	$16,253	$29,986	$53,940	$85,291
Building and occupancy	192	$43,929	$17,922	$24,997	$31,042	$43,524	$51,972	$62,882
Furniture and equipment	173	$10,665	$10,941	$1,242	$3,496	$8,552	$15,187	$24,430
Admin supplies and services	190	$12,693	$7,816	$5,752	$7,690	$10,945	$15,773	$21,840
Prof liability insurance	208	$15,305	$9,757	$6,180	$8,689	$12,708	$18,846	$26,565
Other insurance premiums	183	$2,083	$2,891	$422	$692	$1,324	$2,605	$4,244
Outside professional fees	187	$6,016	$8,443	$1,240	$1,902	$3,820	$6,998	$11,068
Promotion and marketing	189	$3,154	$2,756	$747	$1,339	$2,304	$4,051	$6,792
Clinical laboratory	175	$16,330	$9,944	$4,289	$9,644	$14,940	$21,885	$29,278
Radiology and imaging	164	$13,249	$13,302	$1,518	$3,042	$7,873	$19,342	$31,029
Other ancillary services	95	$10,576	$21,814	$233	$871	$3,053	$11,102	$22,993
Billing purchased services	115	$4,094	$7,065	$172	$772	$1,891	$3,639	$8,275
Management fees paid to MSO	13	$19,447	$15,473	$1,128	$3,343	$21,600	$29,127	$44,445
Misc operating cost	190	$11,901	$11,656	$2,520	$4,772	$8,459	$15,083	$25,118
Cost allocated to prac from par	3	*	*	*	*	*	*	*
Total operating cost	213	$389,705	$130,371	$234,814	$292,267	$378,896	$463,819	$579,550

*See pages 260 and 261 for definition.

Multispecialty — Not Hospital or IDS Owned
(per FTE Physician)

Table 2.4d: Provider Cost

	Count	Mean	Std. Dev.	10th %tile	25th %tile	Median	75th %tile	90th %tile
Total med rev after oper cost	213	$264,291	$104,350	$155,149	$202,077	$256,600	$314,991	$385,927
Total provider cost/physician	213	$265,224	$84,260	$161,688	$204,439	$254,950	$317,432	$379,652
Total NPP cost/physician	199	$22,848	$19,342	$5,510	$9,224	$18,813	$29,005	$46,506
Nonphysician provider comp	185	$18,687	$15,950	$4,927	$7,449	$14,815	$23,463	$39,249
Nonphysician prov benefit cost	170	$4,284	$4,048	$791	$1,412	$3,403	$5,804	$9,405
Provider consultant cost	80	$13,194	$12,656	$1,699	$3,634	$8,707	$20,036	$28,490
Total physician cost/physician	213	$239,683	$79,960	$147,292	$182,281	$224,448	$287,841	$348,720
Total phy compensation	195	$210,211	$73,082	$130,028	$158,621	$194,792	$251,028	$306,882
Total phy benefit cost	192	$32,750	$14,727	$11,941	$21,762	$32,365	$43,031	$50,778

Table 2.4e: Net Income or Loss

	Count	Mean	Std. Dev.	10th %tile	25th %tile	Median	75th %tile	90th %tile
Total cost	213	$654,929	$190,947	$400,910	$517,751	$641,293	$779,356	$908,283
Net nonmedical revenue	173	$8,268	$21,127	-$5,371	$209	$2,485	$9,364	$37,220
Nonmedical revenue	156	$11,924	$20,427	$232	$828	$4,064	$11,652	$42,169
Fin support for oper costs	5	*	*	*	*	*	*	*
Goodwill amortization	26	$2,776	$4,752	$16	$97	$543	$3,781	$11,823
Nonmedical cost	85	$4,610	$8,979	$6	$151	$1,305	$5,521	$16,431
Net inc, prac with fin sup	5	*	*	*	*	*	*	*
Net inc, prac w/o fin sup	195	$8,807	$47,500	-$26,079	-$2,151	$4,207	$21,336	$49,537
Net inc, excl fin supp (all prac)	200	$9,344	$48,904	-$26,152	-$2,537	$4,197	$21,671	$50,979

Table 2.4f: Assets and Liabilities

	Count	Mean	Std. Dev.	10th %tile	25th %tile	Median	75th %tile	90th %tile
Total assets	131	$202,286	$184,952	$45,657	$68,924	$145,611	$271,831	$480,978
Current assets	133	$105,491	$89,026	$7,767	$29,671	$95,831	$165,107	$231,257
Noncurrent assets	133	$93,988	$124,648	$8,158	$21,921	$44,335	$107,589	$283,641
Total liabilities	133	$120,164	$130,087	$13,300	$34,530	$64,789	$160,014	$313,490
Current liabilities	133	$60,207	$60,883	$4,179	$14,771	$40,433	$88,287	$145,624
Noncurrent liabilities	133	$59,957	$89,259	$0	$1,732	$19,035	$78,751	$217,292
Working capital	133	$45,284	$63,947	-$17,736	-$118	$27,207	$76,974	$150,617
Total net worth	133	$79,315	$89,602	$5,696	$13,775	$49,199	$112,627	$187,027

Multispecialty — Not Hospital or IDS Owned
(as a % of Total Medical Revenue)

Table 2.5a: Charges and Revenue

	Count	Mean	Std. Dev.	10th %tile	25th %tile	Median	75th %tile	90th %tile
Net fee-for-service revenue	189	89.74%	18.33%	64.50%	89.93%	97.11%	99.66%	100.00%
Net capitation revenue	72	18.53%	21.00%	.71%	2.99%	9.61%	28.93%	47.12%
Net other medical revenue	139	4.34%	7.40%	.15%	.94%	2.00%	4.39%	10.54%
Total gross charges	**210**	**158.28%**	**33.01%**	**122.07%**	**137.73%**	**155.61%**	**171.70%**	**196.77%**

Table 2.5b: Operating Cost

	Count	Mean	Std. Dev.	10th %tile	25th %tile	Median	75th %tile	90th %tile
Total support staff cost	**213**	**31.32%**	**12.60%**	**23.43%**	**25.83%**	**29.74%**	**33.42%**	**37.56%**
Total empl support staff cost	194	24.66%	9.74%	18.65%	20.52%	23.93%	26.31%	29.66%
General administrative	186	2.98%	2.59%	1.38%	1.75%	2.37%	3.39%	4.81%
Patient accounting	186	3.07%	1.46%	1.65%	2.18%	2.80%	3.57%	4.46%
General accounting	159	.57%	.58%	.20%	.31%	.43%	.66%	.91%
Managed care administrative	88	.71%	.87%	.14%	.24%	.36%	.82%	1.76%
Information technology	127	.65%	.41%	.19%	.38%	.59%	.87%	1.16%
Housekeeping, maint, security	124	.45%	.51%	.09%	.16%	.30%	.60%	.93%
Medical receptionists	182	3.39%	2.00%	1.32%	2.18%	2.98%	3.97%	5.76%
Med secretaries,transcribers	151	1.13%	.88%	.21%	.52%	.96%	1.51%	2.23%
Medical records	170	1.35%	1.07%	.57%	.83%	1.18%	1.58%	2.31%
Other admin support	110	.63%	.88%	.10%	.18%	.33%	.66%	1.57%
*Total administrative supp staff	**110**	**13.49%**	**7.79%**	**9.45%**	**10.39%**	**12.73%**	**14.38%**	**16.19%**
Registered Nurses	166	3.10%	2.98%	.68%	1.32%	2.61%	4.20%	5.86%
Licensed Practical Nurses	157	2.46%	2.15%	.42%	.88%	1.93%	3.44%	4.92%
Med assistants, nurse aides	168	3.26%	2.42%	.73%	1.57%	2.60%	4.58%	6.29%
*Total clinical supp staff	**166**	**7.45%**	**2.55%**	**4.96%**	**5.94%**	**7.07%**	**8.54%**	**10.12%**
Clinical laboratory	157	1.69%	1.30%	.66%	1.09%	1.42%	2.11%	3.04%
Radiology and imaging	162	1.57%	.74%	.69%	.98%	1.64%	2.03%	2.46%
Other medical support serv	119	1.61%	1.69%	.18%	.62%	1.14%	1.86%	3.39%
*Total ancillary supp staff	**139**	**4.27%**	**2.17%**	**1.78%**	**2.90%**	**4.02%**	**5.25%**	**6.83%**
Total empl supp staff benefits	208	6.14%	2.81%	3.59%	4.65%	5.91%	6.89%	8.60%
Tot contracted supp staff	114	.87%	1.66%	.05%	.14%	.38%	1.07%	2.02%
Total general operating cost	**213**	**29.63%**	**8.28%**	**21.99%**	**24.69%**	**28.87%**	**33.11%**	**37.02%**
Information technology	192	1.87%	1.17%	.83%	1.12%	1.62%	2.36%	3.35%
Medical and surgical supply	192	5.91%	3.98%	1.81%	3.07%	4.82%	7.55%	11.21%
Building and occupancy	192	6.84%	2.68%	4.20%	5.06%	6.46%	7.84%	10.17%
Furniture and equipment	173	1.57%	1.44%	.28%	.56%	1.20%	2.19%	3.34%
Admin supplies and services	191	1.93%	1.04%	1.00%	1.27%	1.77%	2.30%	3.22%
Prof liability insurance	208	2.41%	1.39%	.98%	1.43%	2.06%	2.96%	4.33%
Other insurance premiums	181	.28%	.23%	.07%	.11%	.21%	.38%	.61%
Outside professional fees	187	.89%	1.05%	.19%	.30%	.59%	1.06%	1.82%
Promotion and marketing	189	.46%	.36%	.13%	.23%	.37%	.59%	.92%
Clinical laboratory	175	2.58%	1.93%	.73%	1.27%	2.31%	3.30%	5.05%
Radiology and imaging	167	1.82%	1.62%	.25%	.50%	1.31%	2.87%	4.35%
Other ancillary services	95	1.28%	2.23%	.04%	.15%	.56%	1.39%	3.11%
Billing purchased services	115	.72%	1.40%	.03%	.11%	.29%	.58%	1.52%
Management fees paid to MSO	15	4.70%	5.87%	.05%	.51%	3.39%	6.39%	15.88%
Misc operating cost	190	1.77%	1.49%	.46%	.80%	1.33%	2.28%	3.59%
Cost allocated to prac from par	3	*	*	*	*	*	*	*
Total operating cost	**213**	**60.70%**	**16.02%**	**49.11%**	**54.48%**	**59.09%**	**63.09%**	**68.84%**

*See pages 260 and 261 for definition.

Multispecialty — Not Hospital or IDS Owned
(as a % of Total Medical Revenue)

Table 2.5c: Provider Cost

	Count	Mean	Std. Dev.	10th %tile	25th %tile	Median	75th %tile	90th %tile
Total med rev after oper cost	213	40.18%	11.55%	31.42%	37.01%	40.94%	45.63%	51.31%
Total provider cost	213	41.57%	9.50%	32.17%	36.26%	41.00%	45.46%	50.30%
Total NPP cost	199	3.58%	3.33%	.81%	1.53%	2.88%	4.43%	6.93%
Nonphysician provider comp	185	2.88%	2.65%	.69%	1.25%	2.35%	3.52%	5.36%
Nonphysician prov benefit cost	170	.65%	.65%	.12%	.25%	.50%	.86%	1.32%
Provider consultant cost	80	1.80%	1.59%	.23%	.57%	1.32%	2.70%	3.90%
Total physician cost	213	37.64%	8.82%	28.67%	31.98%	37.21%	41.91%	46.72%
Total phy compensation	195	32.31%	7.75%	24.45%	27.40%	31.72%	36.68%	41.05%
Total phy benefit cost	192	5.14%	2.40%	2.04%	3.68%	5.10%	6.41%	7.82%

Table 2.5d: Net Income or Loss

	Count	Mean	Std. Dev.	10th %tile	25th %tile	Median	75th %tile	90th %tile
Total cost	213	102.27%	19.23%	92.70%	97.04%	100.00%	102.41%	108.85%
Net nonmedical revenue	173	1.60%	4.86%	-.87%	.04%	.37%	1.48%	5.50%
Nonmedical revenue	156	2.12%	4.93%	.05%	.14%	.55%	1.75%	6.30%
Fin support for oper costs	5	*	*	*	*	*	*	*
Goodwill amortization	26	.43%	.75%	.00%	.01%	.06%	.53%	2.13%
Nonmedical cost	85	.60%	1.12%	.00%	.03%	.20%	.86%	2.42%
Net inc, prac with fin sup	5	*	*	*	*	*	*	*
Net inc, prac w/o fin sup	195	1.18%	8.77%	-3.70%	-.41%	.66%	3.20%	7.83%
Net inc, excl fin supp (all prac)	200	1.23%	8.83%	-3.91%	-.42%	.66%	3.39%	8.76%

Table 2.5e: Assets and Liabilities

	Count	Mean	Std. Dev.	10th %tile	25th %tile	Median	75th %tile	90th %tile
Total assets	133	29.43%	29.45%	5.58%	10.89%	22.35%	35.13%	62.39%
Current assets	133	15.38%	12.88%	1.54%	4.78%	14.63%	22.99%	29.90%
Noncurrent assets	133	14.05%	20.18%	1.45%	3.45%	6.54%	16.23%	36.97%
Total liabilities	133	17.38%	17.97%	2.46%	5.03%	12.09%	22.49%	45.56%
Current liabilities	133	8.42%	7.32%	.62%	2.72%	6.41%	12.93%	16.72%
Noncurrent liabilities	133	8.96%	13.62%	.00%	.39%	3.19%	11.17%	29.11%
Working capital	133	6.96%	10.28%	-2.73%	-.03%	3.61%	11.44%	20.75%
Total net worth	133	12.05%	16.39%	1.09%	2.46%	7.55%	16.61%	27.70%

Multispecialty — Not Hospital or IDS Owned
(per FTE Provider)

Table 2.6a: Staffing, RVUs, Patients, Procedures and Square Footage

	Count	Mean	Std. Dev.	10th %tile	25th %tile	Median	75th %tile	90th %tile
Total physician FTE/provider	192	.81	.11	.66	.74	.82	.89	.93
Prim care phy/provider	171	.52	.22	.27	.33	.46	.68	.86
Nonsurg phy/provider	122	.24	.16	.05	.12	.22	.33	.45
Surg spec phy/provider	120	.18	.11	.06	.10	.18	.25	.30
Total NPP FTE/provider	192	.19	.11	.07	.11	.18	.26	.34
Total support staff FTE/prov	192	4.34	1.09	3.10	3.62	4.28	4.96	5.76
Total empl supp staff FTE/prov	174	4.35	1.05	3.06	3.60	4.29	4.97	5.68
General administrative	171	.25	.14	.11	.14	.23	.30	.41
Patient accounting	170	.63	.28	.33	.42	.59	.77	1.06
General accounting	151	.07	.04	.03	.05	.06	.09	.13
Managed care administrative	83	.11	.11	.02	.04	.07	.14	.29
Information technology	120	.09	.06	.03	.05	.08	.12	.18
Housekeeping, maint, security	116	.10	.09	.02	.03	.06	.15	.22
Medical receptionists	167	.77	.32	.35	.61	.76	.93	1.13
Med secretaries,transcribers	141	.23	.21	.04	.11	.19	.28	.44
Medical records	158	.35	.18	.13	.22	.32	.45	.57
Other admin support	103	.12	.12	.02	.04	.08	.14	.31
*Total administrative supp staff	108	2.54	.73	1.66	2.05	2.56	3.02	3.39
Registered Nurses	153	.39	.29	.07	.17	.32	.58	.77
Licensed Practical Nurses	147	.44	.38	.07	.16	.35	.67	.89
Med assistants, nurse aides	157	.64	.38	.17	.34	.58	.90	1.19
*Total clinical supp staff	157	1.33	.40	.91	1.08	1.27	1.56	1.84
Clinical laboratory	148	.29	.13	.11	.22	.29	.36	.45
Radiology and imaging	153	.25	.14	.09	.14	.23	.33	.42
Other medical support serv	110	.25	.19	.05	.10	.21	.33	.48
*Total ancillary supp staff	117	.73	.33	.29	.50	.75	.95	1.12
Tot contracted supp staff	75	.13	.14	.01	.02	.08	.18	.33
Tot RVU/provider	74	9,588	4,007	5,383	7,152	9,024	12,167	14,203
Physician work RVU/provider	76	4,508	1,529	2,996	3,646	4,317	5,102	6,183
Patients/provider	96	1,692	1,138	742	947	1,289	2,066	3,229
Tot procedures/provider	145	10,059	3,309	5,975	8,118	9,930	11,614	13,744
Square feet/provider	181	1,725	682	1,005	1,284	1,637	2,026	2,470
Total support staff FTE/phy	213	5.39	1.60	3.64	4.41	5.31	6.20	7.21

*See pages 260 and 261 for definition.

Table 2.6b: Charges, Revenue and Cost

	Count	Mean	Std. Dev.	10th %tile	25th %tile	Median	75th %tile	90th %tile
Total gross charges	190	$851,784	$351,788	$488,518	$597,801	$769,313	$1,028,282	$1,329,452
Total medical revenue	192	$530,617	$165,360	$346,525	$417,539	$509,681	$636,360	$743,391
Net fee-for-service revenue	172	$488,851	$169,958	$288,284	$388,271	$470,471	$604,572	$701,594
Net capitation revenue	64	$102,205	$131,896	$3,607	$13,652	$45,089	$157,332	$295,048
Net other medical revenue	130	$19,652	$27,304	$1,004	$5,330	$12,072	$23,455	$36,209
Total support staff cost/prov	192	$158,603	$49,234	$100,927	$120,838	$157,071	$190,558	$221,605
Total general operating cost	192	$157,699	$67,261	$83,463	$113,763	$145,239	$193,820	$243,380
Total operating cost	192	$316,063	$105,703	$192,799	$235,995	$299,076	$379,737	$444,024
Total med rev after oper cost	192	$216,202	$83,455	$129,873	$166,012	$209,996	$261,481	$319,342
Total provider cost/provider	192	$215,404	$70,889	$130,833	$163,984	$206,515	$257,403	$311,115
Total NPP cost/provider	192	$16,261	$9,973	$5,118	$8,345	$15,518	$21,930	$29,554
Provider consultant cost	74	$10,872	$10,358	$1,557	$3,099	$6,718	$16,048	$22,897
Total physician cost/provider	192	$195,614	$71,955	$108,912	$144,073	$186,473	$234,739	$298,630
Total phy compensation	178	$171,907	$65,571	$94,395	$126,383	$162,982	$202,307	$265,164
Total phy benefit cost	175	$26,438	$12,241	$9,197	$16,215	$26,404	$35,025	$42,075
Total cost	192	$531,466	$158,907	$347,311	$416,712	$506,213	$630,538	$742,259
Net nonmedical revenue	158	$6,484	$17,058	-$4,751	$208	$1,991	$7,192	$28,445
Net inc, prac with fin sup	5	*	*	*	*	*	*	*
Net inc, prac w/o fin sup	174	$6,882	$35,544	-$17,181	-$1,610	$3,381	$16,996	$38,545
Net inc, excl fin supp (all prac)	179	$7,514	$37,175	-$18,454	-$2,333	$3,269	$17,196	$40,658
Total support staff FTE/phy	213	5.39	1.60	3.64	4.41	5.31	6.20	7.21

Multispecialty — Not Hospital or IDS Owned
(per Square Foot)

Table 2.7a: Staffing, RVUs, Patients and Procedures

	Count	Mean	Std. Dev.	10th %tile	25th %tile	Median	75th %tile	90th %tile
Total prov FTE/10,000 sq ft	**181**	**6.88**	**5.17**	**4.05**	**4.94**	**6.11**	**7.79**	**9.95**
Total phy FTE/10,000 sq ft	199	5.67	4.20	3.33	3.95	4.91	6.50	8.71
Prim care phy/10,000 sq ft	175	3.50	2.07	1.39	1.88	3.06	4.62	6.24
Nonsurg phy/10,000 sq ft	124	1.55	1.36	.33	.68	1.29	1.96	2.92
Surg spec phy/10,000 sq ft	122	1.17	.87	.35	.51	1.01	1.51	2.08
Total NPP FTE/10,000 sq ft	181	1.30	1.19	.38	.60	1.12	1.61	2.30
Total supp stf FTE/10,000 sq ft	**199**	**27.41**	**8.23**	**17.71**	**22.05**	**26.69**	**31.52**	**37.50**
Total empl supp stf/10,000 sq ft	178	27.05	7.87	17.65	22.03	26.46	31.28	36.33
General administrative	176	1.59	1.05	.63	.85	1.37	1.91	3.04
Patient accounting	176	3.88	2.29	1.87	2.58	3.40	4.66	6.29
General accounting	149	.46	.34	.18	.29	.39	.53	.79
Managed care administrative	85	.74	.77	.11	.22	.45	1.01	1.83
Information technology	118	.57	.37	.20	.32	.46	.74	1.14
Housekeeping, maint, security	116	.53	.45	.12	.20	.36	.77	1.15
Medical receptionists	172	4.83	2.45	1.80	3.31	4.35	6.12	8.26
Med secretaries,transcribers	143	1.42	1.45	.22	.52	1.04	1.76	2.81
Medical records	159	2.13	1.16	.78	1.28	1.99	2.80	3.69
Other admin support	104	.88	1.31	.14	.25	.44	.88	1.97
*****Total administrative supp staff**	**110**	**14.86**	**4.94**	**9.12**	**11.99**	**14.51**	**17.77**	**20.99**
Registered Nurses	157	2.38	1.72	.48	1.03	2.10	3.34	4.49
Licensed Practical Nurses	152	2.59	2.30	.58	.93	2.02	3.59	4.93
Med assistants, nurse aides	164	4.29	3.25	.93	1.97	3.39	5.58	8.95
*****Total clinical supp staff**	**165**	**8.20**	**3.34**	**4.79**	**5.93**	**7.39**	**9.77**	**11.78**
Clinical laboratory	151	1.73	1.02	.74	1.21	1.58	2.05	2.74
Radiology and imaging	152	1.45	.78	.54	.95	1.38	1.90	2.47
Other medical support serv	109	1.47	1.29	.24	.66	1.09	1.93	3.17
*****Total ancillary supp staff**	**119**	**4.38**	**2.38**	**1.63**	**2.92**	**3.98**	**5.81**	**6.87**
Tot contracted supp staff	80	.98	1.62	.07	.15	.49	1.04	1.99
Tot RVU/sq ft	78	8.48	17.50	3.12	4.55	6.32	7.90	9.88
Physician work RVU/sq ft	79	3.21	3.72	1.70	2.05	2.73	3.27	4.36
Patients/sq ft	96	1.13	.84	.39	.54	.89	1.55	2.37
Tot procedures/sq ft	151	6.37	3.11	3.51	4.45	5.66	7.44	10.10
Total support staff FTE/phy	**213**	**5.39**	**1.60**	**3.64**	**4.41**	**5.31**	**6.20**	**7.21**

*See pages 260 and 261 for definition.

Table 2.7b: Charges, Revenue and Cost

	Count	Mean	Std. Dev.	10th %tile	25th %tile	Median	75th %tile	90th %tile
Total gross charges	197	$569.56	$589.07	$287.34	$377.55	$503.70	$613.52	$838.93
Total medical revenue	199	$350.35	$238.73	$206.10	$253.77	$330.36	$402.29	$481.50
Net fee-for-service revenue	176	$305.39	$124.28	$162.34	$231.20	$293.24	$371.08	$447.94
Net capitation revenue	65	$66.20	$84.66	$3.11	$7.73	$27.11	$92.14	$199.48
Net other medical revenue	130	$13.03	$20.87	$.53	$2.77	$6.82	$15.68	$32.24
Total support staff cost/sq ft	199	$101.27	$37.39	$56.86	$80.23	$96.46	$118.22	$148.36
Total general operating cost	199	$97.85	$41.65	$55.02	$71.02	$91.49	$114.04	$141.35
Total operating cost	199	$199.15	$71.71	$119.22	$151.07	$193.19	$230.20	$271.15
Total med rev after oper cost	199	$151.77	$202.32	$65.28	$100.98	$130.72	$171.98	$209.44
Total provider cost/sq ft	199	$148.79	$166.05	$74.19	$99.44	$130.66	$169.03	$203.41
Total NPP cost/sq ft	187	$11.19	$12.07	$2.68	$4.94	$9.49	$14.26	$20.08
Provider consultant cost	77	$6.07	$6.12	$.88	$1.69	$4.34	$7.53	$14.13
Total physician cost/sq ft	199	$136.38	$157.30	$62.50	$89.57	$117.12	$149.73	$189.58
Total phy compensation	182	$109.73	$49.48	$57.45	$79.31	$104.26	$129.34	$166.13
Total phy benefit cost	180	$17.22	$9.55	$5.41	$10.31	$16.44	$22.27	$30.06
Total cost	199	$347.94	$206.13	$204.30	$258.77	$333.42	$392.21	$481.80
Net nonmedical revenue/sq ft	160	$3.87	$11.99	-$3.47	$.13	$1.11	$3.79	$15.76
Net inc, prac with fin sup	4	*	*	*	*	*	*	*
Net inc, prac w/o fin sup	183	$7.56	$43.26	-$10.51	-$1.32	$2.36	$10.37	$24.73
Net inc, excl fin supp (all prac)	187	$7.59	$43.72	-$12.15	-$1.37	$2.21	$10.37	$24.98
Total support staff FTE/phy	213	5.39	1.60	3.64	4.41	5.31	6.20	7.21

Multispecialty — Not Hospital or IDS Owned
(per Total RVU)

Table 2.8a: Staffing, Patients, Procedures and Square Footage

	Count	Mean	Std. Dev.	10th %tile	25th %tile	Median	75th %tile	90th %tile
Total prov FTE/10,000 tot RVU	74	1.42	1.69	.71	.82	1.11	1.40	1.86
Total phy FTE/10,000 tot RVU	81	1.16	1.33	.52	.70	.88	1.11	1.56
Prim care phy/10,000 tot RVU	74	.77	.92	.23	.35	.54	.83	1.31
Nonsurg phy/10,000 tot RVU	53	.36	.97	.08	.13	.22	.30	.50
Surg spec phy/10,000 tot RVU	49	.18	.11	.05	.09	.17	.23	.34
Total NPP FTE/10,000 tot RVU	74	.29	.40	.07	.12	.20	.32	.44
Total supp stf FTE/10,000 tot RVU	81	5.89	6.55	2.86	3.51	4.53	5.91	7.74
Tot empl supp stf/10,000 tot RVU	76	5.70	6.29	2.96	3.50	4.51	5.82	7.20
General administrative	74	.29	.29	.10	.17	.23	.35	.44
Patient accounting	75	.74	.89	.33	.45	.55	.80	1.12
General accounting	64	.11	.17	.03	.04	.06	.11	.20
Managed care administrative	43	.17	.30	.02	.05	.10	.17	.36
Information technology	50	.14	.17	.03	.05	.10	.16	.25
Housekeeping, maint, security	52	.15	.30	.02	.04	.07	.15	.26
Medical receptionists	73	1.02	1.16	.34	.56	.73	1.21	1.67
Med secretaries,transcribers	61	.28	.38	.04	.12	.18	.29	.74
Medical records	69	.45	.45	.13	.22	.35	.56	.80
Other admin support	47	.27	.66	.02	.04	.08	.18	.46
*Total administrative supp staff	48	3.57	4.45	1.64	1.97	2.71	3.30	5.66
Registered Nurses	72	.52	.53	.11	.22	.41	.58	1.06
Licensed Practical Nurses	67	.47	.72	.04	.12	.24	.49	1.18
Med assistants, nurse aides	70	.88	1.00	.22	.37	.65	1.03	1.66
*Total clinical supp staff	73	1.76	1.97	.68	1.02	1.27	1.85	2.59
Clinical laboratory	67	.34	.26	.15	.20	.26	.41	.61
Radiology and imaging	64	.28	.21	.10	.17	.23	.34	.50
Other medical support serv	51	.39	.77	.05	.10	.21	.43	.83
*Total ancillary supp staff	51	1.10	1.34	.38	.56	.80	1.13	1.65
Tot contracted supp staff	38	.35	.92	.01	.02	.07	.33	.81
Physician work RVU/tot RVU	68	.50	.17	.36	.43	.48	.51	.77
Patients/tot RVU	56	.25	.43	.07	.09	.15	.22	.45
Tot procedures/tot RVU	69	1.34	1.71	.59	.78	.99	1.38	1.98
Square feet/tot RVU	78	.22	.22	.10	.13	.16	.22	.32
Total support staff FTE/phy	213	5.39	1.60	3.64	4.41	5.31	6.20	7.21

*See pages 260 and 261 for definition.

Table 2.8b: Charges, Revenue and Cost

	Count	Mean	Std. Dev.	10th %tile	25th %tile	Median	75th %tile	90th %tile
Total gross charges	80	$115.04	$139.10	$61.17	$73.32	$89.43	$106.58	$164.62
Total medical revenue	81	$72.15	$84.35	$41.29	$47.26	$55.45	$69.20	$98.33
Net fee-for-service revenue	75	$61.35	$71.09	$31.81	$42.76	$47.22	$62.67	$77.84
Net capitation revenue	34	$14.21	$17.45	$.38	$1.97	$8.10	$21.37	$37.90
Net other medical revenue	63	$5.37	$15.53	$.08	$.65	$1.42	$3.15	$14.27
Total supp staff cost/tot RVU	81	$22.45	$23.90	$11.26	$13.96	$16.34	$22.80	$31.86
Total general operating cost	81	$21.25	$29.45	$10.15	$12.35	$15.56	$20.35	$30.28
Total operating cost	81	$43.70	$52.71	$24.40	$25.87	$32.07	$42.40	$59.74
Total med rev after oper cost	81	$28.46	$35.70	$15.23	$17.47	$22.74	$26.90	$37.27
Total provider cost/tot RVU	81	$28.50	$30.53	$16.62	$19.27	$22.26	$26.99	$40.52
Total NPP cost/tot RVU	76	$2.43	$3.31	$.48	$1.05	$1.72	$2.48	$4.14
Provider consultant cost	35	$1.50	$2.26	$.17	$.29	$.88	$1.73	$3.41
Total physician cost/tot RVU	81	$25.75	$26.49	$13.80	$17.15	$20.37	$24.50	$36.32
Total phy compensation	76	$21.49	$24.12	$12.10	$14.59	$17.50	$20.51	$30.05
Total phy benefit cost	76	$3.41	$3.17	$1.20	$2.00	$2.68	$3.73	$5.47
Total cost	67	$72.54	$52.42	$42.97	$54.00	$62.75	$72.69	$107.29
Net nonmedical revenue	64	$.99	$2.83	-$.41	$.03	$.25	$.56	$3.72
Net inc, prac with fin sup	3	*	*	*	*	*	*	*
Net inc, prac w/o fin sup	74	$2.48	$9.43	-$2.05	-$.12	$.43	$1.48	$5.92
Net inc, excl fin supp (all prac)	77	$2.49	$9.47	-$2.22	-$.13	$.42	$1.52	$6.94
Total support staff FTE/phy	213	5.39	1.60	3.64	4.41	5.31	6.20	7.21

Multispecialty — Not Hospital or IDS Owned
(per Work RVU)
Table 2.9a: Staffing, Patients, Procedures and Square Footage

	Count	Mean	Std. Dev.	10th %tile	25th %tile	Median	75th %tile	90th %tile
Total prov FTE/10,000 work RVU	76	**2.76**	**2.83**	**1.62**	**1.96**	**2.32**	**2.74**	**3.34**
Tot phy FTE/10,000 work RVU	82	2.19	2.14	1.30	1.62	1.80	2.13	2.64
Prim care phy/10,000 work RVU	76	1.44	1.32	.50	.70	1.15	1.75	2.42
Nonsurg phy/10,000 work RVU	54	.49	.24	.14	.32	.48	.66	.83
Surg spec phy/10,000 work RVU	52	.38	.22	.12	.21	.38	.48	.64
Total NPP FTE/10,000 work RVU	76	.56	.69	.15	.26	.42	.63	.89
Total supp stf FTE/10,000 wrk RVU	82	**11.41**	**11.16**	**6.01**	**8.26**	**9.71**	**11.78**	**14.30**
Tot empl supp stf/10,000 work RVU	77	11.50	11.18	6.56	8.57	9.69	11.73	14.06
General administrative	75	.63	.55	.27	.37	.50	.78	.96
Patient accounting	75	1.60	1.66	.81	1.02	1.28	1.74	2.32
General accounting	67	.20	.27	.06	.10	.13	.21	.33
Managed care administrative	42	.32	.55	.04	.09	.17	.42	.63
Information technology	54	.28	.31	.07	.13	.24	.33	.42
Housekeeping, maint, security	55	.30	.54	.05	.10	.15	.34	.48
Medical receptionists	75	2.01	1.75	.94	1.28	1.57	2.31	2.95
Med secretaries,transcribers	62	.53	.67	.07	.23	.40	.65	1.00
Medical records	71	.89	.79	.33	.48	.74	1.08	1.50
Other admin support	49	.43	1.03	.04	.08	.15	.32	.82
*****Total administrative supp staff**	51	**6.90**	**7.86**	**3.26**	**4.63**	**5.48**	**6.80**	**8.50**
Registered Nurses	73	1.05	.94	.17	.48	.88	1.30	1.83
Licensed Practical Nurses	68	1.04	1.35	.11	.31	.60	1.39	2.29
Med assistants, nurse aides	71	1.64	1.72	.40	.72	1.26	1.90	2.99
*****Total clinical supp staff**	73	**3.46**	**3.34**	**1.74**	**2.26**	**2.80**	**3.87**	**5.26**
Clinical laboratory	66	.68	.46	.30	.46	.59	.79	1.02
Radiology and imaging	66	.60	.34	.23	.35	.58	.77	.91
Other medical support serv	53	.83	1.42	.11	.29	.54	.96	1.46
*****Total ancillary supp staff**	52	**2.10**	**2.05**	**.90**	**1.27**	**1.82**	**2.34**	**2.95**
Tot contracted supp staff	36	.40	.65	.02	.05	.14	.48	1.23
Tot RVU/work RVU	68	2.86	6.06	1.30	1.95	2.10	2.34	2.81
Patients/work RVU	53	.46	.80	.15	.20	.27	.45	.72
Tot procedures/work RVU	72	2.78	3.24	1.42	1.87	2.16	2.53	3.26
Square feet/work RVU	79	.44	.39	.23	.31	.37	.49	.59
Total support staff FTE/phy	213	**5.39**	**1.60**	**3.64**	**4.41**	**5.31**	**6.20**	**7.21**

*See pages 260 and 261 for definition.

Table 2.9b: Charges, Revenue and Cost

	Count	Mean	Std. Dev.	10th %tile	25th %tile	Median	75th %tile	90th %tile
Total gross charges	81	**$223.25**	**$248.73**	**$123.87**	**$142.51**	**$190.65**	**$225.15**	**$280.30**
Total medical revenue	82	**$144.38**	**$149.74**	**$83.70**	**$98.90**	**$123.23**	**$148.26**	**$172.61**
Net fee-for-service revenue	76	$124.64	$127.18	$67.43	$86.05	$107.94	$128.41	$153.71
Net capitation revenue	32	$31.35	$33.71	$1.39	$4.72	$14.88	$48.22	$97.46
Net other medical revenue	65	$10.96	$29.90	$.17	$1.40	$2.87	$6.32	$24.25
Total supp staff cost/work RVU	82	**$43.37**	**$39.79**	**$22.70**	**$29.58**	**$36.73**	**$48.75**	**$58.43**
Total general operating cost	82	**$43.39**	**$52.94**	**$21.43**	**$26.21**	**$34.48**	**$46.04**	**$63.49**
Total operating cost	82	**$86.76**	**$91.86**	**$49.20**	**$59.33**	**$73.54**	**$93.03**	**$115.29**
Total med rev after oper cost	82	**$57.62**	**$60.07**	**$31.17**	**$40.55**	**$49.97**	**$58.41**	**$71.80**
Total provider cost/work RVU	82	**$56.81**	**$53.65**	**$33.78**	**$41.10**	**$49.79**	**$56.99**	**$68.36**
Total NPP cost/work RVU	78	$4.83	$6.01	$1.12	$2.03	$3.38	$5.49	$8.57
Provider consultant cost	38	$3.13	$4.19	$.47	$.96	$1.73	$4.16	$5.34
Total physician cost/work RVU	82	$51.13	$46.34	$29.47	$38.16	$44.95	$50.02	$60.97
Total phy compensation	77	$44.32	$43.37	$26.90	$31.18	$38.95	$42.84	$49.38
Total phy benefit cost	77	$6.74	$5.13	$2.45	$4.48	$5.97	$7.84	$9.21
Total cost	82	**$143.57**	**$144.54**	**$85.68**	**$102.10**	**$123.28**	**$149.73**	**$174.80**
Net nonmedical revenue	66	$1.94	$4.89	-$.56	$.09	$.65	$1.44	$6.95
Net inc, prac with fin sup	2	*	*	*	*	*	*	*
Net inc, prac w/o fin sup	76	$2.46	$15.58	-$5.33	-$.57	$.98	$3.16	$10.55
Net inc, excl fin supp (all prac)	78	$2.65	$15.94	-$5.82	-$.68	$.98	$3.24	$13.39
Total support staff FTE/phy	213	**5.39**	**1.60**	**3.64**	**4.41**	**5.31**	**6.20**	**7.21**

Multispecialty — Not Hospital or IDS Owned
(per Patient)

Table 2.10a: Staffing, RVUs, Procedures and Square Footage

	Count	Mean	Std. Dev.	10th %tile	25th %tile	Median	75th %tile	90th %tile
Total prov FTE/10,000 patients	96	8.80	9.98	3.10	4.84	7.76	10.56	13.48
Total phy FTE/10,000 pat	104	7.06	8.46	2.46	3.96	6.35	8.71	10.33
Prim care phy/10,000 pat	101	4.19	2.25	1.45	2.66	3.81	5.38	7.61
Nonsurg phy/10,000 pat	69	2.26	3.51	.40	.90	1.52	2.67	4.24
Surg spec phy/10,000 pat	65	2.37	6.17	.25	.54	1.28	2.52	3.34
Total NPP FTE/10,000 pat	96	1.64	1.62	.31	.61	1.16	2.18	3.44
Total supp staff FTE/10,000 pat	104	36.75	32.06	12.34	19.97	31.11	47.40	61.20
Total empl supp staff/10,000 pat	104	36.37	31.93	12.33	19.58	30.77	47.40	61.01
General administrative	100	2.26	3.09	.57	.85	1.61	2.88	4.04
Patient accounting	99	5.36	5.44	1.50	2.39	4.35	6.46	9.40
General accounting	91	.63	.50	.21	.32	.54	.87	1.13
Managed care administrative	53	1.00	1.24	.14	.21	.44	1.29	3.28
Information technology	70	.87	.83	.16	.32	.59	1.16	1.79
Housekeeping, maint, security	65	.80	.89	.09	.18	.47	1.25	2.02
Medical receptionists	99	6.30	5.13	1.77	3.25	5.60	8.25	11.35
Med secretaries,transcribers	83	1.91	2.13	.17	.71	1.29	2.55	3.61
Medical records	91	2.72	1.73	.87	1.40	2.20	4.16	5.49
Other admin support	61	1.47	4.94	.16	.28	.59	1.18	2.21
*Total administrative supp staff	57	24.49	23.64	8.32	13.32	19.53	30.47	38.89
Registered Nurses	93	3.80	6.21	.40	1.15	2.45	4.64	6.67
Licensed Practical Nurses	90	3.49	3.33	.48	1.15	2.10	5.39	8.05
Med assistants, nurse aides	94	4.44	3.16	1.40	2.41	3.59	5.77	9.00
*Total clinical supp staff	88	11.01	9.01	4.02	6.57	9.67	13.52	17.61
Clinical laboratory	87	2.29	1.60	.49	1.08	2.04	3.28	4.23
Radiology and imaging	85	2.27	3.11	.44	.84	1.58	2.96	4.26
Other medical support serv	64	2.30	2.36	.16	.52	1.57	3.30	5.13
*Total ancillary supp staff	60	7.10	6.43	1.50	2.67	5.75	9.74	13.41
Tot contracted supp staff	42	.94	1.28	.08	.20	.44	1.11	2.35
Tot RVU/patient	56	7.99	5.21	2.28	4.54	6.89	10.66	14.98
Physician work RVU/patient	53	3.75	1.97	1.39	2.22	3.67	4.93	6.63
Tot procedures/patient	96	8.29	5.32	2.79	5.16	7.63	11.08	13.48
Square feet/patient	96	1.43	1.40	.42	.65	1.13	1.86	2.53
Total support staff FTE/phy	213	5.39	1.60	3.64	4.41	5.31	6.20	7.21

*See pages 260 and 261 for definition.

Table 2.10b: Charges, Revenue and Cost

	Count	Mean	Std. Dev.	10th %tile	25th %tile	Median	75th %tile	90th %tile
Total gross charges	104	$768.03	$1,070.44	$226.46	$377.29	$572.13	$902.45	$1,385.01
Total medical revenue	104	$479.40	$637.26	$151.04	$236.30	$349.64	$596.44	$831.74
Net fee-for-service revenue	102	$419.02	$614.84	$122.38	$209.18	$304.30	$484.52	$750.76
Net capitation revenue	43	$106.64	$157.33	$1.64	$11.24	$24.14	$153.94	$352.09
Net other medical revenue	79	$22.02	$40.11	$.60	$3.14	$10.33	$22.50	$48.80
Total support staff cost/patient	104	$139.86	$149.78	$47.99	$66.67	$111.24	$170.78	$246.03
Total general operating cost	104	$137.57	$168.83	$43.39	$63.28	$105.08	$159.22	$253.58
Total operating cost	104	$276.43	$316.52	$88.51	$134.82	$211.17	$335.84	$475.81
Total med rev after oper cost	104	$202.97	$327.64	$56.05	$99.10	$144.42	$237.92	$338.05
Total provider cost/patient	104	$199.85	$327.16	$59.61	$97.45	$142.53	$229.48	$325.69
Total NPP cost/patient	99	$13.21	$12.60	$2.35	$4.87	$8.43	$19.23	$28.18
Provider consultant cost	41	$7.86	$7.37	$.63	$2.30	$5.90	$11.36	$17.92
Total physician cost/patient	104	$184.18	$319.06	$53.12	$88.62	$130.97	$203.34	$307.78
Total phy compensation	104	$160.96	$282.45	$44.50	$73.67	$115.72	$175.79	$267.79
Total phy benefit cost	102	$23.64	$38.25	$4.93	$9.81	$18.64	$28.55	$37.93
Total cost	104	$476.28	$638.17	$143.14	$232.29	$355.37	$557.76	$809.27
Net nonmedical revenue	86	$4.78	$21.76	-$4.04	-$.17	$1.17	$4.14	$13.65
Net inc, prac with fin sup	2	*	*	*	*	*	*	*
Net inc, prac w/o fin sup	97	$9.50	$40.28	-$13.37	-$.02	$4.77	$14.80	$35.02
Net inc, excl fin supp (all prac)	99	$9.65	$40.03	-$13.35	-$.04	$4.77	$15.04	$38.05
Total support staff FTE/phy	213	5.39	1.60	3.64	4.41	5.31	6.20	7.21

Multispecialty — Not Hospital or IDS Owned
(Procedure and Charge Data)

Table 2.11a: Activity Charges to Total Gross Charges Ratios

	Count	Mean	Std. Dev.	10th %tile	25th %tile	Median	75th %tile	90th %tile
Total proc gross charges	160	93.11%	6.76%	84.81%	89.58%	95.34%	97.84%	100.00%
Medical proc-inside practice	160	45.73%	18.59%	25.33%	33.09%	41.46%	56.40%	72.45%
Medical proc-outside practice	146	10.02%	8.99%	2.77%	5.42%	8.53%	11.83%	17.96%
Surg proc-inside practice	150	7.22%	5.71%	2.55%	3.81%	5.89%	8.68%	13.91%
Surg proc-outside practice	128	15.11%	11.27%	1.96%	6.93%	14.33%	20.29%	28.32%
Laboratory procedures	156	11.36%	6.93%	2.04%	6.66%	10.88%	14.95%	20.80%
Radiology procedures	150	8.90%	5.35%	1.96%	4.53%	8.54%	12.88%	15.91%
Tot nonproc gross charges	142	8.02%	7.41%	1.77%	3.00%	5.68%	10.93%	16.49%
Total support staff FTE/phy	213	5.39	1.60	3.64	4.41	5.31	6.20	7.21

Table 2.11b: Medical Procedure Data (inside the practice)

	Count	Mean	Std. Dev.	10th %tile	25th %tile	Median	75th %tile	90th %tile
Gross charges/procedure	156	$77.18	$28.81	$52.48	$61.74	$71.74	$85.00	$103.97
Total cost/procedure	138	$60.54	$17.47	$41.42	$48.88	$57.13	$69.98	$82.10
Operating cost/procedure	135	$37.75	$12.94	$23.62	$28.00	$35.81	$44.11	$53.59
Provider cost/procedure	140	$23.07	$7.23	$14.79	$18.07	$22.54	$27.21	$31.22
Procedures/patient	97	3.77	2.18	1.54	2.26	3.57	4.79	5.80
Gross charges/patient	98	$276.06	$175.44	$105.36	$157.54	$243.49	$341.94	$496.89
Procedures/physician	158	6,051	2,443	3,641	4,600	5,709	7,110	8,462
Gross charges/physician	160	$435,149	$157,774	$278,360	$338,555	$409,785	$502,356	$612,610
Procedures/provider	145	4,871	1,997	3,097	3,736	4,597	5,486	6,819
Gross charges/provider	147	$353,613	$136,902	$221,701	$277,164	$330,603	$404,845	$503,741
Gross charge to total cost ratio	138	1.28	.29	.92	1.12	1.26	1.45	1.63
Oper cost to total cost ratio	135	.62	.07	.54	.58	.61	.66	.71
Prov cost to total cost ratio	138	.38	.07	.29	.34	.39	.42	.46
Total support staff FTE/phy	213	5.39	1.60	3.64	4.41	5.31	6.20	7.21

Table 2.11c: Medical Procedure Data (outside the practice)

	Count	Mean	Std. Dev.	10th %tile	25th %tile	Median	75th %tile	90th %tile
Gross charges/procedure	142	$118.43	$34.35	$81.14	$96.65	$113.78	$139.78	$168.47
Total cost/procedure	126	$52.42	$15.78	$35.75	$42.50	$49.65	$61.94	$72.58
Operating cost/procedure	123	$21.39	$8.52	$13.41	$15.78	$19.47	$24.71	$32.30
Provider cost/procedure	128	$30.96	$9.86	$19.81	$25.13	$29.91	$36.07	$44.28
Procedures/patient	90	.68	.79	.11	.25	.49	.85	1.40
Gross charges/patient	91	$81.26	$104.03	$12.61	$27.40	$48.15	$91.67	$196.19
Procedures/physician	143	921	904	238	411	722	1,163	1,572
Gross charges/physician	146	$107,358	$112,762	$29,725	$48,397	$82,667	$111,259	$200,060
Procedures/provider	131	729	614	190	342	590	972	1,364
Gross charges/provider	135	$88,187	$82,728	$26,142	$41,643	$64,724	$100,212	$183,871
Gross charge to total cost ratio	126	2.33	.56	1.71	1.97	2.28	2.59	2.88
Oper cost to total cost ratio	123	.40	.08	.31	.35	.40	.44	.49
Prov cost to total cost ratio	126	.60	.08	.51	.56	.60	.65	.69
Total support staff FTE/phy	213	5.39	1.60	3.64	4.41	5.31	6.20	7.21

Multispecialty — Not Hospital or IDS Owned
(Procedure and Charge Data)

Table 2.11d: Surgery/Anesthesia Procedure Data (inside the practice)

	Count	Mean	Std. Dev.	10th %tile	25th %tile	Median	75th %tile	90th %tile
Gross charges/procedure	148	$146.97	$163.74	$30.66	$57.54	$97.94	$180.52	$290.71
Total cost/procedure	131	$121.40	$122.76	$25.44	$44.38	$82.61	$145.64	$268.17
Operating cost/procedure	128	$75.74	$77.73	$14.25	$26.98	$50.51	$92.25	$174.79
Provider cost/procedure	132	$45.78	$47.24	$9.08	$17.26	$31.15	$55.56	$100.19
Procedures/patient	92	.61	.57	.06	.19	.39	1.00	1.49
Gross charges/patient	92	$59.63	$122.32	$7.84	$15.69	$32.44	$62.02	$112.99
Procedures/physician	149	837	701	136	312	647	1,228	1,674
Gross charges/physician	150	$77,156	$68,391	$15,847	$31,038	$57,725	$99,255	$172,384
Procedures/provider	136	703	594	120	240	584	1,026	1,380
Gross charges/provider	137	$65,887	$60,617	$14,972	$25,227	$46,629	$78,489	$157,158
Gross charge to total cost ratio	131	1.28	.28	.92	1.12	1.26	1.45	1.58
Oper cost to total cost ratio	128	.62	.07	.53	.58	.61	.66	.70
Prov cost to total cost ratio	131	.38	.07	.30	.34	.39	.42	.47
Total support staff FTE/phy	213	5.39	1.60	3.64	4.41	5.31	6.20	7.21

Table 2.11e: Surgery/Anesthesia Procedure Data (outside the practice)

	Count	Mean	Std. Dev.	10th %tile	25th %tile	Median	75th %tile	90th %tile
Gross charges/procedure	125	$812.74	$455.62	$207.69	$401.34	$847.42	$1,076.86	$1,359.40
Total cost/procedure	112	$369.92	$217.19	$86.63	$212.31	$370.14	$487.33	$637.98
Operating cost/procedure	110	$144.76	$95.85	$33.71	$83.03	$135.49	$192.20	$260.18
Provider cost/procedure	113	$224.92	$131.32	$51.29	$114.69	$226.81	$298.89	$378.92
Procedures/patient	78	.28	.48	.01	.06	.11	.27	.57
Gross charges/patient	76	$116.92	$100.94	$8.59	$33.72	$79.47	$210.08	$284.83
Procedures/physician	127	329	508	25	88	210	322	805
Gross charges/physician	128	$181,933	$191,047	$15,948	$55,862	$157,135	$259,253	$336,733
Procedures/provider	118	273	407	14	66	180	272	625
Gross charges/provider	119	$146,247	$142,232	$9,327	$44,411	$128,209	$201,201	$258,251
Gross charge to total cost ratio	112	2.33	.57	1.72	1.98	2.27	2.60	2.89
Oper cost to total cost ratio	110	.40	.08	.31	.35	.39	.44	.48
Prov cost to total cost ratio	112	.60	.08	.52	.56	.61	.65	.69
Total support staff FTE/phy	213	5.39	1.60	3.64	4.41	5.31	6.20	7.21

Multispecialty — Not Hospital or IDS Owned
(Procedure and Charge Data)

Table 2.11f: Clinical Laboratory/Pathology Procedure Data

	Count	Mean	Std. Dev.	10th %tile	25th %tile	Median	75th %tile	90th %tile
Gross charges/procedure	152	$31.01	$15.76	$15.91	$21.55	$29.30	$36.16	$45.69
Total cost/procedure	136	$23.84	$9.83	$13.79	$18.19	$22.37	$27.16	$36.36
Operating cost/procedure	133	$15.49	$6.08	$8.25	$11.69	$14.69	$18.62	$23.34
Provider cost/procedure	138	$8.29	$5.11	$4.13	$5.81	$7.56	$9.48	$12.08
Procedures/patient	95	2.58	1.82	.44	1.13	2.32	3.64	5.13
Gross charges/patient	96	$76.82	$58.24	$10.99	$32.09	$55.64	$108.01	$166.88
Procedures/physician	154	3,887	2,368	956	2,450	3,631	4,871	7,051
Gross charges/physician	156	$118,287	$75,953	$21,206	$67,619	$111,895	$163,506	$204,994
Procedures/provider	141	3,206	1,678	974	2,087	3,064	4,133	5,452
Gross charges/provider	143	$99,739	$59,501	$22,981	$60,875	$97,487	$129,068	$165,225
Gross charge to total cost ratio	136	1.32	.32	.93	1.12	1.31	1.48	1.73
Oper cost to total cost ratio	133	.65	.08	.56	.61	.66	.70	.73
Prov cost to total cost ratio	136	.35	.08	.27	.30	.34	.39	.44
Total support staff FTE/phy	213	5.39	1.60	3.64	4.41	5.31	6.20	7.21

Table 2.11g: Diagnostic Radiology and Imaging Procedure Data

	Count	Mean	Std. Dev.	10th %tile	25th %tile	Median	75th %tile	90th %tile
Gross charges/procedure	148	$170.32	$127.38	$63.76	$94.05	$144.26	$215.16	$292.40
Total cost/procedure	132	$133.38	$106.69	$58.24	$77.92	$106.75	$166.26	$232.10
Operating cost/procedure	130	$87.58	$72.23	$34.34	$48.28	$77.48	$109.08	$151.73
Provider cost/procedure	135	$46.62	$41.07	$15.22	$23.10	$37.03	$60.22	$86.80
Procedures/patient	93	.53	.97	.07	.16	.31	.65	.83
Gross charges/patient	91	$98.58	$225.82	$7.46	$22.45	$44.88	$113.99	$191.67
Procedures/physician	151	646	415	118	395	621	826	1,157
Gross charges/physician	150	$107,737	$90,359	$13,414	$40,116	$85,291	$151,601	$219,163
Procedures/provider	140	532	343	108	355	506	657	866
Gross charges/provider	139	$91,468	$76,906	$14,130	$36,471	$78,076	$123,078	$187,978
Gross charge to total cost ratio	133	1.30	.34	.98	1.11	1.28	1.46	1.67
Oper cost to total cost ratio	131	.66	.10	.52	.60	.66	.72	.78
Prov cost to total cost ratio	133	.34	.10	.23	.28	.34	.40	.48
Total support staff FTE/phy	213	5.39	1.60	3.64	4.41	5.31	6.20	7.21

Table 2.11h: Nonprocedural Gross Charge Data

	Count	Mean	Std. Dev.	10th %tile	25th %tile	Median	75th %tile	90th %tile
Gross charges/patient	88	$80.31	$172.67	$4.28	$12.69	$32.44	$87.78	$189.33
Nonproc gross charges/physician	142	$97,899	$114,071	$10,822	$24,870	$56,160	$142,453	$206,884
Gross charges/provider	131	$86,401	$101,025	$11,131	$22,554	$49,813	$120,312	$195,156
Total support staff FTE/phy	213	5.39	1.60	3.64	4.41	5.31	6.20	7.21

Multispecialty — Hospital or IDS Owned

Table 3.1: Staffing and Practice Data

	Count	Mean	Std. Dev.	10th %tile	25th %tile	Median	75th %tile	90th %tile
Total provider FTE	72	75.39	86.10	9.86	19.89	46.45	101.82	195.29
Total physician FTE	86	55.64	69.10	5.40	13.55	30.94	69.79	132.85
Total nonphysician provider FTE	72	11.98	15.67	1.70	2.40	6.70	14.80	32.43
Total support staff FTE	86	240.42	285.36	25.80	49.73	121.13	297.83	591.39
Number of branch clinics	67	16	20	2	4	10	17	46
Square footage of all facilities	78	110,433	134,869	11,011	22,240	51,013	141,532	302,660

Table 3.2: Accounts Receivable Data, Collection Percentages and Financial Ratios

	Count	Mean	Std. Dev.	10th %tile	25th %tile	Median	75th %tile	90th %tile
Total AR/physician	78	$102,230	$56,299	$45,167	$63,807	$86,459	$132,781	$176,318
Total AR/provider	65	$86,996	$47,065	$41,707	$56,525	$71,926	$107,085	$145,731
0-30 days in AR	78	50.61%	13.01%	32.62%	42.84%	52.21%	59.49%	66.40%
31-60 days in AR	78	15.98%	4.44%	11.35%	12.87%	15.39%	17.83%	20.62%
61-90 days in AR	78	9.01%	2.71%	5.93%	7.13%	8.53%	10.52%	12.27%
91-120 days in AR	78	6.10%	2.02%	3.88%	4.64%	5.93%	7.00%	8.13%
120+ days in AR	78	18.30%	10.57%	6.17%	10.96%	15.46%	23.57%	37.03%
Re-aged: 0-30 days in AR	32	51.39%	13.74%	32.78%	42.09%	51.74%	61.66%	73.04%
Re-aged: 31-60 days in AR	32	16.16%	5.87%	11.02%	12.34%	15.06%	18.24%	21.75%
Re-aged: 61-90 days in AR	32	8.72%	3.51%	5.43%	6.14%	7.85%	10.14%	13.24%
Re-aged: 91-120 days in AR	32	5.89%	2.37%	3.43%	4.20%	5.68%	7.59%	8.78%
Re-aged: 120+ days in AR	32	17.84%	10.29%	4.61%	10.82%	16.38%	23.97%	35.45%
Not re-aged: 0-30 days in AR	42	49.50%	12.99%	30.59%	39.49%	52.21%	57.72%	64.26%
Not re-aged: 31-60 days in AR	42	15.72%	3.23%	11.40%	12.87%	15.92%	17.45%	20.37%
Not re-aged: 61-90 days in AR	42	9.15%	2.03%	6.47%	7.88%	8.78%	10.65%	12.05%
Not re-aged: 91-120 days in AR	42	6.40%	1.74%	4.52%	5.35%	6.33%	7.16%	7.75%
Not re-aged: 120+ days in AR	42	19.24%	11.16%	6.65%	12.11%	15.98%	25.29%	38.57%
Months gross FFS charges in AR	74	1.75	.73	1.08	1.30	1.54	2.04	2.77
Days gross FFS charges in AR	74	53.08	22.11	32.73	39.47	46.98	61.97	84.40
Gross FFS collection %	81	63.18%	10.20%	48.28%	56.95%	64.24%	70.07%	74.82%
Adjusted FFS collection %	80	96.28%	3.29%	92.55%	95.37%	97.02%	98.42%	99.13%
Gross FFS + cap collection %	34	67.96%	20.87%	49.43%	56.62%	65.34%	71.47%	84.25%
Net cap rev % of gross cap chrg	27	76.32%	30.14%	34.77%	58.99%	75.43%	100.00%	114.13%
Current ratio	29	2.07	1.42	.96	1.22	1.66	2.28	4.05
Tot asset turnover ratio	29	3.87	3.05	1.41	2.04	3.38	4.95	7.11
Debt to equity ratio	29	3.91	7.21	.17	.74	1.49	2.83	11.93
Debt ratio	29	56.35%	26.29%	14.29%	41.65%	59.82%	73.88%	92.27%
Return on total assets	30	-15.49%	26.64%	-57.81%	-31.63%	-2.90%	3.07%	10.11%
Return on equity	30	-75.05%	200.57%	-187.15%	-107.07%	-8.05%	8.96%	21.29%

Table 3.3: Breakout of Total Gross Charges by Type of Payer

	Count	Mean	Std. Dev.	10th %tile	25th %tile	Median	75th %tile	90th %tile
Medicare: fee-for-service	79	24.33%	11.61%	8.15%	16.39%	24.00%	32.00%	39.26%
Medicare: managed care FFS	79	1.04%	4.73%	.00%	.00%	.00%	.00%	1.35%
Medicare: capitation	79	.49%	2.06%	.00%	.00%	.00%	.00%	.30%
Medicaid: fee-for-service	79	7.93%	7.19%	1.00%	3.30%	6.59%	10.60%	17.00%
Medicaid: managed care FFS	79	2.42%	8.79%	.00%	.00%	.00%	.60%	7.03%
Medicaid: capitation	79	.60%	2.44%	.00%	.00%	.00%	.00%	.50%
Commercial: fee-for-service	79	33.60%	22.60%	.00%	10.00%	37.70%	50.30%	63.00%
Commercial: managed care FFS	79	16.77%	23.54%	.00%	.00%	.43%	30.00%	56.10%
Commercial: capitation	79	4.92%	13.73%	.00%	.00%	.00%	3.40%	15.00%
Workers' compensation	79	1.15%	1.91%	.00%	.00%	.60%	1.58%	3.00%
Charity care and prof courtesy	79	.48%	.99%	.00%	.00%	.00%	.60%	1.35%
Self-pay	79	5.58%	6.12%	1.51%	2.07%	3.90%	6.63%	11.00%
Other federal government payers	79	.69%	2.86%	.00%	.00%	.00%	.01%	.96%

Multispecialty — Hospital or IDS Owned
(per FTE Physician)

Table 3.4a: Staffing, RVUs, Patients, Procedures and Square Footage

	Count	Mean	Std. Dev.	10th %tile	25th %tile	Median	75th %tile	90th %tile
Total provider FTE/physician	72	**1.22**	**.15**	**1.08**	**1.12**	**1.19**	**1.28**	**1.37**
Prim care phy/physician	74	.77	.21	.45	.60	.82	1.00	1.00
Nonsurg phy/physician	46	.21	.14	.06	.07	.17	.30	.41
Surg spec phy/physician	42	.18	.13	.02	.08	.17	.27	.39
Total NPP FTE/physician	72	.22	.15	.08	.12	.19	.28	.37
Total support staff FTE/phy	86	**4.46**	**1.40**	**2.93**	**3.66**	**4.16**	**5.08**	**6.25**
Total empl support staff FTE	82	4.47	1.39	3.02	3.66	4.17	5.05	6.23
General administrative	75	.29	.18	.10	.14	.26	.39	.58
Patient accounting	63	.58	.37	.09	.33	.57	.78	1.10
General accounting	50	.07	.05	.02	.04	.06	.09	.16
Managed care administrative	27	.11	.20	.01	.01	.04	.08	.32
Information technology	41	.06	.06	.02	.03	.04	.08	.14
Housekeeping, maint, security	33	.08	.09	.01	.02	.04	.13	.24
Medical receptionists	70	1.06	.39	.58	.77	1.07	1.35	1.60
Med secretaries,transcribers	43	.26	.23	.03	.09	.17	.41	.56
Medical records	54	.35	.21	.11	.17	.31	.49	.69
Other admin support	34	.43	.99	.02	.05	.10	.30	1.44
*Total administrative supp staff	32	**2.46**	**.61**	**1.57**	**2.02**	**2.47**	**2.81**	**3.41**
Registered Nurses	64	.46	.40	.08	.14	.30	.66	1.06
Licensed Practical Nurses	65	.53	.38	.07	.18	.46	.81	1.14
Med assistants, nurse aides	69	.72	.48	.20	.36	.60	1.10	1.46
*Total clinical supp staff	61	**1.54**	**.45**	**.95**	**1.25**	**1.54**	**1.81**	**2.20**
Clinical laboratory	42	.23	.16	.04	.08	.21	.33	.48
Radiology and imaging	52	.17	.13	.02	.08	.15	.22	.37
Other medical support serv	35	.35	.73	.03	.04	.14	.31	.73
*Total ancillary supp staff	25	**.62**	**.34**	**.11**	**.44**	**.60**	**.83**	**.95**
Tot contracted supp staff	16	.16	.13	.01	.05	.12	.23	.40
Tot RVU/physician	34	8,959	2,628	5,552	7,558	8,914	10,005	11,785
Physician work RVU/physician	40	4,940	808	4,029	4,485	4,975	5,471	6,098
Patients/physician	33	1,634	677	834	1,110	1,581	2,037	2,405
Tot procedures/physician	63	8,554	3,042	4,434	6,097	8,679	10,245	11,956
Square feet/physician	78	2,074	762	1,286	1,600	1,828	2,463	3,045

*See pages 260 and 261 for definition.

Table 3.4b: Charges and Revenue

	Count	Mean	Std. Dev.	10th %tile	25th %tile	Median	75th %tile	90th %tile
Net fee-for-service revenue	81	$424,387	$147,189	$262,031	$307,382	$401,094	$545,531	$627,254
Gross FFS charges	81	$687,090	$257,334	$393,968	$461,552	$624,481	$896,727	$1,052,224
Adjustments to FFS charges	80	$248,715	$143,872	$99,694	$141,444	$215,009	$323,338	$474,365
Adjusted FFS charges	80	$441,306	$149,157	$275,166	$326,684	$409,948	$563,720	$656,865
Bad debts due to FFS activity	78	$16,055	$13,893	$4,767	$7,504	$11,567	$21,722	$32,012
Net capitation revenue	34	$116,732	$274,379	$3,752	$9,787	$39,357	$94,128	$283,241
Gross capitation charges	27	$100,591	$108,672	$8,393	$14,581	$62,476	$149,528	$289,753
Capitation revenue	32	$227,004	$627,660	$3,561	$9,655	$39,357	$100,151	$630,323
Purch serv for cap patients	6	*	*	*	*	*	*	*
Net other medical revenue	58	$14,369	$19,233	$490	$2,255	$8,833	$20,139	$32,458
Gross rev from other activity	53	$20,848	$31,055	$674	$2,534	$9,541	$22,847	$64,898
Other medical revenue	44	$12,119	$12,101	$460	$1,592	$9,481	$18,168	$30,589
Rev from sale of goods/services	27	$23,623	$36,718	$479	$2,418	$5,032	$25,602	$72,344
Cost of sales	14	$24,117	$37,899	$420	$3,341	$7,831	$38,814	$100,483
Total gross charges	86	**$737,880**	**$255,561**	**$442,151**	**$523,639**	**$674,586**	**$950,189**	**$1,136,930**
Total medical revenue	86	**$493,255**	**$221,059**	**$302,077**	**$348,926**	**$466,985**	**$600,226**	**$665,078**

Multispecialty — Hospital or IDS Owned
(per FTE Physician)

Table 3.4c: Operating Cost

	Count	Mean	Std. Dev.	10th %tile	25th %tile	Median	75th %tile	90th %tile
Total support staff cost/phy	86	$167,919	$57,380	$109,409	$131,781	$157,776	$195,097	$244,731
Total empl supp staff cost/phy	82	$133,132	$44,677	$89,361	$104,382	$120,743	$154,278	$194,799
General administrative	75	$16,255	$9,552	$6,262	$9,707	$13,919	$20,456	$28,127
Patient accounting	64	$15,222	$9,472	$2,129	$8,674	$14,873	$20,927	$28,314
General accounting	50	$3,106	$2,396	$906	$1,499	$2,582	$3,784	$7,109
Managed care administrative	27	$5,006	$10,125	$293	$470	$1,449	$3,565	$15,180
Information technology	40	$2,760	$3,181	$604	$1,184	$2,085	$3,230	$4,746
Housekeeping, maint, security	32	$2,030	$2,170	$70	$380	$1,193	$3,172	$5,345
Medical receptionists	71	$23,800	$10,339	$11,902	$16,305	$24,451	$30,847	$35,718
Med secretaries,transcribers	45	$6,674	$6,372	$741	$1,349	$3,618	$11,085	$15,708
Medical records	54	$7,558	$4,621	$2,036	$3,756	$6,627	$10,885	$15,431
Other admin support	36	$11,795	$23,590	$633	$1,222	$4,587	$7,344	$48,467
***Total administrative supp staff**	29	$68,415	$18,363	$43,780	$53,739	$68,743	$83,796	$88,303
Registered Nurses	65	$18,302	$14,946	$2,489	$6,169	$14,654	$26,306	$39,142
Licensed Practical Nurses	65	$15,174	$10,413	$2,215	$6,147	$13,978	$21,820	$30,954
Med assistants, nurse aides	69	$17,990	$12,306	$4,659	$8,647	$13,904	$26,030	$40,066
***Total clinical supp staff**	63	$47,058	$15,658	$28,186	$35,803	$44,866	$54,363	$72,001
Clinical laboratory	42	$6,910	$5,566	$1,225	$2,268	$5,979	$9,323	$12,295
Radiology and imaging	53	$10,852	$30,797	$658	$3,032	$5,651	$9,173	$14,649
Other medical support serv	36	$11,606	$21,617	$713	$1,449	$3,951	$14,253	$24,794
***Total ancillary supp staff**	33	$18,322	$11,428	$3,269	$7,308	$17,284	$26,350	$35,828
Total empl supp staff benefits	82	$34,785	$14,997	$17,157	$23,382	$31,801	$45,408	$55,527
Tot contracted supp staff	35	$5,435	$5,892	$245	$736	$2,438	$8,015	$13,909
Total general operating cost	86	$151,863	$115,743	$77,795	$93,999	$146,505	$175,455	$219,766
Information technology	79	$8,082	$5,280	$2,690	$4,414	$6,616	$11,483	$15,180
Medical and surgical supply	82	$37,034	$74,304	$8,078	$12,116	$19,894	$37,908	$70,936
Building and occupancy	82	$34,172	$13,135	$18,247	$24,591	$33,706	$42,661	$52,008
Furniture and equipment	66	$8,834	$14,589	$1,498	$3,018	$6,750	$9,954	$14,358
Admin supplies and services	81	$10,983	$7,541	$3,739	$5,668	$9,415	$14,496	$19,627
Prof liability insurance	81	$12,728	$9,381	$4,530	$6,822	$9,338	$16,775	$23,399
Other insurance premiums	48	$2,324	$3,855	$208	$422	$970	$1,789	$6,527
Outside professional fees	66	$7,181	$24,265	$251	$719	$1,655	$4,965	$13,254
Promotion and marketing	68	$1,926	$2,102	$79	$375	$1,283	$3,046	$4,328
Clinical laboratory	57	$11,264	$10,040	$178	$1,091	$10,317	$19,591	$26,154
Radiology and imaging	52	$3,512	$4,690	$143	$518	$2,526	$3,895	$7,856
Other ancillary services	23	$6,091	$7,476	$193	$620	$1,724	$10,734	$20,159
Billing purchased services	45	$8,621	$11,101	$335	$1,104	$3,089	$16,767	$29,109
Management fees paid to MSO	17	$25,475	$18,455	$1,075	$12,585	$23,050	$38,739	$56,927
Misc operating cost	78	$10,235	$13,393	$966	$2,930	$6,566	$13,083	$23,039
Cost allocated to prac from par	32	$17,283	$21,712	$686	$2,783	$12,479	$24,161	$40,314
Total operating cost	86	$320,112	$154,777	$192,802	$229,834	$314,334	$365,740	$433,939

*See pages 260 and 261 for definition.

Multispecialty — Hospital or IDS Owned
(per FTE Physician)

Table 3.4d: Provider Cost

	Count	Mean	Std. Dev.	10th %tile	25th %tile	Median	75th %tile	90th %tile
Total med rev after oper cost	86	$173,140	$104,819	$55,771	$106,792	$159,010	$223,928	$297,339
Total provider cost/physician	86	$248,534	$68,595	$176,783	$197,573	$240,326	$284,613	$320,180
Total NPP cost/physician	71	$19,724	$14,409	$6,863	$9,673	$16,118	$24,667	$35,999
Nonphysician provider comp	69	$16,370	$11,913	$5,395	$7,823	$13,309	$21,093	$30,544
Nonphysician prov benefit cost	65	$3,554	$3,090	$828	$1,488	$2,686	$4,519	$7,817
Provider consultant cost	18	$7,738	$10,724	$873	$1,561	$4,786	$7,945	$19,689
Total physician cost/physician	86	$230,556	$67,145	$159,090	$184,450	$220,192	$267,268	$299,417
Total phy compensation	81	$199,011	$64,524	$137,149	$156,594	$186,525	$229,777	$273,484
Total phy benefit cost	81	$31,733	$10,731	$19,962	$24,733	$30,238	$40,424	$46,555

Table 3.4e: Net Income or Loss

	Count	Mean	Std. Dev.	10th %tile	25th %tile	Median	75th %tile	90th %tile
Total cost	86	$568,646	$188,981	$381,561	$442,967	$554,674	$651,496	$737,106
Net nonmedical revenue	70	$49,151	$102,434	-$2,659	$1,792	$14,824	$66,673	$108,248
Nonmedical revenue	58	$67,833	$443,092	$32	$787	$3,263	$13,307	$24,068
Fin support for oper costs	34	$79,634	$114,276	$7,154	$17,055	$62,413	$85,059	$176,790
Goodwill amortization	22	$6,747	$13,003	$12	$172	$2,949	$8,202	$14,936
Nonmedical cost	17	$179,611	$715,583	$13	$136	$1,412	$4,906	$645,316
Net inc, prac with fin sup	32	-$4,786	$115,370	-$75,594	-$27,932	$0	$6,769	$21,665
Net inc, prac w/o fin sup	51	-$59,567	$69,939	-$129,021	-$105,046	-$70,060	-$21,067	$13,558
Net inc, excl fin supp (all prac)	83	-$68,652	$68,396	-$145,108	-$112,152	-$65,863	-$28,252	$1,986

Table 3.4f: Assets and Liabilities

	Count	Mean	Std. Dev.	10th %tile	25th %tile	Median	75th %tile	90th %tile
Total assets	29	$234,774	$251,747	$71,381	$101,922	$172,385	$247,140	$515,015
Current assets	29	$103,015	$53,813	$49,064	$61,479	$91,552	$142,755	$175,887
Noncurrent assets	29	$131,758	$246,297	$15,094	$28,790	$54,740	$154,097	$297,341
Total liabilities	29	$104,870	$86,463	$24,452	$50,830	$87,227	$135,591	$206,668
Current liabilities	29	$59,346	$28,825	$16,034	$31,137	$61,853	$80,367	$100,547
Noncurrent liabilities	29	$45,524	$73,202	$0	$118	$25,326	$58,751	$129,087
Working capital	29	$43,669	$41,449	-$2,304	$13,723	$33,567	$73,981	$90,113
Total net worth	29	$129,904	$247,346	$4,397	$33,366	$78,989	$110,142	$217,060

Multispecialty — Hospital or IDS Owned
(as a % of Total Medical Revenue)

Table 3.5a: Charges and Revenue

	Count	Mean	Std. Dev.	10th %tile	25th %tile	Median	75th %tile	90th %tile
Net fee-for-service revenue	81	90.67%	16.83%	75.70%	88.21%	98.05%	99.93%	100.00%
Net capitation revenue	34	17.08%	21.31%	.94%	2.72%	8.59%	20.84%	48.64%
Net other medical revenue	58	3.02%	4.44%	.11%	.47%	1.53%	3.71%	7.95%
Total gross charges	**86**	**153.42%**	**26.45%**	**125.74%**	**137.45%**	**150.72%**	**169.72%**	**189.52%**

Table 3.5b: Operating Cost

	Count	Mean	Std. Dev.	10th %tile	25th %tile	Median	75th %tile	90th %tile
Total support staff cost	**86**	**35.78%**	**9.58%**	**24.55%**	**29.45%**	**34.34%**	**41.45%**	**47.90%**
Total empl support staff cost	82	28.42%	7.93%	18.72%	23.58%	27.14%	32.52%	39.27%
General administrative	75	3.61%	2.34%	1.61%	1.93%	2.92%	4.47%	6.17%
Patient accounting	64	3.21%	2.08%	.45%	1.77%	3.24%	4.45%	5.87%
General accounting	50	.69%	.63%	.14%	.24%	.51%	.78%	1.65%
Managed care administrative	27	1.00%	2.33%	.05%	.13%	.33%	.75%	1.88%
Information technology	40	.53%	.65%	.15%	.26%	.43%	.64%	.84%
Housekeeping, maint, security	32	.41%	.60%	.02%	.08%	.18%	.46%	1.40%
Medical receptionists	71	5.76%	3.40%	2.21%	3.29%	5.41%	7.49%	9.85%
Med secretaries,transcribers	45	1.35%	1.52%	.15%	.35%	.77%	1.93%	2.54%
Medical records	54	1.57%	1.18%	.39%	.75%	1.30%	1.97%	3.39%
Other admin support	36	2.32%	4.58%	.08%	.24%	.85%	1.56%	9.29%
*Total administrative supp staff	**29**	**13.84%**	**5.25%**	**8.05%**	**9.41%**	**13.81%**	**16.40%**	**18.48%**
Registered Nurses	65	4.13%	4.16%	.67%	1.33%	2.91%	5.88%	10.30%
Licensed Practical Nurses	65	3.28%	2.53%	.69%	1.45%	2.78%	4.24%	6.53%
Med assistants, nurse aides	69	4.22%	3.06%	.74%	1.77%	3.41%	6.66%	8.38%
*Total clinical supp staff	**63**	**10.53%**	**4.93%**	**5.44%**	**7.47%**	**9.59%**	**12.73%**	**16.49%**
Clinical laboratory	42	1.25%	.98%	.23%	.57%	1.06%	1.64%	2.53%
Radiology and imaging	53	2.07%	6.52%	.14%	.62%	.98%	1.68%	2.54%
Other medical support serv	36	2.16%	4.35%	.12%	.30%	.69%	2.22%	5.39%
*Total ancillary supp staff	**33**	**3.19%**	**1.89%**	**.82%**	**1.67%**	**2.75%**	**4.56%**	**6.28%**
Total empl supp staff benefits	82	7.31%	2.82%	4.17%	5.66%	6.98%	8.49%	10.85%
Tot contracted supp staff	35	1.03%	1.18%	.06%	.14%	.70%	1.71%	2.68%
Total general operating cost	**86**	**30.39%**	**9.73%**	**19.94%**	**24.49%**	**28.90%**	**34.17%**	**41.57%**
Information technology	79	1.73%	1.17%	.53%	1.00%	1.36%	2.20%	4.03%
Medical and surgical supply	82	6.02%	5.16%	1.98%	3.06%	4.55%	6.64%	12.17%
Building and occupancy	82	7.62%	3.58%	3.47%	5.20%	7.33%	9.37%	10.95%
Furniture and equipment	66	1.53%	1.22%	.40%	.62%	1.32%	1.88%	3.16%
Admin supplies and services	81	2.41%	1.73%	.84%	1.18%	1.79%	3.13%	5.21%
Prof liability insurance	81	2.99%	2.48%	.88%	1.26%	2.07%	4.12%	6.08%
Other insurance premiums	48	.51%	.95%	.04%	.10%	.20%	.45%	1.40%
Outside professional fees	66	1.08%	1.85%	.05%	.16%	.33%	1.03%	3.10%
Promotion and marketing	68	.41%	.48%	.02%	.07%	.27%	.57%	.96%
Clinical laboratory	57	1.96%	1.72%	.05%	.26%	1.86%	3.13%	4.14%
Radiology and imaging	52	.57%	.69%	.03%	.11%	.45%	.65%	1.30%
Other ancillary services	23	1.38%	1.89%	.03%	.11%	.38%	2.54%	4.18%
Billing purchased services	45	2.20%	3.06%	.04%	.21%	.54%	4.22%	7.51%
Management fees paid to MSO	17	4.83%	4.16%	.32%	1.89%	3.00%	7.28%	12.35%
Misc operating cost	78	2.17%	2.38%	.16%	.64%	1.59%	2.63%	4.44%
Cost allocated to prac from par	32	3.83%	4.79%	.17%	.84%	2.46%	5.70%	9.26%
Total operating cost	**86**	**66.24%**	**14.57%**	**50.52%**	**58.71%**	**64.12%**	**71.66%**	**83.44%**

*See pages 260 and 261 for definition.

Multispecialty — Hospital or IDS Owned
(as a % of Total Medical Revenue)

Table 3.5c: Provider Cost

	Count	Mean	Std. Dev.	10th %tile	25th %tile	Median	75th %tile	90th %tile
Total med rev after oper cost	86	33.76%	14.57%	16.56%	28.34%	35.88%	41.29%	49.48%
Total provider cost	86	53.59%	12.11%	42.01%	46.28%	51.38%	60.63%	67.69%
Total NPP cost	71	4.26%	3.86%	1.43%	2.05%	2.85%	4.95%	7.94%
Nonphysician provider comp	69	3.55%	3.17%	1.13%	1.69%	2.69%	4.39%	6.83%
Nonphysician prov benefit cost	65	.78%	.81%	.19%	.35%	.53%	.85%	1.60%
Provider consultant cost	18	1.23%	1.71%	.20%	.29%	.68%	1.34%	3.35%
Total physician cost	86	49.80%	12.16%	37.58%	41.76%	47.49%	57.70%	64.16%
Total phy compensation	81	42.90%	10.80%	32.01%	35.90%	41.40%	49.49%	56.94%
Total phy benefit cost	81	7.04%	2.98%	3.90%	5.18%	6.65%	8.28%	11.48%

Table 3.5d: Net Income or Loss

	Count	Mean	Std. Dev.	10th %tile	25th %tile	Median	75th %tile	90th %tile
Total cost	86	119.84%	19.65%	100.75%	105.84%	115.46%	127.37%	144.35%
Net nonmedical revenue	70	12.87%	29.59%	-.43%	.31%	2.63%	17.42%	30.14%
Nonmedical revenue	58	16.31%	108.92%	.01%	.17%	.77%	2.30%	7.07%
Fin support for oper costs	34	21.40%	35.19%	1.06%	4.52%	14.83%	23.05%	44.69%
Goodwill amortization	22	1.13%	1.41%	.00%	.04%	.55%	1.74%	3.22%
Nonmedical cost	17	43.98%	175.88%	.00%	.03%	.37%	1.08%	157.61%
Net inc, prac with fin sup	32	-1.93%	37.35%	-24.24%	-6.77%	.00%	1.25%	4.66%
Net inc, prac w/o fin sup	51	-15.29%	15.79%	-30.45%	-25.55%	-15.32%	-4.43%	2.10%
Net inc, excl fin supp (all prac)	83	-18.21%	18.54%	-40.15%	-26.50%	-15.32%	-6.00%	.32%

Table 3.5e: Assets and Liabilities

	Count	Mean	Std. Dev.	10th %tile	25th %tile	Median	75th %tile	90th %tile
Total assets	29	42.08%	37.95%	14.06%	20.19%	29.61%	49.46%	70.79%
Current assets	29	18.66%	7.85%	8.03%	12.39%	18.74%	24.62%	28.26%
Noncurrent assets	29	23.42%	37.36%	3.20%	4.62%	11.44%	36.03%	46.19%
Total liabilities	29	20.50%	19.81%	5.53%	9.80%	15.24%	25.92%	40.10%
Current liabilities	29	10.90%	5.10%	3.88%	6.31%	11.19%	14.04%	19.32%
Noncurrent liabilities	29	9.61%	16.67%	.00%	.02%	3.86%	11.43%	25.54%
Working capital	29	7.77%	6.54%	-.45%	2.83%	8.34%	11.78%	16.90%
Total net worth	29	21.58%	35.19%	.78%	8.14%	13.88%	21.96%	39.83%

Multispecialty — Hospital or IDS Owned
(per FTE Provider)

Table 3.6a: Staffing, RVUs, Patients, Procedures and Square Footage

	Count	Mean	Std. Dev.	10th %tile	25th %tile	Median	75th %tile	90th %tile
Total physician FTE/provider	72	.83	.09	.73	.78	.84	.90	.92
Prim care phy/provider	62	.62	.19	.35	.51	.62	.78	.89
Nonsurg phy/provider	42	.18	.12	.05	.07	.15	.25	.37
Surg spec phy/provider	38	.14	.09	.02	.06	.13	.21	.27
Total NPP FTE/provider	72	.17	.09	.08	.10	.16	.22	.27
Total support staff FTE/prov	72	3.75	.93	2.55	3.13	3.63	4.35	4.98
Total empl supp staff FTE/prov	69	3.72	.92	2.49	3.12	3.63	4.34	4.91
General administrative	64	.27	.15	.09	.15	.23	.36	.49
Patient accounting	58	.48	.31	.04	.28	.45	.65	.96
General accounting	43	.06	.04	.02	.03	.04	.07	.13
Managed care administrative	24	.10	.18	.00	.01	.03	.08	.35
Information technology	38	.05	.05	.01	.02	.04	.07	.11
Housekeeping, maint, security	31	.07	.07	.01	.02	.04	.11	.22
Medical receptionists	60	.83	.31	.47	.60	.82	1.11	1.26
Med secretaries,transcribers	42	.21	.20	.03	.06	.14	.31	.48
Medical records	51	.29	.18	.09	.15	.26	.40	.60
Other admin support	33	.36	.82	.02	.04	.08	.23	1.37
*Total administrative supp staff	30	2.01	.44	1.33	1.68	2.04	2.41	2.69
Registered Nurses	57	.36	.31	.07	.11	.23	.58	.87
Licensed Practical Nurses	57	.43	.31	.06	.16	.33	.70	.92
Med assistants, nurse aides	60	.62	.40	.14	.28	.51	.98	1.19
*Total clinical supp staff	55	1.27	.33	.81	1.05	1.29	1.45	1.79
Clinical laboratory	40	.19	.12	.03	.09	.18	.27	.36
Radiology and imaging	50	.14	.10	.01	.07	.12	.19	.25
Other medical support serv	32	.22	.44	.02	.04	.09	.24	.37
*Total ancillary supp staff	24	.52	.29	.08	.39	.49	.65	.83
Tot contracted supp staff	15	.14	.12	.01	.04	.11	.20	.36
Tot RVU/provider	26	7,790	1,885	6,098	6,561	7,824	8,330	10,632
Physician work RVU/provider	36	4,135	703	3,217	3,520	4,113	4,701	5,170
Patients/provider	29	1,436	559	725	946	1,421	1,829	2,047
Tot procedures/provider	52	7,266	2,346	4,105	5,266	7,322	9,118	10,129
Square feet/provider	65	1,763	562	1,140	1,389	1,685	2,077	2,458
Total support staff FTE/phy	86	4.46	1.40	2.93	3.66	4.16	5.08	6.25

*See pages 260 and 261 for definition.

Table 3.6b: Charges, Revenue and Cost

	Count	Mean	Std. Dev.	10th %tile	25th %tile	Median	75th %tile	90th %tile
Total gross charges	72	$631,542	$209,226	$375,575	$468,199	$578,689	$793,669	$933,132
Total medical revenue	72	$422,949	$182,805	$268,896	$310,982	$393,341	$509,889	$564,336
Net fee-for-service revenue	69	$361,919	$122,949	$210,175	$267,983	$347,969	$473,611	$529,786
Net capitation revenue	31	$102,765	$235,981	$3,301	$8,295	$36,774	$76,039	$247,219
Net other medical revenue	53	$11,957	$15,670	$254	$1,368	$7,326	$16,171	$28,734
Total support staff cost/prov	72	$141,635	$42,671	$101,079	$115,122	$135,495	$158,774	$196,584
Total general operating cost	72	$133,592	$101,008	$63,792	$83,579	$130,586	$157,899	$182,713
Total operating cost	72	$275,523	$131,086	$172,940	$211,928	$266,015	$310,259	$350,365
Total med rev after oper cost	72	$147,423	$88,882	$49,035	$100,718	$142,518	$187,489	$255,039
Total provider cost/provider	72	$209,370	$48,330	$151,673	$173,753	$205,093	$244,463	$273,489
Total NPP cost/provider	71	$15,206	$8,639	$6,328	$8,774	$13,549	$19,459	$26,589
Provider consultant cost	18	$6,511	$9,527	$785	$1,411	$3,955	$6,896	$16,290
Total physician cost/provider	72	$192,664	$50,228	$125,971	$157,589	$188,704	$229,328	$261,622
Total phy compensation	69	$164,960	$46,616	$106,909	$132,515	$163,319	$196,842	$225,628
Total phy benefit cost	69	$26,377	$8,904	$15,172	$20,129	$25,306	$33,880	$39,273
Total cost	72	$484,893	$150,095	$342,182	$388,483	$486,145	$552,666	$604,144
Net nonmedical revenue	62	$40,921	$89,516	-$2,028	$1,919	$12,469	$52,142	$90,042
Net inc, prac with fin sup	28	-$5,366	$106,270	-$85,563	-$25,115	$1,075	$6,286	$17,607
Net inc, prac w/o fin sup	43	-$43,790	$58,486	-$105,430	-$86,477	-$49,006	-$11,990	$14,381
Net inc, excl fin supp (all prac)	71	-$54,684	$59,738	-$123,392	-$93,481	-$49,006	-$22,491	$4,489
Total support staff FTE/phy	86	4.46	1.40	2.93	3.66	4.16	5.08	6.25

Multispecialty — Hospital or IDS Owned
(per Square Foot)

Table 3.7a: Staffing, RVUs, Patients and Procedures

	Count	Mean	Std. Dev.	10th %tile	25th %tile	Median	75th %tile	90th %tile
Total prov FTE/10,000 sq ft	**65**	**6.22**	**1.95**	**4.07**	**4.82**	**5.93**	**7.20**	**8.77**
Total phy FTE/10,000 sq ft	78	5.43	1.89	3.28	4.06	5.47	6.25	7.78
Prim care phy/10,000 sq ft	67	4.13	1.99	1.87	2.48	3.78	5.50	6.99
Nonsurg phy/10,000 sq ft	41	1.02	.70	.22	.47	.79	1.72	2.12
Surg spec phy/10,000 sq ft	39	1.03	.82	.15	.34	.83	1.33	2.65
Total NPP FTE/10,000 sq ft	65	1.06	.75	.38	.54	.87	1.29	1.86
Total supp stf FTE/10,000 sq ft	**78**	**23.18**	**6.84**	**14.86**	**18.70**	**22.30**	**27.94**	**32.98**
Total empl supp stf/10,000 sq ft	75	22.94	6.82	14.85	18.75	21.88	27.59	32.64
General administrative	69	1.56	1.03	.42	.76	1.41	2.04	2.87
Patient accounting	57	2.95	2.10	.34	1.47	2.56	4.00	5.39
General accounting	45	.38	.32	.10	.18	.31	.51	.75
Managed care administrative	25	.50	.74	.02	.05	.18	.58	1.61
Information technology	40	.30	.25	.07	.15	.27	.37	.58
Housekeeping, maint, security	30	.38	.42	.04	.10	.19	.64	1.07
Medical receptionists	63	5.63	2.93	2.42	3.48	5.22	7.31	10.13
Med secretaries,transcribers	39	1.45	1.67	.14	.41	1.01	1.80	2.86
Medical records	51	1.74	1.07	.55	.97	1.65	2.39	3.71
Other admin support	32	1.80	3.67	.09	.25	.47	1.36	7.36
*Total administrative supp staff	30	12.35	4.10	6.87	9.14	11.94	15.27	19.21
Registered Nurses	58	2.11	1.96	.36	.67	1.51	2.82	4.93
Licensed Practical Nurses	59	2.50	1.78	.67	1.00	2.11	4.06	5.21
Med assistants, nurse aides	62	3.99	2.95	.80	1.58	3.02	5.78	8.57
*Total clinical supp staff	56	7.69	2.85	4.24	5.73	7.41	9.21	12.05
Clinical laboratory	38	1.07	.82	.21	.54	.91	1.44	1.99
Radiology and imaging	47	.83	.64	.10	.50	.75	1.04	1.54
Other medical support serv	32	2.18	5.74	.11	.21	.67	1.46	4.92
*Total ancillary supp staff	24	2.93	1.83	.64	2.00	2.64	3.46	4.97
Tot contracted supp staff	16	.83	.71	.06	.17	.76	.96	2.24
Tot RVU/sq ft	31	5.22	1.71	2.90	4.21	4.88	6.19	8.09
Physician work RVU/sq ft	37	2.69	.87	1.54	2.04	2.54	3.49	3.89
Patients/sq ft	31	.90	.43	.39	.53	.77	1.20	1.56
Tot procedures/sq ft	58	4.54	1.74	2.37	3.16	4.34	5.66	6.90
Total support staff FTE/phy	**86**	**4.46**	**1.40**	**2.93**	**3.66**	**4.16**	**5.08**	**6.25**

*See pages 260 and 261 for definition.

Table 3.7b: Charges, Revenue and Cost

	Count	Mean	Std. Dev.	10th %tile	25th %tile	Median	75th %tile	90th %tile
Total gross charges	78	$388.42	$145.80	$203.35	$287.83	$372.37	$472.03	$588.78
Total medical revenue	78	$257.54	$102.24	$140.31	$192.87	$244.11	$309.84	$376.04
Net fee-for-service revenue	73	$222.28	$84.75	$111.33	$161.74	$223.46	$268.92	$346.12
Net capitation revenue	32	$58.52	$111.06	$1.94	$5.80	$23.32	$53.14	$168.56
Net other medical revenue	52	$7.24	$11.33	$.14	$.98	$3.43	$9.83	$19.93
Total support staff cost/sq ft	78	$88.09	$29.07	$53.89	$72.94	$85.30	$105.58	$128.59
Total general operating cost	78	$76.99	$48.04	$37.29	$54.55	$71.88	$86.92	$114.26
Total operating cost	78	$165.29	$65.77	$100.52	$131.07	$160.48	$189.67	$224.18
Total med rev after oper cost	78	$92.24	$56.14	$31.12	$54.47	$86.63	$128.72	$174.97
Total provider cost/sq ft	78	$131.10	$45.66	$80.68	$95.13	$129.53	$152.28	$184.45
Total NPP cost/sq ft	64	$9.52	$7.27	$3.25	$4.91	$7.77	$12.10	$16.93
Provider consultant cost	17	$3.44	$4.02	$.69	$.91	$2.61	$3.78	$8.29
Total physician cost/sq ft	78	$122.49	$45.54	$70.79	$86.31	$120.39	$144.26	$177.40
Total phy compensation	73	$103.71	$41.42	$58.36	$71.29	$97.47	$124.52	$157.24
Total phy benefit cost	73	$16.39	$6.87	$8.67	$12.15	$15.36	$19.84	$25.59
Total cost	78	$296.39	$92.97	$200.85	$235.52	$283.37	$353.28	$406.02
Net nonmedical revenue/sq ft	63	$26.09	$42.35	-$.61	$1.40	$10.23	$36.79	$76.35
Net inc, prac with fin sup	31	-$8.91	$53.65	-$42.36	-$18.34	$.00	$3.99	$10.69
Net inc, prac w/o fin sup	44	-$27.19	$32.43	-$64.07	-$47.38	-$28.98	-$11.38	$7.64
Net inc, excl fin supp (all prac)	75	-$36.69	$37.12	-$89.74	-$54.03	-$33.32	-$17.83	$1.88
Total support staff FTE/phy	**86**	**4.46**	**1.40**	**2.93**	**3.66**	**4.16**	**5.08**	**6.25**

Multispecialty — Hospital or IDS Owned
(per Total RVU)

Table 3.8a: Staffing, Patients, Procedures and Square Footage

	Count	Mean	Std. Dev.	10th %tile	25th %tile	Median	75th %tile	90th %tile
Total prov FTE/10,000 tot RVU	26	**1.36**	**.37**	**.94**	**1.20**	**1.28**	**1.52**	**1.64**
Total phy FTE/10,000 tot RVU	34	1.24	.49	.85	1.00	1.12	1.32	1.90
Prim care phy/10,000 tot RVU	30	.89	.51	.47	.52	.80	1.12	1.46
Nonsurg phy/10,000 tot RVU	23	.27	.20	.07	.10	.19	.39	.62
Surg spec phy/10,000 tot RVU	18	.19	.14	.03	.08	.16	.28	.41
Total NPP FTE/10,000 tot RVU	26	.23	.11	.08	.15	.22	.30	.37
Total supp stf FTE/10,000 tot RVU	34	**4.85**	**1.83**	**3.24**	**3.81**	**4.58**	**5.22**	**6.77**
Tot empl supp stf/10,000 tot RVU	31	4.85	1.91	3.18	3.78	4.62	5.06	6.85
General administrative	29	.32	.18	.11	.19	.29	.41	.63
Patient accounting	24	.56	.43	.03	.18	.51	.85	1.31
General accounting	21	.07	.04	.02	.03	.07	.09	.13
Managed care administrative	10	.12	.21	.01	.02	.06	.12	.66
Information technology	18	.05	.03	.01	.03	.04	.08	.10
Housekeeping, maint, security	14	.06	.06	.00	.01	.03	.09	.16
Medical receptionists	25	1.36	.60	.73	.91	1.25	1.69	1.91
Med secretaries,transcribers	15	.31	.39	.03	.05	.14	.34	1.10
Medical records	18	.39	.26	.12	.18	.32	.53	.85
Other admin support	14	.30	.66	.01	.05	.09	.21	1.47
***Total administrative supp staff**	12	**2.75**	**1.21**	**1.77**	**1.86**	**2.48**	**3.22**	**5.34**
Registered Nurses	26	.57	.57	.08	.12	.34	.85	1.48
Licensed Practical Nurses	27	.45	.39	.09	.15	.32	.67	1.23
Med assistants, nurse aides	27	.89	.52	.21	.50	.74	1.28	1.59
***Total clinical supp staff**	26	**1.80**	**.66**	**.97**	**1.37**	**1.80**	**2.20**	**2.77**
Clinical laboratory	17	.15	.13	.01	.04	.13	.22	.38
Radiology and imaging	20	.15	.12	.01	.04	.13	.23	.35
Other medical support serv	13	.90	2.81	.03	.05	.09	.22	6.30
***Total ancillary supp staff**	9	*	*	*	*	*	*	*
Tot contracted supp staff	7	*	*	*	*	*	*	*
Physician work RVU/tot RVU	27	.53	.11	.45	.49	.50	.54	.66
Patients/tot RVU	19	.17	.10	.08	.10	.14	.23	.30
Tot procedures/tot RVU	26	.89	.32	.56	.66	.81	1.15	1.29
Square feet/tot RVU	31	.21	.07	.12	.16	.20	.24	.34
Total support staff FTE/phy	86	**4.46**	**1.40**	**2.93**	**3.66**	**4.16**	**5.08**	**6.25**

*See pages 260 and 261 for definition.

Table 3.8b: Charges, Revenue and Cost

	Count	Mean	Std. Dev.	10th %tile	25th %tile	Median	75th %tile	90th %tile
Total gross charges	34	**$83.36**	**$26.86**	**$56.62**	**$61.09**	**$74.35**	**$104.81**	**$126.85**
Total medical revenue	34	**$54.14**	**$17.73**	**$38.81**	**$41.85**	**$49.52**	**$61.71**	**$80.74**
Net fee-for-service revenue	32	$46.30	$15.97	$29.23	$38.29	$42.42	$50.19	$72.65
Net capitation revenue	16	$11.13	$18.74	$.43	$1.39	$4.20	$12.12	$44.76
Net other medical revenue	21	$2.32	$2.79	$.09	$.40	$.95	$4.78	$7.17
Total supp staff cost/tot RVU	34	**$18.96**	**$7.27**	**$11.19**	**$15.53**	**$17.46**	**$20.85**	**$29.37**
Total general operating cost	34	**$16.01**	**$6.99**	**$8.60**	**$11.44**	**$15.46**	**$18.63**	**$25.57**
Total operating cost	34	**$35.06**	**$12.82**	**$22.22**	**$26.34**	**$32.94**	**$37.56**	**$56.93**
Total med rev after oper cost	34	**$19.07**	**$8.84**	**$6.79**	**$12.62**	**$18.61**	**$25.47**	**$30.99**
Total provider cost/tot RVU	34	**$27.96**	**$6.90**	**$20.02**	**$22.42**	**$28.12**	**$31.47**	**$38.69**
Total NPP cost/tot RVU	26	$2.01	$1.02	$.70	$1.31	$1.89	$2.89	$3.38
Provider consultant cost	10	$.56	$.60	$.07	$.13	$.34	$.75	$1.95
Total physician cost/tot RVU	34	$26.26	$7.10	$16.76	$20.87	$27.09	$29.39	$35.56
Total phy compensation	31	$21.74	$6.02	$13.50	$17.37	$22.88	$25.58	$28.36
Total phy benefit cost	31	$3.87	$1.45	$1.82	$2.87	$3.90	$4.97	$5.32
Total cost	26	**$64.24**	**$15.86**	**$47.29**	**$55.53**	**$60.32**	**$67.36**	**$96.32**
Net nonmedical revenue	28	$5.77	$6.44	-$.33	$.86	$3.60	$8.80	$16.33
Net inc, prac with fin sup	18	-$2.97	$5.57	-$9.32	-$5.67	-$.96	$.46	$2.08
Net inc, prac w/o fin sup	16	-$6.55	$5.52	-$14.23	-$11.49	-$5.46	-$1.30	$.24
Net inc, excl fin supp (all prac)	34	-$8.88	$6.77	-$19.13	-$13.65	-$8.50	-$2.50	-$.87
Total support staff FTE/phy	86	**4.46**	**1.40**	**2.93**	**3.66**	**4.16**	**5.08**	**6.25**

Multispecialty — Hospital or IDS Owned
(per Work RVU)

Table 3.9a: Staffing, Patients, Procedures and Square Footage

	Count	Mean	Std. Dev.	10th %tile	25th %tile	Median	75th %tile	90th %tile
Total prov FTE/10,000 work RVU	**36**	**2.49**	**.43**	**1.93**	**2.13**	**2.43**	**2.84**	**3.11**
Tot phy FTE/10,000 work RVU	40	2.09	.42	1.64	1.83	2.01	2.23	2.48
Prim care phy/10,000 work RVU	34	1.48	.46	.84	1.05	1.52	1.83	2.08
Nonsurg phy/10,000 work RVU	25	.47	.35	.11	.20	.41	.56	1.18
Surg spec phy/10,000 work RVU	24	.32	.22	.05	.12	.30	.50	.67
Total NPP FTE/10,000 work RVU	36	.43	.25	.16	.25	.37	.59	.80
Total supp stf FTE/10,000 wrk RVU	**40**	**8.92**	**2.19**	**6.22**	**7.39**	**8.68**	**9.77**	**12.25**
Tot empl supp stf/10,000 work RVU	37	8.90	2.24	6.12	7.17	8.79	9.76	12.38
General administrative	35	.66	.35	.22	.44	.53	.94	1.23
Patient accounting	32	1.08	.73	.08	.49	1.08	1.62	2.13
General accounting	24	.12	.08	.04	.05	.10	.17	.24
Managed care administrative	16	.20	.39	.01	.03	.08	.18	.76
Information technology	21	.10	.06	.03	.05	.09	.16	.20
Housekeeping, maint, security	19	.15	.18	.00	.03	.08	.21	.47
Medical receptionists	33	2.24	.78	1.17	1.55	2.30	2.61	3.41
Med secretaries,transcribers	24	.55	.57	.08	.17	.32	.79	1.52
Medical records	28	.72	.51	.20	.35	.63	.93	1.67
Other admin support	18	.63	1.63	.04	.10	.18	.40	1.36
***Total administrative supp staff**	**19**	**4.91**	**1.28**	**3.51**	**3.68**	**5.08**	**5.83**	**6.48**
Registered Nurses	31	.88	.75	.19	.31	.66	1.34	1.97
Licensed Practical Nurses	31	1.01	.79	.12	.31	.86	1.46	2.43
Med assistants, nurse aides	33	1.71	1.20	.30	.76	1.44	2.63	3.87
***Total clinical supp staff**	**30**	**3.25**	**.97**	**2.02**	**2.71**	**3.14**	**4.21**	**4.55**
Clinical laboratory	23	.37	.34	.03	.10	.26	.56	.98
Radiology and imaging	27	.31	.25	.02	.14	.23	.49	.73
Other medical support serv	16	.22	.21	.03	.07	.13	.35	.61
***Total ancillary supp staff**	**12**	**.94**	**.57**	**.12**	**.36**	**1.00**	**1.43**	**1.72**
Tot contracted supp staff	10	.32	.31	.01	.08	.21	.52	.95
Tot RVU/work RVU	27	1.94	.30	1.52	1.86	1.98	2.04	2.21
Patients/work RVU	20	.32	.12	.15	.24	.31	.36	.50
Tot procedures/work RVU	31	1.79	.60	1.20	1.37	1.76	2.10	2.58
Square feet/work RVU	37	.42	.15	.26	.29	.39	.49	.65
Total support staff FTE/phy	**86**	**4.46**	**1.40**	**2.93**	**3.66**	**4.16**	**5.08**	**6.25**

*See pages 260 and 261 for definition.

Table 3.9b: Charges, Revenue and Cost

	Count	Mean	Std. Dev.	10th %tile	25th %tile	Median	75th %tile	90th %tile
Total gross charges	**40**	**$158.70**	**$41.11**	**$107.71**	**$128.18**	**$148.73**	**$187.17**	**$230.68**
Total medical revenue	**40**	**$101.55**	**$26.40**	**$72.28**	**$84.38**	**$98.69**	**$112.75**	**$136.22**
Net fee-for-service revenue	38	$88.06	$23.85	$62.56	$72.08	$83.52	$101.06	$124.88
Net capitation revenue	19	$21.75	$40.50	$1.02	$2.15	$5.56	$16.46	$68.10
Net other medical revenue	27	$2.60	$3.67	$.02	$.37	$.99	$2.93	$7.79
Total supp staff cost/work RVU	**40**	**$34.31**	**$11.83**	**$22.39**	**$26.76**	**$33.51**	**$36.98**	**$46.56**
Total general operating cost	**40**	**$30.50**	**$11.07**	**$17.13**	**$21.79**	**$30.21**	**$39.57**	**$43.35**
Total operating cost	**40**	**$64.97**	**$20.01**	**$47.06**	**$50.35**	**$64.07**	**$74.49**	**$86.66**
Total med rev after oper cost	**40**	**$36.58**	**$14.50**	**$18.67**	**$27.07**	**$34.80**	**$46.97**	**$56.34**
Total provider cost/work RVU	**40**	**$51.72**	**$9.10**	**$41.92**	**$43.07**	**$50.58**	**$59.01**	**$65.34**
Total NPP cost/work RVU	36	$3.86	$2.61	$1.25	$2.14	$3.35	$5.57	$6.93
Provider consultant cost	11	$1.78	$2.82	$.14	$.26	$.73	$1.49	$8.48
Total physician cost/work RVU	40	$47.76	$9.07	$36.65	$40.70	$46.33	$55.12	$60.98
Total phy compensation	36	$40.05	$8.00	$30.76	$34.64	$38.64	$46.31	$52.70
Total phy benefit cost	36	$6.79	$2.17	$4.19	$4.77	$6.65	$8.74	$9.69
Total cost	**40**	**$116.69**	**$24.97**	**$91.00**	**$97.83**	**$112.73**	**$132.67**	**$144.83**
Net nonmedical revenue	35	$13.07	$26.04	-$.50	$.91	$4.60	$17.06	$33.54
Net inc, prac with fin sup	21	$1.12	$29.28	-$14.32	-$6.06	$.00	$1.06	$4.31
Net inc, prac w/o fin sup	18	-$11.49	$8.51	-$25.75	-$19.54	-$9.82	-$3.90	-$1.60
Net inc, excl fin supp (all prac)	39	-$14.68	$12.51	-$35.97	-$21.34	-$10.71	-$5.16	-$1.96
Total support staff FTE/phy	**86**	**4.46**	**1.40**	**2.93**	**3.66**	**4.16**	**5.08**	**6.25**

Multispecialty — Hospital or IDS Owned
(per Patient)

Table 3.10a: Staffing, RVUs, Procedures and Square Footage

	Count	Mean	Std. Dev.	10th %tile	25th %tile	Median	75th %tile	90th %tile
Total prov FTE/10,000 patients	29	8.17	3.52	4.88	5.47	7.04	10.58	13.80
Total phy FTE/10,000 pat	33	7.15	2.85	4.16	4.91	6.32	9.01	11.99
Prim care phy/10,000 pat	31	4.92	1.86	2.77	3.73	4.75	5.55	7.80
Nonsurg phy/10,000 pat	21	1.93	1.48	.30	.75	1.49	3.13	4.61
Surg spec phy/10,000 pat	21	1.40	1.30	.15	.43	1.02	1.99	3.38
Total NPP FTE/10,000 pat	29	1.34	1.06	.46	.56	1.03	1.87	3.32
Total supp staff FTE/10,000 pat	33	29.69	13.91	16.16	20.29	26.62	38.04	47.55
Total empl supp staff/10,000 pat	33	29.36	13.82	16.13	19.08	24.86	38.04	47.55
General administrative	32	2.34	1.58	.60	1.38	2.03	2.89	4.29
Patient accounting	26	3.56	2.91	.34	1.73	2.84	4.65	8.17
General accounting	23	.49	.40	.10	.15	.29	.85	1.13
Managed care administrative	15	.66	1.16	.02	.06	.24	.65	2.88
Information technology	21	.41	.39	.05	.13	.29	.59	1.05
Housekeeping, maint, security	15	.47	.50	.00	.08	.25	.78	1.34
Medical receptionists	31	7.32	3.20	2.49	5.15	7.24	9.56	11.72
Med secretaries,transcribers	21	1.39	1.79	.12	.23	.75	1.36	5.19
Medical records	24	2.51	2.56	.40	.99	1.36	2.62	7.33
Other admin support	16	.82	.67	.13	.25	.67	1.22	2.00
***Total administrative supp staff**	14	15.01	5.33	6.95	11.79	14.28	18.93	23.74
Registered Nurses	28	2.70	2.42	.37	.66	1.51	4.43	6.86
Licensed Practical Nurses	30	4.11	3.52	.34	1.12	2.43	7.33	9.59
Med assistants, nurse aides	30	4.71	3.13	.89	1.81	4.42	7.01	9.37
***Total clinical supp staff**	24	10.73	5.31	3.29	7.06	9.91	14.85	19.23
Clinical laboratory	21	1.32	1.17	.16	.61	.91	1.45	3.41
Radiology and imaging	23	1.02	.89	.08	.43	.85	1.40	2.75
Other medical support serv	16	1.08	1.18	.13	.26	.77	1.31	3.63
***Total ancillary supp staff**	12	4.18	2.24	.69	2.44	4.00	6.71	6.90
Tot contracted supp staff	11	.98	.94	.02	.23	.63	1.99	2.62
Tot RVU/patient	19	7.25	3.36	3.32	4.39	6.96	9.53	12.17
Physician work RVU/patient	20	3.60	1.51	2.00	2.78	3.25	4.23	6.62
Tot procedures/patient	28	6.18	3.16	2.10	3.74	5.61	8.27	11.39
Square feet/patient	31	1.45	.82	.64	.83	1.30	1.90	2.56
Total support staff FTE/phy	86	4.46	1.40	2.93	3.66	4.16	5.08	6.25

*See pages 260 and 261 for definition.

Table 3.10b: Charges, Revenue and Cost

	Count	Mean	Std. Dev.	10th %tile	25th %tile	Median	75th %tile	90th %tile
Total gross charges	33	$543.66	$318.46	$259.21	$292.89	$456.76	$693.50	$1,149.78
Total medical revenue	33	$358.22	$203.88	$172.04	$208.44	$283.20	$488.18	$702.54
Net fee-for-service revenue	33	$307.87	$195.16	$105.21	$187.20	$237.57	$365.43	$587.70
Net capitation revenue	19	$68.82	$115.09	$2.88	$7.30	$31.44	$55.42	$271.05
Net other medical revenue	25	$14.16	$22.46	$.88	$4.18	$7.77	$17.66	$24.85
Total support staff cost/patient	33	$113.05	$58.63	$62.21	$71.97	$99.99	$131.78	$232.46
Total general operating cost	33	$105.53	$58.41	$40.75	$60.99	$93.29	$141.14	$192.27
Total operating cost	33	$218.60	$109.84	$104.87	$145.33	$198.51	$304.88	$383.43
Total med rev after oper cost	33	$139.61	$110.94	$32.32	$64.37	$115.55	$182.43	$271.79
Total provider cost/patient	33	$183.49	$102.12	$85.26	$100.93	$149.72	$251.81	$373.11
Total NPP cost/patient	29	$11.35	$9.12	$3.02	$4.79	$9.42	$13.41	$30.05
Provider consultant cost	11	$4.71	$6.49	$.41	$.90	$2.92	$5.79	$19.86
Total physician cost/patient	33	$171.95	$95.48	$78.89	$91.01	$147.57	$240.08	$340.82
Total phy compensation	32	$145.86	$83.60	$69.37	$79.85	$126.01	$194.74	$284.40
Total phy benefit cost	32	$23.96	$15.49	$9.06	$13.05	$19.16	$34.24	$51.19
Total cost	33	$402.09	$200.51	$212.30	$244.46	$352.28	$558.09	$715.02
Net nonmedical revenue	29	$26.57	$44.54	-$1.94	$1.48	$10.41	$30.16	$80.22
Net inc, prac with fin sup	15	-$13.75	$40.34	-$82.78	-$16.71	$2.53	$3.81	$11.75
Net inc, prac w/o fin sup	17	-$27.70	$53.36	-$88.48	-$55.08	-$24.65	-$4.70	$28.77
Net inc, excl fin supp (all prac)	32	-$42.53	$58.23	-$138.64	-$63.30	-$27.76	-$14.35	$3.86
Total support staff FTE/phy	86	4.46	1.40	2.93	3.66	4.16	5.08	6.25

Multispecialty — Hospital or IDS Owned
(Procedure and Charge Data)

Table 3.11a: Activity Charges to Total Gross Charges Ratios

	Count	Mean	Std. Dev.	10th %tile	25th %tile	Median	75th %tile	90th %tile
Total proc gross charges	65	93.38%	8.61%	81.34%	91.24%	95.70%	99.40%	100.00%
Medical proc-inside practice	64	54.01%	19.60%	28.33%	37.17%	54.45%	67.36%	82.01%
Medical proc-outside practice	51	10.86%	5.47%	4.21%	6.41%	10.62%	14.88%	19.01%
Surg proc-inside practice	62	7.05%	6.94%	1.92%	3.98%	5.19%	7.89%	13.43%
Surg proc-outside practice	41	17.92%	11.76%	2.58%	7.38%	18.39%	27.28%	35.47%
Laboratory procedures	63	8.10%	7.09%	.69%	1.55%	7.92%	12.77%	18.51%
Radiology procedures	56	4.93%	5.07%	.12%	1.31%	3.78%	5.86%	12.13%
Tot nonproc gross charges	54	7.69%	8.53%	.71%	1.47%	4.92%	9.99%	18.54%
Total support staff FTE/phy	86	4.46	1.40	2.93	3.66	4.16	5.08	6.25

Table 3.11b: Medical Procedure Data (inside the practice)

	Count	Mean	Std. Dev.	10th %tile	25th %tile	Median	75th %tile	90th %tile
Gross charges/procedure	62	$77.37	$19.58	$52.76	$63.98	$76.01	$86.66	$107.75
Total cost/procedure	57	$75.63	$25.34	$49.73	$60.83	$69.08	$84.35	$109.22
Operating cost/procedure	45	$47.49	$23.61	$26.77	$34.40	$42.97	$56.56	$67.75
Provider cost/procedure	58	$29.79	$6.63	$21.45	$25.04	$30.22	$33.51	$38.80
Procedures/patient	28	3.47	1.35	1.29	2.41	3.62	4.59	5.07
Gross charges/patient	28	$251.39	$102.00	$109.52	$182.57	$234.95	$325.85	$406.83
Procedures/physician	63	4,919	1,663	2,746	3,663	4,934	5,746	7,382
Gross charges/physician	64	$365,448	$112,968	$227,323	$283,148	$349,688	$423,182	$495,506
Procedures/provider	52	4,087	1,534	2,205	2,949	3,940	4,776	5,974
Gross charges/provider	54	$297,839	$93,290	$169,893	$231,695	$303,234	$366,752	$397,392
Gross charge to total cost ratio	57	1.08	.35	.77	.94	1.06	1.18	1.26
Oper cost to total cost ratio	45	.60	.07	.52	.55	.59	.65	.66
Prov cost to total cost ratio	57	.41	.08	.34	.37	.42	.46	.49
Total support staff FTE/phy	86	4.46	1.40	2.93	3.66	4.16	5.08	6.25

Table 3.11c: Medical Procedure Data (outside the practice)

	Count	Mean	Std. Dev.	10th %tile	25th %tile	Median	75th %tile	90th %tile
Gross charges/procedure	50	$132.88	$68.96	$80.56	$103.59	$118.18	$154.93	$182.85
Total cost/procedure	45	$75.34	$46.51	$46.12	$56.30	$69.06	$77.56	$103.01
Operating cost/procedure	38	$28.75	$18.00	$13.48	$18.37	$25.80	$32.19	$48.95
Provider cost/procedure	46	$46.98	$30.83	$29.22	$35.35	$43.36	$49.09	$61.18
Procedures/patient	24	.47	.37	.08	.25	.30	.63	1.13
Gross charges/patient	24	$53.18	$38.05	$11.39	$31.28	$40.39	$66.07	$113.86
Procedures/physician	51	697	524	169	373	573	924	1,342
Gross charges/physician	51	$78,182	$43,811	$26,526	$50,467	$69,640	$96,547	$157,061
Procedures/provider	45	569	443	144	307	468	705	1,051
Gross charges/provider	46	$66,210	$36,738	$23,809	$40,464	$58,853	$82,986	$133,653
Gross charge to total cost ratio	45	1.84	.34	1.41	1.58	1.82	2.03	2.27
Oper cost to total cost ratio	38	.37	.06	.29	.32	.36	.42	.45
Prov cost to total cost ratio	45	.63	.06	.54	.58	.64	.68	.71
Total support staff FTE/phy	86	4.46	1.40	2.93	3.66	4.16	5.08	6.25

Multispecialty — Hospital or IDS Owned
(Procedure and Charge Data)

Table 3.11d: Surgery/Anesthesia Procedure Data (inside the practice)

	Count	Mean	Std. Dev.	10th %tile	25th %tile	Median	75th %tile	90th %tile
Gross charges/procedure	60	$113.50	$93.58	$30.95	$56.48	$94.29	$143.82	$196.13
Total cost/procedure	55	$111.62	$86.71	$31.12	$55.52	$84.10	$144.70	$213.31
Operating cost/procedure	44	$72.17	$56.13	$21.67	$37.76	$55.57	$92.72	$141.90
Provider cost/procedure	56	$45.19	$38.68	$15.02	$19.65	$37.15	$58.86	$81.14
Procedures/patient	26	.40	.36	.06	.08	.29	.60	.94
Gross charges/patient	27	$34.81	$32.85	$7.92	$12.22	$23.39	$42.28	$96.33
Procedures/physician	60	574	434	92	237	513	737	1,275
Gross charges/physician	62	$53,352	$61,707	$12,061	$22,457	$41,856	$60,999	$97,551
Procedures/provider	51	500	354	135	234	416	617	1,090
Gross charges/provider	53	$49,104	$58,221	$13,331	$21,998	$36,020	$52,867	$92,590
Gross charge to total cost ratio	55	1.08	.35	.76	.92	1.07	1.19	1.27
Oper cost to total cost ratio	44	.60	.07	.52	.55	.59	.65	.66
Prov cost to total cost ratio	55	.42	.07	.34	.37	.42	.46	.49
Total support staff FTE/phy	86	4.46	1.40	2.93	3.66	4.16	5.08	6.25

Table 3.11e: Surgery/Anesthesia Procedure Data (outside the practice)

	Count	Mean	Std. Dev.	10th %tile	25th %tile	Median	75th %tile	90th %tile
Gross charges/procedure	40	$837.27	$500.75	$167.81	$465.92	$760.47	$1,242.34	$1,511.32
Total cost/procedure	39	$480.50	$297.24	$119.01	$276.45	$455.76	$694.79	$947.03
Operating cost/procedure	32	$184.61	$130.62	$39.71	$82.55	$149.99	$272.12	$382.21
Provider cost/procedure	39	$300.64	$179.17	$84.39	$163.36	$258.69	$419.31	$583.57
Procedures/patient	17	.32	.53	.02	.08	.13	.29	1.09
Gross charges/patient	17	$132.24	$128.28	$15.71	$47.97	$95.61	$210.67	$319.15
Procedures/physician	41	332	673	20	54	134	273	769
Gross charges/physician	41	$142,904	$115,509	$15,225	$61,137	$128,824	$206,549	$302,311
Procedures/provider	35	275	498	18	46	117	217	687
Gross charges/provider	36	$118,452	$95,250	$14,224	$41,466	$94,686	$175,166	$262,417
Gross charge to total cost ratio	39	1.84	.35	1.38	1.58	1.82	2.03	2.31
Oper cost to total cost ratio	32	.36	.06	.28	.32	.36	.41	.45
Prov cost to total cost ratio	39	.63	.06	.54	.59	.65	.68	.71
Total support staff FTE/phy	86	4.46	1.40	2.93	3.66	4.16	5.08	6.25

Multispecialty — Hospital or IDS Owned
(Procedure and Charge Data)

Table 3.11f: Clinical Laboratory/Pathology Procedure Data

	Count	Mean	Std. Dev.	10th %tile	25th %tile	Median	75th %tile	90th %tile
Gross charges/procedure	61	$39.43	$89.21	$11.23	$16.14	$27.11	$38.53	$48.25
Total cost/procedure	55	$32.97	$83.10	$8.81	$15.23	$21.55	$28.92	$34.87
Operating cost/procedure	44	$14.01	$6.47	$6.54	$9.58	$13.17	$18.09	$22.24
Provider cost/procedure	57	$13.25	$27.57	$4.00	$6.61	$8.34	$12.00	$16.21
Procedures/patient	27	1.54	1.57	.12	.30	1.10	2.37	4.04
Gross charges/patient	28	$45.67	$57.95	$2.82	$5.20	$25.86	$56.02	$145.40
Procedures/physician	61	2,054	1,695	274	537	1,691	3,329	4,348
Gross charges/physician	63	$65,428	$64,200	$4,514	$8,483	$57,301	$99,113	$176,187
Procedures/provider	51	1,761	1,202	292	529	1,804	2,844	3,458
Gross charges/provider	53	$60,385	$53,291	$4,862	$9,659	$53,248	$86,727	$147,353
Gross charge to total cost ratio	56	1.25	.37	.91	1.06	1.21	1.39	1.59
Oper cost to total cost ratio	44	.58	.09	.45	.53	.59	.65	.68
Prov cost to total cost ratio	56	.43	.09	.32	.35	.42	.49	.56
Total support staff FTE/phy	86	4.46	1.40	2.93	3.66	4.16	5.08	6.25

Table 3.11g: Diagnostic Radiology and Imaging Procedure Data

	Count	Mean	Std. Dev.	10th %tile	25th %tile	Median	75th %tile	90th %tile
Gross charges/procedure	54	$127.04	$94.35	$64.23	$74.28	$106.77	$139.09	$225.61
Total cost/procedure	49	$124.25	$99.03	$61.68	$68.99	$91.53	$139.30	$201.16
Operating cost/procedure	42	$77.34	$56.28	$37.59	$45.54	$62.74	$84.93	$117.56
Provider cost/procedure	50	$43.15	$26.02	$19.16	$26.47	$34.14	$49.06	$79.25
Procedures/patient	24	.30	.40	.00	.06	.16	.40	1.01
Gross charges/patient	25	$33.91	$47.02	$.48	$3.82	$17.27	$35.99	$141.57
Procedures/physician	54	373	394	5	66	287	499	997
Gross charges/physician	56	$45,536	$59,683	$587	$6,473	$27,406	$44,558	$121,264
Procedures/provider	47	314	304	6	109	264	418	766
Gross charges/provider	49	$39,906	$51,136	$952	$10,953	$24,252	$38,015	$99,756
Gross charge to total cost ratio	49	1.11	.31	.70	.92	1.07	1.36	1.45
Oper cost to total cost ratio	42	.62	.09	.49	.53	.62	.69	.73
Prov cost to total cost ratio	49	.38	.10	.27	.31	.38	.47	.54
Total support staff FTE/phy	86	4.46	1.40	2.93	3.66	4.16	5.08	6.25

Table 3.11h: Nonprocedural Gross Charge Data

	Count	Mean	Std. Dev.	10th %tile	25th %tile	Median	75th %tile	90th %tile
Gross charges/patient	23	$72.65	$104.56	$2.17	$9.33	$28.26	$90.29	$218.03
Nonproc gross charges/physician	54	$68,046	$94,648	$3,739	$9,080	$31,312	$85,699	$186,179
Gross charges/provider	47	$61,980	$83,398	$4,366	$8,563	$24,499	$83,165	$152,402
Total support staff FTE/phy	86	4.46	1.40	2.93	3.66	4.16	5.08	6.25

Multispecialty — Primary Care Only, Not Hospital or IDS Owned

Table 4.1: Staffing and Practice Data

	Count	Mean	Std. Dev.	10th %tile	25th %tile	Median	75th %tile	90th %tile
Total provider FTE	**38**	**22.04**	**29.13**	**6.77**	**9.00**	**12.85**	**24.96**	**43.46**
Total physician FTE	45	15.86	24.03	4.00	5.85	10.50	16.70	23.48
Total nonphysician provider FTE	38	4.67	5.35	.86	1.78	2.46	5.16	12.18
Total support staff FTE	**45**	**74.32**	**92.38**	**21.26**	**28.95**	**45.50**	**87.80**	**148.20**
Number of branch clinics	30	6	8	1	2	4	8	17
Square footage of all facilities	42	26,751	23,528	8,045	14,241	20,379	33,474	47,960

Table 4.2: Accounts Receivable Data, Collection Percentages and Financial Ratios

	Count	Mean	Std. Dev.	10th %tile	25th %tile	Median	75th %tile	90th %tile
Total AR/physician	**40**	**$102,161**	**$48,458**	**$45,110**	**$71,734**	**$84,978**	**$129,697**	**$167,616**
Total AR/provider	**34**	**$75,161**	**$25,520**	**$45,557**	**$57,511**	**$72,044**	**$91,369**	**$118,329**
0-30 days in AR	40	52.81%	14.60%	30.27%	43.78%	55.61%	59.09%	71.42%
31-60 days in AR	40	14.78%	5.68%	8.83%	9.91%	13.92%	18.53%	23.15%
61-90 days in AR	40	8.72%	4.01%	4.51%	6.01%	7.80%	10.86%	12.75%
91-120 days in AR	40	5.43%	2.31%	3.02%	3.84%	4.93%	6.63%	9.05%
120+ days in AR	40	18.26%	12.79%	6.43%	10.99%	15.57%	21.86%	37.05%
Re-aged: 0-30 days in AR	12	56.28%	9.69%	39.46%	52.52%	56.47%	58.92%	72.71%
Re-aged: 31-60 days in AR	12	13.17%	4.28%	9.24%	9.50%	12.20%	15.90%	21.41%
Re-aged: 61-90 days in AR	12	9.36%	3.74%	4.64%	6.01%	9.77%	12.12%	15.65%
Re-aged: 91-120 days in AR	12	5.52%	2.23%	3.23%	3.88%	5.17%	6.51%	9.98%
Re-aged: 120+ days in AR	12	15.67%	7.59%	5.62%	10.03%	14.13%	20.66%	29.57%
Not re-aged: 0-30 days in AR	26	49.53%	15.34%	23.75%	35.89%	54.13%	58.51%	68.61%
Not re-aged: 31-60 days in AR	26	15.47%	6.08%	8.36%	10.37%	14.31%	19.74%	24.20%
Not re-aged: 61-90 days in AR	26	8.65%	4.23%	4.47%	6.39%	7.80%	10.80%	11.93%
Not re-aged: 91-120 days in AR	26	5.55%	2.38%	2.76%	3.79%	5.23%	7.21%	9.26%
Not re-aged: 120+ days in AR	26	20.79%	13.89%	8.26%	12.27%	15.88%	25.13%	42.85%
Months gross FFS charges in AR	36	1.65	.57	1.10	1.30	1.42	2.04	2.44
Days gross FFS charges in AR	36	50.20	17.35	33.48	39.57	43.25	62.14	74.22
Gross FFS collection %	40	68.73%	10.35%	57.30%	61.86%	68.74%	73.30%	86.37%
Adjusted FFS collection %	39	96.09%	6.47%	93.04%	96.11%	97.95%	99.13%	99.77%
Gross FFS + cap collection %	13	72.73%	8.14%	60.89%	67.83%	71.58%	79.49%	85.74%
Net cap rev % of gross cap chrg	12	77.66%	22.71%	45.11%	60.27%	72.35%	99.69%	112.37%
Current ratio	26	9.14	20.29	.54	1.29	2.14	4.73	36.33
Tot asset turnover ratio	26	7.34	6.04	1.79	3.72	5.84	9.61	14.99
Debt to equity ratio	26	2.28	4.47	.15	.27	.95	2.28	5.08
Debt ratio	26	48.01%	25.60%	12.84%	21.17%	48.62%	69.46%	82.14%
Return on total assets	24	30.93%	73.23%	-4.68%	-.70%	6.30%	52.59%	166.75%
Return on equity	24	131.93%	296.02%	-9.69%	-2.01%	8.78%	139.72%	584.17%

Table 4.3: Breakout of Total Gross Charges by Type of Payer

	Count	Mean	Std. Dev.	10th %tile	25th %tile	Median	75th %tile	90th %tile
Medicare: fee-for-service	43	24.20%	14.83%	7.00%	10.00%	22.70%	32.49%	45.72%
Medicare: managed care FFS	43	1.15%	2.78%	.00%	.00%	.00%	.00%	4.60%
Medicare: capitation	43	.04%	.24%	.00%	.00%	.00%	.00%	.00%
Medicaid: fee-for-service	43	7.69%	8.17%	.00%	.83%	5.50%	12.00%	19.05%
Medicaid: managed care FFS	43	2.72%	7.43%	.00%	.00%	.00%	.50%	11.90%
Medicaid: capitation	43	.87%	2.70%	.00%	.00%	.00%	.00%	3.72%
Commercial: fee-for-service	43	33.34%	20.45%	.82%	16.12%	36.30%	46.00%	61.74%
Commercial: managed care FFS	43	16.57%	24.85%	.00%	.00%	4.00%	24.00%	54.60%
Commercial: capitation	43	2.63%	7.74%	.00%	.00%	.00%	.20%	11.65%
Workers' compensation	43	2.63%	6.16%	.00%	.00%	1.00%	2.00%	8.00%
Charity care and prof courtesy	43	.58%	.88%	.00%	.00%	.00%	1.00%	1.80%
Self-pay	43	6.40%	6.33%	.43%	2.00%	4.00%	8.24%	17.40%
Other federal government payers	43	1.16%	4.61%	.00%	.00%	.00%	.80%	2.46%

Multispecialty — Primary Care Only, Not Hospital or IDS Owned
(per FTE Physician)

Table 4.4a: Staffing, RVUs, Patients, Procedures and Square Footage

	Count	Mean	Std. Dev.	10th %tile	25th %tile	Median	75th %tile	90th %tile
Total provider FTE/physician	38	**1.36**	**.32**	**1.07**	**1.12**	**1.29**	**1.51**	**1.88**
Prim care phy/physician	40	.99	.05	1.00	1.00	1.00	1.00	1.00
Nonsurg phy/physician	1	*	*	*	*	*	*	*
Surg spec phy/physician	4	*	*	*	*	*	*	*
Total NPP FTE/physician	38	.36	.32	.07	.12	.29	.51	.88
Total support staff FTE/phy	45	**5.23**	**2.07**	**3.24**	**4.00**	**4.89**	**5.83**	**7.36**
Total empl support staff FTE	41	5.16	2.06	3.08	3.89	4.89	5.81	7.49
General administrative	39	.37	.26	.10	.15	.28	.53	.78
Patient accounting	38	.77	.38	.34	.50	.68	1.00	1.42
General accounting	27	.12	.11	.04	.07	.10	.14	.18
Managed care administrative	10	.19	.15	.06	.09	.14	.26	.50
Information technology	11	.08	.04	.03	.05	.08	.13	.15
Housekeeping, maint, security	17	.19	.29	.02	.03	.07	.23	.70
Medical receptionists	38	1.11	.47	.55	.80	1.08	1.39	1.77
Med secretaries,transcribers	25	.28	.22	.04	.10	.27	.36	.58
Medical records	32	.38	.21	.15	.23	.31	.48	.68
Other admin support	18	.27	.25	.05	.07	.12	.52	.72
*Total administrative supp staff	19	**3.24**	**1.64**	**1.64**	**2.09**	**3.00**	**3.86**	**4.21**
Registered Nurses	30	.48	.47	.05	.15	.39	.71	1.04
Licensed Practical Nurses	31	.70	.54	.14	.29	.49	.98	1.67
Med assistants, nurse aides	34	.98	.62	.36	.61	.81	1.24	1.78
*Total clinical supp staff	32	**1.86**	**.83**	**1.02**	**1.22**	**1.67**	**2.28**	**3.04**
Clinical laboratory	28	.32	.20	.08	.17	.29	.45	.56
Radiology and imaging	27	.24	.15	.08	.13	.21	.36	.49
Other medical support serv	9	*	*	*	*	*	*	*
*Total ancillary supp staff	13	**.67**	**.47**	**.13**	**.19**	**.87**	**1.00**	**1.39**
Tot contracted supp staff	16	.28	.37	.02	.05	.19	.34	1.05
Tot RVU/physician	18	32,935	98,510	2,421	6,181	9,661	12,316	62,547
Physician work RVU/physician	18	5,172	2,160	2,724	4,151	5,113	5,963	8,541
Patients/physician	23	2,151	1,077	1,164	1,326	1,756	2,629	4,069
Tot procedures/physician	39	13,004	8,816	5,302	7,665	11,923	15,022	17,094
Square feet/physician	42	2,437	1,966	1,203	1,495	1,899	2,517	4,070

**See pages 260 and 261 for definition.

Table 4.4b: Charges and Revenue

	Count	Mean	Std. Dev.	10th %tile	25th %tile	Median	75th %tile	90th %tile
Net fee-for-service revenue	40	$522,811	$161,213	$336,243	$378,710	$510,634	$617,771	$774,049
Gross FFS charges	41	$777,410	$294,095	$489,140	$564,701	$744,094	$913,313	$1,091,499
Adjustments to FFS charges	37	$249,682	$163,310	$84,725	$150,143	$234,516	$332,814	$415,433
Adjusted FFS charges	39	$552,365	$175,597	$341,106	$402,095	$531,010	$632,911	$841,109
Bad debts due to FFS activity	34	$14,600	$13,829	$1,781	$5,463	$8,128	$22,997	$38,699
Net capitation revenue	13	$52,012	$43,524	$10,247	$22,285	$30,009	$89,677	$128,830
Gross capitation charges	12	$69,060	$56,788	$13,859	$21,779	$49,806	$106,643	$174,195
Capitation revenue	13	$52,532	$42,949	$14,302	$22,285	$30,009	$89,677	$128,830
Purch serv for cap patients	1	*	*	*	*	*	*	*
Net other medical revenue	22	$46,219	$86,227	$1,723	$6,314	$16,888	$36,532	$177,440
Gross rev from other activity	21	$49,537	$87,325	$3,375	$10,386	$18,050	$38,634	$188,699
Other medical revenue	19	$46,516	$92,757	$2,227	$3,931	$15,191	$37,743	$209,863
Rev from sale of goods/services	12	$44,551	$104,650	$759	$2,380	$10,519	$29,848	$280,066
Cost of sales	2	*	*	*	*	*	*	*
Total gross charges	44	**$761,562**	**$212,354**	**$499,808**	**$577,767**	**$740,869**	**$923,225**	**$1,041,138**
Total medical revenue	45	**$546,775**	**$175,940**	**$355,641**	**$400,403**	**$534,115**	**$625,928**	**$732,226**

Multispecialty — Primary Care Only, Not Hospital or IDS Owned
(per FTE Physician)

Table 4.4c: Operating Cost

	Count	Mean	Std. Dev.	10th %tile	25th %tile	Median	75th %tile	90th %tile
Total support staff cost/phy	45	**$173,707**	**$69,103**	**$105,775**	**$130,372**	**$160,934**	**$200,423**	**$247,889**
Total empl supp staff cost/phy	41	$138,507	$53,873	$89,748	$99,691	$131,608	$163,424	$189,182
General administrative	38	$18,524	$11,430	$7,471	$10,269	$15,054	$25,248	$35,827
Patient accounting	37	$20,064	$10,393	$8,449	$12,449	$19,512	$24,347	$32,363
General accounting	27	$4,070	$2,998	$1,748	$2,221	$3,290	$4,479	$7,781
Managed care administrative	10	$3,931	$3,709	$290	$1,817	$2,654	$5,313	$12,507
Information technology	11	$2,776	$1,140	$1,125	$2,080	$2,502	$4,029	$4,368
Housekeeping, maint, security	17	$3,509	$4,637	$245	$614	$1,497	$5,520	$11,648
Medical receptionists	37	$23,141	$10,503	$7,373	$15,870	$23,240	$31,737	$38,557
Med secretaries,transcribers	24	$6,891	$4,774	$674	$3,602	$6,874	$8,179	$13,457
Medical records	32	$7,312	$4,534	$2,803	$4,382	$6,054	$9,334	$15,436
Other admin support	18	$5,151	$4,613	$948	$1,675	$3,581	$8,607	$12,063
***Total administrative supp staff**	18	**$85,649**	**$37,364**	**$49,019**	**$63,637**	**$79,011**	**$97,409**	**$144,891**
Registered Nurses	29	$15,673	$13,637	$1,642	$5,538	$13,390	$20,772	$35,753
Licensed Practical Nurses	30	$19,224	$13,994	$3,682	$7,826	$14,667	$27,891	$46,377
Med assistants, nurse aides	33	$24,003	$15,965	$8,901	$11,023	$19,869	$32,997	$51,232
***Total clinical supp staff**	29	**$48,797**	**$20,688**	**$24,032**	**$34,485**	**$42,132**	**$59,987**	**$75,515**
Clinical laboratory	27	$9,177	$5,619	$2,339	$4,544	$7,435	$15,457	$16,942
Radiology and imaging	26	$9,269	$7,188	$2,018	$5,054	$7,496	$12,652	$19,341
Other medical support serv	9	*	*	*	*	*	*	*
***Total ancillary supp staff**	19	**$20,622**	**$14,274**	**$4,843**	**$6,043**	**$18,422**	**$31,064**	**$41,584**
Total empl supp staff benefits	43	$32,812	$16,563	$17,955	$22,500	$29,859	$36,412	$58,498
Tot contracted supp staff	20	$7,928	$11,587	$239	$854	$2,965	$11,161	$33,589
Total general operating cost	45	**$158,415**	**$74,734**	**$93,841**	**$109,420**	**$138,937**	**$172,397**	**$241,230**
Information technology	42	$10,087	$5,967	$5,181	$5,789	$9,293	$11,908	$18,633
Medical and surgical supply	42	$23,312	$14,681	$8,804	$12,310	$20,448	$30,152	$41,421
Building and occupancy	42	$41,050	$20,031	$20,988	$26,498	$36,298	$49,773	$66,339
Furniture and equipment	40	$7,057	$6,709	$667	$2,158	$4,778	$10,138	$15,889
Admin supplies and services	40	$11,278	$5,792	$5,550	$7,096	$10,202	$12,815	$20,888
Prof liability insurance	44	$10,940	$5,955	$4,579	$6,629	$9,361	$13,519	$19,982
Other insurance premiums	41	$2,431	$5,083	$270	$564	$1,146	$2,151	$5,633
Outside professional fees	41	$5,367	$7,151	$681	$1,430	$2,738	$6,379	$13,834
Promotion and marketing	42	$2,118	$2,518	$523	$928	$1,357	$2,239	$4,259
Clinical laboratory	36	$17,579	$12,833	$1,569	$5,294	$15,999	$26,739	$34,528
Radiology and imaging	29	$6,595	$5,730	$554	$2,363	$5,429	$8,730	$17,846
Other ancillary services	10	$4,298	$4,897	$290	$380	$1,778	$8,278	$13,910
Billing purchased services	22	$5,813	$9,826	$69	$428	$1,789	$7,068	$23,227
Management fees paid to MSO	3	*	*	*	*	*	*	*
Misc operating cost	41	$10,065	$15,260	$2,211	$3,825	$6,317	$9,285	$16,280
Cost allocated to prac from par	0	*	*	*	*	*	*	*
Total operating cost	45	**$332,122**	**$123,309**	**$207,592**	**$254,745**	**$306,692**	**$382,920**	**$477,161**

*See pages 260 and 261 for definition.

Multispecialty — Primary Care Only, Not Hospital or IDS Owned
(per FTE Physician)

Table 4.4d: Provider Cost

	Count	Mean	Std. Dev.	10th %tile	25th %tile	Median	75th %tile	90th %tile
Total med rev after oper cost	45	$214,659	$111,935	$79,897	$160,442	$226,229	$283,974	$338,253
Total provider cost/physician	45	$217,831	$65,311	$139,973	$158,601	$218,462	$266,593	$308,998
Total NPP cost/physician	40	$29,377	$26,627	$3,881	$8,896	$22,682	$46,136	$61,118
Nonphysician provider comp	39	$24,259	$22,881	$3,237	$8,034	$17,798	$39,238	$56,520
Nonphysician prov benefit cost	38	$4,711	$4,188	$529	$1,341	$3,961	$7,377	$11,577
Provider consultant cost	8	*	*	*	*	*	*	*
Total physician cost/physician	45	$190,151	$51,648	$134,324	$147,210	$186,293	$215,852	$250,085
Total phy compensation	42	$165,020	$45,653	$114,267	$132,870	$163,904	$189,590	$214,125
Total phy benefit cost	42	$26,551	$12,387	$10,369	$15,186	$26,976	$33,866	$42,209

Table 4.4e: Net Income or Loss

	Count	Mean	Std. Dev.	10th %tile	25th %tile	Median	75th %tile	90th %tile
Total cost	45	$549,952	$165,704	$340,430	$425,213	$542,700	$623,693	$747,779
Net nonmedical revenue	29	$10,150	$25,479	-$2,804	$393	$1,740	$6,852	$57,550
Nonmedical revenue	27	$12,573	$25,676	$226	$685	$2,491	$7,646	$58,544
Fin support for oper costs	0	*	*	*	*	*	*	*
Goodwill amortization	2	*	*	*	*	*	*	*
Nonmedical cost	9	*	*	*	*	*	*	*
Net inc, prac with fin sup	0	*	*	*	*	*	*	*
Net inc, prac w/o fin sup	43	$9,718	$70,370	-$21,915	-$963	$4,445	$26,107	$91,593
Net inc, excl fin supp (all prac)	43	$9,718	$70,370	-$21,915	-$963	$4,445	$26,107	$91,593

Table 4.4f: Assets and Liabilities

	Count	Mean	Std. Dev.	10th %tile	25th %tile	Median	75th %tile	90th %tile
Total assets	24	$165,094	$212,458	$52,232	$64,813	$102,165	$163,929	$412,669
Current assets	26	$81,701	$74,626	$7,100	$24,419	$58,224	$123,973	$206,228
Noncurrent assets	26	$71,896	$156,407	$3,913	$14,346	$25,680	$54,675	$187,393
Total liabilities	26	$67,992	$109,768	$9,540	$18,224	$38,932	$76,818	$126,458
Current liabilities	26	$37,316	$54,362	$1,788	$8,530	$25,159	$47,713	$70,960
Noncurrent liabilities	26	$30,677	$58,707	$0	$0	$14,746	$32,873	$81,748
Working capital	26	$44,385	$60,932	-$14,058	$4,315	$20,694	$67,831	$172,249
Total net worth	26	$85,604	$114,981	$7,014	$16,059	$46,596	$93,044	$260,083

Multispecialty — Primary Care Only, Not Hospital or IDS Owned
(as a % of Total Medical Revenue)

Table 4.5a: Charges and Revenue

	Count	Mean	Std. Dev.	10th %tile	25th %tile	Median	75th %tile	90th %tile
Net fee-for-service revenue	40	92.80%	11.28%	72.06%	91.86%	97.55%	100.00%	100.00%
Net capitation revenue	13	11.23%	10.96%	1.85%	4.54%	7.58%	16.39%	33.30%
Net other medical revenue	22	6.51%	9.04%	.44%	1.19%	3.38%	6.71%	27.11%
Total gross charges	**45**	**145.58%**	**25.27%**	**104.24%**	**135.51%**	**144.03%**	**162.83%**	**177.89%**

Table 4.5b: Operating Cost

	Count	Mean	Std. Dev.	10th %tile	25th %tile	Median	75th %tile	90th %tile
Total support staff cost	**45**	**32.55%**	**10.97%**	**23.25%**	**26.74%**	**30.78%**	**34.88%**	**43.18%**
Total empl support staff cost	41	25.22%	5.69%	17.14%	21.04%	25.58%	28.48%	31.94%
General administrative	38	3.38%	1.92%	1.42%	1.66%	3.15%	4.44%	6.27%
Patient accounting	37	3.66%	1.87%	1.83%	2.38%	3.24%	4.04%	7.79%
General accounting	27	.71%	.41%	.37%	.40%	.54%	.91%	1.33%
Managed care administrative	10	.80%	.97%	.06%	.29%	.40%	.91%	3.14%
Information technology	11	.56%	.28%	.22%	.29%	.57%	.76%	1.04%
Housekeeping, maint, security	17	.53%	.52%	.04%	.11%	.40%	.99%	1.50%
Medical receptionists	37	4.28%	2.17%	1.39%	2.70%	3.80%	5.33%	8.01%
Med secretaries,transcribers	24	1.15%	.78%	.14%	.64%	1.13%	1.41%	2.22%
Medical records	32	1.41%	.90%	.59%	.86%	1.29%	1.59%	3.13%
Other admin support	18	.83%	.62%	.17%	.32%	.71%	1.39%	1.80%
***Total administrative supp staff**	**18**	**14.43%**	**4.10%**	**9.85%**	**11.56%**	**14.50%**	**16.27%**	**18.59%**
Registered Nurses	29	2.81%	2.40%	.29%	.96%	2.35%	4.19%	5.84%
Licensed Practical Nurses	30	3.32%	2.30%	1.05%	1.92%	2.79%	4.31%	7.29%
Med assistants, nurse aides	33	4.44%	2.80%	1.56%	2.41%	3.90%	6.30%	8.77%
***Total clinical supp staff**	**29**	**8.76%**	**2.94%**	**5.03%**	**6.99%**	**8.55%**	**10.02%**	**12.57%**
Clinical laboratory	27	1.69%	.99%	.43%	.84%	1.39%	2.61%	3.08%
Radiology and imaging	26	1.52%	.87%	.53%	.92%	1.38%	2.09%	2.90%
Other medical support serv	9	*	*	*	*	*	*	*
***Total ancillary supp staff**	**19**	**3.68%**	**3.21%**	**.85%**	**1.29%**	**3.31%**	**4.54%**	**6.83%**
Total empl supp staff benefits	43	6.13%	2.75%	3.59%	4.25%	5.51%	7.75%	8.82%
Tot contracted supp staff	20	1.68%	3.30%	.04%	.12%	.64%	2.08%	3.04%
Total general operating cost	**45**	**29.49%**	**12.46%**	**21.20%**	**24.15%**	**26.38%**	**30.05%**	**34.37%**
Information technology	42	1.91%	1.15%	.84%	1.19%	1.65%	2.59%	3.11%
Medical and surgical supply	42	4.23%	2.47%	1.81%	2.32%	3.70%	5.12%	8.54%
Building and occupancy	42	7.56%	3.22%	4.08%	5.30%	7.27%	8.57%	11.64%
Furniture and equipment	40	1.35%	1.32%	.10%	.42%	.89%	1.99%	2.98%
Admin supplies and services	41	2.01%	.94%	1.03%	1.47%	1.89%	2.30%	2.95%
Prof liability insurance	44	2.12%	1.03%	.79%	1.41%	1.96%	2.86%	3.80%
Other insurance premiums	40	.28%	.22%	.06%	.10%	.23%	.34%	.64%
Outside professional fees	41	.92%	1.10%	.16%	.25%	.53%	1.30%	2.07%
Promotion and marketing	42	.36%	.36%	.10%	.18%	.29%	.42%	.71%
Clinical laboratory	36	3.18%	2.20%	.39%	1.03%	3.01%	5.05%	6.19%
Radiology and imaging	31	1.43%	1.35%	.15%	.47%	1.14%	1.54%	4.32%
Other ancillary services	10	.77%	.91%	.07%	.09%	.34%	1.40%	2.53%
Billing purchased services	22	1.04%	1.71%	.01%	.05%	.36%	1.02%	4.37%
Management fees paid to MSO	4	*	*	*	*	*	*	*
Misc operating cost	41	1.66%	1.72%	.45%	.69%	1.15%	1.92%	3.12%
Cost allocated to prac from par	0	*	*	*	*	*	*	*
Total operating cost	**45**	**62.04%**	**18.20%**	**47.24%**	**52.26%**	**58.77%**	**63.01%**	**79.28%**

*See pages 260 and 261 for definition.

Multispecialty — Primary Care Only, Not Hospital or IDS Owned
(as a % of Total Medical Revenue)

Table 4.5c: Provider Cost

	Count	Mean	Std. Dev.	10th %tile	25th %tile	Median	75th %tile	90th %tile
Total med rev after oper cost	45	37.96%	18.20%	20.72%	36.99%	41.23%	47.74%	52.76%
Total provider cost	45	40.53%	7.53%	30.17%	36.03%	40.41%	45.65%	49.48%
Total NPP cost	40	4.75%	3.38%	.93%	2.29%	4.32%	6.85%	10.28%
Nonphysician provider comp	39	3.91%	2.88%	.87%	2.01%	3.04%	5.31%	8.88%
Nonphysician prov benefit cost	38	.76%	.55%	.13%	.28%	.69%	1.05%	1.48%
Provider consultant cost	8	*	*	*	*	*	*	*
Total physician cost	45	36.08%	7.85%	23.31%	31.65%	35.83%	40.08%	46.56%
Total phy compensation	42	30.80%	6.90%	19.78%	26.73%	30.25%	34.52%	38.81%
Total phy benefit cost	42	4.92%	2.11%	2.17%	3.12%	5.20%	6.40%	7.42%

Table 4.5d: Net Income or Loss

	Count	Mean	Std. Dev.	10th %tile	25th %tile	Median	75th %tile	90th %tile
Total cost	45	102.57%	19.95%	83.51%	95.64%	99.65%	100.82%	125.04%
Net nonmedical revenue	29	2.17%	5.27%	-.43%	.07%	.36%	1.22%	12.12%
Nonmedical revenue	27	2.66%	5.36%	.05%	.14%	.47%	1.24%	12.60%
Fin support for oper costs	0	*	*	*	*	*	*	*
Goodwill amortization	2	*	*	*	*	*	*	*
Nonmedical cost	9	*	*	*	*	*	*	*
Net inc, prac with fin sup	0	*	*	*	*	*	*	*
Net inc, prac w/o fin sup	43	1.10%	14.41%	-4.14%	-.18%	1.28%	4.59%	19.26%
Net inc, excl fin supp (all prac)	43	1.10%	14.41%	-4.14%	-.18%	1.28%	4.59%	19.26%

Table 4.5e: Assets and Liabilities

	Count	Mean	Std. Dev.	10th %tile	25th %tile	Median	75th %tile	90th %tile
Total assets	26	22.90%	19.18%	7.21%	10.40%	17.12%	26.90%	56.38%
Current assets	26	13.15%	10.04%	1.32%	4.40%	10.82%	21.87%	29.50%
Noncurrent assets	26	9.75%	14.19%	.60%	2.55%	4.61%	9.60%	27.51%
Total liabilities	26	10.05%	10.07%	2.19%	3.47%	7.01%	13.09%	23.31%
Current liabilities	26	5.58%	5.24%	.30%	1.67%	4.55%	7.73%	12.18%
Noncurrent liabilities	26	4.47%	6.11%	.00%	.00%	2.65%	5.59%	14.15%
Working capital	26	7.57%	9.04%	-2.32%	.82%	4.33%	13.15%	22.48%
Total net worth	26	12.85%	12.62%	1.79%	3.26%	9.64%	18.40%	31.69%

Multispecialty — Primary Care Only, Not Hospital or IDS Owned
(per FTE Provider)

Table 4.6a: Staffing, RVUs, Patients, Procedures and Square Footage

	Count	Mean	Std. Dev.	10th %tile	25th %tile	Median	75th %tile	90th %tile
Total physician FTE/provider	**38**	**.77**	**.14**	**.53**	**.66**	**.77**	**.90**	**.94**
Prim care phy/provider	36	.76	.15	.51	.64	.77	.89	.93
Nonsurg phy/provider	1	*	*	*	*	*	*	*
Surg spec phy/provider	3	*	*	*	*	*	*	*
Total NPP FTE/provider	38	.23	.14	.06	.10	.23	.34	.47
Total support staff FTE/prov	**38**	**3.84**	**.91**	**2.69**	**3.27**	**3.71**	**4.49**	**4.92**
Total empl supp staff FTE/prov	37	3.77	.88	2.68	3.14	3.68	4.41	4.92
General administrative	35	.27	.18	.09	.11	.23	.37	.56
Patient accounting	34	.58	.28	.28	.37	.54	.70	.96
General accounting	25	.09	.05	.04	.05	.07	.11	.15
Managed care administrative	9	*	*	*	*	*	*	*
Information technology	10	.07	.03	.03	.04	.06	.09	.14
Housekeeping, maint, security	16	.13	.15	.02	.03	.06	.16	.44
Medical receptionists	34	.81	.32	.30	.62	.81	1.02	1.25
Med secretaries,transcribers	23	.21	.13	.03	.11	.21	.28	.44
Medical records	29	.29	.16	.11	.17	.27	.37	.50
Other admin support	17	.19	.18	.03	.05	.08	.36	.51
***Total administrative supp staff**	**16**	**2.21**	**.68**	**1.48**	**1.64**	**2.08**	**2.68**	**3.29**
Registered Nurses	26	.32	.31	.04	.11	.28	.44	.76
Licensed Practical Nurses	27	.53	.42	.10	.24	.39	.80	1.35
Med assistants, nurse aides	30	.73	.37	.30	.41	.67	1.06	1.26
***Total clinical supp staff**	**26**	**1.35**	**.42**	**.85**	**1.03**	**1.24**	**1.70**	**1.92**
Clinical laboratory	25	.25	.13	.08	.12	.27	.36	.42
Radiology and imaging	25	.18	.11	.06	.11	.14	.24	.34
Other medical support serv	9	*	*	*	*	*	*	*
***Total ancillary supp staff**	**11**	**.42**	**.28**	**.09**	**.12**	**.43**	**.68**	**.86**
Tot contracted supp staff	13	.15	.14	.02	.04	.10	.27	.38
Tot RVU/provider	15	7,439	3,404	2,629	5,463	7,161	9,168	12,686
Physician work RVU/provider	16	3,860	1,570	2,101	2,954	3,686	4,566	5,968
Patients/provider	21	1,507	688	884	1,036	1,282	1,820	2,555
Tot procedures/provider	34	9,052	3,109	5,128	6,366	9,279	10,822	14,024
Square feet/provider	35	1,767	1,034	998	1,165	1,495	1,900	2,840
Total support staff FTE/phy	**45**	**5.23**	**2.07**	**3.24**	**4.00**	**4.89**	**5.83**	**7.36**

*See pages 260 and 261 for definition.

Table 4.6b: Charges, Revenue and Cost

	Count	Mean	Std. Dev.	10th %tile	25th %tile	Median	75th %tile	90th %tile
Total gross charges	**38**	**$583,914**	**$185,443**	**$362,254**	**$493,219**	**$562,546**	**$682,104**	**$743,031**
Total medical revenue	**38**	**$405,069**	**$87,020**	**$294,914**	**$351,755**	**$392,086**	**$454,224**	**$509,892**
Net fee-for-service revenue	35	$379,200	$101,916	$245,785	$319,926	$380,611	$428,963	$505,615
Net capitation revenue	12	$40,147	$34,861	$6,896	$15,696	$27,465	$72,522	$105,836
Net other medical revenue	21	$29,081	$43,039	$1,529	$5,241	$15,209	$31,171	$119,200
Total support staff cost/prov	**38**	**$127,423**	**$33,643**	**$95,657**	**$101,975**	**$120,759**	**$147,796**	**$178,543**
Total general operating cost	**38**	**$115,524**	**$53,627**	**$74,780**	**$85,465**	**$103,014**	**$130,133**	**$144,679**
Total operating cost	**38**	**$242,947**	**$70,731**	**$175,014**	**$190,996**	**$226,531**	**$283,121**	**$330,939**
Total med rev after oper cost	**38**	**$162,126**	**$63,134**	**$93,403**	**$131,990**	**$167,685**	**$193,094**	**$230,843**
Total provider cost/provider	**38**	**$161,608**	**$37,047**	**$119,026**	**$133,313**	**$153,595**	**$182,368**	**$210,218**
Total NPP cost/provider	38	$18,803	$12,883	$3,400	$7,326	$17,333	$28,430	$36,708
Provider consultant cost	5	*	*	*	*	*	*	*
Total physician cost/provider	38	$142,139	$37,952	$96,425	$107,751	$138,190	$164,524	$198,908
Total phy compensation	37	$121,762	$30,545	$85,131	$94,394	$114,949	$146,566	$162,272
Total phy benefit cost	37	$20,345	$10,242	$8,732	$12,337	$18,389	$26,246	$37,508
Total cost	**38**	**$404,555**	**$91,724**	**$298,517**	**$337,719**	**$396,862**	**$454,464**	**$506,313**
Net nonmedical revenue	26	$9,213	$21,577	-$4,297	$288	$1,623	$6,477	$54,580
Net inc, prac with fin sup	0	*	*	*	*	*	*	*
Net inc, prac w/o fin sup	36	$5,766	$51,385	-$11,709	-$975	$2,370	$16,614	$73,077
Net inc, excl fin supp (all prac)	36	$5,766	$51,385	-$11,709	-$975	$2,370	$16,614	$73,077
Total support staff FTE/phy	**45**	**5.23**	**2.07**	**3.24**	**4.00**	**4.89**	**5.83**	**7.36**

Multispecialty — Primary Care Only, Not Hospital or IDS Owned
(per Square Foot)

Table 4.7a: Staffing, RVUs, Patients and Procedures

	Count	Mean	Std. Dev.	10th %tile	25th %tile	Median	75th %tile	90th %tile
Total prov FTE/10,000 sq ft	35	**6.79**	**2.38**	**3.56**	**5.26**	**6.69**	**8.59**	**10.02**
Total phy FTE/10,000 sq ft	42	5.37	2.15	2.53	3.97	5.27	6.69	8.32
Prim care phy/10,000 sq ft	37	5.44	2.17	3.04	3.95	5.31	6.71	8.51
Nonsurg phy/10,000 sq ft	1	*	*	*	*	*	*	*
Surg spec phy/10,000 sq ft	4	*	*	*	*	*	*	*
Total NPP FTE/10,000 sq ft	35	1.52	1.02	.36	.71	1.26	2.06	2.99
Total supp stf FTE/10,000 sq ft	42	**26.09**	**8.09**	**14.29**	**21.43**	**26.03**	**32.20**	**38.42**
Total empl supp stf/10,000 sq ft	38	26.16	7.81	15.05	21.43	25.77	31.96	38.10
General administrative	38	1.82	1.31	.47	.64	1.37	3.19	3.71
Patient accounting	38	4.04	3.00	1.57	2.37	3.40	4.90	6.76
General accounting	26	.55	.31	.22	.37	.48	.58	1.16
Managed care administrative	10	1.22	1.24	.14	.42	.77	1.59	4.11
Information technology	11	.49	.39	.12	.20	.37	.61	1.33
Housekeeping, maint, security	16	.68	.64	.12	.16	.40	1.07	1.77
Medical receptionists	36	5.60	2.93	1.83	3.74	5.31	7.26	10.10
Med secretaries,transcribers	24	1.19	.87	.24	.60	.92	1.73	2.27
Medical records	30	1.96	1.08	.64	1.19	1.89	2.68	3.71
Other admin support	17	1.26	1.38	.21	.37	.62	1.48	4.05
*Total administrative supp staff	17	**12.65**	**4.21**	**6.75**	**9.15**	**13.50**	**15.43**	**17.26**
Registered Nurses	28	2.16	1.92	.36	.64	1.41	3.43	4.51
Licensed Practical Nurses	29	3.42	2.58	.84	1.38	2.68	4.45	7.33
Med assistants, nurse aides	32	5.37	3.45	1.65	2.57	4.22	7.97	11.19
*Total clinical supp staff	30	**8.69**	**3.25**	**4.49**	**5.57**	**8.79**	**11.25**	**13.22**
Clinical laboratory	28	1.54	.80	.53	.87	1.43	1.92	2.96
Radiology and imaging	25	1.24	.79	.27	.56	1.15	1.70	2.42
Other medical support serv	9	*	*	*	*	*	*	*
*Total ancillary supp staff	13	**3.09**	**2.49**	**.32**	**1.18**	**2.79**	**4.35**	**7.80**
Tot contracted supp staff	16	1.29	1.97	.06	.17	.67	1.41	4.42
Tot RVU/sq ft	17	14.10	36.78	1.36	3.73	5.14	8.01	39.16
Physician work RVU/sq ft	16	2.61	.99	1.31	1.87	2.71	3.21	4.33
Patients/sq ft	20	1.20	.73	.50	.68	.94	1.62	2.35
Tot procedures/sq ft	36	6.91	4.17	2.77	4.39	6.02	8.47	11.54
Total support staff FTE/phy	45	**5.23**	**2.07**	**3.24**	**4.00**	**4.89**	**5.83**	**7.36**

*See pages 260 and 261 for definition.

Table 4.7b: Charges, Revenue and Cost

	Count	Mean	Std. Dev.	10th %tile	25th %tile	Median	75th %tile	90th %tile
Total gross charges	42	**$403.46**	**$174.67**	**$205.99**	**$289.17**	**$375.63**	**$510.61**	**$588.92**
Total medical revenue	42	**$276.70**	**$103.49**	**$156.83**	**$208.50**	**$265.28**	**$354.20**	**$408.96**
Net fee-for-service revenue	37	$274.74	$104.99	$137.21	$197.87	$261.79	$366.80	$408.48
Net capitation revenue	11	$28.43	$30.51	$3.46	$7.61	$22.20	$32.69	$91.21
Net other medical revenue	20	$14.92	$18.11	$.98	$3.24	$7.59	$19.14	$47.26
Total support staff cost/sq ft	42	**$87.46**	**$31.45**	**$45.29**	**$61.17**	**$84.90**	**$108.05**	**$129.79**
Total general operating cost	42	**$75.48**	**$28.12**	**$39.79**	**$56.73**	**$73.87**	**$89.95**	**$123.79**
Total operating cost	42	**$162.94**	**$54.38**	**$84.26**	**$133.94**	**$160.44**	**$198.46**	**$229.65**
Total med rev after oper cost	42	**$113.77**	**$66.12**	**$34.68**	**$74.78**	**$109.45**	**$148.25**	**$201.13**
Total provider cost/sq ft	42	**$114.17**	**$50.26**	**$58.17**	**$77.90**	**$112.60**	**$146.79**	**$172.88**
Total NPP cost/sq ft	37	$12.55	$8.63	$1.90	$5.85	$11.02	$17.72	$26.06
Provider consultant cost	8	*	*	*	*	*	*	*
Total physician cost/sq ft	42	$102.37	$47.63	$47.22	$67.12	$99.30	$137.69	$155.55
Total phy compensation	39	$91.13	$41.46	$45.00	$57.45	$86.90	$117.61	$137.53
Total phy benefit cost	39	$14.47	$8.21	$4.78	$8.23	$12.69	$20.94	$26.33
Total cost	42	**$277.11**	**$98.87**	**$159.07**	**$214.04**	**$271.69**	**$347.71**	**$393.23**
Net nonmedical revenue/sq ft	27	$6.52	$17.04	-$.21	$.20	$.82	$2.05	$30.53
Net inc, prac with fin sup	0	*	*	*	*	*	*	*
Net inc, prac w/o fin sup	40	$7.82	$28.99	-$2.66	-$.52	$2.56	$16.02	$36.36
Net inc, excl fin supp (all prac)	40	$7.82	$28.99	-$2.66	-$.52	$2.56	$16.02	$36.36
Total support staff FTE/phy	45	**5.23**	**2.07**	**3.24**	**4.00**	**4.89**	**5.83**	**7.36**

Multispecialty — Primary Care Only, Not Hospital or IDS Owned
(per Total RVU)

Table 4.8a: Staffing, Patients, Procedures and Square Footage

	Count	Mean	Std. Dev.	10th %tile	25th %tile	Median	75th %tile	90th %tile
Total prov FTE/10,000 tot RVU	**15**	**1.97**	**2.15**	**.83**	**1.09**	**1.40**	**1.83**	**5.44**
Total phy FTE/10,000 tot RVU	18	1.55	1.66	.41	.82	1.04	1.62	4.27
Prim care phy/10,000 tot RVU	16	1.47	1.61	.49	.74	1.04	1.49	3.83
Nonsurg phy/10,000 tot RVU	1	*	*	*	*	*	*	*
Surg spec phy/10,000 tot RVU	2	*	*	*	*	*	*	*
Total NPP FTE/10,000 tot RVU	15	.41	.58	.06	.13	.23	.34	1.56
Total supp stf FTE/10,000 tot RVU	**18**	**7.02**	**6.09**	**2.53**	**4.02**	**5.27**	**6.49**	**21.52**
Tot empl supp stf/10,000 tot RVU	17	5.98	4.70	2.26	3.82	4.68	6.10	14.28
General administrative	16	.33	.22	.06	.16	.35	.44	.72
Patient accounting	16	.74	.49	.24	.46	.56	.94	1.71
General accounting	11	.22	.32	.04	.04	.07	.20	.96
Managed care administrative	4	*	*	*	*	*	*	*
Information technology	4	*	*	*	*	*	*	*
Housekeeping, maint, security	7	*	*	*	*	*	*	*
Medical receptionists	15	1.55	2.05	.30	.61	1.27	1.66	4.72
Med secretaries,transcribers	12	.30	.28	.06	.14	.22	.29	.90
Medical records	15	.52	.46	.10	.19	.34	.84	1.36
Other admin support	7	*	*	*	*	*	*	*
***Total administrative supp staff**	**8**	*	*	*	*	*	*	*
Registered Nurses	15	.60	.71	.04	.12	.45	.62	1.92
Licensed Practical Nurses	15	.54	.47	.07	.24	.45	.83	1.44
Med assistants, nurse aides	14	1.18	1.33	.05	.34	.86	1.64	3.67
***Total clinical supp staff**	**14**	**2.38**	**2.16**	**.35**	**1.24**	**1.64**	**2.94**	**6.87**
Clinical laboratory	12	.30	.17	.14	.17	.24	.40	.63
Radiology and imaging	10	.29	.38	.01	.06	.16	.34	1.22
Other medical support serv	3	*	*	*	*	*	*	*
***Total ancillary supp staff**	**3**	*	*	*	*	*	*	*
Tot contracted supp staff	7	*	*	*	*	*	*	*
Physician work RVU/tot RVU	14	.49	.20	.14	.44	.51	.56	.79
Patients/tot RVU	11	.29	.29	.09	.13	.21	.35	.97
Tot procedures/tot RVU	16	1.50	1.27	.38	.85	1.21	1.74	3.78
Square feet/tot RVU	17	.26	.24	.08	.12	.19	.27	.75
Total support staff FTE/phy	**45**	**5.23**	**2.07**	**3.24**	**4.00**	**4.89**	**5.83**	**7.36**

*See pages 260 and 261 for definition.

Table 4.8b: Charges, Revenue and Cost

	Count	Mean	Std. Dev.	10th %tile	25th %tile	Median	75th %tile	90th %tile
Total gross charges	**18**	**$101.62**	**$101.08**	**$28.52**	**$59.34**	**$82.50**	**$95.26**	**$236.79**
Total medical revenue	**18**	**$71.24**	**$71.08**	**$28.29**	**$43.34**	**$54.00**	**$68.07**	**$132.95**
Net fee-for-service revenue	16	$59.24	$51.41	$22.35	$38.22	$49.85	$59.54	$124.37
Net capitation revenue	5	*	*	*	*	*	*	*
Net other medical revenue	10	$8.50	$10.48	$.16	$1.31	$2.63	$16.64	$30.44
Total supp staff cost/tot RVU	**18**	**$24.54**	**$24.10**	**$8.65**	**$13.46**	**$16.46**	**$22.80**	**$77.11**
Total general operating cost	**18**	**$21.56**	**$22.28**	**$8.17**	**$11.60**	**$14.59**	**$19.29**	**$66.15**
Total operating cost	**18**	**$46.11**	**$45.26**	**$16.82**	**$26.57**	**$31.78**	**$39.66**	**$160.74**
Total med rev after oper cost	**18**	**$25.13**	**$40.70**	**-$4.21**	**$14.69**	**$19.41**	**$25.81**	**$63.94**
Total provider cost/tot RVU	**18**	**$27.13**	**$24.39**	**$6.67**	**$17.20**	**$21.96**	**$26.52**	**$60.43**
Total NPP cost/tot RVU	15	$3.18	$3.98	$.39	$1.03	$2.13	$2.64	$12.07
Provider consultant cost	2	*	*	*	*	*	*	*
Total physician cost/tot RVU	18	$24.47	$21.75	$6.67	$14.72	$18.81	$24.10	$58.96
Total phy compensation	17	$19.63	$17.98	$4.83	$12.26	$14.97	$20.13	$42.28
Total phy benefit cost	17	$3.07	$3.24	$.78	$1.43	$2.56	$3.12	$6.55
Total cost	**16**	**$79.33**	**$97.79**	**$16.66**	**$44.88**	**$61.01**	**$69.40**	**$191.47**
Net nonmedical revenue	12	$2.25	$4.27	$.00	$.03	$.21	$3.70	$11.73
Net inc, prac with fin sup	0	*	*	*	*	*	*	*
Net inc, prac w/o fin sup	17	$6.89	$17.33	-$1.00	-$.13	$.39	$3.56	$31.43
Net inc, excl fin supp (all prac)	17	$6.89	$17.33	-$1.00	-$.13	$.39	$3.56	$31.43
Total support staff FTE/phy	**45**	**5.23**	**2.07**	**3.24**	**4.00**	**4.89**	**5.83**	**7.36**

Multispecialty — Primary Care Only, Not Hospital or IDS Owned
(per Work RVU)

Table 4.9a: Staffing, Patients, Procedures and Square Footage

	Count	Mean	Std. Dev.	10th %tile	25th %tile	Median	75th %tile	90th %tile
Total prov FTE/10,000 work RVU	16	3.35	2.86	1.77	2.19	2.71	3.40	6.73
Tot phy FTE/10,000 work RVU	18	2.49	2.07	1.18	1.68	1.96	2.41	4.13
Prim care phy/10,000 work RVU	17	2.56	2.11	1.43	1.73	2.01	2.44	4.83
Nonsurg phy/10,000 work RVU	0	*	*	*	*	*	*	*
Surg spec phy/10,000 work RVU	2	*	*	*	*	*	*	*
Total NPP FTE/10,000 work RVU	16	.75	.86	.11	.26	.41	1.02	2.43
Total supp stf FTE/10,000 wrk RVU	18	11.49	6.65	5.48	7.86	9.49	11.71	25.94
Tot empl supp stf/10,000 work RVU	18	11.30	6.49	5.45	7.86	9.44	11.71	24.61
General administrative	17	.76	.49	.21	.31	.76	1.08	1.61
Patient accounting	16	1.71	.98	.74	1.05	1.29	2.42	3.49
General accounting	12	.36	.46	.07	.09	.15	.40	1.39
Managed care administrative	3	*	*	*	*	*	*	*
Information technology	4	*	*	*	*	*	*	*
Housekeeping, maint, security	8	*	*	*	*	*	*	*
Medical receptionists	16	2.71	2.81	.85	1.25	1.76	3.25	6.57
Med secretaries,transcribers	12	.57	.46	.15	.25	.45	.65	1.53
Medical records	16	.87	.62	.31	.42	.63	1.30	1.91
Other admin support	8	*	*	*	*	*	*	*
*Total administrative supp staff	9	*	*	*	*	*	*	*
Registered Nurses	16	1.14	1.16	.10	.19	.87	1.70	3.45
Licensed Practical Nurses	15	1.45	1.03	.56	.74	.97	1.77	3.56
Med assistants, nurse aides	14	2.11	1.88	.33	.82	1.47	2.62	5.84
*Total clinical supp staff	14	4.18	2.72	1.59	2.36	3.70	4.88	9.51
Clinical laboratory	11	.59	.29	.24	.32	.46	.94	1.03
Radiology and imaging	10	.53	.51	.09	.25	.40	.62	1.77
Other medical support serv	3	*	*	*	*	*	*	*
*Total ancillary supp staff	2	*	*	*	*	*	*	*
Tot contracted supp staff	6	*	*	*	*	*	*	*
Tot RVU/work RVU	14	5.61	13.32	1.29	1.81	1.96	2.27	27.89
Patients/work RVU	12	.51	.38	.23	.29	.33	.66	1.33
Tot procedures/work RVU	17	3.02	2.79	.96	1.67	2.25	2.82	8.79
Square feet/work RVU	16	.49	.39	.23	.31	.37	.54	.99
Total support staff FTE/phy	45	5.23	2.07	3.24	4.00	4.89	5.83	7.36

*See pages 260 and 261 for definition.

Table 4.9b: Charges, Revenue and Cost

	Count	Mean	Std. Dev.	10th %tile	25th %tile	Median	75th %tile	90th %tile
Total gross charges	18	$171.56	$130.32	$109.83	$123.91	$132.09	$174.25	$253.00
Total medical revenue	18	$125.41	$94.43	$79.10	$86.57	$98.58	$123.23	$220.51
Net fee-for-service revenue	17	$109.92	$63.87	$77.32	$85.06	$90.05	$115.37	$173.81
Net capitation revenue	5	*	*	*	*	*	*	*
Net other medical revenue	9	*	*	*	*	*	*	*
Total supp staff cost/work RVU	18	$38.91	$22.93	$18.65	$25.11	$34.22	$45.38	$84.61
Total general operating cost	18	$38.12	$27.78	$20.58	$23.98	$30.12	$35.80	$78.99
Total operating cost	18	$77.03	$47.63	$44.51	$51.02	$64.60	$76.74	$148.26
Total med rev after oper cost	18	$48.39	$51.59	$13.27	$32.60	$40.96	$50.71	$77.70
Total provider cost/work RVU	18	$47.36	$30.58	$28.90	$34.44	$40.30	$47.98	$68.87
Total NPP cost/work RVU	16	$5.84	$6.42	$.78	$1.86	$2.99	$7.81	$20.18
Provider consultant cost	2	*	*	*	*	*	*	*
Total physician cost/work RVU	18	$42.14	$26.41	$26.42	$29.38	$36.84	$41.02	$65.13
Total phy compensation	18	$36.27	$22.52	$22.89	$25.48	$30.77	$36.72	$57.01
Total phy benefit cost	18	$5.87	$4.25	$2.53	$3.83	$5.42	$6.27	$9.12
Total cost	18	$124.39	$75.74	$78.10	$88.46	$105.51	$123.26	$212.02
Net nonmedical revenue	11	$3.89	$6.71	$.02	$.11	$.53	$5.38	$18.69
Net inc, prac with fin sup	0	*	*	*	*	*	*	*
Net inc, prac w/o fin sup	17	$3.61	$29.60	-$40.77	-$1.00	$.59	$2.38	$38.53
Net inc, excl fin supp (all prac)	17	$3.61	$29.60	-$40.77	-$1.00	$.59	$2.38	$38.53
Total support staff FTE/phy	45	5.23	2.07	3.24	4.00	4.89	5.83	7.36

Multispecialty — Primary Care Only, Not Hospital or IDS Owned
(per Patient)

Table 4.10a: Staffing, RVUs, Procedures and Square Footage

	Count	Mean	Std. Dev.	10th %tile	25th %tile	Median	75th %tile	90th %tile
Total prov FTE/10,000 patients	21	7.69	2.70	3.92	5.50	7.80	9.65	11.32
Total phy FTE/10,000 pat	23	5.67	2.31	2.46	3.80	5.69	7.54	8.60
Prim care phy/10,000 pat	23	5.67	2.31	2.46	3.80	5.69	7.54	8.60
Nonsurg phy/10,000 pat	0	*	*	*	*	*	*	*
Surg spec phy/10,000 pat	1	*	*	*	*	*	*	*
Total NPP FTE/10,000 pat	21	1.78	1.24	.30	.61	1.53	2.99	3.46
Total supp staff FTE/10,000 pat	23	27.52	12.78	10.92	16.29	26.25	37.94	47.77
Total empl supp staff/10,000 pat	23	27.22	12.75	10.92	16.29	26.25	35.74	47.77
General administrative	21	2.16	1.66	.39	.66	1.98	3.54	4.99
Patient accounting	20	3.86	2.61	1.76	2.04	3.43	5.39	6.37
General accounting	16	.70	.38	.27	.38	.60	.97	1.37
Managed care administrative	5	*	*	*	*	*	*	*
Information technology	7	*	*	*	*	*	*	*
Housekeeping, maint, security	10	.78	.83	.14	.21	.41	1.18	2.63
Medical receptionists	21	6.17	3.58	1.22	3.38	5.69	8.04	11.99
Med secretaries,transcribers	13	1.95	1.41	.14	.89	1.79	3.12	4.30
Medical records	16	2.10	1.40	.86	1.12	1.62	2.59	5.06
Other admin support	9	*	*	*	*	*	*	*
*Total administrative supp staff	10	16.47	7.30	7.71	10.84	13.72	22.70	28.55
Registered Nurses	18	2.73	3.53	.31	.59	1.84	3.09	5.75
Licensed Practical Nurses	17	4.09	4.16	.99	1.73	2.39	5.28	14.14
Med assistants, nurse aides	21	4.09	2.01	1.83	2.61	4.05	4.77	7.29
*Total clinical supp staff	17	10.00	4.46	5.16	6.19	9.02	12.97	18.22
Clinical laboratory	15	1.43	.89	.39	.67	1.25	2.24	2.76
Radiology and imaging	15	.90	.54	.13	.33	1.05	1.21	1.79
Other medical support serv	5	*	*	*	*	*	*	*
*Total ancillary supp staff	4	*	*	*	*	*	*	*
Tot contracted supp staff	7	*	*	*	*	*	*	*
Tot RVU/patient	11	5.73	3.44	1.11	2.86	4.84	7.64	11.66
Physician work RVU/patient	12	2.66	1.22	.82	1.53	3.07	3.44	4.51
Tot procedures/patient	21	7.54	3.67	2.58	5.09	6.79	10.19	14.30
Square feet/patient	20	1.14	.63	.43	.62	1.06	1.47	2.01
Total support staff FTE/phy	45	5.23	2.07	3.24	4.00	4.89	5.83	7.36

*See pages 260 and 261 for definition.

Table 4.10b: Charges, Revenue and Cost

	Count	Mean	Std. Dev.	10th %tile	25th %tile	Median	75th %tile	90th %tile
Total gross charges	23	$408.10	$174.62	$167.22	$264.98	$422.56	$503.99	$674.46
Total medical revenue	23	$293.27	$116.92	$146.14	$169.45	$285.07	$360.12	$472.54
Net fee-for-service revenue	23	$262.86	$110.43	$137.44	$157.02	$249.90	$307.40	$469.01
Net capitation revenue	9	*	*	*	*	*	*	*
Net other medical revenue	14	$29.26	$40.06	$.69	$6.99	$15.50	$31.15	$115.21
Total support staff cost/patient	23	$90.48	$42.66	$36.73	$55.28	$85.75	$122.53	$158.14
Total general operating cost	23	$85.83	$48.44	$31.34	$43.76	$77.92	$116.01	$128.32
Total operating cost	23	$176.31	$79.58	$69.23	$90.13	$171.73	$244.57	$296.85
Total med rev after oper cost	23	$116.96	$65.27	$61.24	$70.65	$115.81	$156.33	$206.16
Total provider cost/patient	23	$115.50	$56.93	$52.20	$66.68	$105.78	$141.45	$217.80
Total NPP cost/patient	21	$13.69	$10.55	$1.50	$4.51	$11.77	$24.27	$29.22
Provider consultant cost	5	*	*	*	*	*	*	*
Total physician cost/patient	23	$102.43	$51.68	$46.21	$62.52	$92.14	$122.66	$195.47
Total phy compensation	23	$89.12	$47.11	$39.66	$48.64	$78.29	$101.38	$169.83
Total phy benefit cost	23	$13.31	$6.75	$4.43	$7.09	$13.85	$19.18	$22.21
Total cost	23	$291.81	$126.54	$127.99	$151.02	$284.06	$370.24	$478.32
Net nonmedical revenue	16	$4.39	$12.14	-$4.15	$.22	$.64	$3.95	$22.91
Net inc, prac with fin sup	0	*	*	*	*	*	*	*
Net inc, prac w/o fin sup	22	$4.67	$38.92	-$18.50	$.15	$5.40	$20.82	$41.24
Net inc, excl fin supp (all prac)	22	$4.67	$38.92	-$18.50	$.15	$5.40	$20.82	$41.24
Total support staff FTE/phy	45	5.23	2.07	3.24	4.00	4.89	5.83	7.36

Multispecialty — Primary Care Only, Not Hospital or IDS Owned
(Procedure and Charge Data)

Table 4.11a: Activity Charges to Total Gross Charges Ratios

	Count	Mean	Std. Dev.	10th %tile	25th %tile	Median	75th %tile	90th %tile
Total proc gross charges	39	96.26%	3.92%	91.29%	93.80%	97.48%	99.57%	100.00%
Medical proc-inside practice	39	59.34%	21.12%	37.49%	43.29%	61.91%	74.14%	88.18%
Medical proc-outside practice	33	12.98%	15.16%	1.96%	6.27%	10.81%	14.37%	20.98%
Surg proc-inside practice	34	5.29%	2.74%	2.63%	3.11%	4.69%	6.77%	8.93%
Surg proc-outside practice	20	9.32%	14.94%	.22%	1.61%	5.17%	9.82%	27.77%
Laboratory procedures	36	12.78%	8.31%	1.78%	5.53%	13.58%	17.85%	24.09%
Radiology procedures	31	5.96%	4.51%	1.22%	2.83%	4.97%	8.13%	12.26%
Tot nonproc gross charges	30	4.48%	3.11%	.43%	2.01%	3.73%	6.56%	8.71%
Total support staff FTE/phy	45	5.23	2.07	3.24	4.00	4.89	5.83	7.36

Table 4.11b: Medical Procedure Data (inside the practice)

	Count	Mean	Std. Dev.	10th %tile	25th %tile	Median	75th %tile	90th %tile
Gross charges/procedure	38	$75.36	$39.50	$51.73	$55.68	$67.29	$83.45	$96.44
Total cost/procedure	34	$54.96	$15.17	$40.62	$44.03	$50.27	$63.43	$76.77
Operating cost/procedure	33	$33.14	$11.55	$21.47	$25.10	$29.32	$39.15	$49.88
Provider cost/procedure	36	$22.73	$8.47	$15.15	$16.99	$21.06	$26.34	$31.38
Procedures/patient	21	3.55	1.75	1.51	2.00	3.56	4.60	6.32
Gross charges/patient	22	$232.27	$127.14	$81.86	$152.58	$207.27	$316.97	$403.32
Procedures/physician	39	6,413	2,436	3,354	4,113	6,533	7,751	9,132
Gross charges/physician	39	$427,690	$159,849	$233,974	$338,209	$429,110	$512,974	$684,420
Procedures/provider	34	4,779	1,528	3,137	3,553	4,644	5,676	6,982
Gross charges/provider	34	$316,320	$103,409	$199,405	$258,790	$297,217	$398,828	$464,218
Gross charge to total cost ratio	34	1.28	.23	.89	1.14	1.31	1.44	1.58
Oper cost to total cost ratio	33	.60	.07	.51	.55	.59	.65	.70
Prov cost to total cost ratio	34	.40	.06	.30	.36	.42	.45	.49
Total support staff FTE/phy	45	5.23	2.07	3.24	4.00	4.89	5.83	7.36

Table 4.11c: Medical Procedure Data (outside the practice)

	Count	Mean	Std. Dev.	10th %tile	25th %tile	Median	75th %tile	90th %tile
Gross charges/procedure	32	$107.61	$22.59	$80.16	$90.34	$102.74	$124.59	$142.61
Total cost/procedure	29	$49.40	$12.88	$36.59	$38.90	$45.19	$57.67	$69.57
Operating cost/procedure	28	$20.69	$8.89	$13.02	$14.34	$19.18	$23.84	$27.25
Provider cost/procedure	31	$28.25	$7.07	$20.93	$22.99	$26.90	$31.70	$37.56
Procedures/patient	18	.56	.32	.12	.37	.47	.87	1.07
Gross charges/patient	19	$66.18	$52.75	$14.35	$38.94	$50.08	$91.67	$114.19
Procedures/physician	33	749	459	105	341	782	1,124	1,410
Gross charges/physician	33	$105,126	$165,196	$17,698	$38,655	$76,608	$110,347	$147,956
Procedures/provider	30	604	364	77	325	611	890	1,101
Gross charges/provider	30	$74,263	$76,743	$15,961	$40,247	$60,107	$81,110	$125,810
Gross charge to total cost ratio	29	2.24	.43	1.60	1.98	2.20	2.59	2.76
Oper cost to total cost ratio	28	.41	.08	.33	.37	.40	.44	.52
Prov cost to total cost ratio	29	.59	.08	.49	.56	.60	.62	.67
Total support staff FTE/phy	45	5.23	2.07	3.24	4.00	4.89	5.83	7.36

Multispecialty — Primary Care Only, Not Hospital or IDS Owned
(Procedure and Charge Data)

Table 4.11d: Surgery/Anesthesia Procedure Data (inside the practice)

	Count	Mean	Std. Dev.	10th %tile	25th %tile	Median	75th %tile	90th %tile
Gross charges/procedure	34	$95.03	$61.73	$34.45	$47.02	$77.36	$132.76	$204.01
Total cost/procedure	31	$77.39	$58.87	$27.40	$40.12	$62.64	$105.69	$142.51
Operating cost/procedure	30	$47.66	$41.01	$17.28	$21.69	$36.82	$62.81	$84.24
Provider cost/procedure	32	$29.52	$19.91	$8.21	$14.07	$23.77	$41.00	$59.68
Procedures/patient	19	.46	.47	.05	.07	.29	.69	1.46
Gross charges/patient	19	$21.34	$14.30	$5.06	$11.36	$16.42	$33.54	$49.17
Procedures/physician	35	693	629	117	204	440	1,149	1,326
Gross charges/physician	34	$41,335	$24,597	$14,608	$24,462	$38,549	$59,320	$70,227
Procedures/provider	30	545	451	78	183	374	931	1,109
Gross charges/provider	29	$29,594	$16,882	$10,740	$16,222	$22,799	$41,700	$54,966
Gross charge to total cost ratio	31	1.29	.23	.89	1.14	1.33	1.45	1.58
Oper cost to total cost ratio	30	.60	.07	.51	.55	.59	.65	.70
Prov cost to total cost ratio	31	.40	.07	.30	.35	.41	.45	.49
Total support staff FTE/phy	45	5.23	2.07	3.24	4.00	4.89	5.83	7.36

Table 4.11e: Surgery/Anesthesia Procedure Data (outside the practice)

	Count	Mean	Std. Dev.	10th %tile	25th %tile	Median	75th %tile	90th %tile
Gross charges/procedure	20	$890.53	$663.88	$223.96	$322.73	$705.51	$1,163.46	$1,723.30
Total cost/procedure	19	$400.59	$322.96	$83.79	$120.52	$357.20	$535.81	$820.71
Operating cost/procedure	18	$156.16	$154.28	$33.50	$42.75	$114.62	$197.40	$315.95
Provider cost/procedure	20	$247.73	$179.80	$45.60	$86.08	$234.60	$338.22	$567.05
Procedures/patient	10	.04	.03	.00	.01	.05	.08	.09
Gross charges/patient	10	$31.18	$28.38	$1.26	$10.70	$27.21	$42.72	$93.61
Procedures/physician	21	114	138	3	16	74	129	377
Gross charges/physician	20	$83,845	$151,488	$1,585	$11,251	$40,115	$71,979	$237,774
Procedures/provider	19	74	93	1	14	41	90	266
Gross charges/provider	18	$40,261	$48,837	$802	$5,718	$31,213	$46,787	$112,962
Gross charge to total cost ratio	19	2.26	.41	1.73	1.99	2.18	2.58	2.87
Oper cost to total cost ratio	18	.40	.06	.29	.36	.39	.44	.48
Prov cost to total cost ratio	19	.60	.06	.52	.56	.60	.63	.71
Total support staff FTE/phy	45	5.23	2.07	3.24	4.00	4.89	5.83	7.36

Multispecialty — Primary Care Only, Not Hospital or IDS Owned
(Procedure and Charge Data)

Table 4.11f: Clinical Laboratory/Pathology Procedure Data

	Count	Mean	Std. Dev.	10th %tile	25th %tile	Median	75th %tile	90th %tile
Gross charges/procedure	35	$24.46	$7.97	$13.79	$17.97	$24.38	$30.32	$36.24
Total cost/procedure	31	$19.00	$5.58	$12.09	$15.56	$18.03	$23.57	$26.88
Operating cost/procedure	30	$12.46	$4.10	$7.69	$8.87	$12.22	$15.57	$18.41
Provider cost/procedure	33	$6.50	$2.15	$3.71	$4.96	$6.17	$8.09	$9.82
Procedures/patient	19	2.51	1.68	.34	.92	2.38	3.73	5.14
Gross charges/patient	20	$63.63	$47.50	$5.20	$18.47	$54.15	$96.12	$140.66
Procedures/physician	36	3,846	2,554	897	1,598	4,084	4,854	7,394
Gross charges/physician	36	$99,320	$66,349	$14,513	$34,203	$105,971	$135,954	$210,193
Procedures/provider	32	3,090	1,918	819	1,386	3,029	4,218	6,369
Gross charges/provider	31	$78,922	$51,616	$11,328	$31,789	$81,147	$113,233	$158,422
Gross charge to total cost ratio	31	1.34	.27	1.09	1.12	1.31	1.54	1.80
Oper cost to total cost ratio	30	.65	.07	.55	.61	.67	.69	.73
Prov cost to total cost ratio	31	.35	.06	.27	.31	.34	.38	.45
Total support staff FTE/phy	45	5.23	2.07	3.24	4.00	4.89	5.83	7.36

Table 4.11g: Diagnostic Radiology and Imaging Procedure Data

	Count	Mean	Std. Dev.	10th %tile	25th %tile	Median	75th %tile	90th %tile
Gross charges/procedure	31	$115.09	$76.98	$59.30	$70.11	$84.60	$143.82	$209.49
Total cost/procedure	28	$85.59	$41.57	$45.74	$59.51	$74.70	$103.33	$138.53
Operating cost/procedure	27	$59.50	$37.21	$29.00	$39.28	$49.26	$80.79	$97.85
Provider cost/procedure	31	$29.51	$21.48	$14.01	$18.16	$21.77	$35.77	$59.60
Procedures/patient	19	.23	.19	.01	.09	.22	.31	.47
Gross charges/patient	18	$28.80	$29.97	$5.18	$7.53	$23.38	$37.15	$94.53
Procedures/physician	33	518	415	47	183	524	718	1,159
Gross charges/physician	31	$50,079	$42,311	$8,610	$17,321	$36,067	$69,644	$115,535
Procedures/provider	29	382	281	37	172	371	552	615
Gross charges/provider	27	$37,110	$30,579	$6,104	$15,589	$35,724	$47,795	$82,209
Gross charge to total cost ratio	29	1.22	.37	.93	1.04	1.24	1.43	1.66
Oper cost to total cost ratio	28	.68	.12	.50	.62	.67	.78	.83
Prov cost to total cost ratio	29	.32	.12	.18	.23	.32	.38	.50
Total support staff FTE/phy	45	5.23	2.07	3.24	4.00	4.89	5.83	7.36

Table 4.11h: Nonprocedural Gross Charge Data

	Count	Mean	Std. Dev.	10th %tile	25th %tile	Median	75th %tile	90th %tile
Gross charges/patient	17	$18.59	$16.59	$1.54	$7.41	$15.79	$27.88	$46.88
Nonproc gross charges/physician	30	$37,380	$30,427	$3,265	$17,690	$25,744	$52,255	$93,794
Gross charges/provider	26	$28,396	$21,220	$2,831	$12,935	$25,111	$37,690	$66,197
Total support staff FTE/phy	45	5.23	2.07	3.24	4.00	4.89	5.83	7.36

Multispecialty — by Geographic Section, Not Hospital or IDS Owned

Table 5.1: Staffing and Practice Data

	Eastern section		Midwest section		Southern section		Western section	
	Count	Median	Count	Median	Count	Median	Count	Median
Total provider FTE	**38**	**29.65**	**58**	**41.15**	**45**	**33.13**	**51**	**43.00**
Total physician FTE	41	22.71	65	27.00	51	25.00	56	28.61
Total nonphysician provider FTE	38	5.67	58	6.75	45	3.40	51	6.30
Total support staff FTE	**41**	**112.02**	**65**	**144.00**	**51**	**141.00**	**56**	**150.30**
Number of branch clinics	30	4	48	7	37	5	43	4
Square footage of all facilities	39	33,298	58	59,538	49	54,507	53	54,375

Table 5.2: Accounts Receivable Data, Collection Percentages and Financial Ratios

	Eastern section		Midwest section		Southern section		Western section	
	Count	Median	Count	Median	Count	Median	Count	Median
Total AR/physician	37	$108,999	61	$135,220	48	$141,194	51	$107,104
Total AR/provider	35	$93,032	56	$104,149	42	$119,030	47	$102,142
0-30 days in AR	38	53.95%	61	52.00%	48	47.44%	51	49.07%
31-60 days in AR	38	13.62%	61	15.67%	48	12.59%	51	16.79%
61-90 days in AR	38	7.93%	61	7.71%	48	7.51%	51	8.18%
91-120 days in AR	38	4.58%	61	5.19%	48	5.46%	51	5.50%
120+ days in AR	38	16.50%	61	18.63%	48	22.00%	51	16.48%
Re-aged: 0-30 days in AR	17	57.00%	27	52.59%	14	50.46%	20	60.10%
Re-aged: 31-60 days in AR	17	13.73%	27	16.11%	14	12.12%	20	14.84%
Re-aged: 61-90 days in AR	17	7.39%	27	7.97%	14	8.24%	20	6.52%
Re-aged: 91-120 days in AR	17	5.60%	27	5.03%	14	5.40%	20	4.77%
Re-aged: 120+ days in AR	17	15.55%	27	18.63%	14	22.66%	20	14.33%
Not re-aged: 0-30 days in AR	19	51.10%	32	51.40%	31	47.11%	30	42.01%
Not re-aged: 31-60 days in AR	19	14.85%	32	15.64%	31	11.93%	30	17.37%
Not re-aged: 61-90 days in AR	19	8.10%	32	7.77%	31	7.19%	30	9.08%
Not re-aged: 91-120 days in AR	19	4.56%	32	6.03%	31	5.43%	30	6.31%
Not re-aged: 120+ days in AR	19	17.57%	32	17.85%	31	21.96%	30	22.11%
Months gross FFS charges in AR	31	1.44	56	1.79	40	1.56	46	1.73
Days gross FFS charges in AR	31	43.81	56	54.44	40	47.35	46	52.54
Gross FFS collection %	33	60.99%	59	63.92%	43	58.07%	51	64.11%
Adjusted FFS collection %	32	97.32%	57	97.39%	40	97.05%	49	98.00%
Gross FFS + cap collection %	19	63.89%	19	62.87%	11	60.64%	22	66.72%
Net cap rev % of gross cap chrg	16	72.35%	14	72.54%	9	*	21	86.85%
Current ratio	15	1.33	41	1.31	29	1.89	41	2.20
Tot asset turnover ratio	15	6.28	41	3.37	29	5.16	41	3.68
Debt to equity ratio	15	2.48	41	2.03	29	1.86	41	1.52
Debt ratio	15	71.30%	41	66.96%	29	65.03%	41	60.29%
Return on total assets	15	2.97%	38	2.78%	25	4.36%	38	6.22%
Return on equity	15	9.73%	38	8.04%	25	11.31%	38	18.57%

Table 5.3: Breakout of Total Gross Charges by Type of Payer

	Eastern section		Midwest section		Southern section		Western section	
	Count	Median	Count	Median	Count	Median	Count	Median
Medicare: fee-for-service	39	29.70%	55	24.00%	48	31.50%	53	20.00%
Medicare: managed care FFS	39	.00%	55	.00%	48	.00%	53	.00%
Medicare: capitation	39	.00%	55	.00%	48	.00%	53	.00%
Medicaid: fee-for-service	39	3.52%	55	6.00%	48	4.25%	53	2.00%
Medicaid: managed care FFS	39	.00%	55	.00%	48	.00%	53	.00%
Medicaid: capitation	39	.00%	55	.00%	48	.00%	53	.00%
Commercial: fee-for-service	39	25.10%	55	44.50%	48	40.00%	53	39.30%
Commercial: managed care FFS	39	15.00%	55	.00%	48	.00%	53	.00%
Commercial: capitation	39	.00%	55	.00%	48	.00%	53	.00%
Workers' compensation	39	.30%	55	1.00%	48	1.00%	53	1.00%
Charity care and prof courtesy	39	.01%	55	.00%	48	.00%	53	.00%
Self-pay	39	4.00%	55	3.60%	48	3.94%	53	3.80%
Other federal government payers	39	.00%	55	.00%	48	.00%	53	.00%

Multispecialty — by Geographic Section, Not Hospital or IDS Owned
(per FTE Physician)

Table 5.4a: Staffing, RVUs, Patients, Procedures and Square Footage

	Eastern section		Midwest section		Southern section		Western section	
	Count	Median	Count	Median	Count	Median	Count	Median
Total provider FTE/physician	**38**	**1.27**	**58**	**1.30**	**45**	**1.15**	**51**	**1.18**
Prim care phy/physician	34	.71	58	.65	45	.56	50	.71
Nonsurg phy/physician	18	.38	41	.22	35	.22	38	.22
Surg spec phy/physician	16	.27	46	.22	33	.27	35	.21
Total NPP FTE/physician	38	.27	58	.30	45	.15	51	.18
Total support staff FTE/phy	**41**	**4.70**	**65**	**5.63**	**51**	**5.71**	**56**	**4.87**
Total empl support staff FTE	35	4.70	56	5.66	46	5.68	53	4.85
General administrative	34	.28	55	.30	45	.27	51	.26
Patient accounting	34	.62	55	.75	45	.87	50	.59
General accounting	28	.08	43	.08	39	.08	47	.07
Managed care administrative	14	.05	27	.07	17	.09	31	.12
Information technology	16	.06	38	.13	33	.10	38	.11
Housekeeping, maint, security	20	.06	38	.13	29	.09	35	.06
Medical receptionists	32	.93	55	.89	44	.93	51	.95
Med secretaries,transcribers	27	.26	51	.32	36	.19	37	.14
Medical records	31	.32	50	.46	40	.44	48	.38
Other admin support	20	.09	31	.12	27	.11	31	.08
***Total administrative supp staff**	**22**	**2.91**	**37**	**3.38**	**28**	**3.50**	**27**	**3.00**
Registered Nurses	31	.32	51	.67	40	.30	44	.40
Licensed Practical Nurses	27	.42	51	.48	42	.63	40	.21
Med assistants, nurse aides	31	.68	48	.54	43	.68	49	.90
***Total clinical supp staff**	**33**	**1.40**	**52**	**1.71**	**45**	**1.67**	**41**	**1.48**
Clinical laboratory	28	.28	49	.37	38	.36	42	.34
Radiology and imaging	26	.22	50	.27	40	.36	45	.32
Other medical support serv	19	.23	33	.31	30	.24	33	.21
***Total ancillary supp staff**	**23**	**.76**	**37**	**.88**	**30**	**1.00**	**33**	**.89**
Tot contracted supp staff	15	.08	22	.06	20	.15	24	.11
Tot RVU/physician	22	10,529	19	11,316	13	13,798	27	11,216
Physician work RVU/physician	16	4,798	23	5,614	16	6,020	27	5,609
Patients/physician	23	1,579	28	1,399	22	1,624	30	1,870
Tot procedures/physician	30	11,405	41	12,458	40	13,095	48	11,650
Square feet/physician	39	1,696	58	2,316	49	2,308	53	1,817

*See pages 260 and 261 for definition.

Table 5.4b: Charges and Revenue

	Eastern section		Midwest section		Southern section		Western section	
	Count	Median	Count	Median	Count	Median	Count	Median
Net fee-for-service revenue	34	$520,910	60	$618,416	43	$645,544	52	$540,943
Gross FFS charges	34	$779,797	59	$962,486	43	$1,065,482	51	$801,838
Adjustments to FFS charges	30	$360,431	57	$324,872	40	$420,295	47	$265,996
Adjusted FFS charges	32	$540,311	57	$625,635	40	$676,283	49	$559,271
Bad debts due to FFS activity	30	$8,241	51	$16,147	38	$21,435	47	$11,073
Net capitation revenue	19	$28,794	19	$39,925	11	$30,211	23	$144,436
Gross capitation charges	16	$45,745	14	$114,419	9	*	21	$150,267
Capitation revenue	18	$29,091	19	$39,925	11	$30,211	22	$203,635
Purch serv for cap patients	1	*	9	*	2	*	11	$91,199
Net other medical revenue	26	$15,174	46	$25,391	28	$11,695	39	$9,906
Gross rev from other activity	26	$15,174	45	$28,105	28	$18,126	37	$16,054
Other medical revenue	22	$7,710	35	$12,490	21	$8,492	32	$6,310
Rev from sale of goods/services	14	$11,564	28	$19,096	16	$27,239	24	$10,798
Cost of sales	8	*	18	$17,039	12	$21,313	14	$11,563
Total gross charges	**37**	**$744,094**	**64**	**$970,442**	**49**	**$1,026,948**	**53**	**$888,188**
Total medical revenue	**41**	**$564,430**	**65**	**$668,160**	**51**	**$643,091**	**56**	**$636,300**

Multispecialty — by Geographic Section, Not Hospital or IDS Owned
(per FTE Physician)

Table 5.4c: Operating Cost

	Eastern section		Midwest section		Southern section		Western section	
	Count	Median	Count	Median	Count	Median	Count	Median
Total support staff cost/phy	41	$161,655	65	$198,228	51	$184,440	56	$198,688
Total empl supp staff cost/phy	35	$146,594	60	$159,043	46	$146,736	53	$156,133
General administrative	34	$19,195	57	$16,429	44	$14,955	51	$15,598
Patient accounting	34	$17,435	58	$18,808	44	$19,889	50	$17,983
General accounting	28	$2,622	45	$3,272	39	$2,927	47	$2,803
Managed care administrative	14	$2,594	26	$2,242	17	$2,572	31	$4,118
Information technology	16	$3,128	40	$5,233	33	$3,830	38	$4,138
Housekeeping, maint, security	20	$1,585	40	$3,198	29	$2,031	35	$1,874
Medical receptionists	32	$21,300	56	$19,410	43	$18,680	51	$22,286
Med secretaries,transcribers	27	$6,432	52	$8,161	35	$5,534	37	$4,828
Medical records	31	$6,506	51	$8,724	40	$6,748	48	$9,085
Other admin support	20	$2,225	32	$2,742	27	$1,996	31	$1,920
*Total administrative supp staff	20	$78,667	35	$92,481	28	$80,483	27	$92,634
Registered Nurses	31	$13,185	52	$28,347	39	$10,844	44	$18,117
Licensed Practical Nurses	27	$13,025	49	$15,727	41	$17,679	40	$5,957
Med assistants, nurse aides	31	$17,240	46	$12,204	42	$15,014	49	$24,933
*Total clinical supp staff	32	$41,420	49	$55,817	43	$41,860	42	$45,263
Clinical laboratory	28	$7,207	50	$12,196	37	$10,320	42	$10,972
Radiology and imaging	26	$7,589	52	$10,176	39	$10,628	45	$12,586
Other medical support serv	20	$6,984	35	$11,551	31	$7,568	33	$6,447
*Total ancillary supp staff	27	$18,571	42	$30,149	34	$30,653	36	$31,033
Total empl supp staff benefits	41	$27,760	65	$41,164	49	$37,707	53	$39,853
Tot contracted supp staff	19	$1,847	31	$2,773	28	$3,403	36	$1,899
Total general operating cost	41	$169,587	65	$188,924	51	$179,988	56	$172,383
Information technology	35	$10,723	58	$10,399	46	$10,850	53	$9,185
Medical and surgical supply	35	$20,955	58	$32,807	46	$33,516	53	$31,551
Building and occupancy	35	$37,788	58	$41,637	46	$45,629	53	$40,405
Furniture and equipment	31	$7,584	55	$9,982	38	$10,061	49	$4,622
Admin supplies and services	35	$10,988	58	$10,921	46	$10,999	51	$9,739
Prof liability insurance	40	$10,739	63	$11,315	50	$15,998	55	$13,153
Other insurance premiums	33	$1,146	54	$1,682	44	$1,629	52	$932
Outside professional fees	35	$3,104	56	$4,866	44	$4,148	52	$3,185
Promotion and marketing	35	$2,152	57	$2,585	45	$2,644	52	$1,599
Clinical laboratory	29	$13,617	55	$18,988	45	$15,693	46	$10,450
Radiology and imaging	27	$5,429	51	$9,374	41	$13,721	45	$6,767
Other ancillary services	12	$4,125	34	$2,070	26	$2,245	23	$4,912
Billing purchased services	24	$1,823	37	$1,744	28	$2,305	26	$1,649
Management fees paid to MSO	2	*	2	*	2	*	7	*
Misc operating cost	34	$7,260	58	$9,982	46	$6,845	52	$8,233
Cost allocated to prac from par	0	*	1	*	1	*	1	*
Total operating cost	41	$341,075	65	$405,150	51	$376,874	56	$384,826

*See pages 260 and 261 for definition.

Multispecialty — by Geographic Section, Not Hospital or IDS Owned
(per FTE Physician)

Table 5.4d: Provider Cost

	Eastern section		Midwest section		Southern section		Western section	
	Count	Median	Count	Median	Count	Median	Count	Median
Total med rev after oper cost	41	$223,651	65	$279,016	51	$270,245	56	$245,692
Total provider cost/physician	41	$226,435	65	$284,410	51	$254,950	56	$239,874
Total NPP cost/physician	38	$20,516	60	$27,022	47	$11,771	54	$17,597
Nonphysician provider comp	34	$16,854	57	$21,637	42	$9,982	52	$14,424
Nonphysician prov benefit cost	33	$3,095	55	$4,871	36	$1,950	46	$3,333
Provider consultant cost	18	$4,462	28	$13,375	10	$9,545	24	$10,272
Total physician cost/physician	41	$206,818	65	$249,009	51	$224,776	56	$218,391
Total phy compensation	35	$181,680	60	$215,956	46	$208,208	54	$185,573
Total phy benefit cost	35	$30,426	60	$37,490	46	$31,105	51	$29,209

Table 5.4e: Net Income or Loss

	Eastern section		Midwest section		Southern section		Western section	
	Count	Median	Count	Median	Count	Median	Count	Median
Total cost	41	$555,508	65	$724,523	51	$642,870	56	$642,882
Net nonmedical revenue	30	$2,476	59	$4,239	36	$2,489	48	$1,693
Nonmedical revenue	25	$2,672	56	$4,610	33	$3,040	42	$5,042
Fin support for oper costs	2	*	1	*	0	*	2	*
Goodwill amortization	3	*	9	*	9	*	5	*
Nonmedical cost	14	$894	33	$2,752	13	$639	25	$2,388
Net inc, prac with fin sup	2	*	1	*	0	*	2	*
Net inc, prac w/o fin sup	39	$2,447	60	$3,302	45	$704	51	$13,086
Net inc, excl fin supp (all prac)	41	$2,300	61	$2,807	45	$704	53	$13,163

Table 5.4f: Assets and Liabilities

	Eastern section		Midwest section		Southern section		Western section	
	Count	Median	Count	Median	Count	Median	Count	Median
Total assets	18	$59,198	44	$193,002	28	$119,591	41	$183,720
Current assets	18	$26,218	44	$128,894	29	$93,775	42	$114,301
Noncurrent assets	18	$33,637	44	$68,459	29	$31,273	42	$51,339
Total liabilities	18	$38,496	44	$107,179	29	$61,908	42	$64,510
Current liabilities	18	$24,805	44	$72,160	29	$44,097	42	$36,282
Noncurrent liabilities	18	$12,118	44	$36,027	29	$7,221	42	$25,411
Working capital	18	$5,756	44	$29,695	29	$27,690	42	$37,052
Total net worth	18	$16,712	44	$72,213	29	$38,877	42	$59,428
Total support staff FTE/phy	41	4.70	65	5.63	51	5.71	56	4.87

Multispecialty — by Geographic Section, Not Hospital or IDS Owned
(as a % of Total Medical Revenue)

Table 5.5a: Charges and Revenue

	Eastern section		Midwest section		Southern section		Western section	
	Count	Median	Count	Median	Count	Median	Count	Median
Net fee-for-service revenue	34	95.37%	60	97.06%	43	98.55%	52	97.22%
Net capitation revenue	19	6.11%	19	9.77%	11	6.96%	23	21.11%
Net other medical revenue	26	2.79%	46	3.00%	28	1.46%	39	1.58%
Total gross charges	**41**	**162.95%**	**64**	**152.00%**	**51**	**166.53%**	**54**	**149.54%**

Table 5.5b: Operating Cost

	Eastern section		Midwest section		Southern section		Western section	
	Count	Median	Count	Median	Count	Median	Count	Median
Total support staff cost	**41**	**28.64%**	**65**	**30.70%**	**51**	**27.65%**	**56**	**31.71%**
Total empl support staff cost	35	23.76%	60	24.02%	46	22.39%	53	25.25%
General administrative	34	2.89%	57	2.33%	44	2.10%	51	2.52%
Patient accounting	34	2.94%	58	2.80%	44	2.88%	50	2.68%
General accounting	28	.42%	45	.40%	39	.37%	47	.47%
Managed care administrative	14	.34%	26	.30%	17	.31%	31	.65%
Information technology	16	.48%	40	.68%	33	.52%	38	.68%
Housekeeping, maint, security	20	.34%	40	.42%	29	.28%	35	.24%
Medical receptionists	32	3.54%	56	2.74%	43	2.71%	51	3.42%
Med secretaries,transcribers	27	.99%	52	1.11%	35	.82%	37	.66%
Medical records	31	1.01%	51	1.26%	40	.92%	48	1.34%
Other admin support	20	.44%	32	.34%	27	.38%	31	.32%
***Total administrative supp staff**	**20**	**13.20%**	**35**	**12.16%**	**28**	**11.78%**	**27**	**12.69%**
Registered Nurses	31	2.36%	52	3.75%	39	1.53%	44	2.90%
Licensed Practical Nurses	27	2.13%	49	2.06%	41	2.84%	40	.88%
Med assistants, nurse aides	31	2.60%	46	1.64%	42	2.20%	49	3.62%
***Total clinical supp staff**	**32**	**6.89%**	**49**	**7.64%**	**43**	**6.54%**	**42**	**7.11%**
Clinical laboratory	28	1.30%	50	1.49%	37	1.33%	42	1.51%
Radiology and imaging	26	1.18%	52	1.57%	39	1.51%	45	1.85%
Other medical support serv	20	1.03%	35	1.48%	31	1.10%	33	.95%
***Total ancillary supp staff**	**27**	**3.38%**	**42**	**4.08%**	**34**	**4.20%**	**36**	**4.37%**
Total empl supp staff benefits	41	5.03%	65	6.27%	49	5.61%	53	6.26%
Tot contracted supp staff	19	.41%	31	.32%	28	.38%	36	.37%
Total general operating cost	**41**	**29.33%**	**65**	**29.09%**	**51**	**29.91%**	**56**	**27.83%**
Information technology	35	1.70%	58	1.41%	46	1.76%	53	1.43%
Medical and surgical supply	35	3.68%	58	5.34%	46	5.64%	53	4.57%
Building and occupancy	35	7.10%	58	5.77%	46	6.61%	53	6.61%
Furniture and equipment	31	1.18%	55	1.44%	38	1.57%	49	.78%
Admin supplies and services	35	1.94%	58	1.57%	46	1.96%	52	1.65%
Prof liability insurance	40	1.96%	63	1.71%	50	2.71%	55	1.94%
Other insurance premiums	32	.22%	53	.26%	44	.24%	52	.16%
Outside professional fees	35	.53%	56	.75%	44	.61%	52	.45%
Promotion and marketing	35	.35%	57	.38%	45	.43%	52	.25%
Clinical laboratory	29	2.66%	55	2.71%	45	2.32%	46	1.47%
Radiology and imaging	29	.89%	52	1.42%	41	1.85%	45	1.04%
Other ancillary services	12	.62%	34	.30%	26	.30%	23	1.02%
Billing purchased services	24	.21%	37	.26%	28	.31%	26	.31%
Management fees paid to MSO	2	*	2	*	4	*	7	*
Misc operating cost	34	1.34%	58	1.46%	46	.98%	52	1.43%
Cost allocated to prac from par	0	*	1	*	1	*	1	*
Total operating cost	**41**	**60.03%**	**65**	**58.77%**	**51**	**58.72%**	**56**	**59.20%**

*See pages 260 and 261 for definition.

Multispecialty — by Geographic Section, Not Hospital or IDS Owned
(as a % of Total Medical Revenue)

Table 5.5c: Provider Cost

	Eastern section		Midwest section		Southern section		Western section	
	Count	Median	Count	Median	Count	Median	Count	Median
Total med rev after oper cost	41	39.97%	65	41.37%	51	41.28%	56	40.80%
Total provider cost	41	40.93%	65	43.10%	51	40.70%	56	39.53%
Total NPP cost	38	3.09%	60	3.84%	47	1.61%	54	2.67%
Nonphysician provider comp	34	2.47%	57	2.99%	42	1.33%	52	2.17%
Nonphysician prov benefit cost	33	.57%	55	.65%	36	.29%	46	.50%
Provider consultant cost	18	.83%	28	2.01%	10	1.31%	24	1.80%
Total physician cost	41	36.97%	65	38.93%	51	38.60%	56	35.70%
Total phy compensation	35	31.74%	60	32.92%	46	31.85%	54	29.98%
Total phy benefit cost	35	5.40%	60	5.32%	46	5.17%	51	4.78%

Table 5.5d: Net Income or Loss

	Eastern section		Midwest section		Southern section		Western section	
	Count	Median	Count	Median	Count	Median	Count	Median
Total cost	41	99.98%	65	100.56%	51	100.23%	56	98.55%
Net nonmedical revenue	30	.51%	59	.71%	36	.34%	48	.24%
Nonmedical revenue	25	.49%	56	.66%	33	.39%	42	.66%
Fin support for oper costs	2	*	1	*	0	*	2	*
Goodwill amortization	3	*	9	*	9	*	5	*
Nonmedical cost	14	.13%	33	.25%	13	.05%	25	.40%
Net inc, prac with fin sup	2	*	1	*	0	*	2	*
Net inc, prac w/o fin sup	39	.55%	60	.47%	45	.09%	51	1.97%
Net inc, excl fin supp (all prac)	41	.48%	61	.45%	45	.09%	53	2.07%

Table 5.5e: Assets and Liabilities

	Eastern section		Midwest section		Southern section		Western section	
	Count	Median	Count	Median	Count	Median	Count	Median
Total assets	18	12.59%	44	28.03%	29	19.37%	42	27.12%
Current assets	18	4.63%	44	18.98%	29	12.41%	42	15.73%
Noncurrent assets	18	5.57%	44	10.83%	29	4.58%	42	7.26%
Total liabilities	18	5.85%	44	16.77%	29	9.45%	42	13.42%
Current liabilities	18	3.73%	44	11.82%	29	5.86%	42	6.34%
Noncurrent liabilities	18	1.96%	44	6.10%	29	1.43%	42	4.14%
Working capital	18	1.18%	44	4.23%	29	3.61%	42	6.02%
Total net worth	18	2.97%	44	10.16%	29	6.17%	42	9.15%

Multispecialty — by Geographic Section, Not Hospital or IDS Owned
(per FTE Provider)

Table 5.6a: Staffing, RVUs, Patients, Procedures and Square Footage

	Eastern section		Midwest section		Southern section		Western section	
	Count	Median	Count	Median	Count	Median	Count	Median
Total physician FTE/provider	**38**	**.79**	**58**	**.77**	**45**	**.87**	**51**	**.85**
Prim care phy/provider	33	.57	53	.44	40	.46	45	.57
Nonsurg phy/provider	17	.30	38	.19	32	.22	35	.20
Surg spec phy/provider	16	.19	43	.17	29	.21	32	.17
Total NPP FTE/provider	38	.21	58	.23	45	.13	51	.15
Total support staff FTE/prov	**38**	**3.58**	**58**	**4.09**	**45**	**4.83**	**51**	**4.28**
Total empl supp staff FTE/prov	34	3.57	51	4.09	40	5.00	49	4.16
General administrative	33	.23	51	.24	40	.23	47	.20
Patient accounting	33	.52	52	.57	39	.78	46	.52
General accounting	28	.06	42	.06	37	.07	44	.07
Managed care administrative	13	.03	26	.06	15	.08	29	.09
Information technology	16	.05	37	.10	31	.09	36	.09
Housekeeping, maint, security	19	.05	38	.12	26	.06	33	.05
Medical receptionists	31	.77	51	.67	38	.81	47	.82
Med secretaries,transcribers	27	.19	47	.23	32	.18	35	.12
Medical records	31	.25	47	.35	36	.37	44	.32
Other admin support	19	.06	31	.09	24	.08	29	.06
***Total administrative supp staff**	**20**	**2.01**	**35**	**2.52**	**27**	**2.83**	**26**	**2.54**
Registered Nurses	30	.26	47	.48	36	.24	40	.35
Licensed Practical Nurses	27	.34	47	.41	36	.52	37	.16
Med assistants, nurse aides	30	.57	44	.39	38	.58	45	.72
***Total clinical supp staff**	**31**	**1.16**	**47**	**1.32**	**41**	**1.40**	**38**	**1.26**
Clinical laboratory	28	.22	45	.29	36	.32	39	.29
Radiology and imaging	25	.19	47	.21	39	.28	42	.26
Other medical support serv	18	.17	33	.23	28	.21	31	.18
***Total ancillary supp staff**	**21**	**.61**	**36**	**.71**	**29**	**.87**	**31**	**.72**
Tot contracted supp staff	13	.06	20	.05	19	.12	23	.10
Tot RVU/provider	21	7,814	16	8,853	11	10,691	26	8,842
Physician work RVU/provider	15	3,729	21	4,145	14	4,908	26	4,593
Patients/provider	24	1,315	24	1,095	20	1,328	28	1,458
Tot procedures/provider	29	9,532	38	9,454	35	11,151	43	9,769
Square feet/provider	36	1,363	53	1,785	44	1,998	48	1,424
Total support staff FTE/phy	**41**	**4.70**	**65**	**5.63**	**51**	**5.71**	**56**	**4.87**

*See pages 260 and 261 for definition.

Table 5.6b: Charges, Revenue and Cost

	Eastern section		Midwest section		Southern section		Western section	
	Count	Median	Count	Median	Count	Median	Count	Median
Total gross charges	**38**	**$655,836**	**57**	**$762,462**	**45**	**$949,134**	**50**	**$755,702**
Total medical revenue	**38**	**$420,955**	**58**	**$521,019**	**45**	**$572,177**	**51**	**$511,874**
Net fee-for-service revenue	38	$393,632	55	$489,628	37	$547,948	47	$459,515
Net capitation revenue	33	$20,628	17	$48,000	10	$26,828	19	$112,705
Net other medical revenue	25	$11,740	44	$18,899	26	$9,227	35	$8,679
Total support staff cost/prov	**38**	**$123,866**	**58**	**$160,516**	**45**	**$161,424**	**51**	**$163,841**
Total general operating cost	**38**	**$122,861**	**58**	**$148,642**	**45**	**$159,962**	**51**	**$142,856**
Total operating cost	**38**	**$250,383**	**58**	**$309,545**	**45**	**$343,117**	**51**	**$316,391**
Total med rev after oper cost	**38**	**$180,786**	**58**	**$214,957**	**45**	**$212,772**	**51**	**$215,714**
Total provider cost/provider	**38**	**$170,375**	**58**	**$226,221**	**45**	**$211,945**	**51**	**$203,846**
Total NPP cost/provider	38	$16,444	58	$20,881	45	$10,205	51	$14,589
Provider consultant cost	16	$3,916	27	$12,814	9	*	22	$9,122
Total physician cost/provider	38	$149,113	58	$197,225	45	$203,866	51	$183,405
Total phy compensation	34	$130,175	55	$171,435	40	$179,903	49	$162,791
Total phy benefit cost	34	$23,337	55	$28,147	40	$27,754	46	$23,728
Total cost	**38**	**$420,826**	**58**	**$526,764**	**45**	**$562,846**	**51**	**$520,164**
Net nonmedical revenue	28	$2,282	54	$2,227	32	$2,050	44	$1,629
Net inc, prac with fin sup	2	*	1	*	0	*	2	*
Net inc, prac w/o fin sup	36	$2,162	53	$2,297	39	$1,040	46	$9,341
Net inc, excl fin supp (all prac)	38	$2,072	54	$2,072	39	$1,040	48	$11,903
Total support staff FTE/phy	**41**	**4.70**	**65**	**5.63**	**51**	**5.71**	**56**	**4.87**

Multispecialty — by Geographic Section, Not Hospital or IDS Owned
(per Square Foot)

Table 5.7a: Staffing, RVUs, Patients and Procedures

	Eastern section		Midwest section		Southern section		Western section	
	Count	Median	Count	Median	Count	Median	Count	Median
Total prov FTE/10,000 sq ft	36	**7.34**	53	**5.60**	44	**5.01**	48	**7.02**
Total phy FTE/10,000 sq ft	39	5.89	58	4.32	49	4.33	53	5.50
Prim care phy/10,000 sq ft	32	4.26	53	2.59	43	2.34	47	3.71
Nonsurg phy/10,000 sq ft	17	2.00	37	.99	34	1.21	36	1.33
Surg spec phy/10,000 sq ft	15	1.25	42	.96	32	1.06	33	1.11
Total NPP FTE/10,000 sq ft	36	1.38	53	1.23	44	.57	48	1.03
Total supp stf FTE/10,000 sq ft	39	**26.69**	58	**24.47**	49	**26.04**	53	**28.80**
Total empl supp stf/10,000 sq ft	33	26.78	51	23.81	44	25.91	50	28.55
General administrative	33	1.67	51	1.17	43	1.20	49	1.48
Patient accounting	33	3.76	51	3.22	44	3.82	48	3.19
General accounting	27	.42	39	.32	39	.41	44	.39
Managed care administrative	13	.28	25	.39	17	.37	30	.64
Information technology	15	.36	35	.52	32	.46	36	.53
Housekeeping, maint, security	20	.32	35	.73	28	.35	33	.33
Medical receptionists	31	5.52	51	3.66	42	4.09	48	5.79
Med secretaries,transcribers	26	1.24	47	1.28	35	.83	35	.86
Medical records	30	1.96	46	1.99	38	1.93	45	2.61
Other admin support	20	.47	28	.46	25	.45	31	.37
***Total administrative supp staff**	22	**14.29**	35	**13.57**	27	**14.48**	26	**15.55**
Registered Nurses	30	1.99	47	2.76	39	1.18	41	2.41
Licensed Practical Nurses	27	2.47	48	2.15	40	3.06	37	1.07
Med assistants, nurse aides	30	3.71	46	2.04	41	3.13	47	5.15
***Total clinical supp staff**	33	**7.96**	49	**6.93**	44	**7.22**	39	**7.66**
Clinical laboratory	27	1.39	46	1.52	37	1.57	41	1.91
Radiology and imaging	25	1.32	47	1.16	38	1.40	42	1.53
Other medical support serv	18	1.10	31	1.17	29	.92	31	1.31
***Total ancillary supp staff**	22	**3.68**	36	**3.87**	29	**4.12**	32	**3.93**
Tot contracted supp staff	14	.50	22	.38	20	.69	24	.52
Tot RVU/sq ft	22	6.52	18	5.27	13	6.73	25	5.91
Physician work RVU/sq ft	16	2.93	23	2.52	15	2.53	25	2.81
Patients/sq ft	23	1.03	24	.62	21	.70	28	1.08
Tot procedures/sq ft	29	5.66	38	5.22	39	5.40	45	6.41
Total support staff FTE/phy	41	**4.70**	65	**5.63**	51	**5.71**	56	**4.87**

*See pages 260 and 261 for definition.

Table 5.7b: Charges, Revenue and Cost

	Eastern section		Midwest section		Southern section		Western section	
	Count	Median	Count	Median	Count	Median	Count	Median
Total gross charges	39	**$564.71**	58	**$467.63**	49	**$518.27**	51	**$509.57**
Total medical revenue	39	**$341.74**	58	**$319.50**	49	**$295.85**	53	**$373.02**
Net fee-for-service revenue	32	$316.22	54	$272.95	41	$293.11	49	$305.28
Net capitation revenue	17	$22.20	16	$21.81	11	$10.91	21	$66.95
Net other medical revenue	24	$7.71	42	$8.95	27	$4.21	37	$4.38
Total support staff cost/sq ft	39	**$91.23**	58	**$97.91**	49	**$89.21**	53	**$110.63**
Total general operating cost	39	**$89.68**	58	**$89.92**	49	**$91.84**	53	**$99.28**
Total operating cost	39	**$192.42**	58	**$186.90**	49	**$173.73**	53	**$216.97**
Total med rev after oper cost	39	**$142.32**	58	**$120.92**	49	**$119.90**	53	**$152.62**
Total provider cost/sq ft	39	**$145.67**	58	**$125.20**	49	**$122.09**	53	**$138.92**
Total NPP cost/sq ft	36	$10.56	55	$10.75	45	$4.26	51	$9.50
Provider consultant cost	17	$3.14	27	$5.73	10	$4.65	23	$5.61
Total physician cost/sq ft	39	$128.67	58	$112.48	49	$110.16	53	$129.09
Total phy compensation	33	$112.14	54	$99.67	44	$94.65	51	$109.93
Total phy benefit cost	33	$17.77	54	$15.93	44	$14.86	49	$17.81
Total cost	39	**$333.42**	58	**$319.83**	49	**$303.14**	53	**$366.75**
Net nonmedical revenue/sq ft	28	$1.94	52	$1.68	35	$1.10	45	$.76
Net inc, prac with fin sup	2	*	1	*	0	*	1	*
Net inc, prac w/o fin sup	37	$1.67	54	$1.35	43	$.44	49	$6.42
Net inc, excl fin supp (all prac)	39	$.90	55	$1.11	43	$.44	50	$6.82
Total support staff FTE/phy	41	**4.70**	65	**5.63**	51	**5.71**	56	**4.87**

Multispecialty — by Geographic Section, Not Hospital or IDS Owned
(per Total RVU)

Table 5.8a: Staffing, Patients, Procedures and Square Footage

	Eastern section		Midwest section		Southern section		Western section	
	Count	Median	Count	Median	Count	Median	Count	Median
Total prov FTE/10,000 tot RVU	21	1.28	16	1.13	11	.94	26	1.13
Total phy FTE/10,000 tot RVU	22	.95	19	.88	13	.72	27	.89
Prim care phy/10,000 tot RVU	19	.76	18	.52	11	.39	26	.54
Nonsurg phy/10,000 tot RVU	9	*	13	.18	8	*	23	.22
Surg spec phy/10,000 tot RVU	7	*	15	.17	7	*	20	.20
Total NPP FTE/10,000 tot RVU	21	.22	16	.32	11	.12	26	.19
Total supp stf FTE/10,000 tot RVU	22	4.28	19	4.53	13	4.10	27	4.93
Tot empl supp stf/10,000 tot RVU	20	4.33	18	4.40	12	4.05	26	4.91
General administrative	20	.25	18	.20	11	.23	25	.22
Patient accounting	20	.62	18	.54	12	.57	25	.55
General accounting	16	.06	13	.06	10	.05	25	.08
Managed care administrative	9	*	10	.08	5	*	19	.10
Information technology	7	*	13	.11	8	*	22	.14
Housekeeping, maint, security	9	*	13	.15	7	*	23	.07
Medical receptionists	18	.74	18	.67	11	.64	26	.80
Med secretaries,transcribers	16	.24	16	.28	7	*	22	.15
Medical records	18	.28	16	.40	9	*	26	.43
Other admin support	13	.15	8	*	7	*	19	.06
*Total administrative supp staff	12	2.41	12	2.85	6	*	18	2.97
Registered Nurses	18	.35	16	.56	12	.30	26	.43
Licensed Practical Nurses	17	.45	15	.40	11	.27	24	.14
Med assistants, nurse aides	19	.56	15	.37	11	.46	25	.81
*Total clinical supp staff	20	1.26	16	1.31	12	1.01	25	1.36
Clinical laboratory	16	.25	17	.26	9	*	25	.30
Radiology and imaging	14	.19	16	.21	10	.27	24	.29
Other medical support serv	11	.17	11	.24	7	*	22	.21
*Total ancillary supp staff	12	.52	12	.75	6	*	21	.85
Tot contracted supp staff	11	.09	9	*	6	*	12	.07
Physician work RVU/tot RVU	16	.51	15	.45	13	.45	24	.48
Patients/tot RVU	17	.19	12	.11	9	*	18	.14
Tot procedures/tot RVU	19	.95	14	.94	12	.74	24	1.10
Square feet/tot RVU	22	.15	18	.19	13	.15	25	.17
Total support staff FTE/phy	41	4.70	65	5.63	51	5.71	56	4.87

*See pages 260 and 261 for definition.

Table 5.8b: Charges, Revenue and Cost

	Eastern section		Midwest section		Southern section		Western section	
	Count	Median	Count	Median	Count	Median	Count	Median
Total gross charges	22	$92.88	19	$85.68	13	$87.18	26	$91.94
Total medical revenue	22	$51.93	19	$55.88	13	$47.91	27	$64.07
Net fee-for-service revenue	19	$47.17	18	$45.52	12	$43.43	26	$51.70
Net capitation revenue	11	$2.43	6	*	4	*	13	$17.88
Net other medical revenue	14	$1.71	16	$1.93	8	*	25	$1.26
Total supp staff cost/tot RVU	22	$15.32	19	$16.33	13	$14.15	27	$20.54
Total general operating cost	22	$15.99	19	$13.66	13	$13.40	27	$16.68
Total operating cost	22	$32.58	19	$30.74	13	$27.83	27	$39.14
Total med rev after oper cost	22	$21.90	19	$21.71	13	$21.13	27	$25.68
Total provider cost/tot RVU	22	$21.86	19	$21.87	13	$19.42	27	$24.89
Total NPP cost/tot RVU	21	$1.42	17	$2.28	11	$.81	27	$1.84
Provider consultant cost	9	*	8	*	2	*	16	$1.25
Total physician cost/tot RVU	22	$20.37	19	$20.14	13	$19.10	27	$21.42
Total phy compensation	20	$16.74	18	$17.16	12	$15.72	26	$18.90
Total phy benefit cost	20	$2.55	18	$2.54	12	$2.38	26	$3.29
Total cost	17	$63.60	15	$60.99	12	$50.65	23	$66.64
Net nonmedical revenue	14	$.33	16	$.33	9	*	25	$.11
Net inc, prac with fin sup	1	*	1	*	0	*	1	*
Net inc, prac w/o fin sup	21	$.25	16	-$.06	12	$.38	25	$.91
Net inc, excl fin supp (all prac)	22	$.24	17	-$.12	12	$.38	26	$1.07
Total support staff FTE/phy	41	4.70	65	5.63	51	5.71	56	4.87

Multispecialty — by Geographic Section, Not Hospital or IDS Owned
(per Work RVU)

Table 5.9a: Staffing, Patients, Procedures and Square Footage

	Eastern section		Midwest section		Southern section		Western section	
	Count	Median	Count	Median	Count	Median	Count	Median
Total prov FTE/10,000 work RVU	**15**	**2.68**	**21**	**2.41**	**14**	**2.04**	**26**	**2.18**
Tot phy FTE/10,000 work RVU	16	2.08	23	1.78	16	1.66	27	1.78
Prim care phy/10,000 work RVU	14	1.82	22	1.15	14	1.15	26	1.09
Nonsurg phy/10,000 work RVU	6	*	16	.43	10	.46	22	.47
Surg spec phy/10,000 work RVU	4	*	18	.37	9	*	21	.37
Total NPP FTE/10,000 work RVU	15	.44	21	.63	14	.27	26	.35
Total supp stf FTE/10,000 wrk RVU	**16**	**9.24**	**23**	**9.78**	**16**	**9.76**	**27**	**9.83**
Tot empl supp stf/10,000 work RVU	14	9.22	22	10.02	15	9.53	26	9.78
General administrative	14	.49	22	.53	14	.63	25	.46
Patient accounting	14	1.22	22	1.25	14	1.54	25	1.19
General accounting	11	.12	19	.13	12	.12	25	.15
Managed care administrative	7	*	13	.12	6	*	16	.20
Information technology	5	*	17	.29	10	.18	22	.22
Housekeeping, maint, security	6	*	17	.33	9	*	23	.13
Medical receptionists	13	1.57	22	1.58	14	1.43	26	1.68
Med secretaries,transcribers	11	.39	20	.63	9	*	22	.29
Medical records	13	.52	20	.75	12	.74	26	.81
Other admin support	9	*	11	.10	9	*	20	.15
*****Total administrative supp staff**	**10**	**4.67**	**16**	**5.42**	**8**	*****	**17**	**6.11**
Registered Nurses	13	.85	21	1.10	15	.65	24	.82
Licensed Practical Nurses	12	.77	20	1.10	14	.85	22	.35
Med assistants, nurse aides	13	1.11	19	.81	14	1.08	25	1.66
*****Total clinical supp staff**	**14**	**2.53**	**21**	**2.98**	**15**	**2.44**	**23**	**2.62**
Clinical laboratory	11	.48	21	.59	10	.58	24	.59
Radiology and imaging	10	.45	20	.51	13	.69	23	.63
Other medical support serv	8	*	16	.57	9	*	20	.46
*****Total ancillary supp staff**	**9**	*****	**17**	**1.69**	**7**	*****	**19**	**1.93**
Tot contracted supp staff	9	*	8	*	7	*	12	.14
Tot RVU/work RVU	16	1.98	15	2.23	13	2.21	24	2.08
Patients/work RVU	11	.29	13	.21	12	.37	17	.27
Tot procedures/work RVU	14	1.81	18	2.16	15	2.03	25	2.25
Square feet/work RVU	16	.34	23	.40	15	.40	25	.36
Total support staff FTE/phy	**41**	**4.70**	**65**	**5.63**	**51**	**5.71**	**56**	**4.87**

*See pages 260 and 261 for definition.

Table 5.9b: Charges, Revenue and Cost

	Eastern section		Midwest section		Southern section		Western section	
	Count	Median	Count	Median	Count	Median	Count	Median
Total gross charges	**16**	**$167.06**	**23**	**$199.57**	**16**	**$215.58**	**26**	**$190.84**
Total medical revenue	**16**	**$108.32**	**23**	**$127.44**	**16**	**$114.35**	**27**	**$131.98**
Net fee-for-service revenue	13	$90.05	22	$115.63	15	$98.86	26	$112.11
Net capitation revenue	9	*	6	*	5	*	12	$36.57
Net other medical revenue	10	$3.32	21	$5.37	10	$1.61	24	$2.48
Total supp staff cost/work RVU	**16**	**$29.89**	**23**	**$35.51**	**16**	**$34.97**	**27**	**$43.44**
Total general operating cost	**16**	**$31.63**	**23**	**$36.23**	**16**	**$32.84**	**27**	**$35.52**
Total operating cost	**16**	**$66.69**	**23**	**$75.83**	**16**	**$66.87**	**27**	**$75.68**
Total med rev after oper cost	**16**	**$39.37**	**23**	**$50.87**	**16**	**$47.21**	**27**	**$52.10**
Total provider cost/work RVU	**16**	**$38.62**	**23**	**$52.53**	**16**	**$47.76**	**27**	**$52.94**
Total NPP cost/work RVU	15	$2.57	22	$5.42	14	$2.10	27	$3.37
Provider consultant cost	7	*	12	$3.01	3	*	16	$1.77
Total physician cost/work RVU	16	$37.26	23	$44.85	16	$45.02	27	$47.06
Total phy compensation	14	$30.65	22	$39.15	15	$39.05	26	$39.38
Total phy benefit cost	14	$5.06	22	$6.78	15	$5.46	26	$6.98
Total cost	**16**	**$109.46**	**23**	**$130.16**	**16**	**$119.40**	**27**	**$132.77**
Net nonmedical revenue	11	$.83	20	$.90	11	$.65	24	$.37
Net inc, prac with fin sup	0	*	1	*	0	*	1	*
Net inc, prac w/o fin sup	16	$.56	20	$.47	15	$.76	25	$1.66
Net inc, excl fin supp (all prac)	16	$.56	21	$.00	15	$.76	26	$1.83
Total support staff FTE/phy	**41**	**4.70**	**65**	**5.63**	**51**	**5.71**	**56**	**4.87**

Multispecialty — by Geographic Section, Not Hospital or IDS Owned
(per Patient)

Table 5.10a: Staffing, RVUs, Procedures and Square Footage

	Eastern section		Midwest section		Southern section		Western section	
	Count	Median	Count	Median	Count	Median	Count	Median
Total prov FTE/10,000 patients	24	7.61	24	9.13	20	7.59	28	6.87
Total phy FTE/10,000 pat	24	5.70	28	7.15	22	6.26	30	5.35
Prim care phy/10,000 pat	23	3.53	28	3.72	22	3.81	28	3.96
Nonsurg phy/10,000 pat	11	1.68	18	1.35	17	1.91	23	1.50
Surg spec phy/10,000 pat	10	1.36	21	1.53	15	1.61	19	.80
Total NPP FTE/10,000 pat	24	1.11	24	2.08	20	.86	28	1.13
Total supp staff FTE/10,000 pat	24	26.83	28	38.88	22	29.64	30	30.47
Total empl supp staff/10,000 pat	24	26.48	28	37.78	22	29.64	30	29.08
General administrative	23	1.07	27	2.08	21	1.92	29	1.19
Patient accounting	23	3.29	27	5.33	21	4.94	28	2.97
General accounting	21	.47	22	.67	19	.40	29	.44
Managed care administrative	10	.50	14	.23	10	.57	19	.68
Information technology	12	.36	18	.79	17	.55	23	.77
Housekeeping, maint, security	14	.34	16	1.35	13	.57	22	.43
Medical receptionists	22	5.29	27	4.69	21	5.80	29	5.43
Med secretaries,transcribers	19	1.34	25	2.12	16	1.36	23	.86
Medical records	21	1.25	23	3.10	18	2.27	29	2.93
Other admin support	14	.43	15	.76	15	.70	17	.48
*Total administrative supp staff	11	12.74	16	21.91	14	20.85	16	19.26
Registered Nurses	21	1.91	24	4.48	20	1.52	28	2.62
Licensed Practical Nurses	20	1.81	23	3.97	20	4.01	27	1.11
Med assistants, nurse aides	22	3.82	23	3.21	22	3.29	27	5.31
*Total clinical supp staff	21	8.52	23	10.67	20	9.71	24	9.23
Clinical laboratory	20	1.34	24	2.18	16	1.83	27	2.20
Radiology and imaging	17	.94	23	1.72	19	1.89	26	1.51
Other medical support serv	13	1.38	16	2.42	14	1.76	21	1.46
*Total ancillary supp staff	11	4.33	17	6.59	12	6.23	20	6.21
Tot contracted supp staff	11	.41	12	.32	7	*	12	.60
Tot RVU/patient	17	5.37	12	9.18	9	*	18	7.05
Physician work RVU/patient	11	3.41	13	4.77	12	2.71	17	3.68
Tot procedures/patient	23	6.41	23	8.81	22	7.74	28	7.05
Square feet/patient	23	.97	24	1.61	21	1.42	28	.93
Total support staff FTE/phy	41	4.70	65	5.63	51	5.71	56	4.87

*See pages 260 and 261 for definition.

Table 5.10b: Charges, Revenue and Cost

	Eastern section		Midwest section		Southern section		Western section	
	Count	Median	Count	Median	Count	Median	Count	Median
Total gross charges	24	$451.28	28	$638.93	22	$655.18	30	$480.06
Total medical revenue	24	$284.15	28	$436.95	22	$363.65	30	$336.63
Net fee-for-service revenue	24	$257.75	28	$374.89	21	$340.85	29	$262.13
Net capitation revenue	13	$14.89	10	$28.43	5	*	15	$131.00
Net other medical revenue	18	$11.40	22	$18.02	17	$8.22	22	$9.59
Total support staff cost/patient	24	$96.99	28	$127.35	22	$100.83	30	$106.95
Total general operating cost	24	$78.21	28	$113.30	22	$129.60	30	$94.73
Total operating cost	24	$172.84	28	$233.59	22	$225.09	30	$189.69
Total med rev after oper cost	24	$114.15	28	$188.68	22	$160.27	30	$146.77
Total provider cost/patient	24	$116.64	28	$201.03	22	$144.82	30	$131.05
Total NPP cost/patient	24	$7.46	26	$18.30	20	$6.49	29	$8.19
Provider consultant cost	11	$2.67	8	*	6	*	16	$6.35
Total physician cost/patient	24	$102.57	28	$178.39	22	$141.44	30	$119.93
Total phy compensation	24	$89.61	28	$151.08	22	$138.40	30	$100.36
Total phy benefit cost	23	$14.37	28	$21.35	22	$17.19	29	$19.59
Total cost	24	$284.31	28	$436.17	22	$369.67	30	$327.24
Net nonmedical revenue	18	$1.63	25	$2.03	17	$1.20	26	$.83
Net inc, prac with fin sup	1	*	0	*	0	*	1	*
Net inc, prac w/o fin sup	23	$1.77	26	$5.50	20	$5.08	28	$6.65
Net inc, excl fin supp (all prac)	24	$1.40	26	$5.50	20	$5.08	29	$6.69
Total support staff FTE/phy	41	4.70	65	5.63	51	5.71	56	4.87

Multispecialty — by Geographic Section, Not Hospital or IDS Owned
(Procedure and Charge Data)

Table 5.11a: Activity Charges to Total Gross Charges Ratios

	Eastern section		Midwest section		Southern section		Western section	
	Count	Median	Count	Median	Count	Median	Count	Median
Total proc gross charges	29	95.96%	43	95.15%	42	90.71%	46	95.59%
Medical proc-inside practice	29	47.75%	43	35.84%	42	39.42%	46	49.07%
Medical proc-outside practice	27	9.34%	41	8.77%	38	9.08%	40	6.41%
Surg proc-inside practice	26	4.19%	41	6.52%	38	4.49%	45	7.21%
Surg proc-outside practice	19	12.22%	39	18.02%	35	15.90%	35	12.18%
Laboratory procedures	27	10.87%	42	12.38%	42	10.25%	45	9.23%
Radiology procedures	22	4.66%	44	9.29%	41	8.96%	43	8.86%
Tot nonproc gross charges	24	4.38%	39	5.30%	38	10.80%	41	4.91%
Total support staff FTE/phy	41	4.70	65	5.63	51	5.71	56	4.87

Table 5.11b: Medical Procedure Data (inside the practice)

	Eastern section		Midwest section		Southern section		Western section	
	Count	Median	Count	Median	Count	Median	Count	Median
Gross charges/procedure	29	$73.89	42	$68.50	40	$73.82	45	$77.32
Total cost/procedure	26	$55.84	37	$58.45	35	$57.31	40	$57.60
Operating cost/procedure	26	$33.04	36	$36.04	33	$37.26	40	$35.86
Provider cost/procedure	27	$23.32	37	$22.90	36	$20.71	40	$22.43
Procedures/patient	23	2.87	24	3.80	22	3.82	28	3.48
Gross charges/patient	23	$207.30	25	$273.59	22	$240.24	28	$244.13
Procedures/physician	30	5,064	42	5,831	40	6,067	46	5,677
Gross charges/physician	29	$411,321	43	$374,188	42	$461,763	46	$448,881
Procedures/provider	29	4,456	39	4,358	35	5,123	42	4,565
Gross charges/provider	28	$326,363	40	$286,734	37	$383,354	42	$364,600
Gross charge to total cost ratio	26	1.34	37	1.13	35	1.35	40	1.29
Oper cost to total cost ratio	26	.58	36	.61	33	.64	40	.61
Prov cost to total cost ratio	26	.42	37	.38	35	.36	40	.39
Total support staff FTE/phy	41	4.70	65	5.63	51	5.71	56	4.87

Table 5.11c: Medical Procedure Data (outside the practice)

	Eastern section		Midwest section		Southern section		Western section	
	Count	Median	Count	Median	Count	Median	Count	Median
Gross charges/procedure	27	$120.10	39	$108.32	37	$113.49	39	$119.86
Total cost/procedure	24	$50.17	35	$49.43	32	$46.02	35	$52.70
Operating cost/procedure	24	$20.38	34	$19.16	30	$18.60	35	$21.04
Provider cost/procedure	25	$30.04	35	$30.13	33	$26.90	35	$30.90
Procedures/patient	21	.42	23	.59	20	.73	26	.26
Gross charges/patient	21	$48.15	24	$62.56	20	$67.11	26	$29.32
Procedures/physician	28	690	39	813	37	1,009	39	456
Gross charges/physician	27	$93,211	41	$90,805	38	$97,236	40	$56,575
Procedures/provider	27	590	37	618	31	897	36	384
Gross charges/provider	26	$68,816	39	$65,076	33	$86,299	37	$49,260
Gross charge to total cost ratio	24	2.38	35	2.14	32	2.42	35	2.31
Oper cost to total cost ratio	24	.39	34	.40	30	.39	35	.40
Prov cost to total cost ratio	24	.61	35	.60	32	.61	35	.60
Total support staff FTE/phy	41	4.70	65	5.63	51	5.71	56	4.87

Multispecialty — by Geographic Section, Not Hospital or IDS Owned
(Procedure and Charge Data)

Table 5.11d: Surgery/Anesthesia Procedure Data (inside the practice)

	Eastern section		Midwest section		Southern section		Western section	
	Count	Median	Count	Median	Count	Median	Count	Median
Gross charges/procedure	26	$83.46	41	$108.98	37	$104.49	44	$91.46
Total cost/procedure	23	$71.57	36	$87.00	33	$109.62	39	$71.88
Operating cost/procedure	23	$34.89	35	$50.04	31	$70.51	39	$48.50
Provider cost/procedure	24	$30.32	36	$30.87	33	$40.30	39	$30.71
Procedures/patient	21	.21	23	.37	21	.44	27	.49
Gross charges/patient	21	$20.35	23	$52.45	21	$35.57	27	$32.28
Procedures/physician	27	509	41	866	37	488	44	740
Gross charges/physician	26	$38,540	41	$64,928	38	$49,367	45	$59,698
Procedures/provider	26	433	38	593	32	451	40	725
Gross charges/provider	25	$31,975	38	$48,280	33	$44,490	41	$53,100
Gross charge to total cost ratio	23	1.34	36	1.14	33	1.34	39	1.29
Oper cost to total cost ratio	23	.58	35	.61	31	.64	39	.61
Prov cost to total cost ratio	23	.42	36	.39	33	.36	39	.39
Total support staff FTE/phy	41	4.70	65	5.63	51	5.71	56	4.87

Table 5.11e: Surgery/Anesthesia Procedure Data (outside the practice)

	Eastern section		Midwest section		Southern section		Western section	
	Count	Median	Count	Median	Count	Median	Count	Median
Gross charges/procedure	19	$847.42	39	$992.98	33	$865.66	34	$685.96
Total cost/procedure	17	$357.20	35	$418.77	29	$374.45	31	$327.34
Operating cost/procedure	17	$113.22	34	$158.72	28	$146.06	31	$125.28
Provider cost/procedure	18	$227.83	35	$270.67	29	$229.28	31	$197.93
Procedures/patient	15	.11	22	.15	17	.24	24	.10
Gross charges/patient	15	$47.74	20	$106.82	17	$212.55	24	$73.40
Procedures/physician	20	205	39	215	33	210	35	153
Gross charges/physician	19	$150,889	39	$224,922	35	$200,753	35	$120,595
Procedures/provider	19	179	37	171	29	205	33	154
Gross charges/provider	18	$123,234	37	$160,402	31	$161,123	33	$103,856
Gross charge to total cost ratio	17	2.35	35	2.14	29	2.53	31	2.24
Oper cost to total cost ratio	17	.38	34	.40	28	.39	31	.40
Prov cost to total cost ratio	17	.62	35	.60	29	.60	31	.60
Total support staff FTE/phy	41	4.70	65	5.63	51	5.71	56	4.87

Multispecialty — by Geographic Section, Not Hospital or IDS Owned
(Procedure and Charge Data)

Table 5.11f: Clinical Laboratory/Pathology Procedure Data

	Eastern section		Midwest section		Southern section		Western section	
	Count	Median	Count	Median	Count	Median	Count	Median
Gross charges/procedure	27	**$25.93**	40	**$29.49**	40	**$31.40**	45	**$26.76**
Total cost/procedure	24	**$17.81**	36	**$24.60**	35	**$23.20**	41	**$21.64**
Operating cost/procedure	24	$11.49	35	$14.71	33	$15.76	41	$14.68
Provider cost/procedure	25	$6.19	36	$8.66	36	$8.04	41	$6.92
Procedures/patient	22	2.27	23	2.76	22	2.43	28	1.71
Gross charges/patient	22	$57.87	24	$77.49	22	$86.59	28	$51.21
Procedures/physician	28	3,502	40	4,187	40	3,502	46	3,176
Gross charges/physician	27	$98,182	42	$136,113	42	$114,669	45	$93,882
Procedures/provider	27	3,045	38	3,255	35	3,322	41	2,809
Gross charges/provider	26	$80,504	39	$104,255	37	$102,399	41	$75,158
Gross charge to total cost ratio	24	1.41	36	1.22	35	1.41	41	1.29
Oper cost to total cost ratio	24	.64	35	.66	33	.67	41	.66
Prov cost to total cost ratio	24	.36	36	.34	35	.33	41	.34
Total support staff FTE/phy	**41**	**4.70**	**65**	**5.63**	**51**	**5.71**	**56**	**4.87**

Table 5.11g: Diagnostic Radiology and Imaging Procedure Data

	Eastern section		Midwest section		Southern section		Western section	
	Count	Median	Count	Median	Count	Median	Count	Median
Gross charges/procedure	22	**$163.27**	44	**$137.70**	39	**$146.17**	43	**$147.97**
Total cost/procedure	19	**$104.80**	39	**$120.31**	34	**$101.27**	40	**$104.34**
Operating cost/procedure	19	$69.70	38	$78.83	33	$79.01	40	$69.76
Provider cost/procedure	21	$44.09	39	$46.15	35	$38.31	40	$33.54
Procedures/patient	19	.20	25	.47	21	.42	28	.28
Gross charges/patient	17	$18.15	25	$64.73	21	$79.22	28	$44.49
Procedures/physician	24	407	44	662	39	687	44	558
Gross charges/physician	22	$47,218	44	$101,426	41	$113,599	43	$77,519
Procedures/provider	23	255	41	508	35	615	41	481
Gross charges/provider	21	$39,339	41	$88,670	37	$108,778	40	$67,630
Gross charge to total cost ratio	20	1.33	39	1.24	34	1.38	40	1.25
Oper cost to total cost ratio	20	.65	38	.65	33	.65	40	.67
Prov cost to total cost ratio	20	.35	39	.35	34	.34	40	.33
Total support staff FTE/phy	**41**	**4.70**	**65**	**5.63**	**51**	**5.71**	**56**	**4.87**

Table 5.11h: Nonprocedural Gross Charge Data

	Eastern section		Midwest section		Southern section		Western section	
	Count	Median	Count	Median	Count	Median	Count	Median
Gross charges/patient	21	$28.15	21	$35.81	21	$104.67	25	$22.73
Nonproc gross charges/physician	24	$53,990	39	$63,487	38	$99,584	41	$42,976
Gross charges/provider	23	$42,294	37	$52,306	34	$103,391	37	$34,977
Total support staff FTE/phy	**41**	**4.70**	**65**	**5.63**	**51**	**5.71**	**56**	**4.87**

Multispecialty — Practices with 50 or Less FTE Physicians, Not Hospital or IDS Owned

Table 6.1: Staffing and Practice Data

	10 FTE or less		11 to 25 FTE		26 to 50 FTE	
	Count	**Median**	**Count**	**Median**	**Count**	**Median**
Total provider FTE	**35**	**9.10**	**53**	**20.50**	**43**	**46.25**
Total physician FTE	43	6.50	62	18.00	45	38.00
Total nonphysician provider FTE	35	2.00	53	3.00	43	6.91
Total support staff FTE	**43**	**34.00**	**62**	**87.80**	**45**	**189.66**
Number of branch clinics	20	2	44	3	35	5
Square footage of all facilities	42	14,720	58	31,108	39	73,046

Table 6.2: Accounts Receivable Data, Collection Percentages and Financial Ratios

	10 FTE or less		11 to 25 FTE		26 to 50 FTE	
	Count	**Median**	**Count**	**Median**	**Count**	**Median**
Total AR/physician	**39**	**$107,888**	**55**	**$107,104**	**43**	**$157,277**
Total AR/provider	**33**	**$81,550**	**47**	**$87,998**	**41**	**$131,995**
0-30 days in AR	40	53.26%	55	53.49%	43	50.98%
31-60 days in AR	40	15.63%	55	13.40%	43	14.71%
61-90 days in AR	40	7.80%	55	7.50%	43	7.39%
91-120 days in AR	40	5.74%	55	5.02%	43	4.94%
120+ days in AR	40	15.88%	55	18.59%	43	18.63%
Re-aged: 0-30 days in AR	10	52.52%	16	57.84%	19	52.00%
Re-aged: 31-60 days in AR	10	15.53%	16	12.29%	19	14.71%
Re-aged: 61-90 days in AR	10	7.30%	16	8.91%	19	6.63%
Re-aged: 91-120 days in AR	10	5.28%	16	6.08%	19	4.72%
Re-aged: 120+ days in AR	10	15.45%	16	15.03%	19	18.63%
Not re-aged: 0-30 days in AR	29	52.67%	35	46.92%	23	50.98%
Not re-aged: 31-60 days in AR	29	15.58%	35	14.53%	23	13.45%
Not re-aged: 61-90 days in AR	29	7.89%	35	7.50%	23	8.00%
Not re-aged: 91-120 days in AR	29	5.90%	35	4.63%	23	5.31%
Not re-aged: 120+ days in AR	29	15.94%	35	22.04%	23	16.48%
Months gross FFS charges in AR	32	1.59	51	1.54	35	1.65
Days gross FFS charges in AR	32	48.29	51	46.72	35	50.15
Gross FFS collection %	34	65.16%	57	63.93%	37	60.92%
Adjusted FFS collection %	32	97.92%	53	97.73%	36	97.59%
Gross FFS + cap collection %	12	66.38%	17	71.56%	14	61.97%
Net cap rev % of gross cap chrg	11	72.47%	14	83.93%	10	94.20%
Current ratio	17	2.49	38	2.15	29	1.25
Tot asset turnover ratio	17	5.31	38	5.05	29	5.16
Debt to equity ratio	17	.93	38	1.41	29	3.06
Debt ratio	17	48.26%	38	58.44%	29	75.40%
Return on total assets	15	19.22%	34	2.57%	26	3.22%
Return on equity	15	44.41%	34	5.87%	26	16.91%

Table 6.3: Breakout of Total Gross Charges by Type of Payer

	10 FTE or less		11 to 25 FTE		26 to 50 FTE	
	Count	**Median**	**Count**	**Median**	**Count**	**Median**
Medicare: fee-for-service	40	22.00%	57	29.00%	41	28.00%
Medicare: managed care FFS	40	.00%	57	.00%	41	.00%
Medicare: capitation	40	.00%	57	.00%	41	.00%
Medicaid: fee-for-service	40	4.92%	57	5.00%	41	6.00%
Medicaid: managed care FFS	40	.00%	57	.00%	41	.00%
Medicaid: capitation	40	.00%	57	.00%	41	.00%
Commercial: fee-for-service	40	27.24%	57	40.00%	41	39.28%
Commercial: managed care FFS	40	.00%	57	1.40%	41	.00%
Commercial: capitation	40	.00%	57	.00%	41	.00%
Workers' compensation	40	1.00%	57	1.00%	41	.82%
Charity care and prof courtesy	40	.00%	57	.00%	41	.00%
Self-pay	40	4.75%	57	4.00%	41	3.00%
Other federal government payers	40	.00%	57	.00%	41	.00%

Multispecialty — Practices with 50 or Less FTE Physicians, Not Hospital or IDS Owned
(per FTE Physician)

Table 6.4a: Staffing, RVUs, Patients, Procedures and Square Footage

	10 FTE or less		11 to 25 FTE		26 to 50 FTE	
	Count	Median	Count	Median	Count	Median
Total provider FTE/physician	35	1.36	53	1.18	43	1.17
Prim care phy/physician	32	1.00	56	.84	39	.53
Nonsurg phy/physician	10	.21	28	.15	37	.21
Surg spec phy/physician	9	*	31	.16	36	.22
Total NPP FTE/physician	35	.36	53	.18	43	.17
Total support staff FTE/phy	43	5.15	62	4.91	45	5.33
Total empl support staff FTE	34	5.41	55	4.87	40	5.35
General administrative	33	.22	55	.25	38	.27
Patient accounting	33	.83	53	.65	39	.76
General accounting	21	.14	40	.09	38	.08
Managed care administrative	12	.14	20	.09	16	.07
Information technology	9	*	24	.08	34	.08
Housekeeping, maint, security	12	.27	30	.07	30	.06
Medical receptionists	33	.92	55	1.00	38	.97
Med secretaries,transcribers	24	.32	40	.17	35	.21
Medical records	27	.36	47	.36	39	.43
Other admin support	15	.32	27	.09	24	.08
*Total administrative supp staff	23	3.02	25	3.01	26	3.24
Registered Nurses	27	.60	45	.30	36	.39
Licensed Practical Nurses	27	.70	46	.33	31	.56
Med assistants, nurse aides	28	.72	52	.81	33	.68
*Total clinical supp staff	32	1.67	47	1.52	35	1.63
Clinical laboratory	22	.45	44	.38	34	.35
Radiology and imaging	23	.24	41	.22	38	.34
Other medical support serv	9	*	22	.18	30	.20
*Total ancillary supp staff	16	.41	24	.86	29	.97
Tot contracted supp staff	17	.23	18	.11	21	.04
Tot RVU/physician	15	11,668	18	9,805	17	11,517
Physician work RVU/physician	12	5,713	18	5,084	17	5,609
Patients/physician	18	2,497	29	1,862	23	1,563
Tot procedures/physician	29	11,923	48	12,154	33	12,550
Square feet/physician	42	2,036	58	1,877	39	2,099

*See pages 260 and 261 for definition.

Table 6.4b: Charges and Revenue

	10 FTE or less		11 to 25 FTE		26 to 50 FTE	
	Count	Median	Count	Median	Count	Median
Net fee-for-service revenue	34	$543,406	58	$521,816	38	$671,265
Gross FFS charges	35	$838,835	57	$836,855	37	$1,116,992
Adjustments to FFS charges	31	$265,252	51	$265,996	36	$405,439
Adjusted FFS charges	32	$595,762	53	$548,236	36	$723,520
Bad debts due to FFS activity	29	$10,807	49	$10,490	32	$16,813
Net capitation revenue	12	$30,110	17	$37,181	14	$15,141
Gross capitation charges	11	$42,451	14	$66,318	10	$37,187
Capitation revenue	12	$30,110	17	$37,181	12	$17,351
Purch serv for cap patients	1	*	2	*	2	*
Net other medical revenue	19	$14,675	31	$12,285	32	$12,081
Gross rev from other activity	18	$18,276	31	$12,349	32	$14,528
Other medical revenue	17	$7,894	21	$8,188	24	$6,752
Rev from sale of goods/services	10	$10,326	18	$15,597	21	$14,663
Cost of sales	2	*	9	*	14	$9,903
Total gross charges	42	$800,560	61	$837,210	41	$1,026,723
Total medical revenue	43	$580,500	62	$551,930	45	$685,402

Multispecialty — Practices with 50 or Less FTE Physicians, Not Hospital or IDS Owned (per FTE Physician)

Table 6.4c: Operating Cost

	10 FTE or less		11 to 25 FTE		26 to 50 FTE	
	Count	Median	Count	Median	Count	Median
Total support staff cost/phy	43	$171,488	62	$161,035	45	$187,179
Total empl supp staff cost/phy	34	$144,460	59	$130,576	40	$156,690
General administrative	32	$13,038	57	$12,977	38	$15,698
Patient accounting	33	$18,526	55	$18,243	39	$17,821
General accounting	21	$4,871	42	$2,747	38	$2,667
Managed care administrative	12	$4,513	20	$2,130	16	$2,027
Information technology	9	*	26	$3,102	34	$3,373
Housekeeping, maint, security	12	$4,119	32	$1,544	30	$1,623
Medical receptionists	32	$19,996	56	$19,251	38	$19,420
Med secretaries,transcribers	23	$7,391	41	$5,534	35	$6,088
Medical records	26	$7,581	49	$6,779	39	$7,932
Other admin support	15	$7,654	27	$1,981	24	$1,688
*Total administrative supp staff	18	$74,729	26	$74,989	27	$85,339
Registered Nurses	26	$16,207	47	$12,999	36	$12,914
Licensed Practical Nurses	26	$19,807	45	$10,740	31	$15,961
Med assistants, nurse aides	27	$18,317	52	$17,702	32	$15,163
*Total clinical supp staff	30	$48,053	46	$40,964	34	$46,817
Clinical laboratory	21	$15,611	45	$11,370	34	$10,016
Radiology and imaging	22	$8,218	43	$7,707	38	$10,879
Other medical support serv	9	*	24	$6,211	30	$6,310
*Total ancillary supp staff	17	$27,221	34	$23,424	32	$30,134
Total empl supp staff benefits	42	$31,526	59	$31,382	44	$38,528
Tot contracted supp staff	19	$4,083	28	$2,056	24	$1,604
Total general operating cost	43	$156,230	62	$159,538	45	$183,973
Information technology	34	$9,531	58	$7,785	40	$9,854
Medical and surgical supply	34	$20,448	58	$24,209	40	$32,065
Building and occupancy	34	$37,253	58	$37,741	40	$43,450
Furniture and equipment	30	$3,981	49	$5,096	37	$11,326
Admin supplies and services	33	$11,083	57	$9,374	40	$10,666
Prof liability insurance	40	$9,590	61	$13,045	45	$14,424
Other insurance premiums	32	$1,384	57	$1,146	37	$1,349
Outside professional fees	32	$3,929	57	$2,977	39	$4,115
Promotion and marketing	33	$2,080	56	$1,934	40	$2,546
Clinical laboratory	28	$22,573	52	$15,155	36	$15,775
Radiology and imaging	24	$5,557	44	$4,200	37	$13,721
Other ancillary services	11	$1,438	15	$1,109	22	$3,826
Billing purchased services	19	$2,158	33	$2,104	26	$1,683
Management fees paid to MSO	2	*	5	*	2	*
Misc operating cost	34	$7,202	57	$6,436	39	$9,579
Cost allocated to prac from par	0	*	0	*	0	*
Total operating cost	43	$322,459	62	$323,429	45	$379,730

*See pages 260 and 261 for definition.

Multispecialty — Practices with 50 or Less FTE Physicians, Not Hospital or IDS Owned (per FTE Physician)

Table 6.4d: Provider Cost

	10 FTE or less		11 to 25 FTE		26 to 50 FTE	
	Count	Median	Count	Median	Count	Median
Total med rev after oper cost	43	$211,486	62	$222,980	45	$281,563
Total provider cost/physician	43	$201,663	62	$225,235	45	$278,722
Total NPP cost/physician	36	$28,221	57	$14,965	43	$16,396
Nonphysician provider comp	30	$22,226	55	$12,557	39	$12,433
Nonphysician prov benefit cost	28	$5,186	50	$2,353	35	$2,642
Provider consultant cost	8	*	18	$6,823	17	$15,767
Total physician cost/physician	43	$178,027	62	$206,857	45	$255,721
Total phy compensation	35	$149,822	59	$176,425	40	$221,114
Total phy benefit cost	35	$26,907	58	$28,197	38	$40,783

Table 6.4e: Net Income or Loss

	10 FTE or less		11 to 25 FTE		26 to 50 FTE	
	Count	Median	Count	Median	Count	Median
Total cost	43	$567,771	62	$541,336	45	$669,917
Net nonmedical revenue	25	$1,733	45	$3,142	41	$2,742
Nonmedical revenue	19	$2,491	42	$4,282	37	$2,742
Fin support for oper costs	0	*	1	*	2	*
Goodwill amortization	2	*	4	*	3	*
Nonmedical cost	9	*	19	$1,385	19	$1,580
Net inc, prac with fin sup	0	*	1	*	2	*
Net inc, prac w/o fin sup	40	$12,941	57	$26	39	$5,534
Net inc, excl fin supp (all prac)	40	$12,941	58	$21	41	$5,534

Table 6.4f: Assets and Liabilities

	10 FTE or less		11 to 25 FTE		26 to 50 FTE	
	Count	Median	Count	Median	Count	Median
Total assets	18	$112,638	39	$110,835	30	$136,168
Current assets	19	$80,084	40	$64,735	30	$52,547
Noncurrent assets	19	$54,101	40	$28,377	30	$40,697
Total liabilities	19	$47,937	40	$46,943	30	$86,661
Current liabilities	19	$23,165	40	$26,851	30	$47,054
Noncurrent liabilities	19	$24,474	40	$14,402	30	$17,136
Working capital	19	$23,899	40	$26,008	30	$9,769
Total net worth	19	$65,742	40	$37,744	30	$26,684
Total support staff FTE/phy	43	5.15	62	4.91	45	5.33

Multispecialty — Practices with 50 or Less FTE Physicians, Not Hospital or IDS Owned
(as a % of Total Medical Revenue)

Table 6.5a: Charges and Revenue

	10 FTE or less		11 to 25 FTE		26 to 50 FTE	
	Count	Median	Count	Median	Count	Median
Net fee-for-service revenue	34	97.81%	58	98.89%	38	98.15%
Net capitation revenue	12	8.68%	17	8.33%	14	2.31%
Net other medical revenue	19	2.40%	31	2.05%	32	1.60%
Total gross charges	**43**	**151.03%**	**61**	**146.49%**	**45**	**162.25%**

Table 6.5b: Operating Cost

	10 FTE or less		11 to 25 FTE		26 to 50 FTE	
	Count	Median	Count	Median	Count	Median
Total support staff cost	**43**	**31.83%**	**62**	**30.29%**	**45**	**28.64%**
Total empl support staff cost	34	26.06%	59	25.03%	40	22.73%
General administrative	32	2.96%	57	2.27%	38	2.34%
Patient accounting	33	3.37%	55	3.18%	39	2.90%
General accounting	21	.83%	42	.51%	38	.38%
Managed care administrative	12	.83%	20	.40%	16	.28%
Information technology	9	*	26	.53%	34	.42%
Housekeeping, maint, security	12	.81%	32	.28%	30	.21%
Medical receptionists	32	3.70%	56	3.44%	38	2.83%
Med secretaries,transcribers	23	1.16%	41	1.04%	35	.95%
Medical records	26	1.32%	49	1.28%	39	1.17%
Other admin support	15	1.28%	27	.38%	24	.24%
*Total administrative supp staff	18	15.19%	26	12.98%	27	12.50%
Registered Nurses	26	3.05%	47	2.03%	36	1.93%
Licensed Practical Nurses	26	2.95%	45	1.90%	31	2.07%
Med assistants, nurse aides	27	3.57%	52	3.21%	32	2.21%
*Total clinical supp staff	30	9.02%	46	7.55%	34	6.77%
Clinical laboratory	21	2.06%	45	2.13%	34	1.35%
Radiology and imaging	22	1.48%	43	1.41%	38	1.69%
Other medical support serv	9	*	24	1.00%	30	.89%
*Total ancillary supp staff	17	3.72%	34	3.78%	32	3.76%
Total empl supp staff benefits	42	6.07%	59	5.83%	44	5.71%
Tot contracted supp staff	19	1.07%	28	.37%	24	.29%
Total general operating cost	**43**	**27.37%**	**62**	**28.69%**	**45**	**27.10%**
Information technology	34	1.73%	58	1.47%	40	1.40%
Medical and surgical supply	34	3.70%	58	4.27%	40	4.56%
Building and occupancy	34	7.75%	58	6.80%	40	5.84%
Furniture and equipment	30	.73%	49	.92%	37	1.60%
Admin supplies and services	34	2.07%	57	1.78%	40	1.56%
Prof liability insurance	40	1.96%	61	2.22%	45	2.14%
Other insurance premiums	32	.26%	55	.22%	37	.19%
Outside professional fees	32	.69%	57	.53%	39	.56%
Promotion and marketing	33	.42%	56	.32%	40	.40%
Clinical laboratory	28	3.86%	52	2.62%	36	2.21%
Radiology and imaging	26	1.05%	45	.86%	37	1.91%
Other ancillary services	11	.28%	15	.15%	22	.51%
Billing purchased services	19	.41%	33	.37%	26	.21%
Management fees paid to MSO	3	*	6	*	2	*
Misc operating cost	34	1.15%	57	1.33%	39	1.33%
Cost allocated to prac from par	0	*	0	*	0	*
Total operating cost	**43**	**61.50%**	**62**	**57.98%**	**45**	**57.41%**

*See pages 260 and 261 for definition.

Multispecialty — Practices with 50 or Less FTE Physicians, Not Hospital or IDS Owned
(as a % of Total Medical Revenue)

Table 6.5c: Provider Cost

	10 FTE or less		11 to 25 FTE		26 to 50 FTE	
	Count	Median	Count	Median	Count	Median
Total med rev after oper cost	43	38.59%	62	41.91%	45	42.59%
Total provider cost	43	39.07%	62	42.77%	45	41.92%
Total NPP cost	36	4.76%	57	2.88%	43	2.43%
Nonphysician provider comp	30	3.85%	55	2.36%	39	1.72%
Nonphysician prov benefit cost	28	.86%	50	.38%	35	.39%
Provider consultant cost	8	*	18	1.27%	17	2.07%
Total physician cost	43	34.91%	62	39.21%	45	38.24%
Total phy compensation	35	28.79%	59	33.42%	40	33.74%
Total phy benefit cost	35	4.71%	58	5.33%	38	5.80%

Table 6.5d: Net Income or Loss

	10 FTE or less		11 to 25 FTE		26 to 50 FTE	
	Count	Median	Count	Median	Count	Median
Total cost	43	99.35%	62	100.05%	45	100.23%
Net nonmedical revenue	25	.21%	45	.60%	41	.40%
Nonmedical revenue	19	.40%	42	.75%	37	.40%
Fin support for oper costs	0	*	1	*	2	*
Goodwill amortization	2	*	4	*	3	*
Nonmedical cost	9	*	19	.25%	19	.21%
Net inc, prac with fin sup	0	*	1	*	2	*
Net inc, prac w/o fin sup	40	2.40%	57	.00%	39	.62%
Net inc, excl fin supp (all prac)	40	2.40%	58	.00%	41	.62%

Table 6.5e: Assets and Liabilities

	10 FTE or less		11 to 25 FTE		26 to 50 FTE	
	Count	Median	Count	Median	Count	Median
Total assets	19	18.82%	40	19.60%	30	20.18%
Current assets	19	13.22%	40	9.89%	30	11.84%
Noncurrent assets	19	9.41%	40	4.90%	30	5.63%
Total liabilities	19	9.08%	40	8.31%	30	13.46%
Current liabilities	19	5.86%	40	4.62%	30	6.98%
Noncurrent liabilities	19	3.91%	40	2.23%	30	2.43%
Working capital	19	5.82%	40	3.86%	30	1.55%
Total net worth	19	10.48%	40	6.84%	30	4.18%

Multispecialty — Practices with 50 or Less FTE Physicians, Not Hospital or IDS Owned
(per FTE Provider)

Table 6.6a: Staffing, RVUs, Patients, Procedures and Square Footage

	10 FTE or less		11 to 25 FTE		26 to 50 FTE	
	Count	Median	Count	Median	Count	Median
Total physician FTE/provider	35	.73	53	.84	43	.86
Prim care phy/provider	27	.69	48	.64	38	.43
Nonsurg phy/provider	7	*	24	.12	36	.19
Surg spec phy/provider	8	*	25	.12	35	.18
Total NPP FTE/provider	35	.27	53	.16	43	.14
Total support staff FTE/prov	35	3.86	53	4.17	43	4.52
Total empl supp staff FTE/prov	29	4.01	47	4.06	39	4.59
General administrative	29	.16	47	.20	38	.24
Patient accounting	29	.62	45	.53	39	.66
General accounting	20	.11	37	.07	38	.06
Managed care administrative	9	*	18	.08	16	.05
Information technology	8	*	21	.07	34	.07
Housekeeping, maint, security	11	.19	27	.06	30	.05
Medical receptionists	28	.78	47	.79	38	.82
Med secretaries,transcribers	22	.22	34	.17	35	.20
Medical records	24	.27	41	.33	39	.36
Other admin support	13	.21	25	.07	24	.07
*Total administrative supp staff	21	2.39	22	2.46	26	2.84
Registered Nurses	22	.39	39	.19	36	.34
Licensed Practical Nurses	23	.54	39	.27	31	.51
Med assistants, nurse aides	23	.57	45	.70	33	.53
*Total clinical supp staff	26	1.30	41	1.21	35	1.34
Clinical laboratory	20	.32	39	.32	34	.30
Radiology and imaging	20	.16	38	.18	38	.26
Other medical support serv	8	*	20	.10	30	.15
*Total ancillary supp staff	14	.29	22	.67	29	.80
Tot contracted supp staff	13	.21	16	.10	21	.04
Tot RVU/provider	11	9,540	16	7,847	17	8,538
Physician work RVU/provider	9	*	16	4,111	17	4,611
Patients/provider	17	1,816	25	1,511	22	1,256
Tot procedures/provider	24	9,437	42	10,413	32	10,289
Square feet/provider	34	1,606	50	1,466	39	1,674
Total support staff FTE/phy	43	5.15	62	4.91	45	5.33

*See pages 260 and 261 for definition.

Table 6.6b: Charges, Revenue and Cost

	10 FTE or less		11 to 25 FTE		26 to 50 FTE	
	Count	Median	Count	Median	Count	Median
Total gross charges	35	$598,248	52	$687,333	43	$889,718
Total medical revenue	35	$414,787	53	$447,319	43	$557,913
Net fee-for-service revenue	28	$404,644	50	$422,545	37	$541,988
Net capitation revenue	9	*	14	$32,537	14	$11,577
Net other medical revenue	17	$15,209	26	$10,394	32	$10,661
Total support staff cost/prov	35	$131,068	53	$131,442	43	$164,609
Total general operating cost	35	$117,854	53	$123,029	43	$156,924
Total operating cost	35	$243,990	53	$263,290	43	$311,290
Total med rev after oper cost	35	$160,105	53	$180,791	43	$240,435
Total provider cost/provider	35	$150,160	53	$180,983	43	$230,387
Total NPP cost/provider	35	$20,174	53	$12,385	43	$13,439
Provider consultant cost	6	*	15	$5,983	17	$13,018
Total physician cost/provider	35	$132,195	53	$167,663	43	$216,755
Total phy compensation	29	$114,726	51	$137,683	39	$181,026
Total phy benefit cost	29	$16,207	50	$22,359	37	$34,458
Total cost	35	$406,951	53	$448,953	43	$549,381
Net nonmedical revenue	21	$813	38	$2,795	39	$2,010
Net inc, prac with fin sup	0	*	1	*	2	*
Net inc, prac w/o fin sup	32	$10,172	48	$36	37	$3,094
Net inc, excl fin supp (all prac)	32	$10,172	49	$22	39	$3,094
Total support staff FTE/phy	43	5.15	62	4.91	45	5.33

Multispecialty — Practices with 50 or Less FTE Physicians, Not Hospital or IDS Owned (per Square Foot)

Table 6.7a: Staffing, RVUs, Patients and Procedures

	10 FTE or less		11 to 25 FTE		26 to 50 FTE	
	Count	Median	Count	Median	Count	Median
Total prov FTE/10,000 sq ft	34	6.23	50	6.82	39	5.97
Total phy FTE/10,000 sq ft	42	4.91	58	5.33	39	4.76
Prim care phy/10,000 sq ft	31	4.61	53	4.24	34	2.25
Nonsurg phy/10,000 sq ft	10	1.18	27	.85	32	1.11
Surg spec phy/10,000 sq ft	8	*	30	.90	31	1.18
Total NPP FTE/10,000 sq ft	34	1.51	50	.94	39	.88
Total supp stf FTE/10,000 sq ft	42	24.70	58	26.72	39	26.60
Total empl supp stf/10,000 sq ft	33	23.55	52	26.72	35	25.90
General administrative	32	1.23	53	1.26	34	1.38
Patient accounting	32	3.40	52	3.22	35	3.84
General accounting	20	.52	39	.45	34	.36
Managed care administrative	12	.96	20	.40	14	.34
Information technology	9	*	23	.35	30	.42
Housekeeping, maint, security	11	.74	28	.33	28	.27
Medical receptionists	32	4.23	52	5.14	34	4.04
Med secretaries,transcribers	23	1.15	38	1.27	32	1.04
Medical records	26	1.68	44	2.16	35	1.99
Other admin support	14	1.15	25	.40	24	.38
*Total administrative supp staff	23	12.65	23	15.42	25	15.03
Registered Nurses	26	2.65	43	1.57	32	2.01
Licensed Practical Nurses	26	2.91	43	1.65	29	2.63
Med assistants, nurse aides	28	3.41	49	4.28	31	3.53
*Total clinical supp staff	32	7.96	45	7.66	33	7.41
Clinical laboratory	21	1.52	43	1.91	31	1.50
Radiology and imaging	23	1.15	38	1.21	34	1.37
Other medical support serv	9	*	21	.82	27	.85
*Total ancillary supp staff	16	1.81	23	3.38	27	3.98
Tot contracted supp staff	17	.83	18	.63	20	.16
Tot RVU/sq ft	15	5.71	17	4.84	15	6.41
Physician work RVU/sq ft	12	2.75	16	2.67	16	2.81
Patients/sq ft	18	1.20	27	.98	20	.81
Tot procedures/sq ft	29	5.89	46	6.08	29	5.74
Total support staff FTE/phy	43	5.15	62	4.91	45	5.33

*See pages 260 and 261 for definition.

Table 6.7b: Charges, Revenue and Cost

	10 FTE or less		11 to 25 FTE		26 to 50 FTE	
	Count	Median	Count	Median	Count	Median
Total gross charges	42	$371.79	58	$455.70	39	$556.33
Total medical revenue	42	$256.58	58	$301.71	39	$352.01
Net fee-for-service revenue	33	$254.90	54	$274.04	33	$321.50
Net capitation revenue	11	$22.20	16	$23.93	11	$7.86
Net other medical revenue	18	$6.02	29	$6.61	29	$4.26
Total support staff cost/sq ft	42	$85.81	58	$90.26	39	$97.12
Total general operating cost	42	$76.02	58	$86.24	39	$96.35
Total operating cost	42	$166.65	58	$171.33	39	$199.29
Total med rev after oper cost	42	$109.45	58	$117.85	39	$139.24
Total provider cost/sq ft	42	$101.10	58	$123.09	39	$149.13
Total NPP cost/sq ft	35	$11.12	53	$8.33	39	$7.36
Provider consultant cost	8	*	18	$4.28	15	$6.66
Total physician cost/sq ft	42	$93.36	58	$105.00	39	$137.01
Total phy compensation	34	$81.71	55	$91.47	35	$117.03
Total phy benefit cost	34	$11.44	54	$14.41	34	$19.50
Total cost	42	$264.07	58	$301.05	39	$353.72
Net nonmedical revenue/sq ft	24	$.70	42	$1.38	35	$1.10
Net inc, prac with fin sup	0	*	1	*	1	*
Net inc, prac w/o fin sup	40	$5.22	53	$.01	34	$2.36
Net inc, excl fin supp (all prac)	40	$5.22	54	$.01	35	$1.93
Total support staff FTE/phy	43	5.15	62	4.91	45	5.33

Multispecialty — Practices with 50 or Less FTE Physicians, Not Hospital or IDS Owned
(per Total RVU)

Table 6.8a: Staffing, Patients, Procedures and Square Footage

	10 FTE or less		11 to 25 FTE		26 to 50 FTE	
	Count	Median	Count	Median	Count	Median
Total prov FTE/10,000 tot RVU	11	**1.05**	16	**1.27**	17	**1.17**
Total phy FTE/10,000 tot RVU	15	.86	18	1.02	17	.87
Prim care phy/10,000 tot RVU	13	.75	18	.85	14	.51
Nonsurg phy/10,000 tot RVU	4	*	9	*	13	.18
Surg spec phy/10,000 tot RVU	3	*	8	*	13	.21
Total NPP FTE/10,000 tot RVU	11	.22	16	.19	17	.20
Total supp stf FTE/10,000 tot RVU	15	**4.68**	18	**5.31**	17	**4.09**
Tot empl supp stf/10,000 tot RVU	14	4.35	18	4.73	15	4.15
General administrative	13	.21	17	.21	15	.21
Patient accounting	14	.52	17	.61	15	.55
General accounting	8	*	13	.08	15	.07
Managed care administrative	6	*	7	*	8	*
Information technology	2	*	6	*	14	.07
Housekeeping, maint, security	5	*	10	.05	13	.07
Medical receptionists	13	.64	17	.96	15	.66
Med secretaries,transcribers	9	*	15	.25	14	.21
Medical records	11	.19	16	.39	15	.53
Other admin support	8	*	9	*	8	*
***Total administrative supp staff**	9	*	6	*	13	**2.22**
Registered Nurses	13	.55	16	.33	14	.49
Licensed Practical Nurses	11	.58	17	.24	10	.25
Med assistants, nurse aides	12	.62	17	.70	12	.71
***Total clinical supp staff**	13	**2.10**	15	**1.31**	14	**1.21**
Clinical laboratory	7	*	16	.30	15	.27
Radiology and imaging	8	*	13	.20	14	.29
Other medical support serv	5	*	7	*	12	.15
***Total ancillary supp staff**	4	*	6	*	12	**.78**
Tot contracted supp staff	8	*	5	*	9	*
Physician work RVU/tot RVU	11	.51	14	.50	15	.48
Patients/tot RVU	10	.25	14	.20	13	.13
Tot procedures/tot RVU	13	.93	16	1.27	14	1.01
Square feet/tot RVU	15	.18	17	.21	15	.16
Total support staff FTE/phy	43	**5.15**	62	**4.91**	45	**5.33**

*See pages 260 and 261 for definition.

Table 6.8b: Charges, Revenue and Cost

	10 FTE or less		11 to 25 FTE		26 to 50 FTE	
	Count	Median	Count	Median	Count	Median
Total gross charges	15	**$67.76**	18	**$89.47**	17	**$91.54**
Total medical revenue	15	**$45.95**	18	**$52.26**	17	**$56.11**
Net fee-for-service revenue	13	$43.82	18	$47.82	15	$52.02
Net capitation revenue	4	*	9	*	5	*
Net other medical revenue	7	*	13	$1.93	15	$.83
Total supp staff cost/tot RVU	15	**$15.50**	18	**$16.46**	17	**$16.01**
Total general operating cost	15	**$13.40**	18	**$15.12**	17	**$13.66**
Total operating cost	15	**$27.20**	18	**$33.69**	17	**$28.04**
Total med rev after oper cost	15	**$17.10**	18	**$23.37**	17	**$22.83**
Total provider cost/tot RVU	15	**$17.35**	18	**$23.12**	17	**$24.11**
Total NPP cost/tot RVU	11	$1.70	17	$1.37	17	$1.90
Provider consultant cost	1	*	7	*	7	*
Total physician cost/tot RVU	15	$16.94	18	$21.68	17	$21.39
Total phy compensation	14	$13.45	18	$18.20	15	$19.23
Total phy benefit cost	14	$2.12	18	$2.71	15	$2.83
Total cost	13	**$62.68**	16	**$64.35**	14	**$57.34**
Net nonmedical revenue	5	*	14	$.38	15	$.25
Net inc, prac with fin sup	0	*	1	*	0	*
Net inc, prac w/o fin sup	15	$.44	17	$.39	15	$.67
Net inc, excl fin supp (all prac)	15	$.44	18	$.20	15	$.67
Total support staff FTE/phy	43	**5.15**	62	**4.91**	45	**5.33**

Multispecialty — Practices with 50 or Less FTE Physicians, Not Hospital or IDS Owned
(per Work RVU)

Table 6.9a: Staffing, Patients, Procedures and Square Footage

	10 FTE or less		11 to 25 FTE		26 to 50 FTE	
	Count	Median	Count	Median	Count	Median
Total prov FTE/10,000 work RVU	9	*	16	2.44	17	2.17
Tot phy FTE/10,000 work RVU	12	1.75	18	1.97	17	1.78
Prim care phy/10,000 work RVU	11	1.69	18	1.82	14	1.09
Nonsurg phy/10,000 work RVU	3	*	7	*	13	.33
Surg spec phy/10,000 work RVU	2	*	7	*	12	.34
Total NPP FTE/10,000 work RVU	9	*	16	.36	17	.37
Total supp stf FTE/10,000 wrk RVU	12	9.35	18	9.49	17	9.26
Tot empl supp stf/10,000 work RVU	12	9.28	18	9.33	14	10.03
General administrative	11	.48	17	.37	14	.45
Patient accounting	12	1.16	16	1.32	14	1.24
General accounting	7	*	14	.12	14	.15
Managed care administrative	5	*	6	*	7	*
Information technology	2	*	7	*	13	.19
Housekeeping, maint, security	4	*	12	.12	11	.13
Medical receptionists	11	1.40	18	1.90	14	1.62
Med secretaries,transcribers	8	*	13	.35	13	.52
Medical records	9	*	17	.68	14	.82
Other admin support	6	*	11	.15	8	*
*Total administrative supp staff	6	*	9	*	12	5.48
Registered Nurses	12	1.00	16	.63	12	.97
Licensed Practical Nurses	10	1.32	16	.64	9	*
Med assistants, nurse aides	10	1.15	16	1.37	12	1.45
*Total clinical supp staff	10	4.05	15	2.64	13	2.58
Clinical laboratory	6	*	14	.60	14	.62
Radiology and imaging	6	*	14	.43	13	.76
Other medical support serv	4	*	6	*	11	.37
*Total ancillary supp staff	2	*	5	*	12	1.81
Tot contracted supp staff	6	*	4	*	10	.05
Tot RVU/work RVU	11	1.96	14	1.98	15	2.08
Patients/work RVU	8	*	14	.31	11	.23
Tot procedures/work RVU	11	1.70	17	2.35	13	2.34
Square feet/work RVU	12	.36	16	.38	16	.36
Total support staff FTE/phy	43	5.15	62	4.91	45	5.33

*See pages 260 and 261 for definition.

Table 6.9b: Charges, Revenue and Cost

	10 FTE or less		11 to 25 FTE		26 to 50 FTE	
	Count	Median	Count	Median	Count	Median
Total gross charges	12	$125.92	18	$153.74	17	$190.65
Total medical revenue	12	$91.47	18	$98.58	17	$117.33
Net fee-for-service revenue	11	$86.73	18	$90.16	14	$112.11
Net capitation revenue	3	*	8	*	4	*
Net other medical revenue	7	*	11	$3.16	14	$2.13
Total supp staff cost/work RVU	12	$29.94	18	$30.96	17	$35.46
Total general operating cost	12	$22.79	18	$29.76	17	$28.13
Total operating cost	12	$52.64	18	$64.13	17	$63.07
Total med rev after oper cost	12	$39.18	18	$39.82	17	$50.87
Total provider cost/work RVU	12	$40.30	18	$40.70	17	$51.49
Total NPP cost/work RVU	9	*	17	$2.52	17	$3.00
Provider consultant cost	1	*	6	*	7	*
Total physician cost/work RVU	12	$37.15	18	$38.06	17	$47.58
Total phy compensation	12	$29.43	18	$32.72	14	$40.64
Total phy benefit cost	12	$5.06	18	$5.20	14	$6.05
Total cost	12	$94.92	18	$102.56	17	$114.19
Net nonmedical revenue	5	*	13	$.82	14	$.81
Net inc, prac with fin sup	0	*	0	*	0	*
Net inc, prac w/o fin sup	12	$.98	18	$.76	15	$1.83
Net inc, excl fin supp (all prac)	12	$.98	18	$.76	15	$1.83
Total support staff FTE/phy	43	5.15	62	4.91	45	5.33

Multispecialty — Practices with 50 or Less FTE Physicians, Not Hospital or IDS Owned (per Patient)

Table 6.10a: Staffing, RVUs, Procedures and Square Footage

	10 FTE or less		11 to 25 FTE		26 to 50 FTE	
	Count	Median	Count	Median	Count	Median
Total prov FTE/10,000 patients	**17**	**5.51**	**25**	**6.62**	**22**	**7.96**
Total phy FTE/10,000 pat	19	3.92	29	5.37	23	6.40
Prim care phy/10,000 pat	18	3.88	28	4.15	22	3.38
Nonsurg phy/10,000 pat	4	*	14	.94	21	1.47
Surg spec phy/10,000 pat	5	*	12	1.23	21	1.28
Total NPP FTE/10,000 pat	17	1.33	25	.89	22	1.16
Total supp staff FTE/10,000 pat	**19**	**22.32**	**29**	**26.06**	**23**	**34.13**
Total empl supp staff/10,000 pat	19	22.02	29	26.06	23	34.13
General administrative	18	.94	28	1.24	22	1.62
Patient accounting	19	2.78	26	3.92	22	4.88
General accounting	14	.74	23	.54	22	.40
Managed care administrative	9	*	11	.39	12	.32
Information technology	5	*	12	.50	21	.54
Housekeeping, maint, security	7	*	16	.23	19	.32
Medical receptionists	19	3.79	28	5.61	22	5.12
Med secretaries,transcribers	13	1.79	21	1.14	21	2.05
Medical records	14	1.57	25	1.62	22	3.10
Other admin support	8	*	16	.49	15	.34
*Total administrative supp staff	8	*	13	16.00	16	20.02
Registered Nurses	15	1.91	26	1.74	21	3.35
Licensed Practical Nurses	15	3.03	26	1.52	18	3.12
Med assistants, nurse aides	17	2.83	28	4.15	18	3.69
*Total clinical supp staff	14	8.00	26	8.72	18	9.63
Clinical laboratory	12	1.71	23	1.50	21	2.42
Radiology and imaging	12	.99	20	1.24	21	2.09
Other medical support serv	5	*	13	1.05	18	1.04
*Total ancillary supp staff	4	*	12	4.76	17	5.57
Tot contracted supp staff	8	*	7	*	12	.34
Tot RVU/patient	10	4.07	14	5.11	13	7.72
Physician work RVU/patient	8	*	14	3.26	11	4.32
Tot procedures/patient	16	5.48	27	7.27	22	7.93
Square feet/patient	18	.83	27	1.02	20	1.24
Total support staff FTE/phy	**43**	**5.15**	**62**	**4.91**	**45**	**5.33**

*See pages 260 and 261 for definition.

Table 6.10b: Charges, Revenue and Cost

	10 FTE or less		11 to 25 FTE		26 to 50 FTE	
	Count	Median	Count	Median	Count	Median
Total gross charges	**19**	**$336.44**	**29**	**$437.42**	**23**	**$688.17**
Total medical revenue	**19**	**$238.38**	**29**	**$289.75**	**23**	**$431.46**
Net fee-for-service revenue	19	$220.37	29	$271.84	22	$401.90
Net capitation revenue	6	*	14	$15.55	7	*
Net other medical revenue	11	$11.96	18	$8.81	20	$8.18
Total support staff cost/patient	**19**	**$63.25**	**29**	**$86.69**	**23**	**$126.14**
Total general operating cost	**19**	**$55.24**	**29**	**$77.79**	**23**	**$113.88**
Total operating cost	**19**	**$121.63**	**29**	**$166.86**	**23**	**$235.49**
Total med rev after oper cost	**19**	**$80.61**	**29**	**$115.81**	**23**	**$183.28**
Total provider cost/patient	**19**	**$83.86**	**29**	**$116.99**	**23**	**$181.49**
Total NPP cost/patient	17	$8.10	27	$6.39	22	$9.65
Provider consultant cost	4	*	9	*	9	*
Total physician cost/patient	19	$65.72	29	$110.60	23	$164.11
Total phy compensation	19	$58.10	29	$95.94	23	$146.47
Total phy benefit cost	19	$7.94	27	$15.22	23	$20.43
Total cost	**19**	**$227.24**	**29**	**$290.23**	**23**	**$434.96**
Net nonmedical revenue	11	$.45	22	$.62	21	$1.37
Net inc, prac with fin sup	0	*	1	*	0	*
Net inc, prac w/o fin sup	18	$3.89	26	$4.39	22	$5.56
Net inc, excl fin supp (all prac)	18	$3.89	27	$3.43	22	$5.56
Total support staff FTE/phy	**43**	**5.15**	**62**	**4.91**	**45**	**5.33**

Multispecialty — Practices with 50 or Less FTE Physicians, Not Hospital or IDS Owned
(Procedure and Charge Data)

Table 6.11a: Activity Charges to Total Gross Charges Ratios

	10 FTE or less		11 to 25 FTE		26 to 50 FTE	
	Count	Median	Count	Median	Count	Median
Total proc gross charges	**30**	**97.51%**	**49**	**96.32%**	**33**	**94.40%**
Medical proc-inside practice	30	55.03%	49	52.57%	33	34.55%
Medical proc-outside practice	27	10.52%	42	8.38%	30	7.03%
Surg proc-inside practice	27	4.48%	45	5.36%	31	7.44%
Surg proc-outside practice	19	7.36%	35	10.20%	30	18.07%
Laboratory procedures	28	13.16%	48	11.01%	32	10.30%
Radiology procedures	24	4.87%	45	5.33%	33	10.69%
Tot nonproc gross charges	25	3.69%	42	3.99%	28	7.00%
Total support staff FTE/phy	**43**	**5.15**	**62**	**4.91**	**45**	**5.33**

Table 6.11b: Medical Procedure Data (inside the practice)

	10 FTE or less		11 to 25 FTE		26 to 50 FTE	
	Count	Median	Count	Median	Count	Median
Gross charges/procedure	**29**	**$69.95**	**48**	**$68.81**	**32**	**$73.17**
Total cost/procedure	**25**	**$49.87**	**44**	**$52.25**	**27**	**$58.52**
Operating cost/procedure	24	$29.53	43	$32.12	27	$35.20
Provider cost/procedure	25	$22.47	45	$21.00	27	$23.31
Procedures/patient	17	2.68	27	3.56	22	3.21
Gross charges/patient	18	$163.91	27	$224.61	22	$232.83
Procedures/physician	30	6,675	48	5,787	33	5,700
Gross charges/physician	30	$405,335	49	$401,063	33	$389,804
Procedures/provider	25	4,622	42	4,801	32	4,655
Gross charges/provider	25	$300,844	43	$353,091	32	$338,167
Gross charge to total cost ratio	25	1.33	44	1.28	27	1.27
Oper cost to total cost ratio	24	.61	43	.59	27	.60
Prov cost to total cost ratio	25	.39	44	.41	27	.40
Total support staff FTE/phy	**43**	**5.15**	**62**	**4.91**	**45**	**5.33**

Table 6.11c: Medical Procedure Data (outside the practice)

	10 FTE or less		11 to 25 FTE		26 to 50 FTE	
	Count	Median	Count	Median	Count	Median
Gross charges/procedure	**26**	**$107.16**	**41**	**$103.18**	**29**	**$122.61**
Total cost/procedure	**23**	**$44.02**	**37**	**$49.12**	**25**	**$46.78**
Operating cost/procedure	22	$18.56	36	$18.94	25	$18.35
Provider cost/procedure	23	$26.02	38	$26.99	25	$29.22
Procedures/patient	15	.37	23	.34	21	.55
Gross charges/patient	16	$39.57	23	$36.67	21	$52.43
Procedures/physician	27	640	41	672	29	727
Gross charges/physician	27	$76,608	42	$74,243	30	$92,905
Procedures/provider	23	504	36	463	28	608
Gross charges/provider	23	$52,118	37	$57,252	29	$65,076
Gross charge to total cost ratio	23	2.28	37	2.14	25	2.37
Oper cost to total cost ratio	22	.41	36	.40	25	.37
Prov cost to total cost ratio	23	.60	37	.60	25	.63
Total support staff FTE/phy	**43**	**5.15**	**62**	**4.91**	**45**	**5.33**

Multispecialty — Practices with 50 or Less FTE Physicians, Not Hospital or IDS Owned
(Procedure and Charge Data)

Table 6.11d: Surgery/Anesthesia Procedure Data (inside the practice)

	10 FTE or less		11 to 25 FTE		26 to 50 FTE	
	Count	Median	Count	Median	Count	Median
Gross charges/procedure	27	$98.52	44	$79.19	31	$153.50
Total cost/procedure	23	$80.63	41	$64.31	26	$141.41
Operating cost/procedure	22	$49.34	40	$38.19	26	$91.27
Provider cost/procedure	23	$27.33	41	$27.65	26	$49.52
Procedures/patient	15	.29	26	.29	21	.45
Gross charges/patient	15	$14.31	26	$21.57	21	$37.16
Procedures/physician	28	390	44	450	31	666
Gross charges/physician	27	$36,024	45	$40,193	31	$90,412
Procedures/provider	23	308	38	514	30	552
Gross charges/provider	22	$27,578	39	$34,228	30	$71,048
Gross charge to total cost ratio	23	1.30	41	1.29	26	1.28
Oper cost to total cost ratio	22	.61	40	.59	26	.60
Prov cost to total cost ratio	23	.39	41	.41	26	.40
Total support staff FTE/phy	43	5.15	62	4.91	45	5.33

Table 6.11e: Surgery/Anesthesia Procedure Data (outside the practice)

	10 FTE or less		11 to 25 FTE		26 to 50 FTE	
	Count	Median	Count	Median	Count	Median
Gross charges/procedure	19	$382.32	34	$779.10	29	$893.03
Total cost/procedure	18	$194.94	31	$374.45	24	$333.90
Operating cost/procedure	18	$85.86	30	$140.92	24	$138.85
Provider cost/procedure	18	$109.09	31	$229.28	24	$210.67
Procedures/patient	10	.07	19	.08	21	.25
Gross charges/patient	10	$43.86	19	$33.02	20	$126.90
Procedures/physician	20	108	34	102	30	259
Gross charges/physician	19	$55,242	35	$72,133	30	$239,882
Procedures/provider	18	76	29	86	29	238
Gross charges/provider	17	$40,161	30	$64,929	29	$174,784
Gross charge to total cost ratio	18	2.27	31	2.09	24	2.36
Oper cost to total cost ratio	18	.40	30	.39	24	.37
Prov cost to total cost ratio	18	.60	31	.60	24	.63
Total support staff FTE/phy	43	5.15	62	4.91	45	5.33

Multispecialty — Practices with 50 or Less FTE Physicians, Not Hospital or IDS Owned
(Procedure and Charge Data)

Table 6.11f: Clinical Laboratory/Pathology Procedure Data

	10 FTE or less		11 to 25 FTE		26 to 50 FTE	
	Count	Median	Count	Median	Count	Median
Gross charges/procedure	27	$23.96	46	$26.34	31	$29.55
Total cost/procedure	24	$20.77	42	$19.51	27	$21.53
Operating cost/procedure	23	$13.66	41	$13.24	27	$14.08
Provider cost/procedure	24	$6.16	43	$7.09	27	$7.76
Procedures/patient	17	2.18	25	1.67	22	2.55
Gross charges/patient	17	$52.25	26	$46.62	22	$71.94
Procedures/physician	28	3,507	46	3,939	32	3,867
Gross charges/physician	28	$106,393	48	$92,942	32	$108,309
Procedures/provider	23	3,014	41	3,420	32	3,404
Gross charges/provider	23	$88,417	42	$82,235	30	$102,399
Gross charge to total cost ratio	24	1.22	42	1.18	31	1.36
Oper cost to total cost ratio	23	.68	41	.65	27	.64
Prov cost to total cost ratio	24	.32	42	.35	27	.36
Total support staff FTE/phy	43	5.15	62	4.91	45	5.33

Table 6.11g: Diagnostic Radiology and Imaging Procedure Data

	10 FTE or less		11 to 25 FTE		26 to 50 FTE	
	Count	Median	Count	Median	Count	Median
Gross charges/procedure	24	$90.65	44	$102.44	32	$165.67
Total cost/procedure	23	$81.77	40	$82.56	27	$126.42
Operating cost/procedure	23	$49.61	39	$52.84	27	$84.40
Provider cost/procedure	23	$21.77	41	$27.48	27	$41.30
Procedures/patient	16	.22	24	.15	22	.49
Gross charges/patient	15	$23.22	23	$23.55	22	$78.39
Procedures/physician	26	614	44	503	33	689
Gross charges/physician	24	$49,520	45	$42,046	33	$126,928
Procedures/provider	23	404	38	438	32	586
Gross charges/provider	21	$39,339	39	$36,769	32	$101,387
Gross charge to total cost ratio	23	1.28	40	1.28	27	1.27
Oper cost to total cost ratio	23	.68	39	.66	27	.66
Prov cost to total cost ratio	23	.32	40	.33	27	.34
Total support staff FTE/phy	43	5.15	62	4.91	45	5.33

Table 6.11h: Nonprocedural Gross Charge Data

	10 FTE or less		11 to 25 FTE		26 to 50 FTE	
	Count	Median	Count	Median	Count	Median
Gross charges/patient	15	$15.79	23	$14.14	20	$54.44
Nonproc gross charges/physician	25	$25,105	42	$29,614	28	$97,536
Gross charges/provider	20	$22,844	38	$27,891	27	$64,872
Total support staff FTE/phy	43	5.15	62	4.91	45	5.33

Multispecialty — Practices with 51 or More FTE Physicians, Not Hospital or IDS Owned

Table 7.1: Staffing and Practice Data

	51 to 75 FTE		76 to 150 FTE		151 FTE or more	
	Count	Median	Count	Median	Count	Median
Total provider FTE	**24**	**74.88**	**26**	**128.26**	**11**	**228.79**
Total physician FTE	24	64.63	27	102.00	12	176.88
Total nonphysician provider FTE	24	11.30	26	29.80	11	41.70
Total support staff FTE	**24**	**315.66**	**27**	**596.00**	**12**	**958.08**
Number of branch clinics	23	6	25	11	11	14
Square footage of all facilities	22	116,035	26	222,798	12	411,577

Table 7.2: Accounts Receivable Data, Collection Percentages and Financial Ratios

	51 to 75 FTE		76 to 150 FTE		151 FTE or more	
	Count	Median	Count	Median	Count	Median
Total AR/physician	**22**	**$145,158**	**27**	**$177,669**	**11**	**$149,390**
Total AR/provider	**22**	**$120,484**	**26**	**$132,710**	**11**	**$119,280**
0-30 days in AR	22	51.39%	27	44.68%	11	54.25%
31-60 days in AR	22	14.36%	27	16.62%	11	13.75%
61-90 days in AR	22	7.24%	27	8.10%	11	8.62%
91-120 days in AR	22	4.57%	27	5.42%	11	5.98%
120+ days in AR	22	17.11%	27	22.00%	11	18.64%
Re-aged: 0-30 days in AR	10	56.65%	17	49.22%	6	*
Re-aged: 31-60 days in AR	10	13.65%	17	16.62%	6	*
Re-aged: 61-90 days in AR	10	6.90%	17	7.18%	6	*
Re-aged: 91-120 days in AR	10	4.43%	17	4.79%	6	*
Re-aged: 120+ days in AR	10	15.51%	17	19.51%	6	*
Not re-aged: 0-30 days in AR	11	49.51%	9	*	5	*
Not re-aged: 31-60 days in AR	11	15.29%	9	*	5	*
Not re-aged: 61-90 days in AR	11	7.96%	9	*	5	*
Not re-aged: 91-120 days in AR	11	5.40%	9	*	5	*
Not re-aged: 120+ days in AR	11	20.75%	9	*	5	*
Months gross FFS charges in AR	20	1.78	25	1.83	10	1.82
Days gross FFS charges in AR	20	54.08	25	55.75	10	55.51
Gross FFS collection %	22	62.44%	25	61.07%	11	55.46%
Adjusted FFS collection %	21	97.54%	25	96.61%	11	97.10%
Gross FFS + cap collection %	9	*	12	60.84%	7	*
Net cap rev % of gross cap chrg	7	*	11	72.61%	7	*
Current ratio	16	1.73	18	1.27	8	*
Tot asset turnover ratio	16	3.18	18	2.61	8	*
Debt to equity ratio	16	3.11	18	1.63	8	*
Debt ratio	16	75.65%	18	61.95%	8	*
Return on total assets	16	1.55%	18	3.93%	7	*
Return on equity	16	4.03%	18	17.04%	7	*

Table 7.3: Breakout of Total Gross Charges by Type of Payer

	51 to 75 FTE		76 to 150 FTE		151 FTE or more	
	Count	Median	Count	Median	Count	Median
Medicare: fee-for-service	21	28.01%	25	23.00%	11	20.00%
Medicare: managed care FFS	21	.00%	25	.00%	11	.00%
Medicare: capitation	21	.00%	25	.00%	11	.00%
Medicaid: fee-for-service	21	3.50%	25	2.79%	11	4.30%
Medicaid: managed care FFS	21	.00%	25	.00%	11	.00%
Medicaid: capitation	21	.00%	25	.00%	11	.00%
Commercial: fee-for-service	21	42.00%	25	42.36%	11	38.93%
Commercial: managed care FFS	21	.00%	25	.00%	11	.00%
Commercial: capitation	21	.00%	25	.00%	11	3.80%
Workers' compensation	21	.63%	25	1.00%	11	1.00%
Charity care and prof courtesy	21	.00%	25	.00%	11	.00%
Self-pay	21	3.50%	25	3.59%	11	2.90%
Other federal government payers	21	.00%	25	.00%	11	.00%

Multispecialty — Practices with 51 or More FTE Physicians, Not Hospital or IDS Owned
(per FTE Physician)

Table 7.4a: Staffing, RVUs, Patients, Procedures and Square Footage

	51 to 75 FTE		76 to 150 FTE		151 FTE or more	
	Count	Median	Count	Median	Count	Median
Total provider FTE/physician	24	1.19	26	1.27	11	1.20
Prim care phy/physician	24	.41	25	.40	11	.53
Nonsurg phy/physician	22	.32	25	.31	11	.53
Surg spec phy/physician	22	.26	22	.24	10	.24
Total NPP FTE/physician	24	.19	26	.27	11	.20
Total support staff FTE/phy	24	4.99	27	6.08	12	5.33
Total empl support staff FTE	24	4.99	26	5.92	11	5.29
General administrative	22	.27	26	.33	11	.29
Patient accounting	22	.79	26	.76	11	.53
General accounting	21	.07	26	.07	11	.05
Managed care administrative	12	.06	21	.14	8	*
Information technology	22	.10	26	.15	10	.20
Housekeeping, maint, security	19	.07	21	.16	10	.10
Medical receptionists	22	.81	24	.98	10	.77
Med secretaries,transcribers	21	.16	22	.27	9	*
Medical records	22	.41	25	.47	9	*
Other admin support	14	.06	22	.10	7	*
*Total administrative supp staff	12	3.37	21	3.49	7	*
Registered Nurses	22	.36	25	.47	11	.50
Licensed Practical Nurses	20	.29	25	.35	11	.29
Med assistants, nurse aides	22	.84	25	.66	11	.62
*Total clinical supp staff	20	1.54	25	1.58	12	1.35
Clinical laboratory	21	.31	26	.33	10	.29
Radiology and imaging	22	.30	26	.35	11	.32
Other medical support serv	19	.26	25	.32	10	.41
*Total ancillary supp staff	18	.91	26	1.03	10	1.28
Tot contracted supp staff	8	*	10	.10	7	*
Tot RVU/physician	10	12,244	11	13,307	10	11,910
Physician work RVU/physician	11	6,101	14	5,862	10	4,774
Patients/physician	13	1,142	15	1,085	5	*
Tot procedures/physician	19	11,624	22	12,503	8	*
Square feet/physician	22	1,961	26	2,249	12	1,959

*See pages 260 and 261 for definition.

Table 7.4b: Charges and Revenue

	51 to 75 FTE		76 to 150 FTE		151 FTE or more	
	Count	Median	Count	Median	Count	Median
Net fee-for-service revenue	23	$672,430	25	$704,703	11	$592,212
Gross FFS charges	22	$1,116,776	25	$1,104,013	11	$953,726
Adjustments to FFS charges	21	$421,566	25	$344,958	10	$450,060
Adjusted FFS charges	21	$713,310	25	$718,696	11	$597,755
Bad debts due to FFS activity	21	$21,341	24	$14,578	11	$15,882
Net capitation revenue	9	*	12	$217,735	8	*
Gross capitation charges	7	*	11	$339,768	7	*
Capitation revenue	9	*	12	$274,501	8	*
Purch serv for cap patients	4	*	7	*	7	*
Net other medical revenue	23	$15,726	23	$23,192	11	$18,050
Gross rev from other activity	22	$23,268	22	$27,175	11	$53,753
Other medical revenue	19	$14,622	21	$8,724	8	*
Rev from sale of goods/services	12	$26,186	15	$18,706	6	*
Cost of sales	9	*	13	$8,171	5	*
Total gross charges	22	$1,136,618	26	$1,229,028	11	$1,207,812
Total medical revenue	24	$712,030	27	$820,339	12	$751,886

Multispecialty — Practices with 51 or More FTE Physicians, Not Hospital or IDS Owned
(per FTE Physician) (continued)

Table 7.4c: Operating Cost

	51 to 75 FTE		76 to 150 FTE		151 FTE or more	
	Count	Median	Count	Median	Count	Median
Total support staff cost/phy	24	$199,883	27	$247,923	12	$250,984
Total empl supp staff cost/phy	24	$156,883	26	$187,399	11	$191,985
General administrative	22	$15,755	26	$21,071	11	$18,204
Patient accounting	22	$21,136	26	$18,257	11	$19,898
General accounting	21	$2,519	26	$2,652	11	$2,378
Managed care administrative	12	$2,232	20	$3,826	8	*
Information technology	22	$4,045	26	$6,681	10	$9,026
Housekeeping, maint, security	19	$2,016	21	$3,923	10	$2,976
Medical receptionists	22	$19,803	24	$23,437	10	$18,511
Med secretaries,transcribers	21	$5,314	22	$8,003	9	*
Medical records	22	$8,253	25	$10,748	9	*
Other admin support	14	$1,329	22	$2,351	8	*
***Total administrative supp staff**	11	$80,476	20	$100,630	8	*
Registered Nurses	22	$14,285	25	$22,815	10	$28,438
Licensed Practical Nurses	20	$9,160	25	$12,811	10	$7,293
Med assistants, nurse aides	22	$21,572	25	$15,087	10	$16,948
***Total clinical supp staff**	20	$48,038	25	$50,725	11	$48,696
Clinical laboratory	21	$9,973	26	$10,901	10	$11,215
Radiology and imaging	22	$12,349	26	$14,212	11	$12,586
Other medical support serv	21	$6,531	25	$11,294	10	$21,694
***Total ancillary supp staff**	20	$28,980	26	$38,010	10	$51,810
Total empl supp staff benefits	24	$38,222	27	$50,088	12	$50,300
Tot contracted supp staff	14	$1,711	20	$3,374	9	*
Total general operating cost	24	$204,234	27	$244,980	12	$220,435
Information technology	23	$11,108	26	$13,144	11	$24,375
Medical and surgical supply	23	$54,903	26	$53,140	11	$45,937
Building and occupancy	23	$47,529	26	$48,933	11	$37,336
Furniture and equipment	21	$11,182	25	$8,997	11	$10,729
Admin supplies and services	23	$12,401	26	$14,846	11	$13,320
Prof liability insurance	23	$12,080	27	$17,304	12	$16,683
Other insurance premiums	22	$997	24	$2,226	11	$1,020
Outside professional fees	22	$3,488	26	$5,046	11	$5,636
Promotion and marketing	23	$2,923	26	$4,182	11	$2,323
Clinical laboratory	23	$13,502	25	$12,857	11	$12,685
Radiology and imaging	23	$14,663	25	$16,059	11	$7,129
Other ancillary services	17	$1,716	22	$8,561	8	*
Billing purchased services	14	$1,917	18	$1,950	5	*
Management fees paid to MSO	0	*	2	*	2	*
Misc operating cost	23	$8,601	26	$14,246	11	$16,708
Cost allocated to prac from par	1	*	0	*	2	*
Total operating cost	24	$416,902	27	$496,840	12	$476,629

*See pages 260 and 261 for definition.

Multispecialty — Practices with 51 or More FTE Physicians, Not Hospital or IDS Owned
(per FTE Physician)

Table 7.4d: Provider Cost

	51 to 75 FTE		76 to 150 FTE		151 FTE or more	
	Count	Median	Count	Median	Count	Median
Total med rev after oper cost	24	$296,591	27	$327,791	12	$287,624
Total provider cost/physician	24	$298,918	27	$319,985	12	$306,979
Total NPP cost/physician	24	$16,658	27	$23,114	12	$23,424
Nonphysician provider comp	24	$13,772	26	$19,103	11	$19,940
Nonphysician prov benefit cost	21	$3,095	25	$4,162	11	$4,480
Provider consultant cost	13	$11,676	15	$13,053	9	*
Total physician cost/physician	24	$276,850	27	$304,720	12	$272,826
Total phy compensation	24	$243,085	26	$257,896	11	$228,339
Total phy benefit cost	24	$34,568	26	$42,015	11	$42,206

Table 7.4e: Net Income or Loss

	51 to 75 FTE		76 to 150 FTE		151 FTE or more	
	Count	Median	Count	Median	Count	Median
Total cost	24	$734,005	27	$811,972	12	$791,649
Net nonmedical revenue	24	$1,997	27	$4,336	11	$1,206
Nonmedical revenue	22	$3,347	26	$6,580	10	$6,071
Fin support for oper costs	1	*	0	*	1	*
Goodwill amortization	7	*	7	*	3	*
Nonmedical cost	12	$730	21	$2,933	5	*
Net inc, prac with fin sup	1	*	0	*	1	*
Net inc, prac w/o fin sup	23	$2,300	27	$16,059	9	*
Net inc, excl fin supp (all prac)	24	$2,258	27	$16,059	10	$222

Table 7.4f: Assets and Liabilities

	51 to 75 FTE		76 to 150 FTE		151 FTE or more	
	Count	Median	Count	Median	Count	Median
Total assets	17	$211,311	19	$297,528	8	*
Current assets	17	$120,846	19	$150,617	8	*
Noncurrent assets	17	$44,335	19	$139,254	8	*
Total liabilities	17	$71,316	19	$162,415	8	*
Current liabilities	17	$62,325	19	$118,362	8	*
Noncurrent liabilities	17	$29,045	19	$60,831	8	*
Working capital	17	$54,591	19	$38,477	8	*
Total net worth	17	$57,223	19	$114,455	8	*
Total support staff FTE/phy	24	4.99	27	6.08	12	5.33

Multispecialty — Practices with 51 or More FTE Physicians, Not Hospital or IDS Owned
(as a % of Total Medical Revenue)

Table 7.5a: Charges and Revenue

	51 to 75 FTE		76 to 150 FTE		151 FTE or more	
	Count	Median	Count	Median	Count	Median
Net fee-for-service revenue	23	96.88%	25	95.61%	11	69.00%
Net capitation revenue	9	*	12	25.04%	8	*
Net other medical revenue	23	2.19%	23	2.89%	11	3.68%
Total gross charges	**23**	**158.29%**	**27**	**154.53%**	**11**	**159.54%**

Table 7.5b: Operating Cost

	51 to 75 FTE		76 to 150 FTE		151 FTE or more	
	Count	Median	Count	Median	Count	Median
Total support staff cost	**24**	**28.39%**	**27**	**30.07%**	**12**	**31.84%**
Total empl support staff cost	24	22.56%	26	23.46%	11	25.07%
General administrative	22	2.21%	26	2.69%	11	2.25%
Patient accounting	22	2.82%	26	2.38%	11	2.25%
General accounting	21	.36%	26	.36%	11	.34%
Managed care administrative	12	.30%	20	.48%	8	*
Information technology	22	.60%	26	.79%	10	1.16%
Housekeeping, maint, security	19	.27%	21	.45%	10	.39%
Medical receptionists	22	2.90%	24	2.76%	10	2.31%
Med secretaries,transcribers	21	.77%	22	.94%	9	*
Medical records	22	1.03%	25	1.27%	9	*
Other admin support	14	.22%	22	.29%	8	*
*Total administrative supp staff	11	10.09%	20	12.91%	8	*
Registered Nurses	22	2.38%	25	2.93%	10	3.61%
Licensed Practical Nurses	20	1.29%	25	1.27%	10	1.12%
Med assistants, nurse aides	22	2.73%	25	1.71%	10	2.10%
*Total clinical supp staff	20	6.55%	25	6.73%	11	6.33%
Clinical laboratory	21	1.33%	26	1.23%	10	1.43%
Radiology and imaging	22	1.67%	26	1.91%	11	1.69%
Other medical support serv	21	.93%	25	1.28%	10	2.92%
*Total ancillary supp staff	20	3.89%	26	4.27%	10	7.67%
Total empl supp staff benefits	24	5.74%	27	5.96%	12	6.43%
Tot contracted supp staff	14	.32%	20	.38%	9	*
Total general operating cost	**24**	**30.63%**	**27**	**29.60%**	**12**	**28.48%**
Information technology	23	1.66%	26	1.62%	11	3.07%
Medical and surgical supply	23	7.71%	26	6.54%	11	6.17%
Building and occupancy	23	6.53%	26	5.92%	11	5.31%
Furniture and equipment	21	1.92%	25	1.00%	11	1.60%
Admin supplies and services	23	1.79%	26	1.96%	11	1.71%
Prof liability insurance	23	1.49%	27	2.04%	12	2.11%
Other insurance premiums	22	.17%	24	.26%	11	.12%
Outside professional fees	22	.47%	26	.59%	11	.71%
Promotion and marketing	23	.43%	26	.51%	11	.31%
Clinical laboratory	23	1.71%	25	1.57%	11	1.82%
Radiology and imaging	23	1.80%	25	2.13%	11	.75%
Other ancillary services	17	.23%	22	1.02%	8	*
Billing purchased services	14	.25%	18	.28%	5	*
Management fees paid to MSO	0	*	2	*	2	*
Misc operating cost	23	1.20%	26	1.45%	11	2.08%
Cost allocated to prac from par	1	*	0	*	2	*
Total operating cost	**24**	**59.03%**	**27**	**61.64%**	**12**	**60.90%**

*See pages 260 and 261 for definition.

Multispecialty — Practices with 51 or More FTE Physicians, Not Hospital or IDS Owned
(as a % of Total Medical Revenue)

Table 7.5c: Provider Cost

	51 to 75 FTE		76 to 150 FTE		151 FTE or more	
	Count	Median	Count	Median	Count	Median
Total med rev after oper cost	**24**	**40.97%**	**27**	**38.36%**	**12**	**39.10%**
Total provider cost	**24**	**42.45%**	**27**	**39.48%**	**12**	**39.09%**
Total NPP cost	24	2.09%	27	2.84%	12	2.91%
Nonphysician provider comp	24	1.73%	26	2.35%	11	2.69%
Nonphysician prov benefit cost	21	.40%	25	.50%	11	.53%
Provider consultant cost	13	1.44%	15	1.75%	9	*
Total physician cost	24	39.94%	27	35.53%	12	35.83%
Total phy compensation	24	34.80%	26	29.48%	11	29.63%
Total phy benefit cost	24	4.82%	26	4.84%	11	5.38%

Table 7.5d: Net Income or Loss

	51 to 75 FTE		76 to 150 FTE		151 FTE or more	
	Count	Median	Count	Median	Count	Median
Total cost	**24**	**99.98%**	**27**	**99.33%**	**12**	**100.21%**
Net nonmedical revenue	24	.21%	27	.64%	11	.16%
Nonmedical revenue	22	.44%	26	.92%	10	.75%
Fin support for oper costs	1	*	0	*	1	*
Goodwill amortization	7	*	7	*	3	*
Nonmedical cost	12	.10%	21	.40%	5	*
Net inc, prac with fin sup	1	*	0	*	1	*
Net inc, prac w/o fin sup	23	.55%	27	1.84%	9	*
Net inc, excl fin supp (all prac)	24	.42%	27	1.84%	10	.03%

Table 7.5e: Assets and Liabilities

	51 to 75 FTE		76 to 150 FTE		151 FTE or more	
	Count	Median	Count	Median	Count	Median
Total assets	**17**	**30.11%**	**19**	**36.09%**	**8**	*
Current assets	17	22.18%	19	19.37%	8	*
Noncurrent assets	17	5.91%	19	16.33%	8	*
Total liabilities	**17**	**13.13%**	**19**	**22.09%**	**8**	*
Current liabilities	17	5.35%	19	13.31%	8	*
Noncurrent liabilities	17	4.94%	19	8.84%	8	*
Working capital	17	7.70%	19	4.09%	8	*
Total net worth	**17**	**7.66%**	**19**	**11.78%**	**8**	*

Multispecialty — Practices with 51 or More FTE Physicians, Not Hospital or IDS Owned
(per FTE Provider)

Table 7.6a: Staffing, RVUs, Patients, Procedures and Square Footage

	51 to 75 FTE		76 to 150 FTE		151 FTE or more	
	Count	Median	Count	Median	Count	Median
Total physician FTE/provider	24	.84	26	.79	11	.84
Prim care phy/provider	24	.38	24	.32	10	.41
Nonsurg phy/provider	22	.25	24	.27	9	*
Surg spec phy/provider	22	.20	21	.19	9	*
Total NPP FTE/provider	24	.16	26	.21	11	.16
Total support staff FTE/prov	24	4.14	26	4.75	11	4.16
Total empl supp staff FTE/prov	24	4.14	25	4.65	10	4.21
General administrative	22	.24	25	.26	10	.22
Patient accounting	22	.63	25	.56	10	.47
General accounting	21	.06	25	.05	10	.04
Managed care administrative	12	.05	20	.09	8	*
Information technology	22	.08	25	.11	10	.15
Housekeeping, maint, security	19	.06	20	.14	9	*
Medical receptionists	22	.69	23	.77	9	*
Med secretaries,transcribers	21	.12	21	.21	8	*
Medical records	22	.32	24	.34	8	*
Other admin support	14	.04	21	.07	6	*
*Total administrative supp staff	12	2.69	20	2.80	7	*
Registered Nurses	22	.30	24	.40	10	.41
Licensed Practical Nurses	20	.25	24	.30	10	.28
Med assistants, nurse aides	22	.67	24	.45	10	.43
*Total clinical supp staff	20	1.32	24	1.28	11	1.11
Clinical laboratory	21	.26	25	.25	9	*
Radiology and imaging	22	.24	25	.28	10	.26
Other medical support serv	19	.22	24	.23	9	*
*Total ancillary supp staff	18	.77	25	.81	9	*
Tot contracted supp staff	8	*	10	.07	7	*
Tot RVU/provider	10	10,815	11	9,759	9	*
Physician work RVU/provider	11	5,176	14	4,475	9	*
Patients/provider	13	974	14	920	5	*
Tot procedures/provider	19	9,545	21	10,259	7	*
Square feet/provider	22	1,622	25	1,813	11	1,581
Total support staff FTE/phy	24	4.99	27	6.08	12	5.33

*See pages 260 and 261 for definition.

Table 7.6b: Charges, Revenue and Cost

	51 to 75 FTE		76 to 150 FTE		151 FTE or more	
	Count	Median	Count	Median	Count	Median
Total gross charges	23	$989,180	26	$988,283	11	$1,028,062
Total medical revenue	24	$619,563	26	$629,945	11	$572,177
Net fee-for-service revenue	23	$607,933	24	$560,501	10	$491,156
Net capitation revenue	9	*	11	$164,622	7	*
Net other medical revenue	23	$12,006	22	$17,516	10	$14,745
Total support staff cost/prov	24	$171,711	26	$190,685	11	$214,137
Total general operating cost	24	$177,343	26	$193,752	11	$172,811
Total operating cost	24	$350,912	26	$373,509	11	$350,590
Total med rev after oper cost	24	$252,371	26	$252,837	11	$213,041
Total provider cost/provider	24	$256,225	26	$256,931	11	$240,209
Total NPP cost/provider	24	$13,819	26	$18,603	11	$18,417
Provider consultant cost	13	$8,757	15	$10,300	8	*
Total physician cost/provider	24	$222,493	26	$233,280	11	$208,624
Total phy compensation	24	$195,346	25	$192,779	10	$179,903
Total phy benefit cost	24	$27,934	25	$31,590	10	$29,430
Total cost	24	$604,656	26	$618,749	11	$578,315
Net nonmedical revenue	24	$1,560	26	$3,688	10	$1,262
Net inc, prac with fin sup	1	*	0	*	1	*
Net inc, prac w/o fin sup	23	$2,006	26	$10,922	8	*
Net inc, excl fin supp (all prac)	24	$1,866	26	$10,922	9	*
Total support staff FTE/phy	24	4.99	27	6.08	12	5.33

Multispecialty — Practices with 51 or More FTE Physicians, Not Hospital or IDS Owned (per Square Foot)

Table 7.7a: Staffing, RVUs, Patients and Procedures

	51 to 75 FTE		76 to 150 FTE		151 FTE or more	
	Count	Median	Count	Median	Count	Median
Total prov FTE/10,000 sq ft	22	**6.16**	25	**5.52**	11	**6.33**
Total phy FTE/10,000 sq ft	22	5.10	26	4.45	12	5.12
Prim care phy/10,000 sq ft	22	2.28	24	1.65	11	2.61
Nonsurg phy/10,000 sq ft	21	1.43	24	1.40	10	1.32
Surg spec phy/10,000 sq ft	21	1.21	22	1.01	10	1.08
Total NPP FTE/10,000 sq ft	22	1.03	25	1.22	11	1.24
Total supp stf FTE/10,000 sq ft	22	**27.19**	26	**27.26**	12	**26.89**
Total empl supp stf/10,000 sq ft	22	27.03	25	26.80	11	26.95
General administrative	21	1.36	25	1.39	11	1.41
Patient accounting	21	3.83	25	3.19	11	3.12
General accounting	20	.36	25	.34	11	.26
Managed care administrative	11	.32	20	.83	8	*
Information technology	21	.47	25	.69	10	.81
Housekeeping, maint, security	18	.36	21	.54	10	.38
Medical receptionists	21	4.37	23	4.37	10	3.20
Med secretaries,transcribers	20	.84	21	1.25	9	*
Medical records	21	1.84	24	2.20	9	*
Other admin support	13	.30	21	.37	7	*
***Total administrative supp staff**	11	**11.53**	21	**15.23**	7	*
Registered Nurses	21	1.69	24	2.79	11	2.42
Licensed Practical Nurses	19	1.44	24	1.52	11	1.75
Med assistants, nurse aides	21	4.26	24	2.63	11	2.65
***Total clinical supp staff**	19	**7.22**	24	**7.36**	12	**6.71**
Clinical laboratory	21	1.60	25	1.41	10	1.43
Radiology and imaging	21	1.29	25	1.71	11	1.56
Other medical support serv	18	1.03	24	1.35	10	1.87
***Total ancillary supp staff**	18	**4.43**	25	**4.35**	10	**6.64**
Tot contracted supp staff	8	*	10	.38	7	*
Tot RVU/sq ft	10	7.32	11	6.61	10	6.33
Physician work RVU/sq ft	11	2.78	14	2.52	10	2.74
Patients/sq ft	12	.62	14	.53	5	*
Tot procedures/sq ft	18	5.57	21	5.38	8	*
Total support staff FTE/phy	24	**4.99**	27	**6.08**	12	**5.33**

*See pages 260 and 261 for definition.

Table 7.7b: Charges, Revenue and Cost

	51 to 75 FTE		76 to 150 FTE		151 FTE or more	
	Count	Median	Count	Median	Count	Median
Total gross charges	21	**$597.94**	26	**$568.54**	11	**$633.47**
Total medical revenue	22	**$361.00**	26	**$373.71**	12	**$388.23**
Net fee-for-service revenue	21	$347.82	24	$336.42	11	$260.24
Net capitation revenue	7	*	12	$107.11	8	*
Net other medical revenue	21	$6.98	22	$10.51	11	$9.93
Total support staff cost/sq ft	22	**$101.87**	26	**$111.39**	12	**$119.07**
Total general operating cost	22	**$110.68**	26	**$108.00**	12	**$119.41**
Total operating cost	22	**$215.00**	26	**$216.83**	12	**$257.76**
Total med rev after oper cost	22	**$156.90**	26	**$153.95**	12	**$144.93**
Total provider cost/sq ft	22	**$162.82**	26	**$154.28**	12	**$145.82**
Total NPP cost/sq ft	22	$9.11	26	$10.18	12	$11.67
Provider consultant cost	12	$3.60	15	$7.33	9	*
Total physician cost/sq ft	22	$145.13	26	$130.83	12	$127.69
Total phy compensation	22	$124.01	25	$107.56	11	$103.36
Total phy benefit cost	22	$16.84	25	$17.97	11	$20.06
Total cost	22	**$375.16**	26	**$366.56**	12	**$388.25**
Net nonmedical revenue/sq ft	22	$.89	26	$1.95	11	$.59
Net inc, prac with fin sup	1	*	0	*	1	*
Net inc, prac w/o fin sup	21	$1.96	26	$6.11	9	*
Net inc, excl fin supp (all prac)	22	$1.43	26	$6.11	10	$.09
Total support staff FTE/phy	24	**4.99**	27	**6.08**	12	**5.33**

Multispecialty — Practices with 51 or More FTE Physicians, Not Hospital or IDS Owned (per Total RVU)

Table 7.8a: Staffing, Patients, Procedures and Square Footage

	51 to 75 FTE		76 to 150 FTE		151 FTE or more	
	Count	Median	Count	Median	Count	Median
Total prov FTE/10,000 tot RVU	10	.95	11	1.02	9	*
Total phy FTE/10,000 tot RVU	10	.83	11	.75	10	.84
Prim care phy/10,000 tot RVU	10	.39	10	.50	9	*
Nonsurg phy/10,000 tot RVU	9	*	10	.25	8	*
Surg spec phy/10,000 tot RVU	9	*	8	*	8	*
Total NPP FTE/10,000 tot RVU	10	.16	11	.21	9	*
Total supp stf FTE/10,000 tot RVU	10	4.06	11	5.22	10	4.23
Tot empl supp stf/10,000 tot RVU	10	4.05	10	5.15	9	*
General administrative	10	.21	10	.27	9	*
Patient accounting	10	.51	10	.61	9	*
General accounting	9	*	10	.06	9	*
Managed care administrative	6	*	9	*	7	*
Information technology	10	.07	10	.16	8	*
Housekeeping, maint, security	8	*	8	*	8	*
Medical receptionists	10	.70	10	.85	8	*
Med secretaries,transcribers	10	.12	6	*	7	*
Medical records	10	.26	10	.41	7	*
Other admin support	7	*	9	*	6	*
*Total administrative supp staff	5	*	9	*	6	*
Registered Nurses	10	.37	10	.44	9	*
Licensed Practical Nurses	10	.20	10	.19	9	*
Med assistants, nurse aides	10	.69	10	.72	9	*
*Total clinical supp staff	10	1.25	11	1.40	10	1.06
Clinical laboratory	10	.25	10	.26	9	*
Radiology and imaging	10	.18	10	.29	9	*
Other medical support serv	9	*	10	.27	8	*
*Total ancillary supp staff	9	*	11	.91	9	*
Tot contracted supp staff	4	*	6	*	6	*
Physician work RVU/tot RVU	9	*	10	.45	9	*
Patients/tot RVU	7	*	8	*	4	*
Tot procedures/tot RVU	10	.92	10	.91	6	*
Square feet/tot RVU	10	.14	11	.15	10	.16
Total support staff FTE/phy	24	4.99	27	6.08	12	5.33

*See pages 260 and 261 for definition.

Table 7.8b: Charges, Revenue and Cost

	51 to 75 FTE		76 to 150 FTE		151 FTE or more	
	Count	Median	Count	Median	Count	Median
Total gross charges	10	$82.51	11	$105.38	9	*
Total medical revenue	10	$50.37	11	$64.13	10	$56.56
Net fee-for-service revenue	10	$50.03	10	$51.46	9	*
Net capitation revenue	2	*	7	*	7	*
Net other medical revenue	10	$.81	9	*	9	*
Total supp staff cost/tot RVU	10	$14.98	11	$21.15	10	$16.92
Total general operating cost	10	$14.92	11	$19.63	10	$16.83
Total operating cost	10	$28.71	11	$41.19	10	$34.15
Total med rev after oper cost	10	$21.86	11	$25.22	10	$24.40
Total provider cost/tot RVU	10	$22.07	11	$22.32	10	$23.23
Total NPP cost/tot RVU	10	$1.37	11	$1.84	10	$2.02
Provider consultant cost	5	*	8	*	7	*
Total physician cost/tot RVU	10	$20.83	11	$20.31	10	$20.33
Total phy compensation	10	$18.38	10	$17.20	9	*
Total phy benefit cost	10	$2.82	10	$2.61	9	*
Total cost	10	$59.66	9	*	5	*
Net nonmedical revenue	10	$.11	11	$.44	9	*
Net inc, prac with fin sup	1	*	0	*	1	*
Net inc, prac w/o fin sup	9	*	11	$1.13	7	*
Net inc, excl fin supp (all prac)	10	$.05	11	$1.13	8	*
Total support staff FTE/phy	24	4.99	27	6.08	12	5.33

Multispecialty — Practices with 51 or More FTE Physicians, Not Hospital or IDS Owned (per Work RVU)

Table 7.9a: Staffing, Patients, Procedures and Square Footage

	51 to 75 FTE		76 to 150 FTE		151 FTE or more	
	Count	Median	Count	Median	Count	Median
Total prov FTE/10,000 work RVU	11	**1.93**	14	**2.24**	9	*
Tot phy FTE/10,000 work RVU	11	1.64	14	1.71	10	2.09
Prim care phy/10,000 work RVU	11	.76	13	.70	9	*
Nonsurg phy/10,000 work RVU	11	.47	12	.54	8	*
Surg spec phy/10,000 work RVU	11	.42	12	.37	8	*
Total NPP FTE/10,000 work RVU	11	.34	14	.53	9	*
Total supp stf FTE/10,000 wrk RVU	11	**9.69**	14	**11.34**	10	**9.67**
Tot empl supp stf/10,000 work RVU	11	9.69	13	10.56	9	*
General administrative	11	.51	13	.58	9	*
Patient accounting	11	1.62	13	1.38	9	*
General accounting	10	.14	13	.14	9	*
Managed care administrative	6	*	11	.30	7	*
Information technology	11	.20	13	.27	8	*
Housekeeping, maint, security	9	*	11	.33	8	*
Medical receptionists	11	1.53	13	1.89	8	*
Med secretaries,transcribers	11	.32	10	.48	7	*
Medical records	11	.76	13	.82	7	*
Other admin support	7	*	12	.12	5	*
*Total administrative supp staff	7	*	12	6.31	5	*
Registered Nurses	11	.86	13	.85	9	*
Licensed Practical Nurses	11	.42	13	.44	9	*
Med assistants, nurse aides	11	1.53	13	1.12	9	*
*Total clinical supp staff	11	3.03	14	2.84	10	2.50
Clinical laboratory	11	.60	13	.59	8	*
Radiology and imaging	11	.58	13	.69	9	*
Other medical support serv	11	.43	13	.74	8	*
*Total ancillary supp staff	11	1.52	14	2.04	8	*
Tot contracted supp staff	4	*	6	*	6	*
Tot RVU/work RVU	9	*	10	2.24	9	*
Patients/work RVU	8	*	8	*	4	*
Tot procedures/work RVU	11	1.96	13	2.04	7	*
Square feet/work RVU	11	.36	14	.40	10	.37
Total support staff FTE/phy	24	**4.99**	27	**6.08**	12	**5.33**

*See pages 260 and 261 for definition.

Table 7.9b: Charges, Revenue and Cost

	51 to 75 FTE		76 to 150 FTE		151 FTE or more	
	Count	Median	Count	Median	Count	Median
Total gross charges	11	**$196.77**	14	**$225.81**	9	*
Total medical revenue	11	**$127.44**	14	**$147.99**	10	**$141.94**
Net fee-for-service revenue	11	$122.36	13	$143.78	9	*
Net capitation revenue	3	*	6	*	8	*
Net other medical revenue	11	$2.83	13	$4.07	9	*
Total supp staff cost/work RVU	11	**$36.47**	14	**$48.53**	10	**$46.04**
Total general operating cost	11	**$39.48**	14	**$44.66**	10	**$42.44**
Total operating cost	11	**$84.00**	14	**$94.20**	10	**$83.46**
Total med rev after oper cost	11	**$50.30**	14	**$57.30**	10	**$53.68**
Total provider cost/work RVU	11	**$53.02**	14	**$56.67**	10	**$54.80**
Total NPP cost/work RVU	11	$3.04	14	$4.24	10	$3.67
Provider consultant cost	6	*	11	$3.73	7	*
Total physician cost/work RVU	11	$47.79	14	$49.27	10	$47.35
Total phy compensation	11	$40.73	13	$42.18	9	*
Total phy benefit cost	11	$6.96	13	$6.28	9	*
Total cost	11	**$127.42**	14	**$149.35**	10	**$143.04**
Net nonmedical revenue	11	$.42	14	$1.13	9	*
Net inc, prac with fin sup	1	*	0	*	1	*
Net inc, prac w/o fin sup	10	$.17	14	$2.43	7	*
Net inc, excl fin supp (all prac)	11	$.17	14	$2.43	8	*
Total support staff FTE/phy	24	**4.99**	27	**6.08**	12	**5.33**

Multispecialty — Practices with 51 or More FTE Physicians, Not Hospital or IDS Owned (per Patient)

Table 7.10a: Staffing, RVUs, Procedures and Square Footage

	51 to 75 FTE		76 to 150 FTE		151 FTE or more	
	Count	Median	Count	Median	Count	Median
Total prov FTE/10,000 patients	13	10.27	14	10.88	5	*
Total phy FTE/10,000 pat	13	8.76	15	9.22	5	*
Prim care phy/10,000 pat	13	3.26	15	3.91	5	*
Nonsurg phy/10,000 pat	11	2.00	15	2.29	4	*
Surg spec phy/10,000 pat	11	1.28	12	2.02	4	*
Total NPP FTE/10,000 pat	13	.92	14	2.22	5	*
Total supp staff FTE/10,000 pat	13	39.82	15	54.19	5	*
Total empl supp staff/10,000 pat	13	39.82	15	54.19	5	*
General administrative	12	1.87	15	3.14	5	*
Patient accounting	12	7.00	15	6.11	5	*
General accounting	12	.45	15	.68	5	*
Managed care administrative	5	*	12	1.40	4	*
Information technology	12	.54	15	1.22	5	*
Housekeeping, maint, security	9	*	10	.74	4	*
Medical receptionists	12	6.21	14	8.47	4	*
Med secretaries,transcribers	12	1.26	12	.89	4	*
Medical records	12	2.65	14	4.51	4	*
Other admin support	6	*	13	.89	3	*
***Total administrative supp staff**	6	*	11	31.92	3	*
Registered Nurses	12	3.37	14	3.68	5	*
Licensed Practical Nurses	11	3.74	15	2.22	5	*
Med assistants, nurse aides	12	3.88	14	5.38	5	*
***Total clinical supp staff**	11	12.83	14	14.08	5	*
Clinical laboratory	12	1.83	15	2.84	4	*
Radiology and imaging	12	1.90	15	3.76	5	*
Other medical support serv	9	*	15	3.11	4	*
***Total ancillary supp staff**	9	*	15	9.74	3	*
Tot contracted supp staff	3	*	8	*	4	*
Tot RVU/patient	7	*	8	*	4	*
Physician work RVU/patient	8	*	8	*	4	*
Tot procedures/patient	13	10.38	14	11.48	4	*
Square feet/patient	12	1.61	14	1.90	5	*
Total support staff FTE/phy	24	4.99	27	6.08	12	5.33

*See pages 260 and 261 for definition.

Table 7.10b: Charges, Revenue and Cost

	51 to 75 FTE		76 to 150 FTE		151 FTE or more	
	Count	Median	Count	Median	Count	Median
Total gross charges	13	$758.63	15	$1,078.38	5	*
Total medical revenue	13	$523.45	15	$723.99	5	*
Net fee-for-service revenue	13	$479.10	14	$469.80	5	*
Net capitation revenue	4	*	9	*	3	*
Net other medical revenue	13	$15.42	12	$25.60	5	*
Total support staff cost/patient	13	$152.18	15	$218.70	5	*
Total general operating cost	13	$145.58	15	$197.83	5	*
Total operating cost	13	$297.76	15	$433.88	5	*
Total med rev after oper cost	13	$199.78	15	$295.74	5	*
Total provider cost/patient	13	$209.29	15	$277.67	5	*
Total NPP cost/patient	13	$7.25	15	$19.23	5	*
Provider consultant cost	7	*	9	*	3	*
Total physician cost/patient	13	$194.98	15	$252.91	5	*
Total phy compensation	13	$162.99	15	$214.91	5	*
Total phy benefit cost	13	$26.01	15	$28.45	5	*
Total cost	13	$523.36	15	$716.44	5	*
Net nonmedical revenue	13	$1.20	15	$4.07	4	*
Net inc, prac with fin sup	0	*	0	*	1	*
Net inc, prac w/o fin sup	13	$2.98	15	$8.88	3	*
Net inc, excl fin supp (all prac)	13	$2.98	15	$8.88	4	*
Total support staff FTE/phy	24	4.99	27	6.08	12	5.33

Multispecialty — Practices with 51 or More FTE Physicians, Not Hospital or IDS Owned
(Procedure and Charge Data)

Table 7.11a: Activity Charges to Total Gross Charges Ratios

	51 to 75 FTE		76 to 150 FTE		151 FTE or more	
	Count	Median	Count	Median	Count	Median
Total proc gross charges	19	90.75%	22	91.19%	7	*
Medical proc-inside practice	19	34.27%	22	36.00%	7	*
Medical proc-outside practice	19	8.32%	21	7.53%	7	*
Surg proc-inside practice	19	5.63%	22	7.42%	6	*
Surg proc-outside practice	18	16.55%	20	17.83%	6	*
Laboratory procedures	19	11.14%	22	8.70%	7	*
Radiology procedures	19	12.66%	22	12.93%	7	*
Tot nonproc gross charges	19	9.25%	21	9.60%	7	*
Total support staff FTE/phy	24	4.99	27	6.08	12	5.33

Table 7.11b: Medical Procedure Data (inside the practice)

	51 to 75 FTE		76 to 150 FTE		151 FTE or more	
	Count	Median	Count	Median	Count	Median
Gross charges/procedure	18	$76.36	22	$73.74	7	*
Total cost/procedure	16	$65.37	19	$64.40	7	*
Operating cost/procedure	15	$41.64	19	$43.20	7	*
Provider cost/procedure	17	$23.32	19	$23.36	7	*
Procedures/patient	13	4.10	14	5.20	4	*
Gross charges/patient	13	$322.43	14	$438.59	4	*
Procedures/physician	18	4,784	22	5,831	7	*
Gross charges/physician	19	$412,925	22	$434,195	7	*
Procedures/provider	18	3,870	21	4,660	7	*
Gross charges/provider	19	$352,891	21	$330,376	7	*
Gross charge to total cost ratio	16	1.21	19	1.17	7	*
Oper cost to total cost ratio	15	.65	19	.63	7	*
Prov cost to total cost ratio	16	.35	19	.37	7	*
Total support staff FTE/phy	24	4.99	27	6.08	12	5.33

Table 7.11c: Medical Procedure Data (outside the practice)

	51 to 75 FTE		76 to 150 FTE		151 FTE or more	
	Count	Median	Count	Median	Count	Median
Gross charges/procedure	18	$123.22	21	$126.17	7	*
Total cost/procedure	16	$53.85	18	$58.44	7	*
Operating cost/procedure	15	$16.40	18	$23.93	7	*
Provider cost/procedure	17	$33.95	18	$34.97	7	*
Procedures/patient	13	.70	14	.61	4	*
Gross charges/patient	13	$67.68	14	$81.21	4	*
Procedures/physician	18	1,013	21	722	7	*
Gross charges/physician	19	$104,642	21	$94,991	7	*
Procedures/provider	17	764	20	606	7	*
Gross charges/provider	19	$88,148	20	$76,673	7	*
Gross charge to total cost ratio	16	2.30	18	2.27	7	*
Oper cost to total cost ratio	15	.36	18	.42	7	*
Prov cost to total cost ratio	16	.64	18	.58	7	*
Total support staff FTE/phy	24	4.99	27	6.08	12	5.33

Multispecialty — Practices with 51 or More FTE Physicians, Not Hospital or IDS Owned (Procedure and Charge Data)

Table 7.11d: Surgery/Anesthesia Procedure Data (inside the practice)

	51 to 75 FTE		76 to 150 FTE		151 FTE or more	
	Count	Median	Count	Median	Count	Median
Gross charges/procedure	18	$107.58	22	$89.30	6	*
Total cost/procedure	16	$95.00	19	$71.41	6	*
Operating cost/procedure	15	$62.54	19	$43.58	6	*
Provider cost/procedure	17	$29.18	19	$27.30	6	*
Procedures/patient	13	.92	14	.83	3	*
Gross charges/patient	13	$35.57	14	$87.02	3	*
Procedures/physician	18	858	22	1,219	6	*
Gross charges/physician	19	$70,571	22	$102,467	6	*
Procedures/provider	18	672	21	927	6	*
Gross charges/provider	19	$56,247	21	$68,666	6	*
Gross charge to total cost ratio	16	1.21	19	1.17	6	*
Oper cost to total cost ratio	15	.65	19	.63	6	*
Prov cost to total cost ratio	16	.35	19	.37	6	*
Total support staff FTE/phy	24	4.99	27	6.08	12	5.33

Table 7.11e: Surgery/Anesthesia Procedure Data (outside the practice)

	51 to 75 FTE		76 to 150 FTE		151 FTE or more	
	Count	Median	Count	Median	Count	Median
Gross charges/procedure	17	$959.28	20	$968.71	6	*
Total cost/procedure	15	$396.54	18	$389.93	6	*
Operating cost/procedure	14	$123.34	18	$158.72	6	*
Provider cost/procedure	16	$266.68	18	$243.41	6	*
Procedures/patient	12	.15	13	.24	3	*
Gross charges/patient	12	$78.66	12	$209.72	3	*
Procedures/physician	17	242	20	248	6	*
Gross charges/physician	18	$197,756	20	$229,407	6	*
Procedures/provider	17	200	19	200	6	*
Gross charges/provider	18	$170,371	19	$172,768	6	*
Gross charge to total cost ratio	15	2.31	18	2.27	6	*
Oper cost to total cost ratio	14	.35	18	.42	6	*
Prov cost to total cost ratio	15	.64	18	.58	6	*
Total support staff FTE/phy	24	4.99	27	6.08	12	5.33

Multispecialty — Practices with 51 or More FTE Physicians, Not Hospital or IDS Owned
(Procedure and Charge Data)

Table 7.11f: Clinical Laboratory/Pathology Procedure Data

	51 to 75 FTE		76 to 150 FTE		151 FTE or more	
	Count	Median	Count	Median	Count	Median
Gross charges/procedure	19	$37.17	22	$33.99	7	*
Total cost/procedure	17	$26.88	19	$25.84	7	*
Operating cost/procedure	16	$16.92	19	$17.66	7	*
Provider cost/procedure	18	$9.15	19	$8.57	7	*
Procedures/patient	13	3.06	14	3.39	4	*
Gross charges/patient	13	$96.63	14	$119.34	4	*
Procedures/physician	19	3,252	22	3,690	7	*
Gross charges/physician	19	$123,314	22	$122,117	7	*
Procedures/provider	19	2,970	21	2,905	7	*
Gross charges/provider	19	$107,504	21	$103,081	7	*
Gross charge to total cost ratio	17	1.31	19	1.31	7	*
Oper cost to total cost ratio	16	.62	19	.66	7	*
Prov cost to total cost ratio	17	.37	19	.34	7	*
Total support staff FTE/phy	24	4.99	27	6.08	12	5.33

Table 7.11g: Diagnostic Radiology and Imaging Procedure Data

	51 to 75 FTE		76 to 150 FTE		151 FTE or more	
	Count	Median	Count	Median	Count	Median
Gross charges/procedure	19	$180.00	22	$209.63	7	*
Total cost/procedure	16	$149.03	19	$172.83	7	*
Operating cost/procedure	15	$90.96	19	$108.81	7	*
Provider cost/procedure	18	$54.97	19	$58.54	7	*
Procedures/patient	13	.54	14	.70	4	*
Gross charges/patient	13	$92.47	14	$123.36	4	*
Procedures/physician	19	642	22	720	7	*
Gross charges/physician	19	$146,336	22	$162,075	7	*
Procedures/provider	19	528	21	557	7	*
Gross charges/provider	19	$118,517	21	$128,329	7	*
Gross charge to total cost ratio	17	1.28	19	1.23	7	*
Oper cost to total cost ratio	16	.62	19	.67	7	*
Prov cost to total cost ratio	17	.37	19	.33	7	*
Total support staff FTE/phy	24	4.99	27	6.08	12	5.33

Table 7.11h: Nonprocedural Gross Charge Data

	51 to 75 FTE		76 to 150 FTE		151 FTE or more	
	Count	Median	Count	Median	Count	Median
Gross charges/patient	13	$75.51	13	$66.82	4	*
Nonproc gross charges/physician	19	$109,381	21	$108,582	7	*
Gross charges/provider	19	$94,236	20	$90,629	7	*
Total support staff FTE/phy	24	4.99	27	6.08	12	5.33

Multispecialty — by Capitation Revenue Percent, Not Hospital or IDS Owned

Table 8.1: Staffing and Practice Data

	No capitation		10% or less		11% to 50%	
	Count	Median	Count	Median	Count	Median
Total provider FTE	**118**	**30.82**	**28**	**42.37**	**24**	**78.34**
Total physician FTE	127	22.50	32	30.33	27	64.43
Total nonphysician provider FTE	118	4.90	28	5.52	24	12.43
Total support staff FTE	**127**	**135.00**	**32**	**128.96**	**27**	**292.25**
Number of branch clinics	98	5	27	4	24	8
Square footage of all facilities	120	47,996	29	44,000	25	102,196

Table 8.2: Accounts Receivable Data, Collection Percentages and Financial Ratios

	No capitation		10% or less		11% to 50%	
	Count	Median	Count	Median	Count	Median
Total AR/physician	**118**	**$139,023**	**30**	**$126,645**	**23**	**$99,422**
Total AR/provider	**111**	**$106,374**	**26**	**$99,482**	**22**	**$82,701**
0-30 days in AR	118	52.30%	30	52.96%	24	49.28%
31-60 days in AR	118	14.66%	30	13.53%	24	14.44%
61-90 days in AR	118	7.54%	30	7.45%	24	8.34%
91-120 days in AR	118	5.03%	30	5.75%	24	5.55%
120+ days in AR	118	17.85%	30	18.92%	24	20.37%
Re-aged: 0-30 days in AR	50	52.95%	9	*	10	57.32%
Re-aged: 31-60 days in AR	50	13.62%	9	*	10	13.99%
Re-aged: 61-90 days in AR	50	6.94%	9	*	10	7.91%
Re-aged: 91-120 days in AR	50	4.80%	9	*	10	4.57%
Re-aged: 120+ days in AR	50	17.69%	9	*	10	12.23%
Not re-aged: 0-30 days in AR	63	51.51%	20	49.32%	14	42.41%
Not re-aged: 31-60 days in AR	63	15.00%	20	15.08%	14	14.98%
Not re-aged: 61-90 days in AR	63	7.84%	20	7.98%	14	8.92%
Not re-aged: 91-120 days in AR	63	5.31%	20	5.94%	14	6.52%
Not re-aged: 120+ days in AR	63	17.77%	20	19.41%	14	23.20%
Months gross FFS charges in AR	113	1.62	29	1.59	24	1.80
Days gross FFS charges in AR	113	49.37	29	48.44	24	54.74
Gross FFS collection %	120	62.85%	31	60.81%	27	64.62%
Adjusted FFS collection %	115	97.39%	28	97.82%	27	98.00%
Gross FFS + cap collection %	8	*	32	61.38%	26	71.11%
Net cap rev % of gross cap chrg	2	*	28	71.74%	25	81.02%
Current ratio	82	1.79	19	1.36	20	1.37
Tot asset turnover ratio	82	4.68	19	4.59	20	4.30
Debt to equity ratio	82	1.80	19	1.68	20	2.28
Debt ratio	82	64.31%	19	62.70%	20	68.88%
Return on total assets	76	3.16%	18	.13%	18	15.95%
Return on equity	76	9.21%	18	.47%	18	34.96%

Table 8.3: Breakout of Total Gross Charges by Type of Payer

	No capitation		10% or less		11% to 50%	
	Count	Median	Count	Median	Count	Median
Medicare: fee-for-service	115	28.55%	31	28.41%	24	18.65%
Medicare: managed care FFS	115	.00%	31	.00%	24	.00%
Medicare: capitation	115	.00%	31	.00%	24	7.87%
Medicaid: fee-for-service	115	4.83%	31	4.30%	24	1.91%
Medicaid: managed care FFS	115	.00%	31	.00%	24	.00%
Medicaid: capitation	115	.00%	31	.00%	24	.36%
Commercial: fee-for-service	115	46.00%	31	28.90%	24	33.40%
Commercial: managed care FFS	115	.00%	31	11.00%	24	.00%
Commercial: capitation	115	.00%	31	2.23%	24	16.24%
Workers' compensation	115	1.00%	31	1.00%	24	.61%
Charity care and prof courtesy	115	.00%	31	.02%	24	.00%
Self-pay	115	3.87%	31	4.00%	24	3.85%
Other federal government payers	115	.00%	31	.00%	24	.00%

Multispecialty — by Capitation Revenue Percent, Not Hospital or IDS Owned
(per FTE Physician)

Table 8.4a: Staffing, RVUs, Patients, Procedures and Square Footage

	No capitation		10% or less		11% to 50%	
	Count	Median	Count	Median	Count	Median
Total provider FTE/physician	**118**	**1.20**	**28**	**1.27**	**24**	**1.25**
Prim care phy/physician	119	.65	32	.63	27	.57
Nonsurg phy/physician	84	.26	20	.23	22	.26
Surg spec phy/physician	84	.23	20	.21	19	.22
Total NPP FTE/physician	118	.20	28	.27	24	.25
Total support staff FTE/phy	**127**	**5.31**	**32**	**5.21**	**27**	**5.75**
Total empl support staff FTE	122	5.33	32	5.07	27	5.73
General administrative	121	.25	30	.27	25	.34
Patient accounting	118	.77	31	.64	26	.63
General accounting	99	.08	26	.06	23	.08
Managed care administrative	48	.07	17	.09	19	.17
Information technology	81	.10	19	.09	19	.15
Housekeeping, maint, security	74	.09	19	.07	20	.06
Medical receptionists	117	.91	30	.82	27	1.02
Med secretaries,transcribers	100	.27	26	.24	18	.12
Medical records	107	.41	28	.39	25	.46
Other admin support	68	.09	16	.14	18	.12
*Total administrative supp staff	**62**	**3.14**	**12**	**3.10**	**20**	**3.38**
Registered Nurses	104	.40	29	.40	26	.45
Licensed Practical Nurses	104	.44	27	.43	20	.20
Med assistants, nurse aides	112	.70	26	.72	27	.77
*Total clinical supp staff	**100**	**1.60**	**24**	**1.45**	**24**	**1.56**
Clinical laboratory	103	.36	27	.33	21	.31
Radiology and imaging	106	.28	26	.33	21	.33
Other medical support serv	69	.25	20	.22	20	.31
*Total ancillary supp staff	**69**	**.94**	**16**	**1.09**	**19**	**1.01**
Tot contracted supp staff	41	.11	16	.10	16	.08
Tot RVU/physician	44	12,242	16	11,268	14	10,117
Physician work RVU/physician	47	5,759	15	5,334	14	4,721
Patients/physician	64	1,591	16	1,564	15	1,579
Tot procedures/physician	104	12,513	26	11,172	23	11,272
Square feet/physician	120	2,128	29	2,050	25	1,859

*See pages 260 and 261 for definition.

Table 8.4b: Charges and Revenue

	No capitation		10% or less		11% to 50%	
	Count	Median	Count	Median	Count	Median
Net fee-for-service revenue	122	$634,984	32	$532,109	27	$443,423
Gross FFS charges	121	$1,018,052	31	$840,694	27	$660,194
Adjustments to FFS charges	113	$356,078	28	$316,085	25	$249,176
Adjusted FFS charges	115	$675,112	28	$572,113	27	$454,605
Bad debts due to FFS activity	107	$14,734	26	$15,229	27	$7,916
Net capitation revenue	8	*	32	$23,610	27	$206,330
Gross capitation charges	2	*	28	$41,115	25	$214,824
Capitation revenue	7	*	31	$24,799	27	$256,066
Purch serv for cap patients	0	*	6	*	14	$140,642
Net other medical revenue	87	$13,113	22	$15,847	23	$24,262
Gross rev from other activity	84	$18,126	22	$15,867	23	$32,263
Other medical revenue	66	$9,032	16	$11,505	21	$15,354
Rev from sale of goods/services	50	$18,521	18	$10,519	12	$31,417
Cost of sales	31	$13,278	10	$6,453	10	$23,427
Total gross charges	**120**	**$1,005,448**	**32**	**$888,882**	**26**	**$966,001**
Total medical revenue	**127**	**$643,091**	**32**	**$592,103**	**27**	**$686,320**

Multispecialty — by Capitation Revenue Percent, Not Hospital or IDS Owned
(per FTE Physician)

Table 8.4c: Operating Cost

	No capitation		10% or less		11% to 50%	
	Count	Median	Count	Median	Count	Median
Total support staff cost/phy	127	$187,543	32	$190,435	27	$228,083
Total empl supp staff cost/phy	126	$148,145	32	$151,646	27	$181,301
General administrative	122	$14,882	30	$16,239	25	$21,074
Patient accounting	120	$19,298	31	$16,527	26	$17,416
General accounting	101	$2,837	26	$2,594	23	$3,359
Managed care administrative	46	$2,465	18	$2,250	19	$5,309
Information technology	83	$3,822	19	$3,689	19	$6,860
Housekeeping, maint, security	76	$2,270	19	$2,301	20	$1,928
Medical receptionists	117	$19,145	30	$18,164	27	$24,891
Med secretaries,transcribers	100	$6,684	26	$6,260	18	$3,109
Medical records	108	$7,850	28	$7,571	25	$9,880
Other admin support	68	$2,006	17	$3,067	18	$2,465
***Total administrative supp staff**	57	$83,796	14	$81,461	19	$101,886
Registered Nurses	105	$16,847	28	$15,359	26	$19,489
Licensed Practical Nurses	102	$12,918	26	$12,178	20	$5,972
Med assistants, nurse aides	110	$16,511	25	$19,409	27	$20,781
***Total clinical supp staff**	97	$45,993	23	$44,448	23	$46,094
Clinical laboratory	103	$10,857	27	$10,408	21	$9,183
Radiology and imaging	107	$9,568	26	$11,031	21	$12,586
Other medical support serv	73	$8,417	20	$8,033	20	$10,077
***Total ancillary supp staff**	82	$29,496	19	$30,841	20	$35,749
Total empl supp staff benefits	123	$38,088	32	$32,578	27	$45,877
Tot contracted supp staff	62	$2,155	18	$2,371	23	$2,074
Total general operating cost	127	$183,973	32	$167,203	27	$190,229
Information technology	124	$10,128	32	$9,329	27	$12,970
Medical and surgical supply	124	$31,424	32	$25,742	27	$29,264
Building and occupancy	124	$42,710	32	$37,590	27	$45,064
Furniture and equipment	113	$8,469	30	$9,048	24	$5,569
Admin supplies and services	122	$10,889	32	$10,656	27	$13,320
Prof liability insurance	123	$13,231	32	$10,823	26	$12,502
Other insurance premiums	117	$1,202	32	$1,352	25	$1,027
Outside professional fees	121	$3,848	32	$3,303	25	$4,284
Promotion and marketing	122	$2,559	32	$2,398	26	$2,205
Clinical laboratory	117	$16,013	27	$14,940	23	$11,410
Radiology and imaging	107	$9,171	28	$6,833	21	$6,700
Other ancillary services	60	$2,307	17	$4,801	15	$3,746
Billing purchased services	73	$1,943	24	$1,935	14	$1,710
Management fees paid to MSO	6	*	3	*	3	*
Misc operating cost	123	$8,319	32	$6,376	27	$9,689
Cost allocated to prac from par	1	*	0	*	1	*
Total operating cost	127	$379,730	32	$359,916	27	$427,981

*See pages 260 and 261 for definition.

Multispecialty — by Capitation Revenue Percent, Not Hospital or IDS Owned
(per FTE Physician)

Table 8.4d: Provider Cost

	No capitation		10% or less		11% to 50%	
	Count	Median	Count	Median	Count	Median
Total med rev after oper cost	127	$268,083	32	$223,351	27	$270,284
Total provider cost/physician	127	$267,542	32	$229,848	27	$271,614
Total NPP cost/physician	121	$17,507	30	$16,513	25	$20,058
Nonphysician provider comp	121	$14,469	30	$13,115	25	$16,305
Nonphysician prov benefit cost	110	$3,047	28	$3,401	24	$3,829
Provider consultant cost	40	$11,146	16	$8,547	16	$6,466
Total physician cost/physician	127	$233,914	32	$210,605	27	$230,455
Total phy compensation	127	$202,755	32	$180,123	27	$195,040
Total phy benefit cost	124	$34,469	32	$29,097	27	$31,805

Table 8.4e: Net Income or Loss

	No capitation		10% or less		11% to 50%	
	Count	Median	Count	Median	Count	Median
Total cost	127	$642,870	32	$582,088	27	$657,259
Net nonmedical revenue	102	$2,488	29	$3,129	23	$2,096
Nonmedical revenue	98	$3,938	28	$4,246	23	$4,065
Fin support for oper costs	2	*	1	*	1	*
Goodwill amortization	16	$339	3	*	4	*
Nonmedical cost	56	$1,240	13	$1,305	13	$3,070
Net inc, prac with fin sup	2	*	1	*	1	*
Net inc, prac w/o fin sup	118	$3,655	29	$899	23	$16,059
Net inc, excl fin supp (all prac)	120	$3,655	30	$596	24	$16,168

Table 8.4f: Assets and Liabilities

	No capitation		10% or less		11% to 50%	
	Count	Median	Count	Median	Count	Median
Total assets	86	$122,887	20	$133,440	20	$189,488
Current assets	87	$89,073	21	$80,084	20	$90,746
Noncurrent assets	87	$39,037	21	$39,336	20	$80,105
Total liabilities	87	$58,909	21	$93,308	20	$96,714
Current liabilities	87	$35,525	21	$40,433	20	$40,003
Noncurrent liabilities	87	$18,384	21	$19,035	20	$40,741
Working capital	87	$27,207	21	$27,355	20	$16,596
Total net worth	87	$37,527	21	$52,965	20	$63,688
Total support staff FTE/phy	127	5.31	32	5.21	27	5.75

Multispecialty — by Capitation Revenue Percent, Not Hospital or IDS Owned
(as a % of Total Medical Revenue)

Table 8.5a: Charges and Revenue

	No capitation		10% or less		11% to 50%	
	Count	Median	Count	Median	Count	Median
Net fee-for-service revenue	122	98.86%	32	92.92%	27	66.66%
Net capitation revenue	8	*	32	4.34%	27	25.35%
Net other medical revenue	87	1.86%	22	2.65%	23	3.21%
Total gross charges	**125**	**157.90%**	**32**	**159.24%**	**26**	**139.04%**

Table 8.5b: Operating Cost

	No capitation		10% or less		11% to 50%	
	Count	Median	Count	Median	Count	Median
Total support staff cost	**127**	**28.98%**	**32**	**30.86%**	**27**	**31.98%**
Total empl support staff cost	126	22.96%	32	25.04%	27	25.71%
General administrative	122	2.28%	30	2.93%	25	2.75%
Patient accounting	120	2.92%	31	2.71%	26	2.46%
General accounting	101	.43%	26	.37%	23	.41%
Managed care administrative	46	.35%	18	.28%	19	.91%
Information technology	83	.54%	19	.53%	19	.85%
Housekeeping, maint, security	76	.30%	19	.41%	20	.28%
Medical receptionists	117	2.97%	30	2.78%	27	3.22%
Med secretaries,transcribers	100	1.05%	26	1.02%	18	.48%
Medical records	108	1.16%	28	1.22%	25	1.21%
Other admin support	68	.32%	17	.52%	18	.28%
*Total administrative supp staff	57	12.16%	14	12.99%	19	13.20%
Registered Nurses	105	2.15%	28	2.38%	26	2.99%
Licensed Practical Nurses	102	1.92%	26	2.12%	20	1.18%
Med assistants, nurse aides	110	2.34%	25	2.97%	27	2.96%
*Total clinical supp staff	97	6.94%	23	7.52%	23	7.05%
Clinical laboratory	103	1.46%	27	1.57%	21	1.14%
Radiology and imaging	107	1.51%	26	1.82%	21	1.69%
Other medical support serv	73	1.14%	20	1.14%	20	1.38%
*Total ancillary supp staff	82	4.18%	19	4.44%	20	3.89%
Total empl supp staff benefits	123	5.88%	32	6.10%	27	6.11%
Tot contracted supp staff	62	.37%	18	.42%	23	.32%
Total general operating cost	**127**	**28.83%**	**32**	**29.88%**	**27**	**26.35%**
Information technology	124	1.52%	32	1.73%	27	2.04%
Medical and surgical supply	124	4.88%	32	4.69%	27	4.21%
Building and occupancy	124	6.12%	32	6.52%	27	6.68%
Furniture and equipment	113	1.20%	30	1.50%	24	.89%
Admin supplies and services	123	1.66%	32	2.00%	27	1.85%
Prof liability insurance	123	2.08%	32	1.81%	26	1.98%
Other insurance premiums	116	.20%	31	.27%	25	.24%
Outside professional fees	121	.62%	32	.52%	25	.53%
Promotion and marketing	122	.41%	32	.35%	26	.28%
Clinical laboratory	117	2.41%	27	2.54%	23	1.52%
Radiology and imaging	109	1.51%	29	1.16%	21	1.05%
Other ancillary services	60	.30%	17	.74%	15	.56%
Billing purchased services	73	.26%	24	.32%	14	.29%
Management fees paid to MSO	7	*	3	*	4	*
Misc operating cost	123	1.26%	32	1.34%	27	1.49%
Cost allocated to prac from par	1	*	0	*	1	*
Total operating cost	**127**	**57.98%**	**32**	**61.37%**	**27**	**58.24%**

*See pages 260 and 261 for definition.

Multispecialty — by Capitation Revenue Percent, Not Hospital or IDS Owned
(as a % of Total Medical Revenue)

Table 8.5c: Provider Cost

	No capitation		10% or less		11% to 50%	
	Count	Median	Count	Median	Count	Median
Total med rev after oper cost	127	41.99%	32	39.10%	27	41.76%
Total provider cost	127	41.42%	32	40.75%	27	39.37%
Total NPP cost	121	2.78%	30	3.24%	25	2.88%
Nonphysician provider comp	121	2.34%	30	2.68%	25	2.28%
Nonphysician prov benefit cost	110	.44%	28	.57%	24	.53%
Provider consultant cost	40	1.86%	16	1.51%	16	.86%
Total physician cost	127	38.93%	32	35.80%	27	36.28%
Total phy compensation	127	33.27%	32	30.41%	27	29.63%
Total phy benefit cost	124	5.23%	32	5.21%	27	4.78%

Table 8.5d: Net Income or Loss

	No capitation		10% or less		11% to 50%	
	Count	Median	Count	Median	Count	Median
Total cost	127	100.02%	32	100.10%	27	98.03%
Net nonmedical revenue	102	.36%	29	.57%	23	.26%
Nonmedical revenue	98	.52%	28	.78%	23	.53%
Fin support for oper costs	2	*	1	*	1	*
Goodwill amortization	16	.04%	3	*	4	*
Nonmedical cost	56	.18%	13	.20%	13	.41%
Net inc, prac with fin sup	2	*	1	*	1	*
Net inc, prac w/o fin sup	118	.61%	29	.18%	23	1.97%
Net inc, excl fin supp (all prac)	120	.61%	30	.11%	24	2.37%

Table 8.5e: Assets and Liabilities

	No capitation		10% or less		11% to 50%	
	Count	Median	Count	Median	Count	Median
Total assets	87	20.98%	21	21.60%	20	23.26%
Current assets	87	14.44%	21	12.18%	20	12.64%
Noncurrent assets	87	5.64%	21	7.20%	20	13.65%
Total liabilities	87	9.83%	21	13.05%	20	14.45%
Current liabilities	87	6.24%	21	8.02%	20	6.60%
Noncurrent liabilities	87	2.99%	21	3.84%	20	5.10%
Working capital	87	3.61%	21	4.06%	20	2.43%
Total net worth	87	6.09%	21	8.55%	20	10.64%

Multispecialty — by Capitation Revenue Percent, Not Hospital or IDS Owned
(per FTE Provider)

Table 8.6a: Staffing, RVUs, Patients, Procedures and Square Footage

	No capitation		10% or less		11% to 50%	
	Count	Median	Count	Median	Count	Median
Total physician FTE/provider	118	.83	28	.79	24	.80
Prim care phy/provider	111	.46	28	.51	24	.49
Nonsurg phy/provider	80	.22	18	.20	19	.20
Surg spec phy/provider	79	.17	18	.17	17	.18
Total NPP FTE/provider	118	.17	28	.21	24	.20
Total support staff FTE/prov	118	4.27	28	4.08	24	4.85
Total empl supp staff FTE/prov	114	4.29	28	3.87	24	4.76
General administrative	114	.21	26	.23	23	.27
Patient accounting	112	.62	27	.50	23	.55
General accounting	97	.07	24	.05	22	.07
Managed care administrative	47	.06	14	.07	18	.14
Information technology	79	.08	17	.06	19	.12
Housekeeping, maint, security	71	.07	18	.07	19	.05
Medical receptionists	110	.74	26	.66	24	.86
Med secretaries,transcribers	95	.21	24	.16	16	.10
Medical records	102	.33	25	.32	23	.41
Other admin support	66	.08	15	.10	16	.10
*Total administrative supp staff	60	2.61	12	2.33	20	2.72
Registered Nurses	99	.32	25	.28	23	.36
Licensed Practical Nurses	97	.35	24	.37	18	.15
Med assistants, nurse aides	106	.57	22	.58	24	.65
*Total clinical supp staff	95	1.27	21	1.18	22	1.25
Clinical laboratory	99	.29	24	.28	20	.25
Radiology and imaging	103	.21	23	.25	20	.27
Other medical support serv	67	.20	19	.16	19	.24
*Total ancillary supp staff	68	.77	16	.88	18	.84
Tot contracted supp staff	40	.06	12	.13	16	.07
Tot RVU/provider	42	9,367	14	9,024	12	8,192
Physician work RVU/provider	45	4,570	13	4,137	12	4,244
Patients/provider	61	1,282	13	1,348	15	1,131
Tot procedures/provider	97	10,212	23	9,512	20	9,697
Square feet/provider	113	1,727	25	1,598	22	1,526
Total support staff FTE/phy	127	5.31	32	5.21	27	5.75

*See pages 260 and 261 for definition.

Table 8.6b: Charges, Revenue and Cost

	No capitation		10% or less		11% to 50%	
	Count	Median	Count	Median	Count	Median
Total gross charges	116	$789,553	28	$733,842	24	$809,664
Total medical revenue	118	$512,821	28	$449,204	24	$571,453
Net fee-for-service revenue	113	$507,962	28	$421,515	24	$378,531
Net capitation revenue	8	*	28	$17,523	24	$162,264
Net other medical revenue	84	$10,394	19	$15,209	21	$20,810
Total support staff cost/prov	118	$158,418	28	$141,830	24	$198,738
Total general operating cost	118	$146,985	28	$137,675	24	$164,766
Total operating cost	118	$300,170	28	$288,515	24	$366,345
Total med rev after oper cost	118	$215,831	28	$174,013	24	$210,254
Total provider cost/provider	118	$219,576	28	$190,218	24	$208,635
Total NPP cost/provider	118	$14,533	28	$15,392	24	$16,038
Provider consultant cost	39	$8,725	14	$7,753	15	$5,363
Total physician cost/provider	118	$196,406	28	$168,968	24	$183,931
Total phy compensation	118	$169,956	28	$142,974	24	$159,520
Total phy benefit cost	115	$27,787	28	$24,904	24	$23,885
Total cost	118	$517,116	28	$475,629	24	$551,007
Net nonmedical revenue	96	$1,860	26	$2,606	21	$1,751
Net inc, prac with fin sup	2	*	1	*	1	*
Net inc, prac w/o fin sup	109	$2,818	25	$778	20	$16,019
Net inc, excl fin supp (all prac)	111	$2,818	26	$480	21	$16,930
Total support staff FTE/phy	127	5.31	32	5.21	27	5.75

Multispecialty — by Capitation Revenue Percent, Not Hospital or IDS Owned
(per Square Foot)

Table 8.7a: Staffing, RVUs, Patients and Procedures

	No capitation		10% or less		11% to 50%	
	Count	Median	Count	Median	Count	Median
Total prov FTE/10,000 sq ft	113	5.79	25	6.26	22	6.57
Total phy FTE/10,000 sq ft	120	4.70	29	4.88	25	5.38
Prim care phy/10,000 sq ft	113	2.81	29	3.26	25	3.37
Nonsurg phy/10,000 sq ft	79	1.29	18	1.11	21	1.31
Surg spec phy/10,000 sq ft	80	.98	18	1.21	18	1.00
Total NPP FTE/10,000 sq ft	113	1.00	25	1.28	22	1.19
Total supp stf FTE/10,000 sq ft	120	25.56	29	26.98	25	28.57
Total empl supp stf/10,000 sq ft	116	25.32	29	26.56	25	27.95
General administrative	116	1.23	28	1.47	24	1.55
Patient accounting	114	3.56	29	2.93	25	3.12
General accounting	96	.40	24	.33	21	.36
Managed care administrative	47	.36	15	.84	18	1.08
Information technology	77	.43	17	.36	18	.72
Housekeeping, maint, security	72	.39	18	.50	18	.31
Medical receptionists	112	4.13	28	4.55	25	5.52
Med secretaries,transcribers	97	1.12	24	1.01	16	.56
Medical records	102	1.95	26	2.00	23	2.07
Other admin support	65	.40	16	.51	17	.50
*Total administrative supp staff	60	13.93	12	13.77	18	15.51
Registered Nurses	100	1.94	27	2.38	24	2.26
Licensed Practical Nurses	100	1.89	26	2.44	18	1.15
Med assistants, nurse aides	108	3.03	25	3.75	25	4.83
*Total clinical supp staff	96	7.21	24	8.51	22	7.45
Clinical laboratory	100	1.65	25	1.57	21	1.42
Radiology and imaging	101	1.35	24	1.48	19	1.44
Other medical support serv	66	1.07	18	1.09	19	1.33
*Total ancillary supp staff	67	4.02	14	5.23	19	4.35
Tot contracted supp staff	41	.48	15	.69	16	.38
Tot RVU/sq ft	43	6.33	15	5.82	13	5.41
Physician work RVU/sq ft	46	2.73	14	2.35	13	2.38
Patients/sq ft	60	.84	14	1.29	15	.91
Tot procedures/sq ft	99	5.64	24	5.83	22	5.57
Total support staff FTE/phy	127	5.31	32	5.21	27	5.75

*See pages 260 and 261 for definition.

Table 8.7b: Charges, Revenue and Cost

	No capitation		10% or less		11% to 50%	
	Count	Median	Count	Median	Count	Median
Total gross charges	119	$496.79	29	$503.70	24	$494.97
Total medical revenue	120	$318.00	29	$334.11	25	$349.09
Net fee-for-service revenue	115	$305.28	29	$308.80	25	$208.38
Net capitation revenue	7	*	29	$10.91	25	$92.10
Net other medical revenue	84	$6.64	19	$5.03	21	$10.62
Total support staff cost/sq ft	120	$90.55	29	$101.32	25	$106.91
Total general operating cost	120	$90.11	29	$87.32	25	$94.33
Total operating cost	120	$183.93	29	$193.19	25	$206.97
Total med rev after oper cost	120	$126.08	29	$133.74	25	$142.32
Total provider cost/sq ft	120	$127.47	29	$135.62	25	$145.69
Total NPP cost/sq ft	115	$8.50	27	$9.75	23	$10.61
Provider consultant cost	40	$4.77	14	$6.27	15	$2.81
Total physician cost/sq ft	120	$115.27	29	$128.37	25	$124.12
Total phy compensation	120	$103.18	29	$107.56	25	$106.15
Total phy benefit cost	118	$16.05	29	$17.51	25	$17.97
Total cost	120	$316.81	29	$333.42	25	$342.43
Net nonmedical revenue/sq ft	96	$1.11	26	$1.19	21	$.81
Net inc, prac with fin sup	1	*	1	*	1	*
Net inc, prac w/o fin sup	112	$1.73	26	$.35	21	$7.23
Net inc, excl fin supp (all prac)	113	$1.70	27	$.10	22	$7.62
Total support staff FTE/phy	127	5.31	32	5.21	27	5.75

Multispecialty — by Capitation Revenue Percent, Not Hospital or IDS Owned
(per Total RVU)

Table 8.8a: Staffing, Patients, Procedures and Square Footage

	No capitation		10% or less		11% to 50%	
	Count	Median	Count	Median	Count	Median
Total prov FTE/10,000 tot RVU	42	1.07	14	1.11	12	1.22
Total phy FTE/10,000 tot RVU	44	.82	16	.89	14	.99
Prim care phy/10,000 tot RVU	42	.51	16	.52	14	.65
Nonsurg phy/10,000 tot RVU	29	.19	12	.20	11	.24
Surg spec phy/10,000 tot RVU	29	.18	10	.18	10	.16
Total NPP FTE/10,000 tot RVU	42	.19	14	.23	12	.17
Total supp stf FTE/10,000 tot RVU	44	4.18	16	4.42	14	5.65
Tot empl supp stf/10,000 tot RVU	44	4.18	16	4.26	14	5.64
General administrative	44	.19	16	.25	12	.28
Patient accounting	44	.60	16	.51	13	.53
General accounting	34	.07	15	.06	13	.06
Managed care administrative	20	.07	11	.10	11	.17
Information technology	28	.08	11	.07	9	*
Housekeeping, maint, security	28	.07	11	.07	11	.06
Medical receptionists	41	.65	16	.71	14	1.03
Med secretaries,transcribers	37	.20	13	.20	10	.11
Medical records	40	.34	15	.33	12	.54
Other admin support	26	.07	8	*	11	.09
*Total administrative supp staff	26	2.32	5	*	11	3.10
Registered Nurses	41	.36	16	.33	13	.53
Licensed Practical Nurses	40	.24	15	.38	10	.20
Med assistants, nurse aides	40	.62	14	.50	14	.92
*Total clinical supp staff	40	1.26	13	1.23	13	1.40
Clinical laboratory	40	.28	14	.24	11	.27
Radiology and imaging	38	.23	13	.22	11	.34
Other medical support serv	28	.20	12	.17	10	.27
*Total ancillary supp staff	28	.75	9	*	9	*
Tot contracted supp staff	17	.06	9	*	10	.08
Physician work RVU/tot RVU	36	.48	15	.47	13	.48
Patients/tot RVU	33	.15	10	.14	11	.22
Tot procedures/tot RVU	39	.93	14	1.05	14	1.07
Square feet/tot RVU	43	.16	15	.17	13	.18
Total support staff FTE/phy	127	5.31	32	5.21	27	5.75

*See pages 260 and 261 for definition.

Table 8.8b: Charges, Revenue and Cost

	No capitation		10% or less		11% to 50%	
	Count	Median	Count	Median	Count	Median
Total gross charges	44	$87.83	16	$81.69	13	$94.32
Total medical revenue	44	$52.60	16	$50.44	14	$70.28
Net fee-for-service revenue	43	$51.39	16	$45.42	14	$42.03
Net capitation revenue	3	*	16	$2.32	14	$21.65
Net other medical revenue	37	$.98	13	$1.52	12	$2.31
Total supp staff cost/tot RVU	44	$15.25	16	$16.25	14	$25.25
Total general operating cost	44	$14.02	16	$15.12	14	$16.89
Total operating cost	44	$28.78	16	$32.15	14	$42.92
Total med rev after oper cost	44	$22.87	16	$18.11	14	$27.86
Total provider cost/tot RVU	44	$21.81	16	$19.84	14	$25.69
Total NPP cost/tot RVU	42	$1.55	15	$1.46	13	$1.86
Provider consultant cost	15	$.95	10	$.99	9	*
Total physician cost/tot RVU	44	$20.29	16	$18.38	14	$21.36
Total phy compensation	44	$17.54	16	$15.41	14	$19.07
Total phy benefit cost	44	$2.69	16	$2.61	14	$3.25
Total cost	39	$60.56	13	$61.14	13	$68.92
Net nonmedical revenue	33	$.20	15	$.41	11	$.20
Net inc, prac with fin sup	1	*	1	*	1	*
Net inc, prac w/o fin sup	41	$.39	15	$.00	11	$1.41
Net inc, excl fin supp (all prac)	42	$.34	16	-$.06	12	$1.43
Total support staff FTE/phy	127	5.31	32	5.21	27	5.75

Multispecialty — by Capitation Revenue Percent, Not Hospital or IDS Owned
(per Work RVU)

Table 8.9a: Staffing, Patients, Procedures and Square Footage

	No capitation		10% or less		11% to 50%	
	Count	Median	Count	Median	Count	Median
Total prov FTE/10,000 work RVU	45	**2.19**	13	**2.42**	12	**2.36**
Tot phy FTE/10,000 work RVU	47	1.74	15	1.87	14	2.12
Prim care phy/10,000 work RVU	46	1.20	15	1.02	14	1.21
Nonsurg phy/10,000 work RVU	30	.44	11	.37	12	.53
Surg spec phy/10,000 work RVU	31	.38	9	*	11	.35
Total NPP FTE/10,000 work RVU	45	.38	13	.56	12	.31
Total supp stf FTE/10,000 wrk RVU	47	**9.35**	15	**9.91**	14	**12.11**
Tot empl supp stf/10,000 work RVU	47	9.35	15	9.35	14	11.66
General administrative	47	.46	15	.50	12	.57
Patient accounting	46	1.34	15	1.18	13	1.16
General accounting	39	.13	14	.11	13	.17
Managed care administrative	19	.12	11	.16	11	.39
Information technology	32	.20	11	.18	10	.33
Housekeeping, maint, security	32	.20	10	.14	12	.12
Medical receptionists	45	1.55	15	1.57	14	2.02
Med secretaries,transcribers	38	.48	12	.43	11	.18
Medical records	44	.70	14	.70	12	1.04
Other admin support	30	.15	8	*	11	.19
*Total administrative supp staff	30	5.28	5	*	11	6.71
Registered Nurses	43	.85	15	.71	14	1.21
Licensed Practical Nurses	42	.62	14	.74	11	.50
Med assistants, nurse aides	43	1.26	13	1.07	14	1.67
*Total clinical supp staff	42	2.62	12	2.65	13	3.12
Clinical laboratory	41	.59	13	.58	12	.60
Radiology and imaging	40	.50	13	.62	12	.70
Other medical support serv	29	.47	12	.51	11	.54
*Total ancillary supp staff	29	1.68	9	*	10	1.88
Tot contracted supp staff	16	.12	9	*	9	*
Tot RVU/work RVU	36	2.10	15	2.12	13	2.08
Patients/work RVU	32	.30	9	*	11	.26
Tot procedures/work RVU	44	2.11	13	2.20	14	2.34
Square feet/work RVU	46	.37	14	.43	13	.42
Total support staff FTE/phy	127	**5.31**	32	**5.21**	27	**5.75**

*See pages 260 and 261 for definition.

Table 8.9b: Charges, Revenue and Cost

	No capitation		10% or less		11% to 50%	
	Count	Median	Count	Median	Count	Median
Total gross charges	47	**$182.64**	15	**$179.93**	13	**$200.40**
Total medical revenue	47	**$117.47**	15	**$115.66**	14	**$142.88**
Net fee-for-service revenue	46	$115.79	15	$105.81	14	$83.47
Net capitation revenue	2	*	15	$5.15	14	$47.21
Net other medical revenue	38	$2.48	13	$3.10	13	$4.39
Total supp staff cost/work RVU	47	**$34.85**	15	**$36.79**	14	**$50.52**
Total general operating cost	47	**$33.98**	15	**$37.92**	14	**$41.87**
Total operating cost	47	**$68.73**	15	**$75.68**	14	**$85.69**
Total med rev after oper cost	47	**$50.30**	15	**$38.41**	14	**$54.39**
Total provider cost/work RVU	47	**$49.01**	15	**$49.63**	14	**$54.00**
Total NPP cost/work RVU	45	$3.10	14	$3.72	13	$3.37
Provider consultant cost	17	$2.30	9	*	10	$1.25
Total physician cost/work RVU	47	$44.82	15	$42.09	14	$47.92
Total phy compensation	47	$39.05	15	$38.44	14	$41.50
Total phy benefit cost	47	$5.87	15	$5.62	14	$7.05
Total cost	47	**$117.72**	15	**$123.34**	14	**$142.20**
Net nonmedical revenue	36	$.68	14	$.82	12	$.42
Net inc, prac with fin sup	1	*	0	*	1	*
Net inc, prac w/o fin sup	44	$1.03	15	$.00	11	$2.87
Net inc, excl fin supp (all prac)	45	$1.02	15	$.00	12	$3.00
Total support staff FTE/phy	127	**5.31**	32	**5.21**	27	**5.75**

Multispecialty — by Capitation Revenue Percent, Not Hospital or IDS Owned (per Patient)

Table 8.10a: Staffing, RVUs, Procedures and Square Footage

	No capitation		10% or less		11% to 50%	
	Count	Median	Count	Median	Count	Median
Total prov FTE/10,000 patients	61	7.80	13	7.42	15	8.84
Total phy FTE/10,000 pat	64	6.29	16	6.39	16	6.33
Prim care phy/10,000 pat	61	3.38	16	3.90	16	4.40
Nonsurg phy/10,000 pat	44	1.56	8	*	12	1.93
Surg spec phy/10,000 pat	41	1.30	8	*	10	1.63
Total NPP FTE/10,000 pat	61	1.13	13	.92	15	1.77
Total supp staff FTE/10,000 pat	64	30.17	16	28.77	16	34.69
Total empl supp staff/10,000 pat	64	30.17	16	28.16	16	34.52
General administrative	63	1.34	15	1.33	14	2.55
Patient accounting	61	4.89	15	3.15	15	4.40
General accounting	55	.54	13	.41	15	.57
Managed care administrative	27	.39	9	*	12	1.30
Information technology	44	.55	8	*	12	1.11
Housekeeping, maint, security	38	.47	7	*	12	.31
Medical receptionists	61	5.47	15	4.04	16	6.39
Med secretaries,transcribers	53	1.53	12	1.47	12	.70
Medical records	55	2.05	13	1.95	15	3.78
Other admin support	37	.53	6	*	12	.74
*Total administrative supp staff	35	20.65	5	*	14	20.37
Registered Nurses	57	2.05	14	1.98	15	4.03
Licensed Practical Nurses	56	2.00	14	2.55	12	1.44
Med assistants, nurse aides	59	3.35	13	3.39	16	5.33
*Total clinical supp staff	54	9.28	13	8.52	15	10.69
Clinical laboratory	54	2.10	14	1.44	13	2.72
Radiology and imaging	55	1.58	11	1.09	12	2.46
Other medical support serv	38	1.60	9	*	12	2.00
*Total ancillary supp staff	37	6.06	7	*	11	8.11
Tot contracted supp staff	21	.48	8	*	11	.73
Tot RVU/patient	33	6.84	10	6.98	11	4.54
Physician work RVU/patient	32	3.37	9	*	11	3.79
Tot procedures/patient	60	7.74	14	6.57	16	8.73
Square feet/patient	60	1.18	14	.81	15	1.10
Total support staff FTE/phy	127	5.31	32	5.21	27	5.75

*See pages 260 and 261 for definition.

Table 8.10b: Charges, Revenue and Cost

	No capitation		10% or less		11% to 50%	
	Count	Median	Count	Median	Count	Median
Total gross charges	64	$616.26	16	$435.85	16	$533.68
Total medical revenue	64	$353.54	16	$306.02	16	$417.82
Net fee-for-service revenue	63	$342.68	16	$260.00	16	$279.95
Net capitation revenue	6	*	16	$13.36	16	$142.47
Net other medical revenue	51	$9.00	10	$13.02	12	$17.93
Total support staff cost/patient	64	$110.05	16	$99.07	16	$133.61
Total general operating cost	64	$110.60	16	$90.40	16	$105.49
Total operating cost	64	$211.17	16	$196.66	16	$231.97
Total med rev after oper cost	64	$151.14	16	$113.59	16	$182.96
Total provider cost/patient	64	$143.98	16	$117.18	16	$165.10
Total NPP cost/patient	61	$8.19	15	$6.68	15	$16.23
Provider consultant cost	21	$7.25	9	*	9	*
Total physician cost/patient	64	$136.17	16	$103.60	16	$142.81
Total phy compensation	64	$119.81	16	$88.75	16	$119.34
Total phy benefit cost	63	$19.59	15	$13.28	16	$21.36
Total cost	64	$361.21	16	$317.12	16	$381.33
Net nonmedical revenue	52	$1.21	15	$.40	13	$.86
Net inc, prac with fin sup	0	*	1	*	1	*
Net inc, prac w/o fin sup	60	$3.35	15	$.01	15	$13.23
Net inc, excl fin supp (all prac)	60	$3.35	16	-$.01	16	$14.75
Total support staff FTE/phy	127	5.31	32	5.21	27	5.75

Multispecialty — by Capitation Revenue Percent, Not Hospital or IDS Owned
(Procedure and Charge Data)

Table 8.11a: Activity Charges to Total Gross Charges Ratios

	No capitation		10% or less		11% to 50%	
	Count	Median	Count	Median	Count	Median
Total proc gross charges	**105**	**95.09%**	**26**	**95.45%**	**22**	**95.08%**
Medical proc-inside practice	105	39.19%	26	48.48%	22	48.17%
Medical proc-outside practice	95	9.19%	24	8.90%	20	5.92%
Surg proc-inside practice	97	5.36%	26	5.51%	20	9.92%
Surg proc-outside practice	84	16.90%	21	8.39%	16	12.31%
Laboratory procedures	103	10.90%	25	11.71%	21	9.23%
Radiology procedures	101	8.63%	24	8.05%	18	9.20%
Tot nonproc gross charges	94	6.12%	23	5.54%	19	6.20%
Total support staff FTE/phy	**127**	**5.31**	**32**	**5.21**	**27**	**5.75**

Table 8.11b: Medical Procedure Data (inside the practice)

	No capitation		10% or less		11% to 50%	
	Count	Median	Count	Median	Count	Median
Gross charges/procedure	**101**	**$71.78**	**26**	**$73.34**	**22**	**$72.50**
Total cost/procedure	**88**	**$57.42**	**22**	**$56.97**	**21**	**$58.24**
Operating cost/procedure	87	$36.40	22	$34.63	19	$36.51
Provider cost/procedure	89	$22.72	23	$20.48	21	$24.09
Procedures/patient	60	3.35	14	3.43	16	4.30
Gross charges/patient	61	$231.31	14	$216.28	16	$306.40
Procedures/physician	103	5,646	26	5,579	22	5,749
Gross charges/physician	105	$389,804	26	$413,173	22	$457,929
Procedures/provider	96	4,472	23	4,534	20	4,768
Gross charges/provider	98	$321,330	23	$311,731	20	$372,572
Gross charge to total cost ratio	88	1.27	22	1.30	21	1.26
Oper cost to total cost ratio	87	.61	22	.62	19	.62
Prov cost to total cost ratio	88	.39	22	.38	21	.38
Total support staff FTE/phy	**127**	**5.31**	**32**	**5.21**	**27**	**5.75**

Table 8.11c: Medical Procedure Data (outside the practice)

	No capitation		10% or less		11% to 50%	
	Count	Median	Count	Median	Count	Median
Gross charges/procedure	**92**	**$112.38**	**23**	**$108.03**	**20**	**$125.63**
Total cost/procedure	**80**	**$47.40**	**20**	**$49.90**	**19**	**$61.17**
Operating cost/procedure	79	$18.63	20	$21.83	17	$29.03
Provider cost/procedure	81	$29.49	21	$27.40	19	$33.19
Procedures/patient	56	.62	13	.36	14	.31
Gross charges/patient	57	$54.81	13	$45.09	14	$39.16
Procedures/physician	93	905	23	683	20	456
Gross charges/physician	95	$92,727	24	$79,767	20	$62,062
Procedures/provider	87	681	20	562	18	367
Gross charges/provider	90	$71,547	21	$60,782	18	$51,722
Gross charge to total cost ratio	80	2.31	20	2.23	19	2.05
Oper cost to total cost ratio	79	.37	20	.43	17	.46
Prov cost to total cost ratio	80	.63	20	.57	19	.54
Total support staff FTE/phy	**127**	**5.31**	**32**	**5.21**	**27**	**5.75**

Multispecialty — by Capitation Revenue Percent, Not Hospital or IDS Owned
(Procedure and Charge Data)

Table 8.11d: Surgery/Anesthesia Procedure Data (inside the practice)

	No capitation		10% or less		11% to 50%	
	Count	Median	Count	Median	Count	Median
Gross charges/procedure	95	$88.68	26	$138.24	20	$107.43
Total cost/procedure	83	$73.38	22	$129.45	19	$102.38
Operating cost/procedure	82	$47.38	22	$82.12	17	$44.11
Provider cost/procedure	83	$29.18	23	$41.23	19	$36.83
Procedures/patient	56	.41	14	.34	15	1.06
Gross charges/patient	56	$28.17	14	$30.66	15	$58.16
Procedures/physician	96	656	26	475	20	1,309
Gross charges/physician	97	$57,353	26	$45,432	20	$103,702
Procedures/provider	89	568	23	422	18	1,092
Gross charges/provider	90	$46,365	23	$36,240	18	$91,527
Gross charge to total cost ratio	83	1.26	22	1.30	19	1.26
Oper cost to total cost ratio	82	.61	22	.62	17	.62
Prov cost to total cost ratio	83	.39	22	.38	19	.38
Total support staff FTE/phy	127	5.31	32	5.21	27	5.75

Table 8.11e: Surgery/Anesthesia Procedure Data (outside the practice)

	No capitation		10% or less		11% to 50%	
	Count	Median	Count	Median	Count	Median
Gross charges/procedure	81	$888.26	21	$463.46	16	$761.71
Total cost/procedure	73	$375.72	17	$233.40	15	$362.96
Operating cost/procedure	72	$141.89	17	$88.25	14	$143.38
Provider cost/procedure	73	$231.82	18	$148.31	15	$226.81
Procedures/patient	50	.17	10	.11	11	.09
Gross charges/patient	48	$108.56	10	$55.49	11	$71.34
Procedures/physician	83	235	21	122	16	123
Gross charges/physician	84	$192,832	21	$56,467	16	$94,815
Procedures/provider	78	187	19	100	15	103
Gross charges/provider	79	$153,517	19	$47,709	15	$77,647
Gross charge to total cost ratio	73	2.31	17	2.17	15	2.05
Oper cost to total cost ratio	72	.37	17	.44	14	.44
Prov cost to total cost ratio	73	.63	17	.56	15	.54
Total support staff FTE/phy	127	5.31	32	5.21	27	5.75

Multispecialty — by Capitation Revenue Percent, Not Hospital or IDS Owned
(Procedure and Charge Data)

Table 8.11f: Clinical Laboratory/Pathology Procedure Data

	No capitation		10% or less		11% to 50%	
	Count	Median	Count	Median	Count	Median
Gross charges/procedure	99	$29.55	25	$24.38	21	$31.22
Total cost/procedure	87	$22.37	22	$19.67	20	$24.10
Operating cost/procedure	86	$14.67	22	$13.19	18	$16.05
Provider cost/procedure	88	$8.00	23	$6.04	20	$7.97
Procedures/patient	58	2.33	14	2.44	16	2.32
Gross charges/patient	59	$55.69	14	$50.40	16	$74.95
Procedures/physician	101	3,714	25	3,998	21	3,308
Gross charges/physician	103	$117,445	25	$101,873	21	$98,249
Procedures/provider	94	3,107	22	3,379	19	2,659
Gross charges/provider	96	$99,242	22	$86,163	19	$81,627
Gross charge to total cost ratio	87	1.29	22	1.28	20	1.29
Oper cost to total cost ratio	86	.65	22	.68	18	.65
Prov cost to total cost ratio	87	.35	22	.32	20	.33
Total support staff FTE/phy	127	5.31	32	5.21	27	5.75

Table 8.11g: Diagnostic Radiology and Imaging Procedure Data

	No capitation		10% or less		11% to 50%	
	Count	Median	Count	Median	Count	Median
Gross charges/procedure	99	$138.04	24	$138.09	18	$167.15
Total cost/procedure	89	$103.00	20	$84.83	17	$140.26
Operating cost/procedure	88	$77.48	20	$61.64	16	$106.35
Provider cost/procedure	90	$37.14	21	$24.25	17	$41.30
Procedures/patient	60	.32	13	.28	13	.58
Gross charges/patient	60	$42.57	11	$46.71	13	$101.64
Procedures/physician	101	655	25	614	18	557
Gross charges/physician	101	$91,882	24	$67,444	18	$106,070
Procedures/provider	95	528	22	410	17	498
Gross charges/provider	95	$78,127	21	$52,139	17	$91,756
Gross charge to total cost ratio	89	1.32	20	1.21	17	1.22
Oper cost to total cost ratio	88	.65	20	.69	16	.68
Prov cost to total cost ratio	89	.35	20	.31	17	.33
Total support staff FTE/phy	127	5.31	32	5.21	27	5.75

Table 8.11h: Nonprocedural Gross Charge Data

	No capitation		10% or less		11% to 50%	
	Count	Median	Count	Median	Count	Median
Gross charges/patient	54	$36.23	14	$24.41	14	$33.45
Nonproc gross charges/physician	94	$68,449	23	$42,889	19	$68,218
Gross charges/provider	89	$53,101	20	$33,277	17	$53,258
Total support staff FTE/phy	127	5.31	32	5.21	27	5.75

THIS PAGE INTENTIONALLY LEFT BLANK

Primary Care Single Specialty Practices by Ownership

Primary Care Single Specialty Practices by Ownership — Family Practice, Not Hospital or IDS Owned and All Owner Types

Table 9.1: Staffing and Practice Data

	Family Practice - Not Hospital Owned				Family Practice - All			
	Count	25th %tile	Median	75th %tile	Count	25th %tile	Median	75th %tile
Total provider FTE	**43**	**6.00**	**7.75**	**13.80**	**77**	**5.51**	**7.50**	**12.05**
Total physician FTE	60	4.00	5.40	9.94	102	4.00	5.00	8.00
Total nonphysician provider FTE	43	1.50	2.00	3.15	77	1.00	2.00	3.00
Total support staff FTE	**60**	**19.13**	**30.25**	**49.03**	**102**	**17.10**	**24.63**	**39.55**
Number of branch clinics	19	1	3	6	25	1	3	6
Square footage of all facilities	58	9,333	11,800	19,917	99	7,800	11,300	17,890

Table 9.2: Accounts Receivable Data, Collection Percentages and Financial Ratios

	Family Practice - Not Hospital Owned				Family Practice - All			
	Count	25th %tile	Median	75th %tile	Count	25th %tile	Median	75th %tile
Total AR/physician	**58**	**$61,729**	**$76,802**	**$107,746**	**98**	**$61,729**	**$85,901**	**$113,589**
Total AR/provider	**42**	**$43,650**	**$55,558**	**$77,496**	**75**	**$44,511**	**$61,611**	**$78,143**
0-30 days in AR	58	43.32%	53.50%	64.19%	98	48.74%	56.48%	66.43%
31-60 days in AR	58	12.88%	15.11%	18.43%	98	11.46%	14.07%	17.93%
61-90 days in AR	58	6.22%	7.90%	9.85%	98	6.07%	7.53%	9.20%
91-120 days in AR	58	3.54%	5.24%	6.26%	98	3.68%	4.99%	6.19%
120+ days in AR	58	7.79%	13.32%	20.06%	98	8.75%	13.59%	20.92%
Re-aged: 0-30 days in AR	20	49.77%	56.86%	73.95%	36	49.27%	56.93%	71.27%
Re-aged: 31-60 days in AR	20	10.13%	14.35%	16.91%	36	9.69%	12.75%	15.13%
Re-aged: 61-90 days in AR	20	4.61%	7.18%	9.63%	36	5.12%	6.34%	7.95%
Re-aged: 91-120 days in AR	20	2.71%	4.29%	6.08%	36	3.17%	4.17%	5.66%
Re-aged: 120+ days in AR	20	4.80%	11.73%	18.76%	36	8.98%	12.92%	21.20%
Not re-aged: 0-30 days in AR	36	43.12%	51.24%	62.39%	60	47.73%	54.60%	63.71%
Not re-aged: 31-60 days in AR	36	13.44%	16.14%	19.39%	60	12.99%	15.50%	19.52%
Not re-aged: 61-90 days in AR	36	6.53%	7.93%	9.79%	60	6.70%	7.86%	9.48%
Not re-aged: 91-120 days in AR	36	3.91%	5.38%	6.46%	60	3.97%	5.47%	6.46%
Not re-aged: 120+ days in AR	36	8.82%	15.80%	21.89%	60	7.93%	14.93%	19.24%
Months gross FFS charges in AR	54	1.20	1.41	1.69	92	1.24	1.44	1.71
Days gross FFS charges in AR	54	36.59	42.84	51.38	92	37.66	43.82	51.93
Gross FFS collection %	55	65.89%	69.98%	76.26%	95	66.42%	69.81%	75.65%
Adjusted FFS collection %	52	96.69%	98.59%	99.39%	92	97.00%	97.89%	99.02%
Gross FFS + cap collection %	14	66.08%	76.25%	81.85%	22	67.21%	77.90%	81.66%
Net cap rev % of gross cap chrg	12	54.32%	76.74%	81.73%	20	66.44%	76.74%	87.23%
Current ratio	28	1.10	1.57	3.26	31	1.08	1.61	3.46
Tot asset turnover ratio	28	5.32	9.37	15.27	31	5.12	7.58	13.89
Debt to equity ratio	28	.65	1.49	2.31	31	.64	1.52	2.35
Debt ratio	28	39.28%	59.78%	69.77%	31	39.07%	60.27%	70.15%
Return on total assets	24	-.44%	5.28%	41.77%	27	-.56%	7.06%	32.98%
Return on equity	24	-1.45%	8.97%	69.84%	27	-1.72%	10.12%	70.29%

Table 9.3: Breakout of Total Gross Charges by Type of Payer

	Family Practice - Not Hospital Owned				Family Practice - All			
	Count	25th %tile	Median	75th %tile	Count	25th %tile	Median	75th %tile
Medicare: fee-for-service	56	11.00%	16.00%	27.53%	96	12.35%	18.12%	28.00%
Medicare: managed care FFS	56	.00%	.00%	1.62%	96	.00%	.00%	.00%
Medicare: capitation	56	.00%	.00%	.00%	96	.00%	.00%	.00%
Medicaid: fee-for-service	56	1.00%	1.79%	7.76%	96	1.00%	3.05%	8.46%
Medicaid: managed care FFS	56	.00%	.00%	.75%	96	.00%	.00%	.00%
Medicaid: capitation	56	.00%	.00%	.00%	96	.00%	.00%	.00%
Commercial: fee-for-service	56	10.00%	40.44%	56.30%	96	8.50%	40.74%	56.30%
Commercial: managed care FFS	56	.00%	17.41%	50.00%	96	.00%	14.53%	51.06%
Commercial: capitation	56	.00%	.00%	.00%	96	.00%	.00%	.00%
Workers' compensation	56	.00%	.50%	1.00%	96	.00%	.50%	1.01%
Charity care and prof courtesy	56	.00%	.00%	.98%	96	.00%	.00%	1.00%
Self-pay	56	2.00%	3.90%	7.15%	96	1.58%	3.49%	7.00%
Other federal government payers	56	.00%	.00%	.79%	96	.00%	.00%	.32%

Primary Care Single Specialty Practices by Ownership — Family Practice, Not Hospital or IDS Owned and All Owner Types (per FTE Physician)

Table 9.4a: Staffing, RVUs, Patients, Procedures and Square Footage

	Family Practice - Not Hospital Owned				Family Practice - All			
	Count	25th %tile	Median	75th %tile	Count	25th %tile	Median	75th %tile
Total provider FTE/physician	43	**1.20**	**1.36**	**1.51**	77	**1.19**	**1.33**	**1.51**
Prim care phy/physician	53	1.00	1.00	1.00	93	1.00	1.00	1.00
Nonsurg phy/physician	0	*	*	*	0	*	*	*
Surg spec phy/physician	0	*	*	*	0	*	*	*
Total NPP FTE/physician	43	.20	.36	.51	77	.19	.33	.51
Total support staff FTE/phy	60	**4.02**	**5.03**	**5.93**	102	**3.79**	**4.60**	**5.55**
Total empl support staff FTE	53	4.06	5.00	5.86	93	3.91	4.60	5.51
General administrative	54	.19	.25	.34	93	.19	.25	.30
Patient accounting	54	.45	.70	.91	68	.48	.76	1.00
General accounting	30	.07	.12	.17	34	.06	.12	.17
Managed care administrative	15	.10	.13	.31	18	.10	.14	.25
Information technology	14	.05	.15	.34	16	.06	.15	.36
Housekeeping, maint, security	8	*	*	*	11	.04	.13	.33
Medical receptionists	52	.85	1.08	1.35	75	.90	1.12	1.40
Med secretaries,transcribers	32	.22	.29	.43	47	.22	.29	.40
Medical records	46	.26	.40	.63	62	.26	.39	.61
Other admin support	22	.04	.09	.53	33	.05	.20	.37
*Total administrative supp staff	20	**2.40**	**2.86**	**3.60**	27	**2.20**	**2.76**	**3.42**
Registered Nurses	40	.21	.42	.68	62	.23	.39	.69
Licensed Practical Nurses	42	.21	.48	.76	71	.28	.63	1.09
Med assistants, nurse aides	52	.45	.83	1.21	85	.59	.90	1.31
*Total clinical supp staff	44	**1.27**	**1.52**	**2.20**	63	**1.29**	**1.63**	**2.17**
Clinical laboratory	32	.25	.35	.47	49	.21	.33	.46
Radiology and imaging	29	.12	.19	.25	47	.15	.22	.31
Other medical support serv	16	.06	.13	.40	34	.06	.26	1.56
*Total ancillary supp staff	14	**.38**	**.59**	**1.28**	17	**.46**	**.69**	**1.56**
Tot contracted supp staff	11	.05	.15	.64	14	.07	.14	.31
Tot RVU/physician	16	7,595	9,928	11,999	20	7,714	9,650	11,498
Physician work RVU/physician	14	3,760	4,608	5,675	20	4,035	4,608	5,564
Patients/physician	23	1,407	2,483	3,563	40	1,731	2,145	3,056
Tot procedures/physician	46	9,190	11,320	12,932	85	8,681	11,518	15,202
Square feet/physician	58	1,413	2,000	2,458	99	1,561	2,126	2,528

*See pages 260 and 261 for definition.

Table 9.4b: Charges and Revenue

	Family Practice - Not Hospital Owned				Family Practice - All			
	Count	25th %tile	Median	75th %tile	Count	25th %tile	Median	75th %tile
Net fee-for-service revenue	55	$417,222	$475,534	$581,305	95	$403,165	$473,097	$567,434
Gross FFS charges	56	$531,587	$677,821	$842,742	96	$526,349	$685,558	$832,039
Adjustments to FFS charges	52	$121,706	$194,197	$258,022	92	$123,873	$201,194	$266,517
Adjusted FFS charges	53	$410,036	$488,996	$589,318	93	$393,561	$482,082	$575,988
Bad debts due to FFS activity	49	$3,754	$6,548	$11,767	88	$4,503	$8,359	$15,367
Net capitation revenue	14	$8,346	$64,719	$130,237	22	$23,706	$54,660	$108,162
Gross capitation charges	12	$29,147	$89,090	$187,754	20	$32,974	$77,576	$149,071
Capitation revenue	14	$8,346	$64,719	$132,560	22	$23,706	$52,102	$108,162
Purch serv for cap patients	1	*	*	*	1	*	*	*
Net other medical revenue	30	$1,520	$5,167	$15,838	56	$3,416	$13,755	$31,085
Gross rev from other activity	29	$1,771	$6,111	$15,852	55	$4,314	$13,969	$31,143
Other medical revenue	26	$1,239	$4,304	$13,584	52	$3,408	$13,358	$31,085
Rev from sale of goods/services	9	*	*	*	10	$675	$1,773	$10,599
Cost of sales	2	*	*	*	2	*	*	*
Total gross charges	60	**$564,446**	**$691,888**	**$857,342**	102	**$556,468**	**$691,888**	**$836,667**
Total medical revenue	60	**$428,558**	**$508,226**	**$597,141**	102	**$425,279**	**$501,146**	**$582,312**

Primary Care Single Specialty Practices by Ownership — Family Practice, Not Hospital or IDS Owned and All Owner Types (per FTE Physician)

Table 9.4c: Operating Cost

	Family Practice - Not Hospital Owned				Family Practice - All			
	Count	25th %tile	Median	75th %tile	Count	25th %tile	Median	75th %tile
Total support staff cost/phy	60	$132,393	$164,599	$187,639	102	$129,198	$160,312	$189,080
Total empl supp staff cost/phy	54	$114,230	$132,853	$158,362	94	$108,168	$130,677	$154,280
General administrative	55	$11,188	$15,402	$20,337	93	$10,229	$13,072	$18,177
Patient accounting	55	$13,105	$18,788	$25,412	68	$14,413	$19,878	$27,488
General accounting	31	$2,187	$3,655	$5,985	34	$2,216	$3,740	$6,263
Managed care administrative	16	$3,253	$4,184	$8,133	19	$3,211	$3,767	$7,114
Information technology	14	$1,201	$4,925	$8,785	16	$1,780	$4,925	$10,787
Housekeeping, maint, security	10	$1,771	$3,173	$5,928	13	$1,506	$2,805	$6,179
Medical receptionists	53	$19,005	$24,460	$29,620	76	$19,494	$25,780	$31,800
Med secretaries,transcribers	32	$4,366	$6,858	$10,102	46	$4,597	$7,029	$10,238
Medical records	47	$4,000	$7,132	$12,749	62	$4,282	$7,155	$12,654
Other admin support	22	$1,040	$2,322	$14,889	33	$1,435	$4,845	$13,494
*Total administrative supp staff	22	$62,881	$74,064	$91,970	32	$62,965	$73,361	$91,628
Registered Nurses	40	$6,607	$13,046	$20,682	61	$7,767	$13,000	$21,685
Licensed Practical Nurses	42	$6,252	$11,609	$20,145	70	$8,043	$16,027	$28,649
Med assistants, nurse aides	53	$11,137	$20,432	$31,176	85	$14,416	$21,477	$34,603
*Total clinical supp staff	46	$36,076	$45,448	$56,185	68	$37,212	$45,816	$60,446
Clinical laboratory	34	$6,464	$11,620	$17,371	51	$5,750	$11,423	$16,601
Radiology and imaging	30	$3,432	$7,279	$9,243	48	$4,778	$7,958	$12,966
Other medical support serv	16	$1,671	$4,797	$10,000	34	$2,051	$9,419	$40,033
*Total ancillary supp staff	17	$12,393	$20,578	$33,322	26	$16,060	$21,903	$41,814
Total empl supp staff benefits	58	$22,229	$29,492	$34,533	100	$24,053	$29,552	$35,660
Tot contracted supp staff	19	$1,127	$2,227	$5,217	44	$1,852	$4,430	$7,407
Total general operating cost	60	$105,627	$131,654	$170,266	102	$105,394	$132,033	$165,053
Information technology	56	$7,234	$9,306	$14,520	95	$5,242	$8,160	$11,496
Medical and surgical supply	55	$15,821	$20,329	$26,145	95	$15,336	$19,624	$23,969
Building and occupancy	56	$25,727	$35,683	$46,527	95	$25,751	$35,309	$44,879
Furniture and equipment	50	$2,356	$3,987	$8,594	86	$2,273	$4,154	$7,663
Admin supplies and services	56	$8,319	$12,576	$16,525	96	$6,528	$9,279	$15,070
Prof liability insurance	60	$7,251	$10,333	$15,224	97	$3,845	$8,123	$13,801
Other insurance premiums	53	$891	$1,520	$2,315	70	$587	$1,203	$2,165
Outside professional fees	56	$1,567	$2,971	$5,382	75	$1,470	$2,993	$6,163
Promotion and marketing	56	$631	$1,401	$2,663	84	$497	$1,121	$2,000
Clinical laboratory	48	$3,578	$14,867	$21,574	80	$4,413	$8,657	$18,391
Radiology and imaging	37	$2,012	$3,494	$6,441	53	$1,575	$2,522	$4,774
Other ancillary services	11	$761	$3,685	$8,184	19	$599	$840	$8,184
Billing purchased services	21	$951	$1,724	$2,234	53	$1,014	$2,542	$31,943
Management fees paid to MSO	4	*	*	*	32	$21,023	$22,755	$28,063
Misc operating cost	55	$3,293	$6,033	$12,912	90	$3,500	$7,512	$15,798
Cost allocated to prac from par	0	*	*	*	4	*	*	*
Total operating cost	60	$250,136	$292,794	$359,796	102	$245,230	$290,545	$357,029

*See pages 260 and 261 for definition.

Primary Care Single Specialty Practices by Ownership — Family Practice, Not Hospital or IDS Owned and All Owner Types (per FTE Physician)

Table 9.4d: Provider Cost

	Family Practice - Not Hospital Owned				Family Practice - All			
	Count	25th %tile	Median	75th %tile	Count	25th %tile	Median	75th %tile
Total med rev after oper cost	60	$176,871	$215,569	$261,541	102	$169,899	$210,549	$258,923
Total provider cost/physician	60	$178,156	$201,171	$236,269	102	$183,294	$206,685	$239,852
Total NPP cost/physician	47	$14,701	$28,787	$46,100	82	$13,788	$26,639	$43,949
Nonphysician provider comp	41	$11,120	$24,339	$39,975	74	$11,999	$23,743	$39,760
Nonphysician prov benefit cost	40	$1,828	$3,558	$6,535	73	$1,824	$3,458	$6,083
Provider consultant cost	7	*	*	*	7	*	*	*
Total physician cost/physician	60	$149,107	$184,593	$203,545	102	$160,398	$186,844	$215,056
Total phy compensation	53	$128,850	$155,556	$176,455	93	$141,413	$159,362	$196,516
Total phy benefit cost	52	$20,066	$28,780	$36,064	88	$17,813	$26,909	$34,398

Table 9.4e: Net Income or Loss

	Family Practice - Not Hospital Owned				Family Practice - All			
	Count	25th %tile	Median	75th %tile	Count	25th %tile	Median	75th %tile
Total cost	60	$426,775	$505,664	$591,466	102	$443,262	$506,065	$580,690
Net nonmedical revenue	32	$52	$753	$8,632	52	$126	$3,692	$45,650
Nonmedical revenue	28	$130	$1,163	$8,404	36	$115	$1,078	$6,520
Fin support for oper costs	1	*	*	*	14	$40,245	$63,448	$122,985
Goodwill amortization	0	*	*	*	2	*	*	*
Nonmedical cost	12	$164	$1,036	$7,172	14	$122	$922	$7,172
Net inc, prac with fin sup	1	*	*	*	9	*	*	*
Net inc, prac w/o fin sup	55	-$243	$2,620	$28,822	76	-$2,684	$4,521	$30,659
Net inc, excl fin supp (all prac)	56	-$515	$2,562	$27,887	85	-$7,424	$2,444	$25,125

Table 9.4f: Assets and Liabilities

	Family Practice - Not Hospital Owned				Family Practice - All			
	Count	25th %tile	Median	75th %tile	Count	25th %tile	Median	75th %tile
Total assets	33	$29,299	$58,337	$89,141	37	$29,437	$64,883	$100,485
Current assets	33	$11,549	$27,421	$67,089	37	$13,190	$27,686	$67,523
Noncurrent assets	33	$7,691	$19,009	$37,276	37	$8,581	$22,372	$38,999
Total liabilities	33	$11,386	$26,331	$47,108	37	$9,733	$26,331	$49,242
Current liabilities	33	$2,244	$10,000	$28,360	37	$2,244	$10,000	$32,320
Noncurrent liabilities	33	$314	$6,366	$21,086	37	$0	$6,077	$21,086
Working capital	33	$1,792	$10,906	$25,928	37	$1,792	$12,419	$35,764
Total net worth	33	$11,018	$23,446	$40,276	37	$11,716	$25,349	$59,256

Primary Care Single Specialty Practices by Ownership — Family Practice, Not Hospital or IDS Owned and All Owner Types (as a % of Total Medical Revenue)

Table 9.5a: Charges and Revenue

	Family Practice - Not Hospital Owned				Family Practice - All			
	Count	25th %tile	Median	75th %tile	Count	25th %tile	Median	75th %tile
Net fee-for-service revenue	55	95.45%	99.63%	100.00%	95	93.14%	98.84%	100.00%
Net capitation revenue	14	1.80%	12.29%	32.14%	22	4.73%	12.29%	29.42%
Net other medical revenue	30	.39%	.95%	2.53%	56	.62%	2.75%	5.39%
Total gross charges	**60**	**127.58%**	**139.47%**	**149.73%**	**102**	**128.24%**	**138.38%**	**149.63%**

Table 9.5b: Operating Cost

	Family Practice - Not Hospital Owned				Family Practice - All			
	Count	25th %tile	Median	75th %tile	Count	25th %tile	Median	75th %tile
Total support staff cost	**60**	**28.53%**	**31.94%**	**35.05%**	**102**	**28.39%**	**31.93%**	**34.98%**
Total empl support staff cost	54	23.47%	26.00%	28.96%	94	22.81%	25.84%	28.37%
General administrative	55	2.16%	2.91%	3.88%	93	2.01%	2.73%	3.46%
Patient accounting	55	2.57%	3.49%	4.81%	68	2.64%	3.96%	5.38%
General accounting	31	.48%	.79%	1.05%	34	.51%	.76%	1.08%
Managed care administrative	16	.73%	.86%	1.74%	19	.73%	.83%	1.71%
Information technology	14	.30%	1.04%	1.57%	16	.34%	1.04%	1.57%
Housekeeping, maint, security	10	.41%	.69%	.85%	13	.34%	.64%	.89%
Medical receptionists	53	3.44%	4.59%	5.85%	76	3.69%	5.09%	6.62%
Med secretaries,transcribers	32	.94%	1.31%	1.96%	46	.97%	1.41%	1.94%
Medical records	47	.87%	1.63%	2.23%	62	.95%	1.66%	2.27%
Other admin support	22	.26%	.47%	1.91%	33	.32%	1.05%	2.25%
*Total administrative supp staff	22	12.76%	15.67%	18.56%	32	12.63%	13.88%	17.86%
Registered Nurses	40	1.26%	2.67%	3.79%	61	1.37%	2.72%	4.10%
Licensed Practical Nurses	42	1.22%	2.38%	3.97%	70	1.44%	3.24%	5.36%
Med assistants, nurse aides	53	2.20%	4.02%	5.97%	85	2.68%	4.54%	6.14%
*Total clinical supp staff	46	7.37%	8.46%	9.98%	68	7.64%	8.79%	11.14%
Clinical laboratory	34	1.33%	2.10%	2.90%	51	1.19%	2.01%	2.72%
Radiology and imaging	30	.75%	1.21%	1.53%	48	.85%	1.33%	2.13%
Other medical support serv	16	.36%	.87%	1.92%	34	.48%	1.78%	6.88%
*Total ancillary supp staff	17	2.44%	4.23%	5.56%	26	2.92%	4.23%	6.42%
Total empl supp staff benefits	58	4.53%	5.71%	6.61%	100	5.03%	5.71%	6.78%
Tot contracted supp staff	19	.24%	.38%	.84%	44	.33%	.70%	1.13%
Total general operating cost	**60**	**23.17%**	**26.03%**	**29.34%**	**102**	**23.06%**	**27.29%**	**30.43%**
Information technology	56	1.32%	2.03%	2.73%	95	1.04%	1.60%	2.36%
Medical and surgical supply	55	3.00%	4.11%	5.41%	95	2.84%	4.06%	4.99%
Building and occupancy	56	5.38%	7.14%	8.63%	95	5.52%	6.74%	8.18%
Furniture and equipment	50	.50%	.77%	1.58%	86	.45%	.81%	1.32%
Admin supplies and services	56	1.61%	2.13%	3.31%	96	1.32%	1.79%	3.04%
Prof liability insurance	60	1.34%	2.08%	2.96%	97	.85%	1.61%	2.81%
Other insurance premiums	53	.17%	.32%	.44%	70	.12%	.25%	.38%
Outside professional fees	56	.28%	.58%	1.14%	75	.27%	.60%	1.17%
Promotion and marketing	56	.14%	.26%	.48%	84	.09%	.22%	.43%
Clinical laboratory	48	.64%	2.89%	3.89%	80	.75%	1.69%	3.55%
Radiology and imaging	37	.37%	.75%	1.30%	53	.24%	.56%	.92%
Other ancillary services	11	.15%	.63%	1.17%	19	.12%	.17%	1.17%
Billing purchased services	21	.16%	.26%	.49%	53	.19%	.60%	5.86%
Management fees paid to MSO	4	*	*	*	32	3.87%	4.24%	5.16%
Misc operating cost	55	.69%	1.30%	2.60%	90	.80%	1.51%	3.06%
Cost allocated to prac from par	0	*	*	*	4	*	*	*
Total operating cost	**60**	**53.77%**	**57.81%**	**61.63%**	**102**	**53.92%**	**58.78%**	**63.44%**

*See pages 260 and 261 for definition.

Primary Care Single Specialty Practices by Ownership — Family Practice Not Hospital or IDS Owned and All Owner Types (as a % of Total Medical Revenue)

Table 9.5c: Provider Cost

	Family Practice - Not Hospital Owned				Family Practice - All			
	Count	25th %tile	Median	75th %tile	Count	25th %tile	Median	75th %tile
Total med rev after oper cost	60	38.37%	42.19%	46.23%	102	36.56%	41.22%	46.08%
Total provider cost	60	35.95%	40.45%	45.41%	102	38.10%	42.32%	47.82%
Total NPP cost	47	3.07%	5.66%	7.32%	82	3.12%	5.55%	7.33%
Nonphysician provider comp	41	2.43%	4.64%	6.73%	74	2.67%	4.60%	6.70%
Nonphysician prov benefit cost	40	.42%	.66%	1.30%	73	.38%	.61%	1.10%
Provider consultant cost	7	*	*	*	7	*	*	*
Total physician cost	60	30.01%	35.74%	42.31%	102	32.45%	36.60%	44.53%
Total phy compensation	53	25.93%	31.07%	36.41%	93	28.30%	32.84%	38.69%
Total phy benefit cost	52	4.02%	5.41%	7.02%	88	3.20%	5.23%	6.66%

Table 9.5d: Net Income or Loss

	Family Practice - Not Hospital Owned				Family Practice - All			
	Count	25th %tile	Median	75th %tile	Count	25th %tile	Median	75th %tile
Total cost	60	95.26%	99.76%	101.27%	102	96.47%	100.00%	102.29%
Net nonmedical revenue	32	.01%	.17%	1.84%	52	.03%	.95%	11.99%
Nonmedical revenue	28	.03%	.17%	2.21%	36	.02%	.12%	1.69%
Fin support for oper costs	1	*	*	*	14	9.68%	16.02%	36.20%
Goodwill amortization	0	*	*	*	2	*	*	*
Nonmedical cost	12	.03%	.20%	.72%	14	.03%	.19%	.72%
Net inc, prac with fin sup	1	*	*	*	9	*	*	*
Net inc, prac w/o fin sup	55	-.06%	.46%	5.13%	76	-.50%	.69%	5.10%
Net inc, excl fin supp (all prac)	56	-.10%	.46%	5.10%	85	-1.42%	.42%	4.76%

Table 9.5e: Assets and Liabilities

	Family Practice - Not Hospital Owned				Family Practice - All			
	Count	25th %tile	Median	75th %tile	Count	25th %tile	Median	75th %tile
Total assets	33	6.09%	9.98%	18.68%	37	6.14%	10.87%	20.42%
Current assets	33	2.73%	4.89%	13.81%	37	2.92%	5.77%	14.07%
Noncurrent assets	33	1.76%	3.59%	5.41%	37	1.93%	3.86%	7.26%
Total liabilities	33	2.25%	5.34%	8.35%	37	2.00%	5.34%	10.58%
Current liabilities	33	.60%	1.89%	5.58%	37	.60%	1.89%	6.22%
Noncurrent liabilities	33	.08%	1.45%	4.06%	37	.00%	1.00%	4.06%
Working capital	33	.35%	2.26%	5.77%	37	.35%	2.33%	8.06%
Total net worth	33	1.98%	4.84%	8.65%	37	2.07%	5.48%	11.33%

Primary Care Single Specialty Practices by Ownership — Family Practice, Not Hospital or IDS Owned and All Owner Types (per FTE Provider)

Table 9.6a: Staffing, RVUs, Patients, Procedures and Square Footage

	Family Practice - Not Hospital Owned				Family Practice - All			
	Count	25th %tile	Median	75th %tile	Count	25th %tile	Median	75th %tile
Total physician FTE/provider	43	.66	.73	.83	77	.66	.75	.84
Prim care phy/provider	37	.66	.73	.84	69	.66	.75	.83
Nonsurg phy/provider	0	*	*	*	0	*	*	*
Surg spec phy/provider	0	*	*	*	0	*	*	*
Total NPP FTE/provider	43	.17	.27	.34	77	.16	.25	.34
Total support staff FTE/prov	43	2.92	3.50	4.19	77	2.93	3.42	4.02
Total empl supp staff FTE/prov	37	3.12	3.50	4.25	69	3.00	3.44	4.05
General administrative	37	.15	.19	.31	69	.14	.18	.23
Patient accounting	37	.28	.52	.68	46	.30	.52	.71
General accounting	21	.04	.09	.11	25	.04	.09	.11
Managed care administrative	10	.08	.11	.21	13	.07	.11	.19
Information technology	11	.04	.13	.34	13	.05	.13	.30
Housekeeping, maint, security	5	*	*	*	8	*	*	*
Medical receptionists	36	.61	.80	1.02	55	.67	.84	1.13
Med secretaries,transcribers	24	.13	.20	.27	36	.14	.20	.26
Medical records	32	.18	.31	.46	44	.17	.29	.46
Other admin support	15	.04	.07	.40	25	.05	.18	.31
*Total administrative supp staff	13	1.76	2.11	2.76	19	1.59	1.96	2.59
Registered Nurses	26	.17	.34	.49	47	.17	.29	.50
Licensed Practical Nurses	31	.21	.38	.55	53	.23	.45	.74
Med assistants, nurse aides	36	.37	.68	.85	66	.43	.68	.92
*Total clinical supp staff	30	.96	1.14	1.48	47	1.00	1.20	1.60
Clinical laboratory	21	.19	.27	.38	34	.18	.26	.38
Radiology and imaging	21	.07	.13	.17	37	.10	.16	.21
Other medical support serv	11	.04	.14	.27	24	.08	.39	1.20
*Total ancillary supp staff	10	.26	.41	.93	13	.29	.51	1.24
Tot contracted supp staff	4	*	*	*	7	*	*	*
Tot RVU/provider	14	5,609	7,315	9,343	17	6,010	7,302	8,597
Physician work RVU/provider	13	2,948	3,664	4,109	17	3,117	3,664	4,109
Patients/provider	17	1,108	1,792	2,268	30	1,312	1,677	2,308
Tot procedures/provider	32	6,695	8,117	10,173	63	6,553	8,248	12,047
Square feet/provider	41	1,151	1,367	1,670	74	1,224	1,435	2,000
Total support staff FTE/phy	60	4.02	5.03	5.93	102	3.79	4.60	5.55

*See pages 260 and 261 for definition.

Table 9.6b: Charges, Revenue and Cost

	Family Practice - Not Hospital Owned				Family Practice - All			
	Count	25th %tile	Median	75th %tile	Count	25th %tile	Median	75th %tile
Total gross charges	43	$420,749	$496,362	$646,659	77	$412,222	$523,297	$629,594
Total medical revenue	43	$322,593	$369,313	$436,721	77	$319,122	$377,249	$438,980
Net fee-for-service revenue	38	$282,281	$367,071	$418,178	70	$285,921	$367,491	$428,499
Net capitation revenue	13	$5,058	$38,206	$120,129	19	$12,124	$38,206	$94,081
Net other medical revenue	23	$1,749	$3,638	$12,364	47	$3,229	$12,364	$22,087
Total support staff cost/prov	43	$97,442	$116,437	$147,198	77	$104,383	$119,682	$143,524
Total general operating cost	43	$78,368	$92,919	$122,575	77	$76,324	$100,742	$125,230
Total operating cost	43	$181,431	$213,863	$268,578	77	$187,227	$221,671	$268,566
Total med rev after oper cost	43	$134,668	$150,608	$179,969	77	$129,461	$152,301	$190,885
Total provider cost/provider	43	$127,413	$150,925	$175,116	77	$134,810	$156,121	$181,505
Total NPP cost/provider	43	$11,320	$19,940	$28,142	77	$11,500	$18,887	$28,879
Provider consultant cost	6	*	*	*	6	*	*	*
Total physician cost/provider	43	$105,098	$117,600	$151,490	77	$108,982	$134,139	$161,272
Total phy compensation	38	$91,219	$103,277	$134,060	70	$95,688	$118,341	$144,372
Total phy benefit cost	37	$14,994	$22,142	$24,267	69	$10,835	$19,389	$25,897
Total cost	43	$308,309	$365,581	$436,845	77	$342,967	$392,880	$439,201
Net nonmedical revenue	24	$18	$1,686	$7,272	38	$45	$2,747	$34,264
Net inc, prac with fin sup	1	*	*	*	5	*	*	*
Net inc, prac w/o fin sup	40	-$202	$1,489	$19,993	59	-$407	$2,232	$20,953
Net inc, excl fin supp (all prac)	41	-$310	$1,437	$19,400	64	-$4,541	$1,855	$19,993
Total support staff FTE/phy	60	4.02	5.03	5.93	102	3.79	4.60	5.55

Primary Care Single Specialty Practices by Ownership — Family Practice, Not Hospital or IDS Owned and All Owner Types (per Square Foot)

Table 9.7a: Staffing, RVUs, Patients and Procedures

	Family Practice - Not Hospital Owned				Family Practice - All			
	Count	25th %tile	Median	75th %tile	Count	25th %tile	Median	75th %tile
Total prov FTE/10,000 sq ft	**41**	**5.99**	**7.32**	**8.69**	**74**	**5.00**	**6.97**	**8.17**
Total phy FTE/10,000 sq ft	58	4.07	5.00	7.08	99	3.96	4.70	6.41
Prim care phy/10,000 sq ft	51	4.09	5.12	7.18	90	3.90	4.66	6.47
Nonsurg phy/10,000 sq ft	0	*	*	*	0	*	*	*
Surg spec phy/10,000 sq ft	0	*	*	*	0	*	*	*
Total NPP FTE/10,000 sq ft	41	1.03	1.79	2.50	74	1.01	1.50	2.28
Total supp stf FTE/10,000 sq ft	**58**	**20.81**	**25.70**	**30.38**	**99**	**17.66**	**23.23**	**28.88**
Total empl supp stf/10,000 sq ft	51	21.00	25.82	32.02	90	17.58	23.49	28.90
General administrative	52	.85	1.47	2.05	90	.72	1.17	1.86
Patient accounting	52	2.05	3.43	4.99	66	2.07	3.81	5.63
General accounting	29	.43	.60	.83	33	.39	.57	.81
Managed care administrative	14	.66	.92	1.10	17	.58	.76	1.00
Information technology	13	.44	.91	1.46	15	.39	.91	1.55
Housekeeping, maint, security	8	*	*	*	11	.27	.68	1.14
Medical receptionists	50	3.44	5.64	7.71	73	3.53	5.85	7.52
Med secretaries,transcribers	32	.63	1.65	2.45	47	.67	1.36	2.09
Medical records	44	1.26	2.01	3.19	60	1.20	1.93	3.10
Other admin support	21	.22	.49	2.16	32	.32	.72	1.70
*Total administrative supp staff	19	11.66	15.18	18.14	26	11.16	14.89	17.78
Registered Nurses	39	1.00	2.11	3.80	60	.88	1.86	3.56
Licensed Practical Nurses	41	1.26	1.88	3.38	69	1.43	2.37	4.62
Med assistants, nurse aides	50	2.23	4.50	6.61	82	1.98	4.39	6.60
*Total clinical supp staff	42	6.22	7.82	10.32	60	5.88	8.06	10.37
Clinical laboratory	30	1.30	1.74	2.48	47	1.00	1.60	2.29
Radiology and imaging	28	.48	.87	1.41	46	.52	1.01	1.42
Other medical support serv	14	.34	.49	1.05	31	.34	1.04	4.18
*Total ancillary supp staff	13	2.06	2.42	3.87	16	2.18	3.22	5.85
Tot contracted supp staff	9	*	*	*	12	.38	.93	1.59
Tot RVU/sq ft	15	4.60	5.18	5.90	19	3.67	4.83	5.45
Physician work RVU/sq ft	13	2.26	2.60	3.17	19	2.23	2.56	2.87
Patients/sq ft	23	.75	1.36	1.75	41	.84	1.09	1.63
Tot procedures/sq ft	44	4.15	5.74	7.36	82	3.69	5.41	7.23
Total support staff FTE/phy	**60**	**4.02**	**5.03**	**5.93**	**102**	**3.79**	**4.60**	**5.55**

*See pages 260 and 261 for definition.

Table 9.7b: Charges, Revenue and Cost

	Family Practice - Not Hospital Owned				Family Practice - All			
	Count	25th %tile	Median	75th %tile	Count	25th %tile	Median	75th %tile
Total gross charges	58	$306.28	$369.01	$462.76	99	$274.23	$344.98	$426.72
Total medical revenue	58	$222.23	$260.05	$324.28	99	$200.06	$250.28	$307.74
Net fee-for-service revenue	53	$203.62	$250.85	$307.19	92	$187.24	$231.95	$289.72
Net capitation revenue	14	$4.06	$42.37	$102.25	22	$10.83	$33.15	$60.81
Net other medical revenue	30	$.84	$2.27	$7.89	55	$1.89	$6.17	$10.17
Total support staff cost/sq ft	58	$66.38	$86.96	$96.16	99	$61.39	$81.83	$94.67
Total general operating cost	58	$58.10	$69.44	$83.84	99	$51.49	$67.07	$80.85
Total operating cost	58	$123.83	$157.74	$182.45	99	$115.21	$148.65	$175.07
Total med rev after oper cost	58	$90.21	$108.50	$133.66	99	$74.84	$103.00	$127.10
Total provider cost/sq ft	58	$80.43	$103.10	$130.20	99	$80.78	$103.14	$126.83
Total NPP cost/sq ft	45	$8.23	$14.60	$18.21	79	$7.63	$11.98	$17.33
Provider consultant cost	7	*	*	*	7	*	*	*
Total physician cost/sq ft	58	$75.09	$85.83	$118.09	99	$73.85	$88.73	$117.38
Total phy compensation	51	$60.91	$73.72	$110.33	90	$59.89	$76.46	$105.04
Total phy benefit cost	50	$9.32	$12.53	$19.81	85	$7.83	$11.58	$18.28
Total cost	58	$210.64	$261.07	$314.58	99	$200.53	$252.46	$314.13
Net nonmedical revenue/sq ft	32	$.02	$.62	$6.10	52	$.07	$1.99	$25.62
Net inc, prac with fin sup	1	*	*	*	9	*	*	*
Net inc, prac w/o fin sup	53	-$.15	$1.78	$9.98	73	-$.25	$1.78	$10.29
Net inc, excl fin supp (all prac)	54	-$.21	$1.77	$9.55	82	-$3.20	$1.33	$9.37
Total support staff FTE/phy	**60**	**4.02**	**5.03**	**5.93**	**102**	**3.79**	**4.60**	**5.55**

Primary Care Single Specialty Practices by Ownership — Family Practice, Not Hospital or IDS Owned and All Owner Types (per Total RVU)

Table 9.8a: Staffing, Patients, Procedures and Square Footage

	Family Practice - Not Hospital Owned				Family Practice - All			
	Count	25th %tile	Median	75th %tile	Count	25th %tile	Median	75th %tile
Total prov FTE/10,000 tot RVU	14	1.08	1.37	1.78	17	1.16	1.37	1.67
Total phy FTE/10,000 tot RVU	16	.83	1.01	1.32	20	.87	1.04	1.30
Prim care phy/10,000 tot RVU	15	.83	1.02	1.32	19	.86	1.05	1.30
Nonsurg phy/10,000 tot RVU	0	*	*	*	0	*	*	*
Surg spec phy/10,000 tot RVU	0	*	*	*	0	*	*	*
Total NPP FTE/10,000 tot RVU	14	.18	.34	.46	17	.19	.31	.42
Total supp stf FTE/10,000 tot RVU	16	3.85	5.11	5.77	20	4.24	5.11	5.85
Tot empl supp stf/10,000 tot RVU	15	4.35	5.09	5.78	19	4.35	5.09	5.88
General administrative	15	.16	.28	.39	19	.13	.27	.34
Patient accounting	15	.45	.68	.87	17	.46	.68	.87
General accounting	10	.11	.13	.16	10	.11	.13	.16
Managed care administrative	5	*	*	*	6	*	*	*
Information technology	3	*	*	*	3	*	*	*
Housekeeping, maint, security	2	*	*	*	2	*	*	*
Medical receptionists	14	.60	.94	1.26	18	.63	.94	1.33
Med secretaries,transcribers	11	.11	.32	.46	13	.13	.32	.42
Medical records	14	.34	.47	.68	18	.34	.53	.68
Other admin support	8	*	*	*	11	.10	.26	.34
*Total administrative supp staff	5	*	*	*	5	*	*	*
Registered Nurses	10	.10	.36	.77	13	.12	.34	.57
Licensed Practical Nurses	13	.18	.47	.59	17	.22	.51	.83
Med assistants, nurse aides	14	.36	.92	1.43	16	.43	1.03	1.36
*Total clinical supp staff	11	1.10	1.62	2.07	13	1.10	1.69	2.14
Clinical laboratory	9	*	*	*	11	.32	.37	.45
Radiology and imaging	7	*	*	*	8	*	*	*
Other medical support serv	4	*	*	*	5	*	*	*
*Total ancillary supp staff	3	*	*	*	3	*	*	*
Tot contracted supp staff	2	*	*	*	2	*	*	*
Physician work RVU/tot RVU	13	.44	.48	.50	16	.46	.49	.52
Patients/tot RVU	11	.14	.25	.37	13	.15	.25	.37
Tot procedures/tot RVU	15	.94	1.10	1.17	19	.86	1.00	1.15
Square feet/tot RVU	15	.17	.19	.22	19	.18	.21	.27
Total support staff FTE/phy	60	4.02	5.03	5.93	102	3.79	4.60	5.55

*See pages 260 and 261 for definition.

Table 9.8b: Charges, Revenue and Cost

	Family Practice - Not Hospital Owned				Family Practice - All			
	Count	25th %tile	Median	75th %tile	Count	25th %tile	Median	75th %tile
Total gross charges	16	$53.46	$63.90	$71.98	20	$53.46	$63.33	$69.41
Total medical revenue	16	$40.45	$50.69	$55.77	20	$40.45	$50.43	$55.37
Net fee-for-service revenue	15	$39.92	$50.43	$54.72	19	$39.92	$49.19	$51.98
Net capitation revenue	3	*	*	*	5	*	*	*
Net other medical revenue	9	*	*	*	13	$.20	$.63	$1.98
Total supp staff cost/tot RVU	16	$14.13	$16.54	$19.06	20	$15.32	$17.44	$19.36
Total general operating cost	16	$11.55	$13.09	$15.78	20	$10.93	$12.74	$15.78
Total operating cost	16	$24.71	$29.86	$35.21	20	$27.38	$30.51	$32.89
Total med rev after oper cost	16	$16.77	$19.39	$22.92	20	$13.16	$18.44	$22.92
Total provider cost/tot RVU	16	$17.48	$20.40	$24.57	20	$17.83	$20.79	$25.56
Total NPP cost/tot RVU	15	$1.44	$3.32	$4.26	19	$1.54	$3.21	$4.26
Provider consultant cost	4	*	*	*	4	*	*	*
Total physician cost/tot RVU	16	$14.34	$16.67	$23.54	20	$15.43	$17.17	$24.82
Total phy compensation	15	$12.10	$13.76	$20.49	19	$13.15	$14.39	$20.49
Total phy benefit cost	15	$1.86	$3.06	$3.94	19	$2.05	$3.57	$4.14
Total cost	14	$44.38	$52.85	$56.71	18	$43.15	$52.80	$56.71
Net nonmedical revenue	11	$.01	$.18	$1.32	15	$.01	$.18	$1.72
Net inc, prac with fin sup	1	*	*	*	1	*	*	*
Net inc, prac w/o fin sup	14	-$.55	$.02	$1.35	16	-$.75	$.02	$1.11
Net inc, excl fin supp (all prac)	15	-$.85	$.01	$1.29	17	-$.87	$.01	$.92
Total support staff FTE/phy	60	4.02	5.03	5.93	102	3.79	4.60	5.55

Primary Care Single Specialty Practices by Ownership — Family Practice, Not Hospital or IDS Owned and All Owner Types (per Work RVU)

Table 9.9a: Staffing, Patients, Procedures and Square Footage

	Family Practice - Not Hospital Owned				Family Practice - All			
	Count	25th %tile	Median	75th %tile	Count	25th %tile	Median	75th %tile
Total prov FTE/10,000 work RVU	13	2.44	2.73	3.39	17	2.44	2.73	3.21
Tot phy FTE/10,000 work RVU	14	1.77	2.17	2.66	20	1.80	2.17	2.48
Prim care phy/10,000 work RVU	13	1.73	2.27	2.68	19	1.79	2.27	2.48
Nonsurg phy/10,000 work RVU	0	*	*	*	0	*	*	*
Surg spec phy/10,000 work RVU	0	*	*	*	0	*	*	*
Total NPP FTE/10,000 work RVU	13	.42	.64	.89	17	.42	.62	.89
Total supp stf FTE/10,000 wrk RVU	14	8.66	10.27	11.47	20	7.99	10.27	11.73
Tot empl supp stf/10,000 work RVU	13	9.35	10.28	11.72	19	8.41	10.28	11.87
General administrative	13	.42	.64	.96	18	.26	.55	.76
Patient accounting	13	1.07	1.70	1.89	16	1.00	1.54	1.94
General accounting	8	*	*	*	9	*	*	*
Managed care administrative	4	*	*	*	5	*	*	*
Information technology	2	*	*	*	3	*	*	*
Housekeeping, maint, security	1	*	*	*	1	*	*	*
Medical receptionists	12	1.23	1.94	2.39	18	1.37	2.07	2.76
Med secretaries,transcribers	9	*	*	*	12	.29	.66	.84
Medical records	12	.78	1.27	1.41	17	.67	1.23	1.40
Other admin support	7	*	*	*	11	.13	.51	.70
*Total administrative supp staff	4	*	*	*	5	*	*	*
Registered Nurses	10	.27	.69	1.55	13	.23	.66	1.16
Licensed Practical Nurses	11	.38	.93	1.39	15	.58	1.18	1.65
Med assistants, nurse aides	12	.67	1.52	3.03	16	1.11	1.92	3.28
*Total clinical supp staff	10	2.18	3.30	3.93	13	2.39	3.73	4.21
Clinical laboratory	10	.65	.80	.89	12	.65	.80	.92
Radiology and imaging	6	*	*	*	9	*	*	*
Other medical support serv	4	*	*	*	5	*	*	*
*Total ancillary supp staff	3	*	*	*	3	*	*	*
Tot contracted supp staff	1	*	*	*	1	*	*	*
Tot RVU/work RVU	13	1.99	2.06	2.25	16	1.94	2.04	2.18
Patients/work RVU	9	*	*	*	10	.32	.45	.68
Tot procedures/work RVU	13	1.94	2.20	2.83	19	1.71	2.19	2.76
Square feet/work RVU	13	.32	.38	.44	19	.35	.39	.45
Total support staff FTE/phy	60	4.02	5.03	5.93	102	3.79	4.60	5.55

*See pages 260 and 261 for definition.

Table 9.9b: Charges, Revenue and Cost

	Family Practice - Not Hospital Owned				Family Practice - All			
	Count	25th %tile	Median	75th %tile	Count	25th %tile	Median	75th %tile
Total gross charges	14	$120.95	$132.18	$167.56	20	$111.71	$126.65	$161.94
Total medical revenue	14	$99.51	$104.85	$124.35	20	$82.19	$102.73	$119.85
Net fee-for-service revenue	13	$88.81	$101.47	$116.81	19	$79.59	$94.12	$111.29
Net capitation revenue	2	*	*	*	4	*	*	*
Net other medical revenue	7	*	*	*	11	$.64	$2.19	$3.44
Total supp staff cost/work RVU	14	$30.46	$37.28	$43.73	20	$28.63	$37.28	$43.99
Total general operating cost	14	$26.00	$31.94	$42.40	20	$23.77	$29.04	$34.99
Total operating cost	14	$59.90	$66.66	$82.36	20	$58.33	$62.51	$77.96
Total med rev after oper cost	14	$34.14	$41.24	$48.29	20	$23.78	$38.83	$46.46
Total provider cost/work RVU	14	$35.02	$42.52	$50.45	20	$35.25	$44.78	$52.88
Total NPP cost/work RVU	14	$3.38	$5.27	$7.64	19	$3.45	$5.94	$8.96
Provider consultant cost	3	*	*	*	3	*	*	*
Total physician cost/work RVU	14	$28.62	$37.58	$46.29	20	$29.33	$39.15	$47.23
Total phy compensation	13	$23.62	$32.09	$38.74	19	$24.70	$32.43	$39.45
Total phy benefit cost	13	$5.39	$7.35	$8.13	19	$4.99	$7.35	$8.22
Total cost	14	$99.39	$109.95	$131.98	20	$98.75	$109.95	$124.00
Net nonmedical revenue	10	$.01	$.47	$3.41	15	$.01	$.58	$28.09
Net inc, prac with fin sup	1	*	*	*	2	*	*	*
Net inc, prac w/o fin sup	12	-$.65	$.28	$2.94	15	-$1.76	$.05	$3.04
Net inc, excl fin supp (all prac)	13	-$1.31	$.05	$2.83	17	-$7.55	-$.01	$2.83
Total support staff FTE/phy	60	4.02	5.03	5.93	102	3.79	4.60	5.55

Primary Care Single Specialty Practices by Ownership — Family Practice, Not Hospital or IDS Owned and All Owner Types (per Patient)

Table 9.10a: Staffing, RVUs, Procedures and Square Footage

	Family Practice - Not Hospital Owned				Family Practice - All			
	Count	25th %tile	Median	75th %tile	Count	25th %tile	Median	75th %tile
Total prov FTE/10,000 patients	17	4.41	5.58	9.06	30	4.33	5.97	7.62
Total phy FTE/10,000 pat	23	2.81	4.03	7.11	41	3.07	4.63	5.72
Prim care phy/10,000 pat	21	2.84	4.03	6.47	39	3.27	4.63	5.62
Nonsurg phy/10,000 pat	0	*	*	*	0	*	*	*
Surg spec phy/10,000 pat	0	*	*	*	0	*	*	*
Total NPP FTE/10,000 pat	17	.74	.98	1.87	30	.76	1.05	1.76
Total supp staff FTE/10,000 pat	23	15.25	21.31	31.61	41	14.82	21.76	27.23
Total empl supp staff/10,000 pat	22	13.67	21.16	26.33	40	14.10	21.71	25.28
General administrative	23	.65	1.01	2.04	41	.66	1.05	1.58
Patient accounting	23	1.68	2.91	4.29	30	2.03	3.61	10.77
General accounting	14	.29	.34	.75	14	.29	.34	.75
Managed care administrative	8	*	*	*	9	*	*	*
Information technology	6	*	*	*	6	*	*	*
Housekeeping, maint, security	5	*	*	*	6	*	*	*
Medical receptionists	22	2.59	3.68	5.55	34	2.92	4.71	6.95
Med secretaries,transcribers	16	.75	1.15	1.42	20	.82	1.21	1.62
Medical records	20	1.04	1.59	2.76	27	.82	1.46	2.91
Other admin support	13	.16	.26	2.44	20	.25	.76	1.93
*Total administrative supp staff	8	*	*	*	10	6.74	12.47	15.32
Registered Nurses	16	1.00	1.64	2.99	24	.79	1.47	2.72
Licensed Practical Nurses	20	1.08	1.99	2.85	32	1.51	2.50	4.47
Med assistants, nurse aides	22	1.21	3.36	6.75	35	2.05	3.83	6.56
*Total clinical supp staff	19	4.43	6.44	9.45	24	4.47	6.58	9.94
Clinical laboratory	16	.81	1.45	2.69	26	.71	1.61	2.31
Radiology and imaging	15	.54	.73	1.46	22	.51	.84	1.54
Other medical support serv	7	*	*	*	12	.14	.29	1.34
*Total ancillary supp staff	6	*	*	*	6	*	*	*
Tot contracted supp staff	3	*	*	*	4	*	*	*
Tot RVU/patient	11	2.73	4.05	7.20	13	2.74	4.05	6.82
Physician work RVU/patient	9	*	*	*	10	1.47	2.24	3.13
Tot procedures/patient	22	2.74	4.57	8.72	40	2.86	5.06	8.65
Square feet/patient	23	.57	.74	1.33	41	.61	.92	1.20
Total support staff FTE/phy	60	4.02	5.03	5.93	102	3.79	4.60	5.55

*See pages 260 and 261 for definition.

Table 9.10b: Charges, Revenue and Cost

	Family Practice - Not Hospital Owned				Family Practice - All			
	Count	25th %tile	Median	75th %tile	Count	25th %tile	Median	75th %tile
Total gross charges	23	$157.11	$294.52	$434.01	41	$211.00	$311.82	$422.69
Total medical revenue	23	$147.99	$212.89	$324.70	41	$149.41	$227.24	$300.87
Net fee-for-service revenue	23	$134.51	$194.05	$324.64	41	$138.82	$210.41	$286.61
Net capitation revenue	7	*	*	*	11	$3.32	$30.08	$43.69
Net other medical revenue	14	$.26	$2.50	$9.27	25	$.95	$6.74	$16.86
Total support staff cost/patient	23	$37.52	$67.62	$103.70	41	$48.79	$70.73	$93.75
Total general operating cost	23	$33.66	$60.24	$103.64	41	$37.80	$60.30	$84.30
Total operating cost	23	$64.04	$133.59	$201.65	41	$84.83	$133.59	$177.96
Total med rev after oper cost	23	$61.57	$95.77	$124.61	41	$62.55	$101.68	$121.99
Total provider cost/patient	23	$59.09	$100.13	$130.00	41	$62.49	$103.99	$127.51
Total NPP cost/patient	18	$5.31	$8.69	$15.45	31	$5.77	$9.45	$14.20
Provider consultant cost	5	*	*	*	5	*	*	*
Total physician cost/patient	23	$49.38	$76.61	$110.81	41	$53.66	$99.21	$111.16
Total phy compensation	22	$44.89	$73.88	$94.71	40	$47.00	$85.21	$98.64
Total phy benefit cost	21	$8.29	$13.22	$21.06	35	$8.31	$14.58	$19.83
Total cost	23	$118.57	$219.99	$343.78	41	$148.39	$236.70	$307.17
Net nonmedical revenue	15	$.02	$1.41	$7.66	24	$.04	$2.09	$9.05
Net inc, prac with fin sup	1	*	*	*	4	*	*	*
Net inc, prac w/o fin sup	21	-$.14	$2.48	$8.92	26	-$.09	$2.24	$9.10
Net inc, excl fin supp (all prac)	22	-$.48	$2.24	$7.67	30	-$2.53	$1.54	$6.90
Total support staff FTE/phy	60	4.02	5.03	5.93	102	3.79	4.60	5.55

Primary Care Single Specialty Practices by Ownership — Family Practice, Not Hospital or IDS Owned and All Owner Types (Procedure and Charge Data)

Table 9.11a: Activity Charges to Total Gross Charges Ratios

	Family Practice - Not Hospital Owned				Family Practice - All			
	Count	25th %tile	Median	75th %tile	Count	25th %tile	Median	75th %tile
Total proc gross charges	50	95.50%	98.30%	100.00%	89	94.83%	97.29%	99.12%
Medical proc-inside practice	50	53.74%	62.81%	70.46%	89	58.77%	67.23%	79.82%
Medical proc-outside practice	45	4.48%	7.04%	12.07%	62	2.99%	6.51%	12.06%
Surg proc-inside practice	46	4.09%	6.91%	9.08%	83	3.39%	5.26%	8.01%
Surg proc-outside practice	23	1.25%	4.90%	7.18%	32	.22%	3.63%	7.86%
Laboratory procedures	48	7.19%	12.32%	20.28%	87	3.89%	10.69%	17.16%
Radiology procedures	39	1.40%	3.65%	6.23%	66	2.13%	3.88%	5.72%
Tot nonproc gross charges	34	1.37%	2.89%	5.07%	71	1.68%	3.29%	5.49%
Total support staff FTE/phy	60	4.02	5.03	5.93	102	3.79	4.60	5.55

Table 9.11b: Medical Procedure Data (inside the practice)

	Family Practice - Not Hospital Owned				Family Practice - All			
	Count	25th %tile	Median	75th %tile	Count	25th %tile	Median	75th %tile
Gross charges/procedure	46	$57.96	$66.81	$77.77	85	$59.28	$66.88	$81.42
Total cost/procedure	42	$44.67	$54.17	$63.00	81	$46.02	$55.58	$68.12
Operating cost/procedure	42	$27.51	$30.44	$37.93	61	$27.41	$30.75	$39.68
Provider cost/procedure	42	$18.55	$21.72	$27.21	81	$19.15	$23.12	$28.73
Procedures/patient	22	1.64	2.82	3.66	40	1.76	2.94	3.40
Gross charges/patient	22	$98.62	$172.20	$278.77	40	$122.06	$210.02	$287.27
Procedures/physician	47	5,143	6,198	7,635	86	5,482	6,396	8,059
Gross charges/physician	50	$369,051	$438,466	$506,789	89	$377,562	$452,800	$564,748
Procedures/provider	33	3,879	5,049	5,995	64	4,352	5,094	6,341
Gross charges/provider	34	$266,763	$323,678	$385,866	65	$281,750	$357,437	$442,097
Gross charge to total cost ratio	42	1.13	1.31	1.45	81	1.11	1.31	1.40
Oper cost to total cost ratio	42	.56	.59	.62	61	.56	.59	.62
Prov cost to total cost ratio	42	.38	.41	.44	81	.39	.41	.45
Total support staff FTE/phy	60	4.02	5.03	5.93	102	3.79	4.60	5.55

Table 9.11c: Medical Procedure Data (outside the practice)

	Family Practice - Not Hospital Owned				Family Practice - All			
	Count	25th %tile	Median	75th %tile	Count	25th %tile	Median	75th %tile
Gross charges/procedure	42	$85.40	$98.71	$118.46	59	$85.22	$98.96	$119.96
Total cost/procedure	38	$41.85	$47.70	$53.59	55	$41.97	$49.90	$61.25
Operating cost/procedure	38	$15.61	$19.66	$25.24	43	$15.87	$20.67	$25.39
Provider cost/procedure	38	$24.75	$28.13	$31.29	55	$24.94	$28.95	$33.08
Procedures/patient	21	.12	.22	.38	30	.05	.19	.34
Gross charges/patient	21	$15.61	$21.44	$35.73	30	$4.07	$18.64	$31.03
Procedures/physician	43	280	462	979	60	191	416	920
Gross charges/physician	45	$29,426	$42,850	$84,671	62	$20,435	$41,478	$78,332
Procedures/provider	31	210	421	772	42	134	395	752
Gross charges/provider	32	$18,603	$37,358	$63,341	43	$15,578	$37,317	$54,836
Gross charge to total cost ratio	38	1.85	2.08	2.34	55	1.76	2.02	2.28
Oper cost to total cost ratio	38	.37	.42	.47	43	.37	.42	.46
Prov cost to total cost ratio	38	.53	.58	.63	55	.54	.58	.63
Total support staff FTE/phy	60	4.02	5.03	5.93	102	3.79	4.60	5.55

Primary Care Single Specialty Practices by Ownership — Family Practice, Not Hospital or IDS Owned and All Owner Types (Procedure and Charge Data)

Table 9.11d: Surgery/Anesthesia Procedure Data (inside the practice)

	Family Practice - Not Hospital Owned				Family Practice - All			
	Count	25th %tile	Median	75th %tile	Count	25th %tile	Median	75th %tile
Gross charges/procedure	44	$48.93	$92.85	$113.89	81	$50.85	$94.91	$115.55
Total cost/procedure	40	$37.04	$74.95	$100.84	77	$38.63	$75.48	$98.75
Operating cost/procedure	40	$23.22	$44.62	$59.57	57	$20.44	$39.93	$58.28
Provider cost/procedure	40	$14.68	$27.56	$42.14	77	$16.08	$30.44	$43.27
Procedures/patient	21	.10	.23	.83	37	.08	.16	.32
Gross charges/patient	21	$10.59	$16.68	$35.08	37	$10.04	$15.72	$29.33
Procedures/physician	45	234	472	1,145	82	230	366	938
Gross charges/physician	46	$27,304	$47,975	$70,338	83	$21,488	$36,166	$58,895
Procedures/provider	32	190	361	861	61	173	300	686
Gross charges/provider	33	$21,579	$36,493	$52,701	62	$17,136	$26,722	$45,445
Gross charge to total cost ratio	40	1.13	1.31	1.44	77	1.11	1.31	1.40
Oper cost to total cost ratio	40	.56	.59	.62	57	.56	.59	.62
Prov cost to total cost ratio	40	.38	.41	.44	77	.39	.41	.45
Total support staff FTE/phy	60	4.02	5.03	5.93	102	3.79	4.60	5.55

Table 9.11e: Surgery/Anesthesia Procedure Data (outside the practice)

	Family Practice - Not Hospital Owned				Family Practice - All			
	Count	25th %tile	Median	75th %tile	Count	25th %tile	Median	75th %tile
Gross charges/procedure	22	$214.10	$504.94	$711.01	31	$214.00	$451.74	$697.61
Total cost/procedure	21	$104.04	$244.23	$426.81	30	$101.77	$236.30	$426.51
Operating cost/procedure	21	$45.14	$104.45	$161.63	23	$43.29	$104.45	$173.04
Provider cost/procedure	21	$51.88	$126.01	$264.36	30	$57.59	$133.71	$256.01
Procedures/patient	14	.00	.01	.04	19	.00	.01	.03
Gross charges/patient	13	$1.21	$7.31	$16.26	18	$.13	$6.06	$15.01
Procedures/physician	23	16	40	90	32	6	31	87
Gross charges/physician	23	$9,390	$32,138	$52,670	32	$1,218	$26,540	$53,490
Procedures/provider	16	12	42	97	23	10	36	59
Gross charges/provider	16	$11,416	$24,389	$41,985	23	$3,758	$24,141	$42,012
Gross charge to total cost ratio	21	1.84	2.02	2.31	30	1.69	1.98	2.26
Oper cost to total cost ratio	21	.36	.42	.46	23	.37	.42	.45
Prov cost to total cost ratio	21	.54	.58	.64	30	.55	.59	.63
Total support staff FTE/phy	60	4.02	5.03	5.93	102	3.79	4.60	5.55

Primary Care Single Specialty Practices by Ownership — Family Practice, Not Hospital or IDS Owned and All Owner Types (Procedure and Charge Data)

Table 9.11f: Clinical Laboratory/Pathology Procedure Data

	Family Practice - Not Hospital Owned				Family Practice - All			
	Count	25th %tile	Median	75th %tile	Count	25th %tile	Median	75th %tile
Gross charges/procedure	45	$15.65	$24.54	$29.93	84	$15.01	$23.59	$29.18
Total cost/procedure	41	$13.10	$19.07	$24.99	80	$11.88	$18.16	$22.46
Operating cost/procedure	41	$7.56	$12.74	$16.41	60	$7.34	$11.73	$15.78
Provider cost/procedure	41	$4.70	$6.58	$8.70	80	$4.70	$6.70	$8.55
Procedures/patient	21	.60	1.60	2.68	39	.50	1.61	3.39
Gross charges/patient	21	$12.84	$34.93	$75.35	39	$7.77	$30.41	$60.54
Procedures/physician	45	1,893	3,555	5,592	84	1,148	3,463	5,748
Gross charges/physician	48	$39,077	$86,941	$175,330	87	$17,909	$72,219	$158,561
Procedures/provider	32	1,075	2,244	4,662	63	861	2,224	4,612
Gross charges/provider	33	$22,694	$57,458	$121,584	64	$13,983	$49,835	$87,246
Gross charge to total cost ratio	41	1.12	1.34	1.50	80	1.09	1.35	1.53
Oper cost to total cost ratio	41	.58	.63	.71	60	.59	.63	.70
Prov cost to total cost ratio	41	.29	.37	.42	80	.30	.37	.44
Total support staff FTE/phy	60	4.02	5.03	5.93	102	3.79	4.60	5.55

Table 9.11g: Diagnostic Radiology and Imaging Procedure Data

	Family Practice - Not Hospital Owned				Family Practice - All			
	Count	25th %tile	Median	75th %tile	Count	25th %tile	Median	75th %tile
Gross charges/procedure	37	$63.94	$77.89	$104.42	64	$64.32	$76.54	$96.02
Total cost/procedure	34	$53.86	$73.73	$89.74	61	$47.35	$68.35	$84.44
Operating cost/procedure	34	$31.40	$47.53	$62.82	47	$29.44	$42.16	$58.24
Provider cost/procedure	34	$17.35	$21.78	$32.66	61	$17.16	$21.11	$26.91
Procedures/patient	17	.08	.21	.38	30	.14	.22	.32
Gross charges/patient	17	$8.08	$15.82	$41.12	30	$10.08	$15.92	$27.71
Procedures/physician	37	79	343	617	64	132	418	630
Gross charges/physician	39	$8,531	$23,334	$49,867	66	$11,252	$29,372	$48,020
Procedures/provider	26	76	231	410	46	115	316	490
Gross charges/provider	27	$7,093	$15,897	$34,588	47	$11,650	$19,146	$32,862
Gross charge to total cost ratio	34	1.03	1.26	1.44	61	1.03	1.24	1.48
Oper cost to total cost ratio	34	.60	.67	.74	47	.58	.66	.72
Prov cost to total cost ratio	34	.26	.33	.40	61	.27	.34	.42
Total support staff FTE/phy	60	4.02	5.03	5.93	102	3.79	4.60	5.55

Table 9.11h: Nonprocedural Gross Charge Data

	Family Practice - Not Hospital Owned				Family Practice - All			
	Count	25th %tile	Median	75th %tile	Count	25th %tile	Median	75th %tile
Gross charges/patient	16	$7.30	$10.04	$14.05	33	$8.62	$11.52	$20.72
Nonproc gross charges/physician	34	$9,711	$19,513	$40,475	71	$12,351	$22,658	$41,082
Gross charges/provider	24	$5,882	$11,113	$19,956	53	$8,323	$14,307	$25,908
Total support staff FTE/phy	60	4.02	5.03	5.93	102	3.79	4.60	5.55

Primary Care Single Specialty Practices by Ownership — Internal Medicine, Not Hospital or IDS Owned and All Owner Types

Table 10.1: Staffing and Practice Data

	Internal Medicine - Not Hospital Owned				Internal Medicine - All			
	Count	25th %tile	Median	75th %tile	Count	25th %tile	Median	75th %tile
Total provider FTE	8	*	*	*	18	4.95	7.15	15.98
Total physician FTE	14	4.00	6.50	14.50	31	4.00	5.00	8.00
Total nonphysician provider FTE	8	*	*	*	18	.83	1.00	1.50
Total support staff FTE	14	21.29	29.05	63.83	31	15.20	22.00	36.10
Number of branch clinics	5	*	*	*	7	*	*	*
Square footage of all facilities	14	7,145	11,693	21,688	30	5,313	9,668	15,052

Table 10.2: Accounts Receivable Data, Collection Percentages and Financial Ratios

	Internal Medicine - Not Hospital Owned				Internal Medicine - All			
	Count	25th %tile	Median	75th %tile	Count	25th %tile	Median	75th %tile
Total AR/physician	12	$54,801	$74,402	$81,788	29	$63,467	$77,382	$104,205
Total AR/provider	7	*	*	*	17	$64,325	$77,340	$114,002
0-30 days in AR	12	41.17%	59.00%	65.84%	29	42.43%	55.40%	66.37%
31-60 days in AR	12	12.90%	15.00%	17.88%	29	12.40%	15.29%	18.30%
61-90 days in AR	12	5.33%	8.43%	13.33%	29	5.65%	7.70%	10.44%
91-120 days in AR	12	3.75%	5.09%	6.28%	29	3.60%	5.20%	6.65%
120+ days in AR	12	8.37%	10.95%	18.49%	29	7.10%	12.92%	26.23%
Re-aged: 0-30 days in AR	5	*	*	*	9	*	*	*
Re-aged: 31-60 days in AR	5	*	*	*	9	*	*	*
Re-aged: 61-90 days in AR	5	*	*	*	9	*	*	*
Re-aged: 91-120 days in AR	5	*	*	*	9	*	*	*
Re-aged: 120+ days in AR	5	*	*	*	9	*	*	*
Not re-aged: 0-30 days in AR	7	*	*	*	20	42.39%	52.60%	63.70%
Not re-aged: 31-60 days in AR	7	*	*	*	20	13.22%	15.51%	18.33%
Not re-aged: 61-90 days in AR	7	*	*	*	20	5.97%	9.01%	10.86%
Not re-aged: 91-120 days in AR	7	*	*	*	20	3.75%	5.32%	6.68%
Not re-aged: 120+ days in AR	7	*	*	*	20	7.61%	14.73%	30.71%
Months gross FFS charges in AR	12	.96	1.18	2.04	29	1.14	1.38	1.88
Days gross FFS charges in AR	12	29.18	35.93	61.92	29	34.75	42.07	57.12
Gross FFS collection %	14	62.95%	67.08%	72.94%	31	61.15%	66.50%	71.78%
Adjusted FFS collection %	11	98.68%	98.99%	99.88%	28	96.93%	97.75%	98.97%
Gross FFS + cap collection %	2	*	*	*	3	*	*	*
Net cap rev % of gross cap chrg	2	*	*	*	3	*	*	*
Current ratio	6	*	*	*	11	1.37	2.79	24.66
Tot asset turnover ratio	6	*	*	*	11	.03	3.08	7.91
Debt to equity ratio	6	*	*	*	11	.05	.16	1.84
Debt ratio	6	*	*	*	11	4.65%	13.70%	64.80%
Return on total assets	6	*	*	*	12	-.32%	.04%	11.12%
Return on equity	6	*	*	*	12	-.34%	.05%	14.35%

Table 10.3: Breakout of Total Gross Charges by Type of Payer

	Internal Medicine - Not Hospital Owned				Internal Medicine - All			
	Count	25th %tile	Median	75th %tile	Count	25th %tile	Median	75th %tile
Medicare: fee-for-service	13	26.42%	54.80%	62.13%	29	27.08%	37.40%	56.00%
Medicare: managed care FFS	13	.00%	.00%	.00%	29	.00%	.00%	.00%
Medicare: capitation	13	.00%	.00%	.00%	29	.00%	.00%	.00%
Medicaid: fee-for-service	13	.01%	.68%	1.46%	29	.01%	.70%	2.05%
Medicaid: managed care FFS	13	.00%	.00%	.71%	29	.00%	.00%	.00%
Medicaid: capitation	13	.00%	.00%	.00%	29	.00%	.00%	.00%
Commercial: fee-for-service	13	11.92%	25.00%	43.00%	29	4.47%	33.00%	51.15%
Commercial: managed care FFS	13	.00%	.00%	24.00%	29	.00%	.00%	33.33%
Commercial: capitation	13	.00%	.00%	.00%	29	.00%	.00%	.00%
Workers' compensation	13	.00%	.01%	.65%	29	.00%	.10%	1.00%
Charity care and prof courtesy	13	.00%	.00%	.57%	29	.00%	.00%	.35%
Self-pay	13	1.31%	2.00%	9.15%	29	1.02%	2.00%	4.50%
Other federal government payers	13	.00%	.00%	.35%	29	.00%	.00%	.00%

Primary Care Single Specialty Practices by Ownership — Internal Medicine, Not Hospital or IDS Owned and All Owner Types (per FTE Physician)

Table 10.4a: Staffing, RVUs, Patients, Procedures and Square Footage

	Internal Medicine - Not Hospital Owned				Internal Medicine - All			
	Count	25th %tile	Median	75th %tile	Count	25th %tile	Median	75th %tile
Total provider FTE/physician	8	*	*	*	18	**1.13**	**1.17**	**1.25**
Prim care phy/physician	12	.65	1.00	1.00	28	1.00	1.00	1.00
Nonsurg phy/physician	7	*	*	*	9	*	*	*
Surg spec phy/physician	0	*	*	*	0	*	*	*
Total NPP FTE/physician	8	*	*	*	18	.13	.17	.25
Total support staff FTE/phy	14	**3.75**	**4.38**	**5.96**	31	**3.45**	**4.36**	**5.12**
Total empl support staff FTE	14	3.60	4.38	5.77	31	3.38	4.36	4.99
General administrative	13	.17	.20	.25	28	.17	.23	.36
Patient accounting	13	.54	.75	.82	19	.52	.75	1.00
General accounting	6	*	*	*	7	*	*	*
Managed care administrative	2	*	*	*	2	*	*	*
Information technology	5	*	*	*	5	*	*	*
Housekeeping, maint, security	0	*	*	*	2	*	*	*
Medical receptionists	11	.62	.76	1.25	24	.66	1.05	1.43
Med secretaries,transcribers	5	*	*	*	12	.15	.32	.49
Medical records	11	.20	.29	.48	20	.20	.27	.43
Other admin support	6	*	*	*	12	.10	.20	.44
*Total administrative supp staff	4	*	*	*	11	2.00	2.07	2.70
Registered Nurses	7	*	*	*	18	.14	.44	.68
Licensed Practical Nurses	8	*	*	*	23	.23	.40	.78
Med assistants, nurse aides	12	.67	1.00	1.22	28	.64	.82	1.23
*Total clinical supp staff	7	*	*	*	20	1.27	1.64	2.19
Clinical laboratory	10	.26	.39	.75	18	.28	.37	.50
Radiology and imaging	9	*	*	*	16	.13	.23	.33
Other medical support serv	4	*	*	*	7	*	*	*
*Total ancillary supp staff	3	*	*	*	4	*	*	*
Tot contracted supp staff	5	*	*	*	11	.13	.19	.23
Tot RVU/physician	3	*	*	*	6	*	*	*
Physician work RVU/physician	3	*	*	*	5	*	*	*
Patients/physician	5	*	*	*	10	970	1,307	1,760
Tot procedures/physician	12	6,317	10,787	13,999	29	7,374	11,354	15,193
Square feet/physician	14	1,426	1,597	1,800	30	1,397	1,569	1,896

*See pages 260 and 261 for definition.

Table 10.4b: Charges and Revenue

	Internal Medicine - Not Hospital Owned				Internal Medicine - All			
	Count	25th %tile	Median	75th %tile	Count	25th %tile	Median	75th %tile
Net fee-for-service revenue	14	$391,538	$528,562	$814,855	31	$395,023	$463,481	$571,521
Gross FFS charges	14	$576,745	$748,583	$1,142,023	31	$594,024	$759,742	$864,337
Adjustments to FFS charges	11	$179,198	$223,505	$440,000	28	$181,556	$250,176	$329,761
Adjusted FFS charges	11	$400,287	$463,843	$645,975	28	$404,941	$486,252	$584,207
Bad debts due to FFS activity	10	$1,116	$5,432	$7,574	27	$5,264	$9,143	$17,564
Net capitation revenue	2	*	*	*	3	*	*	*
Gross capitation charges	2	*	*	*	3	*	*	*
Capitation revenue	2	*	*	*	3	*	*	*
Purch serv for cap patients	0	*	*	*	0	*	*	*
Net other medical revenue	5	*	*	*	18	$8,570	$31,712	$40,062
Gross rev from other activity	5	*	*	*	18	$8,570	$31,712	$40,062
Other medical revenue	4	*	*	*	17	$7,114	$32,780	$40,125
Rev from sale of goods/services	1	*	*	*	2	*	*	*
Cost of sales	0	*	*	*	0	*	*	*
Total gross charges	14	$576,745	$783,047	$1,142,023	31	$594,024	$759,742	$864,337
Total medical revenue	14	$412,999	$559,907	$814,855	31	$409,975	$518,029	$608,078

Primary Care Single Specialty Practices by Ownership — Internal Medicine, Not Hospital or IDS Owned and All Owner Types (per FTE Physician)

Table 10.4c: Operating Cost

	Internal Medicine - Not Hospital Owned				Internal Medicine - All			
	Count	25th %tile	Median	75th %tile	Count	25th %tile	Median	75th %tile
Total support staff cost/phy	14	$122,803	$164,036	$210,289	31	$122,745	$143,565	$187,226
Total empl supp staff cost/phy	14	$102,522	$135,232	$185,452	31	$94,564	$113,653	$151,521
General administrative	13	$8,824	$14,346	$18,521	28	$9,688	$14,701	$19,992
Patient accounting	13	$14,172	$21,760	$26,567	19	$14,890	$21,111	$26,733
General accounting	6	*	*	*	7	*	*	*
Managed care administrative	2	*	*	*	2	*	*	*
Information technology	5	*	*	*	5	*	*	*
Housekeeping, maint, security	0	*	*	*	2	*	*	*
Medical receptionists	11	$13,558	$16,984	$33,400	24	$15,139	$22,675	$37,972
Med secretaries,transcribers	5	*	*	*	12	$4,648	$9,163	$15,184
Medical records	11	$3,636	$6,278	$9,107	20	$3,388	$5,847	$8,542
Other admin support	6	*	*	*	12	$2,362	$4,450	$9,963
*Total administrative supp staff	2	*	*	*	10	$51,075	$53,869	$67,239
Registered Nurses	7	*	*	*	18	$5,634	$14,692	$26,088
Licensed Practical Nurses	8	*	*	*	23	$7,372	$11,567	$22,038
Med assistants, nurse aides	12	$15,127	$26,236	$37,704	28	$14,666	$20,166	$33,160
*Total clinical supp staff	6	*	*	*	19	$36,511	$48,365	$57,026
Clinical laboratory	10	$10,802	$12,522	$21,638	18	$9,217	$12,871	$15,887
Radiology and imaging	9	*	*	*	16	$5,167	$9,809	$11,943
Other medical support serv	4	*	*	*	7	*	*	*
*Total ancillary supp staff	3	*	*	*	8	*	*	*
Total empl supp staff benefits	12	$16,717	$31,061	$39,201	28	$17,693	$28,476	$35,671
Tot contracted supp staff	6	*	*	*	17	$2,385	$5,344	$10,441
Total general operating cost	14	$117,978	$148,592	$251,985	31	$114,369	$137,299	$183,459
Information technology	13	$8,414	$11,960	$14,349	30	$3,329	$6,019	$11,988
Medical and surgical supply	13	$5,320	$13,585	$23,766	30	$6,428	$11,696	$18,896
Building and occupancy	13	$30,407	$35,336	$44,979	29	$25,132	$32,683	$43,014
Furniture and equipment	9	*	*	*	19	$2,913	$5,512	$7,473
Admin supplies and services	13	$7,538	$12,064	$20,597	30	$7,461	$14,416	$20,416
Prof liability insurance	13	$6,195	$9,373	$14,150	29	$3,269	$7,405	$9,468
Other insurance premiums	12	$356	$987	$2,697	13	$383	$974	$2,395
Outside professional fees	13	$1,905	$5,851	$14,044	22	$750	$3,365	$9,452
Promotion and marketing	12	$406	$2,478	$4,522	23	$360	$682	$2,826
Clinical laboratory	10	$13,281	$22,914	$29,096	21	$6,345	$19,873	$24,421
Radiology and imaging	9	*	*	*	17	$855	$1,864	$9,624
Other ancillary services	4	*	*	*	8	*	*	*
Billing purchased services	5	*	*	*	16	$2,498	$21,920	$34,031
Management fees paid to MSO	0	*	*	*	10	$14,427	$17,462	$26,226
Misc operating cost	13	$3,017	$7,288	$43,414	29	$2,569	$7,288	$27,129
Cost allocated to prac from par	0	*	*	*	5	*	*	*
Total operating cost	14	$245,167	$313,420	$447,231	31	$234,061	$292,776	$352,861

*See pages 260 and 261 for definition.

Primary Care Single Specialty Practices by Ownership — Internal Medicine, Not Hospital or IDS Owned and All Owner Types (per FTE Physician)

Table 10.4d: Provider Cost

	Internal Medicine - Not Hospital Owned				Internal Medicine - All			
	Count	25th %tile	Median	75th %tile	Count	25th %tile	Median	75th %tile
Total med rev after oper cost	14	$168,670	$213,697	$338,796	31	$167,740	$213,618	$287,435
Total provider cost/physician	13	$161,814	$212,822	$344,987	30	$196,787	$227,520	$269,901
Total NPP cost/physician	8	*	*	*	19	$7,514	$11,383	$16,770
Nonphysician provider comp	7	*	*	*	18	$6,118	$10,947	$15,121
Nonphysician prov benefit cost	6	*	*	*	17	$963	$1,711	$3,451
Provider consultant cost	1	*	*	*	1	*	*	*
Total physician cost/physician	14	$161,422	$193,575	$334,919	31	$182,985	$216,851	$252,847
Total phy compensation	13	$147,618	$177,582	$287,448	30	$160,603	$193,089	$238,747
Total phy benefit cost	12	$14,538	$25,266	$39,577	29	$17,793	$26,285	$35,058

Table 10.4e: Net Income or Loss

	Internal Medicine - Not Hospital Owned				Internal Medicine - All			
	Count	25th %tile	Median	75th %tile	Count	25th %tile	Median	75th %tile
Total cost	13	$393,526	$573,489	$835,108	30	$443,738	$533,678	$612,476
Net nonmedical revenue	8	*	*	*	18	$13,047	$28,989	$52,912
Nonmedical revenue	8	*	*	*	11	$782	$3,670	$25,073
Fin support for oper costs	0	*	*	*	9	*	*	*
Goodwill amortization	0	*	*	*	0	*	*	*
Nonmedical cost	3	*	*	*	8	*	*	*
Net inc, prac with fin sup	0	*	*	*	8	*	*	*
Net inc, prac w/o fin sup	13	$408	$15,780	$33,494	18	$602	$15,780	$27,398
Net inc, excl fin supp (all prac)	13	$408	$15,780	$33,494	26	-$38,035	$2,263	$20,055

Table 10.4f: Assets and Liabilities

	Internal Medicine - Not Hospital Owned				Internal Medicine - All			
	Count	25th %tile	Median	75th %tile	Count	25th %tile	Median	75th %tile
Total assets	7	*	*	*	12	$69,136	$218,610	$12,818,638
Current assets	7	*	*	*	12	$22,564	$195,379	$14,687,899
Noncurrent assets	7	*	*	*	12	-$1,869,261	$12,177	$57,514
Total liabilities	7	*	*	*	12	$27,439	$82,350	$737,074
Current liabilities	7	*	*	*	12	$23,429	$66,803	$595,685
Noncurrent liabilities	7	*	*	*	12	$0	$0	$6,950
Working capital	7	*	*	*	12	$2,781	$157,948	$14,092,214
Total net worth	7	*	*	*	12	$17,941	$168,805	$12,222,953

Primary Care Single Specialty Practices by Ownership — Internal Medicine, Not Hospital or IDS Owned and All Owner Types (as a % of Total Medical Revenue)

Table 10.5a: Charges and Revenue

	Internal Medicine - Not Hospital Owned				Internal Medicine - All			
	Count	25th %tile	Median	75th %tile	Count	25th %tile	Median	75th %tile
Net fee-for-service revenue	14	92.56%	100.00%	100.00%	31	93.23%	98.23%	100.00%
Net capitation revenue	2	*	*	*	3	*	*	*
Net other medical revenue	5	*	*	*	18	1.75%	6.26%	7.68%
Total gross charges	**14**	**131.49%**	**142.85%**	**153.68%**	**31**	**135.23%**	**140.88%**	**158.06%**

Table 10.5b: Operating Cost

	Internal Medicine - Not Hospital Owned				Internal Medicine - All			
	Count	25th %tile	Median	75th %tile	Count	25th %tile	Median	75th %tile
Total support staff cost	**14**	**27.18%**	**30.44%**	**32.99%**	**31**	**26.60%**	**30.50%**	**34.06%**
Total empl support staff cost	14	21.02%	23.52%	29.26%	31	21.14%	23.64%	27.55%
General administrative	13	1.32%	2.23%	3.02%	28	1.87%	2.86%	3.85%
Patient accounting	13	2.78%	3.58%	4.40%	19	2.74%	3.58%	5.27%
General accounting	6	*	*	*	7	*	*	*
Managed care administrative	2	*	*	*	2	*	*	*
Information technology	5	*	*	*	5	*	*	*
Housekeeping, maint, security	0	*	*	*	2	*	*	*
Medical receptionists	11	2.23%	4.04%	5.57%	24	3.27%	4.78%	6.62%
Med secretaries,transcribers	5	*	*	*	12	.95%	2.00%	2.75%
Medical records	11	.68%	1.05%	1.18%	20	.70%	1.06%	1.30%
Other admin support	6	*	*	*	12	.43%	.85%	2.77%
*Total administrative supp staff	2	*	*	*	10	10.65%	11.64%	13.37%
Registered Nurses	7	*	*	*	18	1.48%	3.00%	5.23%
Licensed Practical Nurses	8	*	*	*	23	1.20%	2.56%	4.82%
Med assistants, nurse aides	12	2.84%	4.11%	7.48%	28	2.73%	3.91%	6.44%
*Total clinical supp staff	6	*	*	*	19	8.00%	8.98%	12.12%
Clinical laboratory	10	1.35%	2.62%	3.86%	18	1.43%	2.45%	3.14%
Radiology and imaging	9	*	*	*	16	.98%	1.46%	1.78%
Other medical support serv	4	*	*	*	7	*	*	*
*Total ancillary supp staff	3	*	*	*	8	*	*	*
Total empl supp staff benefits	12	3.62%	5.54%	6.16%	28	3.95%	5.67%	6.34%
Tot contracted supp staff	6	*	*	*	17	.46%	.79%	2.44%
Total general operating cost	**14**	**24.10%**	**30.46%**	**35.76%**	**31**	**23.55%**	**29.02%**	**34.66%**
Information technology	13	1.21%	1.97%	2.78%	30	.59%	1.34%	1.98%
Medical and surgical supply	13	1.52%	2.51%	3.88%	30	1.66%	2.47%	3.45%
Building and occupancy	13	5.00%	5.72%	8.11%	29	4.63%	6.24%	8.26%
Furniture and equipment	9	*	*	*	19	.52%	.98%	1.53%
Admin supplies and services	13	.95%	2.07%	3.17%	30	1.34%	2.86%	4.06%
Prof liability insurance	13	.84%	1.60%	2.74%	29	.75%	1.29%	1.96%
Other insurance premiums	12	.08%	.20%	.46%	13	.09%	.20%	.41%
Outside professional fees	13	.44%	.86%	2.08%	22	.21%	.71%	1.51%
Promotion and marketing	12	.06%	.41%	1.11%	23	.09%	.16%	.58%
Clinical laboratory	10	2.25%	4.07%	5.86%	21	1.11%	3.26%	4.92%
Radiology and imaging	9	*	*	*	17	.21%	.37%	1.19%
Other ancillary services	4	*	*	*	8	*	*	*
Billing purchased services	5	*	*	*	16	.64%	4.89%	5.85%
Management fees paid to MSO	0	*	*	*	10	3.25%	3.70%	4.27%
Misc operating cost	13	.69%	1.33%	5.45%	29	.57%	1.33%	5.38%
Cost allocated to prac from par	0	*	*	*	5	*	*	*
Total operating cost	**14**	**53.64%**	**59.51%**	**65.41%**	**31**	**53.04%**	**59.45%**	**65.91%**

**See pages 260 and 261 for definition.

Primary Care Single Specialty Practices by Ownership — Internal Medicine, Not Hospital or IDS Owned and All Owner Types (as a % of Total Medical Revenue)

Table 10.5c: Provider Cost

	Internal Medicine - Not Hospital Owned				Internal Medicine - All			
	Count	25th %tile	Median	75th %tile	Count	25th %tile	Median	75th %tile
Total med rev after oper cost	14	34.59%	40.49%	46.36%	31	34.08%	40.55%	46.96%
Total provider cost	13	36.48%	40.94%	43.09%	30	39.89%	43.49%	53.32%
Total NPP cost	8	*	*	*	19	.98%	2.44%	4.18%
Nonphysician provider comp	7	*	*	*	18	1.32%	2.14%	3.42%
Nonphysician prov benefit cost	6	*	*	*	17	.17%	.42%	.70%
Provider consultant cost	1	*	*	*	1	*	*	*
Total physician cost	14	35.57%	39.20%	41.60%	31	38.06%	41.66%	49.09%
Total phy compensation	13	31.07%	34.16%	38.13%	30	33.21%	37.28%	43.10%
Total phy benefit cost	12	3.07%	5.03%	7.08%	29	4.54%	5.55%	7.09%

Table 10.5d: Net Income or Loss

	Internal Medicine - Not Hospital Owned				Internal Medicine - All			
	Count	25th %tile	Median	75th %tile	Count	25th %tile	Median	75th %tile
Total cost	13	96.76%	99.85%	100.69%	30	98.96%	100.69%	109.60%
Net nonmedical revenue	8	*	*	*	18	1.76%	5.44%	12.22%
Nonmedical revenue	8	*	*	*	11	.17%	.39%	4.93%
Fin support for oper costs	0	*	*	*	9	*	*	*
Goodwill amortization	0	*	*	*	0	*	*	*
Nonmedical cost	3	*	*	*	8	*	*	*
Net inc, prac with fin sup	0	*	*	*	8	*	*	*
Net inc, prac w/o fin sup	13	.08%	1.78%	4.97%	18	.12%	2.20%	4.17%
Net inc, excl fin supp (all prac)	13	.08%	1.78%	4.97%	26	-8.05%	.32%	3.81%

Table 10.5e: Assets and Liabilities

	Internal Medicine - Not Hospital Owned				Internal Medicine - All			
	Count	25th %tile	Median	75th %tile	Count	25th %tile	Median	75th %tile
Total assets	7	*	*	*	12	9.46%	27.15%	2948.68%
Current assets	7	*	*	*	12	4.35%	25.61%	3378.67%
Noncurrent assets	7	*	*	*	12	-429.99%	2.86%	8.09%
Total liabilities	7	*	*	*	12	6.68%	11.75%	151.00%
Current liabilities	7	*	*	*	12	4.27%	11.61%	137.03%
Noncurrent liabilities	7	*	*	*	12	.00%	.00%	1.63%
Working capital	7	*	*	*	12	.24%	18.78%	3241.64%
Total net worth	7	*	*	*	12	2.70%	20.18%	2811.66%

Primary Care Single Specialty Practices by Ownership — Internal Medicine, Not Hospital or IDS Owned and All Owner Types (per FTE Provider)

Table 10.6a: Staffing, RVUs, Patients, Procedures and Square Footage

	Internal Medicine - Not Hospital Owned				Internal Medicine - All			
	Count	25th %tile	Median	75th %tile	Count	25th %tile	Median	75th %tile
Total physician FTE/provider	8	*	*	*	18	.80	.85	.89
Prim care phy/provider	7	*	*	*	16	.62	.81	.88
Nonsurg phy/provider	5	*	*	*	6	*	*	*
Surg spec phy/provider	0	*	*	*	0	*	*	*
Total NPP FTE/provider	8	*	*	*	18	.11	.15	.20
Total support staff FTE/prov	8	*	*	*	18	3.38	4.06	4.53
Total empl supp staff FTE/prov	8	*	*	*	18	3.25	3.95	4.48
General administrative	8	*	*	*	16	.14	.19	.32
Patient accounting	8	*	*	*	11	.57	.60	.83
General accounting	5	*	*	*	6	*	*	*
Managed care administrative	2	*	*	*	2	*	*	*
Information technology	5	*	*	*	5	*	*	*
Housekeeping, maint, security	0	*	*	*	1	*	*	*
Medical receptionists	7	*	*	*	15	.59	1.00	1.19
Med secretaries,transcribers	4	*	*	*	9	*	*	*
Medical records	8	*	*	*	13	.17	.25	.45
Other admin support	5	*	*	*	8	*	*	*
*Total administrative supp staff	2	*	*	*	7	*	*	*
Registered Nurses	6	*	*	*	12	.10	.51	.63
Licensed Practical Nurses	5	*	*	*	15	.21	.50	.83
Med assistants, nurse aides	7	*	*	*	17	.55	.73	1.01
*Total clinical supp staff	5	*	*	*	13	1.22	1.35	2.09
Clinical laboratory	8	*	*	*	13	.23	.32	.41
Radiology and imaging	6	*	*	*	11	.11	.20	.27
Other medical support serv	3	*	*	*	5	*	*	*
*Total ancillary supp staff	3	*	*	*	4	*	*	*
Tot contracted supp staff	3	*	*	*	7	*	*	*
Tot RVU/provider	3	*	*	*	6	*	*	*
Physician work RVU/provider	3	*	*	*	4	*	*	*
Patients/provider	2	*	*	*	4	*	*	*
Tot procedures/provider	6	*	*	*	16	9,279	11,263	13,920
Square feet/provider	8	*	*	*	18	1,247	1,458	1,918
Total support staff FTE/phy	14	3.75	4.38	5.96	31	3.45	4.36	5.12

*See pages 260 and 261 for definition.

Table 10.6b: Charges, Revenue and Cost

	Internal Medicine - Not Hospital Owned				Internal Medicine - All			
	Count	25th %tile	Median	75th %tile	Count	25th %tile	Median	75th %tile
Total gross charges	8	*	*	*	18	$557,143	$646,869	$808,813
Total medical revenue	8	*	*	*	18	$384,677	$438,460	$544,093
Net fee-for-service revenue	8	*	*	*	18	$351,608	$417,234	$507,045
Net capitation revenue	1	*	*	*	1	*	*	*
Net other medical revenue	4	*	*	*	13	$9,718	$29,306	$35,671
Total support staff cost/prov	8	*	*	*	18	$111,432	$141,301	$172,651
Total general operating cost	8	*	*	*	18	$103,518	$118,858	$152,532
Total operating cost	8	*	*	*	18	$229,425	$259,721	$329,553
Total med rev after oper cost	8	*	*	*	18	$137,909	$178,063	$271,730
Total provider cost/provider	8	*	*	*	18	$170,671	$196,123	$261,499
Total NPP cost/provider	8	*	*	*	18	$6,712	$11,194	$14,907
Provider consultant cost	1	*	*	*	1	*	*	*
Total physician cost/provider	8	*	*	*	18	$158,272	$183,418	$254,164
Total phy compensation	8	*	*	*	18	$131,171	$162,941	$228,442
Total phy benefit cost	8	*	*	*	18	$16,712	$23,769	$30,397
Total cost	8	*	*	*	18	$407,159	$471,971	$549,244
Net nonmedical revenue	7	*	*	*	12	$956	$23,616	$29,146
Net inc, prac with fin sup	0	*	*	*	5	*	*	*
Net inc, prac w/o fin sup	8	*	*	*	11	-$188	$3,661	$19,002
Net inc, excl fin supp (all prac)	8	*	*	*	16	-$30,219	-$85	$17,186
Total support staff FTE/phy	14	3.75	4.38	5.96	31	3.45	4.36	5.12

Primary Care Single Specialty Practices by Ownership — Internal Medicine, Not Hospital or IDS Owned and All Owner Types (per Square Foot)

Table 10.7a: Staffing, RVUs, Patients and Procedures

	Internal Medicine - Not Hospital Owned				Internal Medicine - All			
	Count	25th %tile	Median	75th %tile	Count	25th %tile	Median	75th %tile
Total prov FTE/10,000 sq ft	8	*	*	*	18	5.22	6.86	8.02
Total phy FTE/10,000 sq ft	14	5.56	6.27	7.03	30	5.29	6.37	7.17
Prim care phy/10,000 sq ft	12	3.77	5.47	7.48	27	4.15	5.73	7.70
Nonsurg phy/10,000 sq ft	7	*	*	*	9	*	*	*
Surg spec phy/10,000 sq ft	0	*	*	*	0	*	*	*
Total NPP FTE/10,000 sq ft	8	*	*	*	18	.60	.92	1.42
Total supp stf FTE/10,000 sq ft	14	24.50	29.22	34.35	30	22.50	27.02	31.62
Total empl supp stf/10,000 sq ft	14	23.30	27.97	32.78	30	21.66	27.02	30.37
General administrative	13	.82	1.36	2.18	27	1.10	1.39	2.80
Patient accounting	13	3.09	4.53	5.25	19	3.13	4.38	5.46
General accounting	6	*	*	*	7	*	*	*
Managed care administrative	2	*	*	*	2	*	*	*
Information technology	5	*	*	*	5	*	*	*
Housekeeping, maint, security	0	*	*	*	2	*	*	*
Medical receptionists	11	3.99	6.73	9.09	24	4.28	7.54	9.02
Med secretaries,transcribers	5	*	*	*	12	1.22	1.50	2.21
Medical records	11	1.34	2.21	3.03	20	.90	1.85	2.67
Other admin support	6	*	*	*	12	.60	1.11	2.73
*Total administrative supp staff	4	*	*	*	11	13.71	14.78	21.21
Registered Nurses	7	*	*	*	17	1.21	2.67	4.49
Licensed Practical Nurses	8	*	*	*	23	.98	2.77	5.02
Med assistants, nurse aides	12	3.69	6.36	9.15	28	3.56	4.50	9.15
*Total clinical supp staff	7	*	*	*	20	7.63	9.63	14.22
Clinical laboratory	10	1.68	1.83	4.48	18	1.76	1.95	2.52
Radiology and imaging	9	*	*	*	16	.66	1.06	2.10
Other medical support serv	4	*	*	*	6	*	*	*
*Total ancillary supp staff	3	*	*	*	4	*	*	*
Tot contracted supp staff	5	*	*	*	11	.60	1.23	1.67
Tot RVU/sq ft	3	*	*	*	6	*	*	*
Physician work RVU/sq ft	3	*	*	*	5	*	*	*
Patients/sq ft	5	*	*	*	10	.64	.80	1.03
Tot procedures/sq ft	12	5.06	6.46	7.52	28	5.06	7.45	9.26
Total support staff FTE/phy	14	3.75	4.38	5.96	31	3.45	4.36	5.12

*See pages 260 and 261 for definition.

Table 10.7b: Charges, Revenue and Cost

	Internal Medicine - Not Hospital Owned				Internal Medicine - All			
	Count	25th %tile	Median	75th %tile	Count	25th %tile	Median	75th %tile
Total gross charges	14	$364.00	$480.48	$685.64	30	$326.34	$460.32	$641.36
Total medical revenue	14	$260.21	$337.46	$449.79	30	$250.24	$312.17	$433.50
Net fee-for-service revenue	14	$254.70	$322.35	$449.79	30	$230.93	$292.71	$413.57
Net capitation revenue	2	*	*	*	3	*	*	*
Net other medical revenue	5	*	*	*	17	$6.12	$18.88	$22.05
Total support staff cost/sq ft	14	$83.32	$105.50	$123.92	30	$82.53	$96.59	$121.21
Total general operating cost	14	$74.20	$94.39	$132.90	30	$65.85	$88.64	$117.73
Total operating cost	14	$176.85	$202.00	$244.93	30	$151.35	$193.39	$223.25
Total med rev after oper cost	14	$99.39	$139.19	$213.88	30	$87.67	$121.45	$176.61
Total provider cost/sq ft	13	$98.67	$139.85	$208.62	29	$100.52	$139.85	$194.42
Total NPP cost/sq ft	8	*	*	*	19	$4.17	$5.73	$10.70
Provider consultant cost	1	*	*	*	1	*	*	*
Total physician cost/sq ft	14	$96.75	$126.84	$203.61	30	$98.40	$132.68	$184.53
Total phy compensation	13	$87.93	$109.60	$179.81	29	$91.15	$114.50	$163.14
Total phy benefit cost	12	$8.79	$14.49	$23.72	28	$12.39	$16.00	$23.72
Total cost	13	$302.43	$341.06	$438.62	29	$279.62	$326.26	$412.95
Net nonmedical revenue/sq ft	8	*	*	*	18	$8.99	$18.02	$60.02
Net inc, prac with fin sup	0	*	*	*	8	*	*	*
Net inc, prac w/o fin sup	13	$.27	$8.77	$16.62	17	$.27	$8.55	$14.05
Net inc, excl fin supp (all prac)	13	$.27	$8.77	$16.62	25	-$44.32	$.52	$10.49
Total support staff FTE/phy	14	3.75	4.38	5.96	31	3.45	4.36	5.12

Primary Care Single Specialty Practices by Ownership — Internal Medicine, Not Hospital or IDS Owned and All Owner Types (per Total RVU)

Table 10.8a: Staffing, Patients, Procedures and Square Footage

	Internal Medicine - Not Hospital Owned				Internal Medicine - All			
	Count	25th %tile	Median	75th %tile	Count	25th %tile	Median	75th %tile
Total prov FTE/10,000 tot RVU	3	*	*	*	6	*	*	*
Total phy FTE/10,000 tot RVU	3	*	*	*	6	*	*	*
Prim care phy/10,000 tot RVU	2	*	*	*	5	*	*	*
Nonsurg phy/10,000 tot RVU	2	*	*	*	2	*	*	*
Surg spec phy/10,000 tot RVU	0	*	*	*	0	*	*	*
Total NPP FTE/10,000 tot RVU	3	*	*	*	6	*	*	*
Total supp stf FTE/10,000 tot RVU	3	*	*	*	6	*	*	*
Tot empl supp stf/10,000 tot RVU	3	*	*	*	6	*	*	*
General administrative	3	*	*	*	6	*	*	*
Patient accounting	3	*	*	*	4	*	*	*
General accounting	2	*	*	*	2	*	*	*
Managed care administrative	0	*	*	*	0	*	*	*
Information technology	2	*	*	*	2	*	*	*
Housekeeping, maint, security	0	*	*	*	0	*	*	*
Medical receptionists	3	*	*	*	6	*	*	*
Med secretaries,transcribers	2	*	*	*	3	*	*	*
Medical records	3	*	*	*	4	*	*	*
Other admin support	2	*	*	*	3	*	*	*
*Total administrative supp staff	1	*	*	*	4	*	*	*
Registered Nurses	3	*	*	*	4	*	*	*
Licensed Practical Nurses	3	*	*	*	6	*	*	*
Med assistants, nurse aides	3	*	*	*	6	*	*	*
*Total clinical supp staff	3	*	*	*	6	*	*	*
Clinical laboratory	3	*	*	*	4	*	*	*
Radiology and imaging	1	*	*	*	3	*	*	*
Other medical support serv	0	*	*	*	0	*	*	*
*Total ancillary supp staff	0	*	*	*	0	*	*	*
Tot contracted supp staff	2	*	*	*	3	*	*	*
Physician work RVU/tot RVU	3	*	*	*	3	*	*	*
Patients/tot RVU	2	*	*	*	2	*	*	*
Tot procedures/tot RVU	3	*	*	*	6	*	*	*
Square feet/tot RVU	3	*	*	*	6	*	*	*
Total support staff FTE/phy	14	3.75	4.38	5.96	31	3.45	4.36	5.12

*See pages 260 and 261 for definition.

Table 10.8b: Charges, Revenue and Cost

	Internal Medicine - Not Hospital Owned				Internal Medicine - All			
	Count	25th %tile	Median	75th %tile	Count	25th %tile	Median	75th %tile
Total gross charges	3	*	*	*	6	*	*	*
Total medical revenue	3	*	*	*	6	*	*	*
Net fee-for-service revenue	3	*	*	*	6	*	*	*
Net capitation revenue	0	*	*	*	0	*	*	*
Net other medical revenue	2	*	*	*	5	*	*	*
Total supp staff cost/tot RVU	3	*	*	*	6	*	*	*
Total general operating cost	3	*	*	*	6	*	*	*
Total operating cost	3	*	*	*	6	*	*	*
Total med rev after oper cost	3	*	*	*	6	*	*	*
Total provider cost/tot RVU	3	*	*	*	6	*	*	*
Total NPP cost/tot RVU	3	*	*	*	6	*	*	*
Provider consultant cost	0	*	*	*	0	*	*	*
Total physician cost/tot RVU	3	*	*	*	6	*	*	*
Total phy compensation	3	*	*	*	6	*	*	*
Total phy benefit cost	3	*	*	*	6	*	*	*
Total cost	3	*	*	*	6	*	*	*
Net nonmedical revenue	3	*	*	*	6	*	*	*
Net inc, prac with fin sup	0	*	*	*	3	*	*	*
Net inc, prac w/o fin sup	3	*	*	*	3	*	*	*
Net inc, excl fin supp (all prac)	3	*	*	*	6	*	*	*
Total support staff FTE/phy	14	3.75	4.38	5.96	31	3.45	4.36	5.12

Primary Care Single Specialty Practices by Ownership — Internal Medicine, Not Hospital or IDS Owned and All Owner Types (per Work RVU)

Table 10.9a: Staffing, Patients, Procedures and Square Footage

	Internal Medicine - Not Hospital Owned				Internal Medicine - All			
	Count	25th %tile	Median	75th %tile	Count	25th %tile	Median	75th %tile
Total prov FTE/10,000 work RVU	3	*	*	*	4	*	*	*
Tot phy FTE/10,000 work RVU	3	*	*	*	5	*	*	*
Prim care phy/10,000 work RVU	2	*	*	*	4	*	*	*
Nonsurg phy/10,000 work RVU	2	*	*	*	2	*	*	*
Surg spec phy/10,000 work RVU	0	*	*	*	0	*	*	*
Total NPP FTE/10,000 work RVU	3	*	*	*	4	*	*	*
Total supp stf FTE/10,000 wrk RVU	3	*	*	*	5	*	*	*
Tot empl supp stf/10,000 work RVU	3	*	*	*	5	*	*	*
General administrative	3	*	*	*	5	*	*	*
Patient accounting	3	*	*	*	3	*	*	*
General accounting	2	*	*	*	2	*	*	*
Managed care administrative	0	*	*	*	0	*	*	*
Information technology	2	*	*	*	2	*	*	*
Housekeeping, maint, security	0	*	*	*	0	*	*	*
Medical receptionists	3	*	*	*	5	*	*	*
Med secretaries,transcribers	2	*	*	*	4	*	*	*
Medical records	3	*	*	*	4	*	*	*
Other admin support	2	*	*	*	4	*	*	*
***Total administrative supp staff**	1	*	*	*	1	*	*	*
Registered Nurses	3	*	*	*	3	*	*	*
Licensed Practical Nurses	3	*	*	*	4	*	*	*
Med assistants, nurse aides	3	*	*	*	5	*	*	*
***Total clinical supp staff**	3	*	*	*	3	*	*	*
Clinical laboratory	3	*	*	*	3	*	*	*
Radiology and imaging	1	*	*	*	1	*	*	*
Other medical support serv	0	*	*	*	0	*	*	*
***Total ancillary supp staff**	0	*	*	*	0	*	*	*
Tot contracted supp staff	2	*	*	*	2	*	*	*
Tot RVU/work RVU	3	*	*	*	3	*	*	*
Patients/work RVU	2	*	*	*	2	*	*	*
Tot procedures/work RVU	3	*	*	*	5	*	*	*
Square feet/work RVU	3	*	*	*	5	*	*	*
Total support staff FTE/phy	14	3.75	4.38	5.96	31	3.45	4.36	5.12

*See pages 260 and 261 for definition.

Table 10.9b: Charges, Revenue and Cost

	Internal Medicine - Not Hospital Owned				Internal Medicine - All			
	Count	25th %tile	Median	75th %tile	Count	25th %tile	Median	75th %tile
Total gross charges	3	*	*	*	5	*	*	*
Total medical revenue	3	*	*	*	5	*	*	*
Net fee-for-service revenue	3	*	*	*	5	*	*	*
Net capitation revenue	0	*	*	*	0	*	*	*
Net other medical revenue	2	*	*	*	4	*	*	*
Total supp staff cost/work RVU	3	*	*	*	5	*	*	*
Total general operating cost	3	*	*	*	5	*	*	*
Total operating cost	3	*	*	*	5	*	*	*
Total med rev after oper cost	3	*	*	*	5	*	*	*
Total provider cost/work RVU	3	*	*	*	5	*	*	*
Total NPP cost/work RVU	3	*	*	*	4	*	*	*
Provider consultant cost	0	*	*	*	0	*	*	*
Total physician cost/work RVU	3	*	*	*	5	*	*	*
Total phy compensation	3	*	*	*	5	*	*	*
Total phy benefit cost	3	*	*	*	5	*	*	*
Total cost	3	*	*	*	5	*	*	*
Net nonmedical revenue	3	*	*	*	5	*	*	*
Net inc, prac with fin sup	0	*	*	*	2	*	*	*
Net inc, prac w/o fin sup	3	*	*	*	3	*	*	*
Net inc, excl fin supp (all prac)	3	*	*	*	5	*	*	*
Total support staff FTE/phy	14	3.75	4.38	5.96	31	3.45	4.36	5.12

Primary Care Single Specialty Practices by Ownership — Internal Medicine, Not Hospital or IDS Owned and All Owner Types (per Patient)

Table 10.10a: Staffing, RVUs, Procedures and Square Footage

	Internal Medicine - Not Hospital Owned				Internal Medicine - All			
	Count	25th %tile	Median	75th %tile	Count	25th %tile	Median	75th %tile
Total prov FTE/10,000 patients	2	*	*	*	4	*	*	*
Total phy FTE/10,000 pat	5	*	*	*	10	5.68	7.65	10.39
Prim care phy/10,000 pat	4	*	*	*	9	*	*	*
Nonsurg phy/10,000 pat	2	*	*	*	3	*	*	*
Surg spec phy/10,000 pat	0	*	*	*	0	*	*	*
Total NPP FTE/10,000 pat	2	*	*	*	4	*	*	*
Total supp staff FTE/10,000 pat	5	*	*	*	10	25.64	33.76	37.12
Total empl supp staff/10,000 pat	5	*	*	*	10	25.64	32.94	37.12
General administrative	4	*	*	*	9	*	*	*
Patient accounting	4	*	*	*	6	*	*	*
General accounting	1	*	*	*	1	*	*	*
Managed care administrative	0	*	*	*	0	*	*	*
Information technology	1	*	*	*	1	*	*	*
Housekeeping, maint, security	0	*	*	*	1	*	*	*
Medical receptionists	3	*	*	*	7	*	*	*
Med secretaries,transcribers	1	*	*	*	3	*	*	*
Medical records	3	*	*	*	7	*	*	*
Other admin support	1	*	*	*	2	*	*	*
***Total administrative supp staff**	2	*	*	*	4	*	*	*
Registered Nurses	3	*	*	*	8	*	*	*
Licensed Practical Nurses	3	*	*	*	8	*	*	*
Med assistants, nurse aides	4	*	*	*	9	*	*	*
***Total clinical supp staff**	3	*	*	*	8	*	*	*
Clinical laboratory	2	*	*	*	5	*	*	*
Radiology and imaging	0	*	*	*	4	*	*	*
Other medical support serv	0	*	*	*	0	*	*	*
***Total ancillary supp staff**	0	*	*	*	0	*	*	*
Tot contracted supp staff	2	*	*	*	5	*	*	*
Tot RVU/patient	2	*	*	*	2	*	*	*
Physician work RVU/patient	2	*	*	*	2	*	*	*
Tot procedures/patient	5	*	*	*	10	4.69	7.03	11.88
Square feet/patient	5	*	*	*	10	.97	1.26	1.58
Total support staff FTE/phy	14	3.75	4.38	5.96	31	3.45	4.36	5.12

*See pages 260 and 261 for definition.

Table 10.10b: Charges, Revenue and Cost

	Internal Medicine - Not Hospital Owned				Internal Medicine - All			
	Count	25th %tile	Median	75th %tile	Count	25th %tile	Median	75th %tile
Total gross charges	5	*	*	*	10	$411.13	$480.01	$649.17
Total medical revenue	5	*	*	*	10	$312.61	$338.13	$514.04
Net fee-for-service revenue	5	*	*	*	10	$287.74	$311.12	$443.22
Net capitation revenue	1	*	*	*	2	*	*	*
Net other medical revenue	3	*	*	*	6	*	*	*
Total support staff cost/patient	5	*	*	*	10	$99.37	$113.37	$131.69
Total general operating cost	5	*	*	*	10	$69.93	$92.48	$143.64
Total operating cost	5	*	*	*	10	$174.38	$200.65	$275.33
Total med rev after oper cost	5	*	*	*	10	$113.97	$137.32	$192.33
Total provider cost/patient	4	*	*	*	9	*	*	*
Total NPP cost/patient	2	*	*	*	4	*	*	*
Provider consultant cost	0	*	*	*	0	*	*	*
Total physician cost/patient	5	*	*	*	10	$116.69	$142.72	$200.32
Total phy compensation	4	*	*	*	9	*	*	*
Total phy benefit cost	4	*	*	*	9	*	*	*
Total cost	4	*	*	*	9	*	*	*
Net nonmedical revenue	3	*	*	*	5	*	*	*
Net inc, prac with fin sup	0	*	*	*	0	*	*	*
Net inc, prac w/o fin sup	4	*	*	*	6	*	*	*
Net inc, excl fin supp (all prac)	4	*	*	*	6	*	*	*
Total support staff FTE/phy	14	3.75	4.38	5.96	31	3.45	4.36	5.12

Primary Care Single Specialty Practices by Ownership — Internal Medicine, Not Hospital or IDS Owned and All Owner Types (Procedure and Charge Data)

Table 10.11a: Activity Charges to Total Gross Charges Ratios

	Internal Medicine - Not Hospital Owned				Internal Medicine - All			
	Count	25th %tile	Median	75th %tile	Count	25th %tile	Median	75th %tile
Total proc gross charges	13	90.95%	97.57%	100.00%	30	93.64%	97.75%	99.22%
Medical proc-inside practice	13	36.24%	53.36%	64.93%	30	41.88%	54.65%	76.13%
Medical proc-outside practice	12	9.50%	15.96%	20.07%	21	8.27%	16.92%	27.57%
Surg proc-inside practice	12	1.82%	2.36%	4.69%	27	1.28%	2.21%	4.33%
Surg proc-outside practice	7	*	*	*	9	*	*	*
Laboratory procedures	11	9.80%	14.58%	17.86%	27	3.48%	13.43%	17.97%
Radiology procedures	11	3.57%	5.12%	18.99%	22	2.79%	5.06%	7.83%
Tot nonproc gross charges	9	*	*	*	23	1.95%	2.45%	8.87%
Total support staff FTE/phy	14	3.75	4.38	5.96	31	3.45	4.36	5.12

Table 10.11b: Medical Procedure Data (inside the practice)

	Internal Medicine - Not Hospital Owned				Internal Medicine - All			
	Count	25th %tile	Median	75th %tile	Count	25th %tile	Median	75th %tile
Gross charges/procedure	13	$69.75	$80.34	$87.48	30	$65.52	$81.28	$96.85
Total cost/procedure	10	$42.93	$59.02	$83.84	27	$51.08	$62.22	$79.40
Operating cost/procedure	10	$26.29	$33.11	$54.51	19	$29.85	$39.14	$48.20
Provider cost/procedure	10	$15.35	$24.07	$31.54	27	$20.75	$27.93	$32.37
Procedures/patient	5	*	*	*	10	2.50	3.23	3.56
Gross charges/patient	5	*	*	*	10	$240.92	$279.60	$334.15
Procedures/physician	13	3,450	4,324	7,154	30	3,465	4,845	7,076
Gross charges/physician	13	$244,977	$366,941	$428,791	30	$332,692	$384,695	$471,539
Procedures/provider	7	*	*	*	17	3,611	4,905	6,055
Gross charges/provider	7	*	*	*	17	$279,202	$344,895	$417,596
Gross charge to total cost ratio	10	.98	1.30	1.56	27	1.05	1.26	1.45
Oper cost to total cost ratio	10	.54	.61	.69	19	.55	.59	.63
Prov cost to total cost ratio	10	.31	.39	.46	27	.39	.42	.46
Total support staff FTE/phy	14	3.75	4.38	5.96	31	3.45	4.36	5.12

Table 10.11c: Medical Procedure Data (outside the practice)

	Internal Medicine - Not Hospital Owned				Internal Medicine - All			
	Count	25th %tile	Median	75th %tile	Count	25th %tile	Median	75th %tile
Gross charges/procedure	12	$83.16	$116.50	$158.36	21	$80.82	$105.04	$129.50
Total cost/procedure	9	*	*	*	18	$38.30	$54.83	$74.22
Operating cost/procedure	9	*	*	*	13	$13.99	$23.98	$30.49
Provider cost/procedure	9	*	*	*	18	$23.01	$31.89	$50.97
Procedures/patient	5	*	*	*	7	*	*	*
Gross charges/patient	5	*	*	*	7	*	*	*
Procedures/physician	12	399	988	1,916	21	405	1,032	2,312
Gross charges/physician	12	$56,950	$99,519	$183,447	21	$58,909	$122,793	$240,885
Procedures/provider	7	*	*	*	12	478	906	1,860
Gross charges/provider	7	*	*	*	12	$61,839	$98,854	$181,515
Gross charge to total cost ratio	9	*	*	*	18	1.76	2.05	2.16
Oper cost to total cost ratio	9	*	*	*	13	.37	.40	.43
Prov cost to total cost ratio	9	*	*	*	18	.58	.61	.64
Total support staff FTE/phy	14	3.75	4.38	5.96	31	3.45	4.36	5.12

Primary Care Single Specialty Practices by Ownership — Internal Medicine, Not Hospital or IDS Owned and All Owner Types (Procedure and Charge Data)

Table 10.11d: Surgery/Anesthesia Procedure Data (inside the practice)

	Internal Medicine - Not Hospital Owned				Internal Medicine - All			
	Count	25th %tile	Median	75th %tile	Count	25th %tile	Median	75th %tile
Gross charges/procedure	12	$16.75	$94.98	$138.14	27	$16.70	$71.98	$125.71
Total cost/procedure	9	*	*	*	24	$12.36	$56.77	$104.36
Operating cost/procedure	9	*	*	*	17	$6.94	$26.66	$65.97
Provider cost/procedure	9	*	*	*	24	$4.96	$22.67	$47.68
Procedures/patient	5	*	*	*	9	*	*	*
Gross charges/patient	5	*	*	*	9	*	*	*
Procedures/physician	12	94	264	1,883	27	80	361	1,719
Gross charges/physician	12	$10,232	$17,894	$36,471	27	$9,105	$11,963	$32,218
Procedures/provider	7	*	*	*	16	90	699	1,665
Gross charges/provider	7	*	*	*	16	$8,915	$20,694	$31,647
Gross charge to total cost ratio	9	*	*	*	24	1.03	1.24	1.40
Oper cost to total cost ratio	9	*	*	*	17	.55	.59	.62
Prov cost to total cost ratio	9	*	*	*	24	.39	.43	.47
Total support staff FTE/phy	14	3.75	4.38	5.96	31	3.45	4.36	5.12

Table 10.11e: Surgery/Anesthesia Procedure Data (outside the practice)

	Internal Medicine - Not Hospital Owned				Internal Medicine - All			
	Count	25th %tile	Median	75th %tile	Count	25th %tile	Median	75th %tile
Gross charges/procedure	7	*	*	*	9	*	*	*
Total cost/procedure	5	*	*	*	7	*	*	*
Operating cost/procedure	5	*	*	*	6	*	*	*
Provider cost/procedure	5	*	*	*	7	*	*	*
Procedures/patient	2	*	*	*	4	*	*	*
Gross charges/patient	2	*	*	*	4	*	*	*
Procedures/physician	7	*	*	*	9	*	*	*
Gross charges/physician	7	*	*	*	9	*	*	*
Procedures/provider	5	*	*	*	5	*	*	*
Gross charges/provider	5	*	*	*	5	*	*	*
Gross charge to total cost ratio	5	*	*	*	7	*	*	*
Oper cost to total cost ratio	5	*	*	*	6	*	*	*
Prov cost to total cost ratio	5	*	*	*	7	*	*	*
Total support staff FTE/phy	14	3.75	4.38	5.96	31	3.45	4.36	5.12

Primary Care Single Specialty Practices by Ownership — Internal Medicine, Not Hospital or IDS Owned and All Owner Types (Procedure and Charge Data)

Table 10.11f: Clinical Laboratory/Pathology Procedure Data

	Internal Medicine - Not Hospital Owned				Internal Medicine - All			
	Count	25th %tile	Median	75th %tile	Count	25th %tile	Median	75th %tile
Gross charges/procedure	11	$19.85	$26.45	$34.42	27	$15.05	$23.90	$35.80
Total cost/procedure	9	*	*	*	25	$14.53	$22.30	$28.52
Operating cost/procedure	9	*	*	*	18	$10.30	$14.17	$18.00
Provider cost/procedure	9	*	*	*	25	$6.49	$8.44	$11.93
Procedures/patient	3	*	*	*	8	*	*	*
Gross charges/patient	3	*	*	*	8	*	*	*
Procedures/physician	11	2,326	3,995	5,968	27	1,711	4,261	6,599
Gross charges/physician	11	$74,385	$112,685	$185,059	27	$25,290	$97,171	$185,059
Procedures/provider	7	*	*	*	17	3,321	3,919	6,019
Gross charges/provider	7	*	*	*	17	$56,076	$95,847	$176,662
Gross charge to total cost ratio	9	*	*	*	25	1.09	1.23	1.36
Oper cost to total cost ratio	9	*	*	*	18	.61	.66	.69
Prov cost to total cost ratio	9	*	*	*	25	.32	.35	.46
Total support staff FTE/phy	14	3.75	4.38	5.96	31	3.45	4.36	5.12

Table 10.11g: Diagnostic Radiology and Imaging Procedure Data

	Internal Medicine - Not Hospital Owned				Internal Medicine - All			
	Count	25th %tile	Median	75th %tile	Count	25th %tile	Median	75th %tile
Gross charges/procedure	11	$96.12	$150.00	$157.20	22	$72.60	$139.59	$160.98
Total cost/procedure	8	*	*	*	19	$64.59	$108.74	$165.77
Operating cost/procedure	8	*	*	*	15	$40.92	$58.21	$77.87
Provider cost/procedure	8	*	*	*	19	$22.51	$38.63	$50.53
Procedures/patient	3	*	*	*	7	*	*	*
Gross charges/patient	3	*	*	*	7	*	*	*
Procedures/physician	11	96	517	1,397	22	138	356	747
Gross charges/physician	11	$14,851	$65,042	$197,483	22	$14,968	$41,853	$70,515
Procedures/provider	7	*	*	*	15	77	199	599
Gross charges/provider	7	*	*	*	15	$11,781	$29,319	$50,038
Gross charge to total cost ratio	8	*	*	*	19	1.12	1.22	1.42
Oper cost to total cost ratio	8	*	*	*	15	.60	.64	.68
Prov cost to total cost ratio	8	*	*	*	19	.34	.37	.46
Total support staff FTE/phy	14	3.75	4.38	5.96	31	3.45	4.36	5.12

Table 10.11h: Nonprocedural Gross Charge Data

	Internal Medicine - Not Hospital Owned				Internal Medicine - All			
	Count	25th %tile	Median	75th %tile	Count	25th %tile	Median	75th %tile
Gross charges/patient	3	*	*	*	8	*	*	*
Nonproc gross charges/physician	9	*	*	*	23	$14,840	$23,392	$74,751
Gross charges/provider	6	*	*	*	14	$11,929	$27,588	$99,880
Total support staff FTE/phy	14	3.75	4.38	5.96	31	3.45	4.36	5.12

Primary Care Single Specialty Practices by Ownership — Pediatrics, Not Hospital or IDS Owned and All Owner Types

Table 11.1: Staffing and Practice Data

	Pediatrics - Not Hospital Owned				Pediatrics - All			
	Count	25th %tile	Median	75th %tile	Count	25th %tile	Median	75th %tile
Total provider FTE	**53**	**6.75**	**9.00**	**15.15**	**62**	**6.65**	**9.00**	**14.20**
Total physician FTE	71	4.96	6.70	9.80	89	4.25	6.00	9.40
Total nonphysician provider FTE	53	1.00	2.00	3.38	62	1.00	2.00	3.23
Total support staff FTE	**71**	**18.50**	**25.90**	**47.00**	**89**	**17.25**	**25.60**	**46.20**
Number of branch clinics	1	*	*	*	5	*	*	*
Square footage of all facilities	70	6,000	10,065	16,179	87	6,000	10,500	16,893

Table 11.2: Accounts Receivable Data, Collection Percentages and Financial Ratios

	Pediatrics - Not Hospital Owned				Pediatrics - All			
	Count	25th %tile	Median	75th %tile	Count	25th %tile	Median	75th %tile
Total AR/physician	**59**	**$58,773**	**$73,110**	**$109,000**	**77**	**$62,494**	**$81,059**	**$113,047**
Total AR/provider	**44**	**$48,709**	**$61,480**	**$83,851**	**53**	**$52,117**	**$64,024**	**$89,793**
0-30 days in AR	59	49.53%	60.86%	66.53%	77	49.54%	62.05%	65.64%
31-60 days in AR	59	11.10%	15.34%	18.65%	77	11.74%	15.55%	18.60%
61-90 days in AR	59	5.00%	6.24%	8.51%	77	5.22%	6.81%	8.91%
91-120 days in AR	59	3.28%	4.13%	5.56%	77	3.51%	4.37%	5.99%
120+ days in AR	59	6.43%	11.66%	20.68%	77	6.48%	12.12%	20.28%
Re-aged: 0-30 days in AR	23	47.06%	63.42%	69.32%	27	49.24%	63.41%	66.53%
Re-aged: 31-60 days in AR	23	9.91%	14.73%	16.57%	27	10.50%	14.12%	16.41%
Re-aged: 61-90 days in AR	23	5.27%	6.05%	8.16%	27	5.09%	6.04%	7.73%
Re-aged: 91-120 days in AR	23	3.14%	3.84%	4.89%	27	3.28%	3.99%	4.61%
Re-aged: 120+ days in AR	23	4.69%	11.81%	30.89%	27	6.60%	12.22%	26.77%
Not re-aged: 0-30 days in AR	36	49.65%	57.76%	65.31%	50	49.55%	56.87%	65.27%
Not re-aged: 31-60 days in AR	36	12.24%	16.77%	19.45%	50	13.59%	16.77%	19.60%
Not re-aged: 61-90 days in AR	36	4.98%	6.50%	8.73%	50	5.34%	7.58%	9.02%
Not re-aged: 91-120 days in AR	36	3.39%	4.36%	6.23%	50	3.80%	4.96%	6.41%
Not re-aged: 120+ days in AR	36	6.46%	11.60%	19.64%	50	6.09%	12.02%	20.08%
Months gross FFS charges in AR	6	*	*	*	21	1.27	1.59	2.18
Days gross FFS charges in AR	6	*	*	*	21	38.58	48.42	66.42
Gross FFS collection %	6	*	*	*	21	67.91%	72.37%	75.50%
Adjusted FFS collection %	6	*	*	*	21	97.00%	97.08%	98.30%
Gross FFS + cap collection %	3	*	*	*	6	*	*	*
Net cap rev % of gross cap chrg	2	*	*	*	5	*	*	*
Current ratio	2	*	*	*	4	*	*	*
Tot asset turnover ratio	2	*	*	*	4	*	*	*
Debt to equity ratio	2	*	*	*	4	*	*	*
Debt ratio	2	*	*	*	4	*	*	*
Return on total assets	3	*	*	*	5	*	*	*
Return on equity	3	*	*	*	5	*	*	*

Table 11.3: Breakout of Total Gross Charges by Type of Payer

	Pediatrics - Not Hospital Owned				Pediatrics - All			
	Count	25th %tile	Median	75th %tile	Count	25th %tile	Median	75th %tile
Medicare: fee-for-service	67	.00%	.00%	.00%	84	.00%	.00%	.00%
Medicare: managed care FFS	67	.00%	.00%	.00%	84	.00%	.00%	.00%
Medicare: capitation	67	.00%	.00%	.00%	84	.00%	.00%	.00%
Medicaid: fee-for-service	67	.00%	2.00%	5.20%	84	.00%	2.50%	9.21%
Medicaid: managed care FFS	67	.00%	2.10%	10.00%	84	.00%	.25%	10.00%
Medicaid: capitation	67	.00%	.00%	.00%	84	.00%	.00%	.00%
Commercial: fee-for-service	67	5.00%	20.00%	51.50%	84	1.86%	25.05%	59.00%
Commercial: managed care FFS	67	15.00%	42.00%	70.00%	84	5.00%	39.13%	70.00%
Commercial: capitation	67	.00%	.00%	6.00%	84	.00%	.00%	5.00%
Workers' compensation	67	.00%	.00%	.00%	84	.00%	.00%	.00%
Charity care and prof courtesy	67	.00%	.20%	1.00%	84	.00%	.00%	1.45%
Self-pay	67	1.20%	4.00%	8.00%	84	1.05%	3.95%	6.93%
Other federal government payers	67	.00%	.00%	1.00%	84	.00%	.00%	.45%

Primary Care Single Specialty Practices by Ownership — Pediatrics, Not Hospital or IDS Owned and All Owner Types (per FTE Physician)

Table 11.4a: Staffing, RVUs, Patients, Procedures and Square Footage

	Pediatrics - Not Hospital Owned				Pediatrics - All			
	Count	25th %tile	Median	75th %tile	Count	25th %tile	Median	75th %tile
Total provider FTE/physician	53	**1.13**	**1.32**	**1.50**	62	**1.14**	**1.33**	**1.50**
Prim care phy/physician	3	*	*	*	15	1.00	1.00	1.00
Nonsurg phy/physician	0	*	*	*	4	*	*	*
Surg spec phy/physician	0	*	*	*	0	*	*	*
Total NPP FTE/physician	53	.13	.32	.50	62	.14	.33	.50
Total support staff FTE/phy	71	**3.25**	**4.00**	**4.99**	89	**3.28**	**3.89**	**4.81**
Total empl support staff FTE	6	*	*	*	22	3.52	3.70	4.75
General administrative	7	*	*	*	21	.18	.33	.33
Patient accounting	7	*	*	*	8	*	*	*
General accounting	2	*	*	*	2	*	*	*
Managed care administrative	1	*	*	*	1	*	*	*
Information technology	1	*	*	*	1	*	*	*
Housekeeping, maint, security	0	*	*	*	0	*	*	*
Medical receptionists	6	*	*	*	16	1.01	1.33	1.50
Med secretaries,transcribers	0	*	*	*	4	*	*	*
Medical records	3	*	*	*	3	*	*	*
Other admin support	2	*	*	*	5	*	*	*
*Total administrative supp staff	68	**1.67**	**2.11**	**2.67**	71	**1.67**	**2.11**	**2.61**
Registered Nurses	4	*	*	*	18	.64	.83	1.16
Licensed Practical Nurses	5	*	*	*	16	.17	.40	.69
Med assistants, nurse aides	6	*	*	*	19	.36	.83	1.01
*Total clinical supp staff	68	**1.34**	**1.71**	**2.22**	79	**1.36**	**1.71**	**2.25**
Clinical laboratory	2	*	*	*	8	*	*	*
Radiology and imaging	0	*	*	*	0	*	*	*
Other medical support serv	0	*	*	*	4	*	*	*
*Total ancillary supp staff	18	**.30**	**.37**	**.58**	19	**.32**	**.38**	**.52**
Tot contracted supp staff	9	*	*	*	12	.05	.11	.44
Tot RVU/physician	20	8,253	10,644	13,147	21	8,457	11,355	13,066
Physician work RVU/physician	17	4,777	5,823	10,102	19	5,011	5,823	10,271
Patients/physician	1	*	*	*	8	*	*	*
Tot procedures/physician	7	*	*	*	22	9,840	12,567	17,670
Square feet/physician	70	1,134	1,519	1,858	87	1,154	1,519	1,857

*See pages 260 and 261 for definition.

Table 11.4b: Charges and Revenue

	Pediatrics - Not Hospital Owned				Pediatrics - All			
	Count	25th %tile	Median	75th %tile	Count	25th %tile	Median	75th %tile
Net fee-for-service revenue	7	*	*	*	22	$477,971	$526,904	$628,913
Gross FFS charges	6	*	*	*	21	$649,785	$723,922	$852,170
Adjustments to FFS charges	6	*	*	*	21	$153,711	$182,642	$245,386
Adjusted FFS charges	6	*	*	*	21	$495,507	$530,528	$624,519
Bad debts due to FFS activity	5	*	*	*	20	$5,229	$15,468	$19,461
Net capitation revenue	3	*	*	*	6	*	*	*
Gross capitation charges	2	*	*	*	5	*	*	*
Capitation revenue	3	*	*	*	6	*	*	*
Purch serv for cap patients	0	*	*	*	0	*	*	*
Net other medical revenue	1	*	*	*	11	$18,132	$20,559	$28,637
Gross rev from other activity	1	*	*	*	11	$18,132	$20,559	$28,637
Other medical revenue	1	*	*	*	11	$18,132	$20,559	$28,637
Rev from sale of goods/services	0	*	*	*	0	*	*	*
Cost of sales	0	*	*	*	0	*	*	*
Total gross charges	70	**$615,672**	**$735,785**	**$904,723**	88	**$621,541**	**$731,393**	**$903,010**
Total medical revenue	71	**$454,556**	**$525,058**	**$632,850**	88	**$456,349**	**$525,668**	**$636,007**

Primary Care Single Specialty Practices by Ownership — Pediatrics, Not Hospital or IDS Owned and All Owner Types (per FTE Physician)

Table 11.4c: Operating Cost

	Pediatrics - Not Hospital Owned				Pediatrics - All			
	Count	25th %tile	Median	75th %tile	Count	25th %tile	Median	75th %tile
Total support staff cost/phy	71	$107,716	$147,972	$174,165	89	$114,735	$147,972	$175,155
Total empl supp staff cost/phy	7	*	*	*	23	$103,350	$125,180	$144,228
General administrative	7	*	*	*	21	$10,575	$16,264	$20,367
Patient accounting	6	*	*	*	7	*	*	*
General accounting	1	*	*	*	1	*	*	*
Managed care administrative	1	*	*	*	1	*	*	*
Information technology	1	*	*	*	1	*	*	*
Housekeeping, maint, security	0	*	*	*	0	*	*	*
Medical receptionists	6	*	*	*	16	$24,288	$30,557	$39,422
Med secretaries,transcribers	0	*	*	*	4	*	*	*
Medical records	3	*	*	*	3	*	*	*
Other admin support	2	*	*	*	5	*	*	*
*Total administrative supp staff	68	$46,766	$62,756	$77,541	72	$47,143	$62,125	$77,235
Registered Nurses	4	*	*	*	18	$26,389	$33,294	$50,311
Licensed Practical Nurses	6	*	*	*	17	$5,235	$12,690	$24,306
Med assistants, nurse aides	6	*	*	*	19	$9,515	$20,791	$27,600
*Total clinical supp staff	68	$43,431	$54,216	$64,881	80	$44,383	$54,846	$66,102
Clinical laboratory	2	*	*	*	8	*	*	*
Radiology and imaging	0	*	*	*	0	*	*	*
Other medical support serv	0	*	*	*	4	*	*	*
*Total ancillary supp staff	18	$7,186	$12,623	$19,209	19	$7,955	$12,715	$18,906
Total empl supp staff benefits	61	$16,594	$24,371	$35,168	79	$19,699	$25,691	$34,007
Tot contracted supp staff	10	$1,904	$5,003	$11,503	23	$970	$2,850	$9,750
Total general operating cost	71	$146,470	$180,121	$225,615	89	$141,662	$175,482	$217,297
Information technology	7	*	*	*	23	$3,493	$5,783	$6,624
Medical and surgical supply	7	*	*	*	23	$31,745	$52,572	$63,029
Building and occupancy	7	*	*	*	23	$31,473	$34,542	$39,000
Furniture and equipment	4	*	*	*	19	$1,879	$3,202	$7,333
Admin supplies and services	6	*	*	*	22	$3,713	$5,889	$11,265
Prof liability insurance	71	$6,645	$9,518	$12,515	89	$4,232	$7,874	$11,777
Other insurance premiums	7	*	*	*	10	$1,087	$1,366	$2,192
Outside professional fees	7	*	*	*	18	$93	$565	$2,838
Promotion and marketing	5	*	*	*	13	$505	$1,199	$2,428
Clinical laboratory	4	*	*	*	15	$2,995	$5,500	$6,556
Radiology and imaging	1	*	*	*	2	*	*	*
Other ancillary services	1	*	*	*	4	*	*	*
Billing purchased services	5	*	*	*	19	$5,000	$30,770	$41,487
Management fees paid to MSO	3	*	*	*	12	$11,591	$23,900	$28,334
Misc operating cost	6	*	*	*	22	$3,381	$9,882	$20,042
Cost allocated to prac from par	0	*	*	*	6	*	*	*
Total operating cost	71	$264,044	$325,867	$376,235	89	$266,958	$308,854	$374,064

*See pages 260 and 261 for definition.

Primary Care Single Specialty Practices by Ownership — Pediatrics, Not Hospital or IDS Owned and All Owner Types (per FTE Physician)

Table 11.4d: Provider Cost

	Pediatrics - Not Hospital Owned				Pediatrics - All			
	Count	25th %tile	Median	75th %tile	Count	25th %tile	Median	75th %tile
Total med rev after oper cost	71	$174,077	$218,851	$285,462	89	$171,326	$219,567	$286,513
Total provider cost/physician	70	$160,962	$203,927	$248,434	88	$167,838	$213,934	$266,944
Total NPP cost/physician	53	$9,778	$23,111	$35,718	63	$9,885	$24,269	$37,066
Nonphysician provider comp	3	*	*	*	12	$8,446	$25,788	$52,524
Nonphysician prov benefit cost	3	*	*	*	12	$1,813	$4,067	$5,867
Provider consultant cost	3	*	*	*	3	*	*	*
Total physician cost/physician	71	$149,000	$185,831	$233,317	89	$157,158	$197,107	$235,962
Total phy compensation	3	*	*	*	19	$170,000	$201,536	$216,616
Total phy benefit cost	3	*	*	*	19	$15,125	$23,861	$36,852

Table 11.4e: Net Income or Loss

	Pediatrics - Not Hospital Owned				Pediatrics - All			
	Count	25th %tile	Median	75th %tile	Count	25th %tile	Median	75th %tile
Total cost	70	$433,013	$518,987	$619,955	88	$446,638	$523,024	$632,001
Net nonmedical revenue	33	$378	$1,757	$6,045	39	$398	$1,938	$8,595
Nonmedical revenue	1	*	*	*	3	*	*	*
Fin support for oper costs	0	*	*	*	3	*	*	*
Goodwill amortization	0	*	*	*	0	*	*	*
Nonmedical cost	1	*	*	*	2	*	*	*
Net inc, prac with fin sup	0	*	*	*	3	*	*	*
Net inc, prac w/o fin sup	67	$96	$5,091	$13,293	78	$70	$5,283	$16,715
Net inc, excl fin supp (all prac)	67	$96	$5,091	$13,293	81	$0	$5,091	$15,303

Table 11.4f: Assets and Liabilities

	Pediatrics - Not Hospital Owned				Pediatrics - All			
	Count	25th %tile	Median	75th %tile	Count	25th %tile	Median	75th %tile
Total assets	2	*	*	*	5	*	*	*
Current assets	2	*	*	*	5	*	*	*
Noncurrent assets	2	*	*	*	5	*	*	*
Total liabilities	2	*	*	*	5	*	*	*
Current liabilities	2	*	*	*	5	*	*	*
Noncurrent liabilities	2	*	*	*	5	*	*	*
Working capital	2	*	*	*	5	*	*	*
Total net worth	2	*	*	*	5	*	*	*

Primary Care Single Specialty Practices by Ownership — Pediatrics, Not Hospital or IDS Owned and All Owner Types (as a % of Total Medical Revenue)

Table 11.5a: Charges and Revenue

	Pediatrics - Not Hospital Owned				Pediatrics - All			
	Count	25th %tile	Median	75th %tile	Count	25th %tile	Median	75th %tile
Net fee-for-service revenue	7	*	*	*	22	94.35%	96.12%	100.00%
Net capitation revenue	3	*	*	*	6	*	*	*
Net other medical revenue	1	*	*	*	11	2.98%	3.93%	4.35%
Total gross charges	**71**	**129.20%**	**139.64%**	**155.82%**	**89**	**127.88%**	**138.37%**	**152.35%**

Table 11.5b: Operating Cost

	Pediatrics - Not Hospital Owned				Pediatrics - All			
	Count	25th %tile	Median	75th %tile	Count	25th %tile	Median	75th %tile
Total support staff cost	**71**	**22.77%**	**26.51%**	**31.12%**	**89**	**23.49%**	**27.08%**	**31.23%**
Total empl support staff cost	7	*	*	*	23	20.77%	22.58%	24.71%
General administrative	7	*	*	*	21	1.52%	3.18%	3.54%
Patient accounting	6	*	*	*	7	*	*	*
General accounting	1	*	*	*	1	*	*	*
Managed care administrative	1	*	*	*	1	*	*	*
Information technology	1	*	*	*	1	*	*	*
Housekeeping, maint, security	0	*	*	*	0	*	*	*
Medical receptionists	6	*	*	*	16	4.39%	6.09%	6.98%
Med secretaries,transcribers	0	*	*	*	4	*	*	*
Medical records	3	*	*	*	3	*	*	*
Other admin support	2	*	*	*	5	*	*	*
*Total administrative supp staff	68	9.21%	11.70%	14.40%	72	9.21%	11.70%	14.25%
Registered Nurses	4	*	*	*	18	5.03%	6.19%	8.15%
Licensed Practical Nurses	6	*	*	*	17	.90%	2.40%	3.64%
Med assistants, nurse aides	6	*	*	*	19	1.86%	4.06%	4.58%
*Total clinical supp staff	68	8.19%	10.58%	12.50%	80	8.29%	10.66%	12.50%
Clinical laboratory	2	*	*	*	8	*	*	*
Radiology and imaging	0	*	*	*	0	*	*	*
Other medical support serv	0	*	*	*	4	*	*	*
*Total ancillary supp staff	18	1.49%	2.07%	3.20%	19	1.62%	2.10%	3.16%
Total empl supp staff benefits	61	3.32%	4.30%	6.70%	79	3.40%	4.68%	6.15%
Tot contracted supp staff	10	.33%	1.19%	2.69%	23	.19%	.50%	2.17%
Total general operating cost	**71**	**27.80%**	**33.72%**	**38.95%**	**89**	**27.73%**	**31.35%**	**38.44%**
Information technology	7	*	*	*	23	.65%	.82%	1.35%
Medical and surgical supply	7	*	*	*	23	6.01%	10.88%	12.67%
Building and occupancy	7	*	*	*	23	4.31%	6.32%	7.52%
Furniture and equipment	4	*	*	*	19	.36%	.58%	1.19%
Admin supplies and services	6	*	*	*	22	.68%	1.01%	1.86%
Prof liability insurance	71	1.26%	1.71%	2.25%	89	.92%	1.57%	1.98%
Other insurance premiums	7	*	*	*	10	.16%	.23%	.41%
Outside professional fees	7	*	*	*	18	.02%	.13%	.53%
Promotion and marketing	5	*	*	*	13	.06%	.30%	.51%
Clinical laboratory	4	*	*	*	15	.57%	.99%	1.16%
Radiology and imaging	1	*	*	*	2	*	*	*
Other ancillary services	1	*	*	*	4	*	*	*
Billing purchased services	5	*	*	*	19	.95%	5.92%	5.98%
Management fees paid to MSO	3	*	*	*	12	2.10%	4.20%	4.46%
Misc operating cost	6	*	*	*	22	.51%	1.51%	2.84%
Cost allocated to prac from par	0	*	*	*	6	*	*	*
Total operating cost	**71**	**53.21%**	**60.82%**	**66.28%**	**89**	**53.16%**	**60.04%**	**65.39%**

*See pages 260 and 261 for definition.

Primary Care Single Specialty Practices by Ownership — Pediatrics, Not Hospital or IDS Owned and All Owner Types (as a % of Total Medical Revenue)

Table 11.5c: Provider Cost

	Pediatrics - Not Hospital Owned				Pediatrics - All			
	Count	25th %tile	Median	75th %tile	Count	25th %tile	Median	75th %tile
Total med rev after oper cost	71	33.72%	39.37%	46.89%	89	34.61%	40.35%	47.00%
Total provider cost	70	33.42%	38.57%	43.61%	88	34.08%	39.99%	45.82%
Total NPP cost	53	1.83%	3.97%	6.00%	63	1.85%	4.14%	6.23%
Nonphysician provider comp	3	*	*	*	12	1.68%	4.54%	7.33%
Nonphysician prov benefit cost	3	*	*	*	12	.31%	.66%	1.02%
Provider consultant cost	3	*	*	*	3	*	*	*
Total physician cost	71	30.03%	34.94%	40.12%	89	30.96%	35.66%	42.58%
Total phy compensation	3	*	*	*	19	29.69%	35.51%	40.38%
Total phy benefit cost	3	*	*	*	19	2.51%	5.43%	6.52%

Table 11.5d: Net Income or Loss

	Pediatrics - Not Hospital Owned				Pediatrics - All			
	Count	25th %tile	Median	75th %tile	Count	25th %tile	Median	75th %tile
Total cost	70	97.71%	99.49%	100.22%	88	97.65%	99.59%	100.47%
Net nonmedical revenue	33	.07%	.23%	1.11%	39	.08%	.34%	1.68%
Nonmedical revenue	1	*	*	*	3	*	*	*
Fin support for oper costs	0	*	*	*	3	*	*	*
Goodwill amortization	0	*	*	*	0	*	*	*
Nonmedical cost	1	*	*	*	2	*	*	*
Net inc, prac with fin sup	0	*	*	*	3	*	*	*
Net inc, prac w/o fin sup	67	.02%	.91%	2.54%	78	.01%	.93%	2.74%
Net inc, excl fin supp (all prac)	67	.02%	.91%	2.54%	81	.00%	.91%	2.64%

Table 11.5e: Assets and Liabilities

	Pediatrics - Not Hospital Owned				Pediatrics - All			
	Count	25th %tile	Median	75th %tile	Count	25th %tile	Median	75th %tile
Total assets	2	*	*	*	5	*	*	*
Current assets	2	*	*	*	5	*	*	*
Noncurrent assets	2	*	*	*	5	*	*	*
Total liabilities	2	*	*	*	5	*	*	*
Current liabilities	2	*	*	*	5	*	*	*
Noncurrent liabilities	2	*	*	*	5	*	*	*
Working capital	2	*	*	*	5	*	*	*
Total net worth	2	*	*	*	5	*	*	*

Primary Care Single Specialty Practices by Ownership — Pediatrics, Not Hospital or IDS Owned and All Owner Types (per FTE Provider)

Table 11.6a: Staffing, RVUs, Patients, Procedures and Square Footage

	Pediatrics - Not Hospital Owned				Pediatrics - All			
	Count	25th %tile	Median	75th %tile	Count	25th %tile	Median	75th %tile
Total physician FTE/provider	53	.67	.76	.89	62	.67	.75	.88
Prim care phy/provider	2	*	*	*	6	*	*	*
Nonsurg phy/provider	0	*	*	*	4	*	*	*
Surg spec phy/provider	0	*	*	*	0	*	*	*
Total NPP FTE/provider	53	.11	.24	.33	62	.12	.25	.33
Total support staff FTE/prov	53	2.94	3.40	4.15	62	2.87	3.33	4.03
Total empl supp staff FTE/prov	3	*	*	*	11	2.72	3.01	3.54
General administrative	3	*	*	*	10	.10	.19	.25
Patient accounting	3	*	*	*	3	*	*	*
General accounting	1	*	*	*	1	*	*	*
Managed care administrative	0	*	*	*	0	*	*	*
Information technology	1	*	*	*	1	*	*	*
Housekeeping, maint, security	0	*	*	*	0	*	*	*
Medical receptionists	2	*	*	*	7	*	*	*
Med secretaries,transcribers	0	*	*	*	1	*	*	*
Medical records	1	*	*	*	1	*	*	*
Other admin support	2	*	*	*	3	*	*	*
***Total administrative supp staff**	51	1.40	1.87	2.20	52	1.40	1.86	2.20
Registered Nurses	2	*	*	*	10	.49	.66	.97
Licensed Practical Nurses	3	*	*	*	10	.16	.37	.48
Med assistants, nurse aides	3	*	*	*	9	*	*	*
***Total clinical supp staff**	52	1.18	1.41	1.80	58	1.19	1.43	1.81
Clinical laboratory	2	*	*	*	5	*	*	*
Radiology and imaging	0	*	*	*	0	*	*	*
Other medical support serv	0	*	*	*	3	*	*	*
***Total ancillary supp staff**	15	.21	.29	.34	15	.21	.29	.34
Tot contracted supp staff	6	*	*	*	7	*	*	*
Tot RVU/provider	15	6,440	8,630	9,292	16	6,723	8,784	9,287
Physician work RVU/provider	13	3,614	4,908	8,028	15	3,686	4,908	8,120
Patients/provider	0	*	*	*	3	*	*	*
Tot procedures/provider	3	*	*	*	11	8,076	10,029	12,543
Square feet/provider	52	1,034	1,226	1,500	61	1,042	1,226	1,507
Total support staff FTE/phy	71	3.25	4.00	4.99	89	3.28	3.89	4.81

*See pages 260 and 261 for definition.

Table 11.6b: Charges, Revenue and Cost

	Pediatrics - Not Hospital Owned				Pediatrics - All			
	Count	25th %tile	Median	75th %tile	Count	25th %tile	Median	75th %tile
Total gross charges	53	$508,454	$588,980	$739,003	62	$511,662	$586,801	$736,126
Total medical revenue	53	$374,545	$434,129	$488,385	62	$374,647	$428,833	$485,562
Net fee-for-service revenue	3	*	*	*	11	$346,596	$385,124	$460,634
Net capitation revenue	1	*	*	*	2	*	*	*
Net other medical revenue	1	*	*	*	8	*	*	*
Total support staff cost/prov	53	$104,323	$115,544	$139,835	62	$105,026	$115,104	$137,312
Total general operating cost	53	$121,467	$148,936	$173,214	62	$112,848	$139,238	$169,687
Total operating cost	53	$234,448	$268,739	$296,052	62	$224,829	$261,679	$295,190
Total med rev after oper cost	53	$142,112	$179,858	$204,920	62	$140,647	$180,086	$207,698
Total provider cost/provider	53	$138,355	$175,404	$199,988	62	$139,676	$175,945	$203,390
Total NPP cost/provider	53	$8,818	$19,259	$24,719	62	$8,937	$19,762	$25,135
Provider consultant cost	3	*	*	*	3	*	*	*
Total physician cost/provider	53	$116,839	$153,242	$181,144	62	$117,336	$157,044	$189,428
Total phy compensation	2	*	*	*	10	$108,904	$139,505	$184,262
Total phy benefit cost	2	*	*	*	10	$9,247	$14,974	$29,581
Total cost	53	$386,124	$431,301	$480,481	62	$377,246	$431,647	$480,268
Net nonmedical revenue	28	$411	$1,363	$4,786	30	$509	$1,569	$5,703
Net inc, prac with fin sup	0	*	*	*	1	*	*	*
Net inc, prac w/o fin sup	50	$63	$3,620	$11,138	56	$29	$3,739	$12,059
Net inc, excl fin supp (all prac)	50	$63	$3,620	$11,138	57	$6	$3,697	$11,929
Total support staff FTE/phy	71	3.25	4.00	4.99	89	3.28	3.89	4.81

Primary Care Single Specialty Practices by Ownership — Pediatrics, Not Hospital or IDS Owned and All Owner Types (per Square Foot)

Table 11.7a: Staffing, RVUs, Patients and Procedures

	Pediatrics - Not Hospital Owned				Pediatrics - All			
	Count	25th %tile	Median	75th %tile	Count	25th %tile	Median	75th %tile
Total prov FTE/10,000 sq ft	52	6.66	8.16	9.67	61	6.64	8.16	9.60
Total phy FTE/10,000 sq ft	70	5.38	6.58	8.82	87	5.38	6.58	8.67
Prim care phy/10,000 sq ft	3	*	*	*	14	5.54	6.70	7.57
Nonsurg phy/10,000 sq ft	0	*	*	*	4	*	*	*
Surg spec phy/10,000 sq ft	0	*	*	*	0	*	*	*
Total NPP FTE/10,000 sq ft	52	.87	1.72	2.69	61	.89	1.89	2.67
Total supp stf FTE/10,000 sq ft	70	21.91	27.39	31.71	87	21.66	27.14	30.75
Total empl supp stf/10,000 sq ft	6	*	*	*	21	19.97	23.50	29.39
General administrative	7	*	*	*	21	1.07	1.78	2.36
Patient accounting	7	*	*	*	8	*	*	*
General accounting	2	*	*	*	2	*	*	*
Managed care administrative	1	*	*	*	1	*	*	*
Information technology	1	*	*	*	1	*	*	*
Housekeeping, maint, security	0	*	*	*	0	*	*	*
Medical receptionists	6	*	*	*	16	6.38	7.50	14.18
Med secretaries,transcribers	0	*	*	*	4	*	*	*
Medical records	3	*	*	*	3	*	*	*
Other admin support	2	*	*	*	5	*	*	*
*Total administrative supp staff	67	11.40	14.18	18.18	70	11.39	14.17	17.99
Registered Nurses	4	*	*	*	18	4.17	5.78	6.24
Licensed Practical Nurses	5	*	*	*	16	1.10	2.27	4.08
Med assistants, nurse aides	6	*	*	*	19	3.07	4.62	5.83
*Total clinical supp staff	67	9.09	11.19	14.29	78	9.07	11.18	14.27
Clinical laboratory	2	*	*	*	8	*	*	*
Radiology and imaging	0	*	*	*	0	*	*	*
Other medical support serv	0	*	*	*	4	*	*	*
*Total ancillary supp staff	18	1.89	2.70	4.30	19	1.96	2.78	3.38
Tot contracted supp staff	9	*	*	*	12	.28	1.13	2.56
Tot RVU/sq ft	19	5.32	7.26	9.68	20	5.33	7.51	10.16
Physician work RVU/sq ft	16	3.31	4.45	5.27	18	3.25	4.45	5.49
Patients/sq ft	1	*	*	*	9	*	*	*
Tot procedures/sq ft	7	*	*	*	22	5.84	8.09	10.06
Total support staff FTE/phy	71	3.25	4.00	4.99	89	3.28	3.89	4.81

*See pages 260 and 261 for definition.

Table 11.7b: Charges, Revenue and Cost

	Pediatrics - Not Hospital Owned				Pediatrics - All			
	Count	25th %tile	Median	75th %tile	Count	25th %tile	Median	75th %tile
Total gross charges	70	$411.27	$485.80	$683.10	87	$397.37	$476.04	$627.58
Total medical revenue	70	$291.96	$347.75	$443.08	87	$291.08	$342.37	$434.24
Net fee-for-service revenue	7	*	*	*	22	$263.81	$300.90	$415.49
Net capitation revenue	3	*	*	*	6	*	*	*
Net other medical revenue	1	*	*	*	11	$7.91	$10.59	$15.44
Total support staff cost/sq ft	70	$74.38	$93.87	$125.52	87	$75.85	$93.69	$114.66
Total general operating cost	70	$84.22	$116.31	$153.61	87	$83.57	$112.77	$143.07
Total operating cost	70	$178.05	$204.57	$266.01	87	$172.83	$199.70	$256.67
Total med rev after oper cost	70	$105.70	$149.80	$203.27	87	$105.85	$147.74	$194.96
Total provider cost/sq ft	69	$102.64	$146.21	$172.16	86	$104.57	$144.04	$176.56
Total NPP cost/sq ft	52	$6.86	$13.53	$20.64	62	$7.01	$14.86	$20.86
Provider consultant cost	3	*	*	*	3	*	*	*
Total physician cost/sq ft	70	$91.78	$130.26	$162.15	87	$96.15	$129.65	$162.31
Total phy compensation	3	*	*	*	18	$90.86	$106.12	$168.96
Total phy benefit cost	3	*	*	*	18	$6.95	$18.77	$25.28
Total cost	69	$286.02	$333.62	$434.07	86	$288.86	$330.10	$432.65
Net nonmedical revenue/sq ft	33	$.28	$.79	$3.84	39	$.34	$1.25	$4.86
Net inc, prac with fin sup	0	*	*	*	3	*	*	*
Net inc, prac w/o fin sup	66	$.11	$3.09	$8.53	76	$.06	$3.14	$10.71
Net inc, excl fin supp (all prac)	66	$.11	$3.09	$8.53	79	$.00	$3.09	$10.04
Total support staff FTE/phy	71	3.25	4.00	4.99	89	3.28	3.89	4.81

Primary Care Single Specialty Practices by Ownership — Pediatrics, Not Hospital or IDS Owned and All Owner Types (per Total RVU)

Table 11.8a: Staffing, Patients, Procedures and Square Footage

	Pediatrics - Not Hospital Owned				Pediatrics - All			
	Count	25th %tile	Median	75th %tile	Count	25th %tile	Median	75th %tile
Total prov FTE/10,000 tot RVU	15	1.08	1.16	1.55	16	1.08	1.14	1.49
Total phy FTE/10,000 tot RVU	20	.76	.94	1.21	21	.77	.88	1.19
Prim care phy/10,000 tot RVU	1	*	*	*	1	*	*	*
Nonsurg phy/10,000 tot RVU	0	*	*	*	1	*	*	*
Surg spec phy/10,000 tot RVU	0	*	*	*	0	*	*	*
Total NPP FTE/10,000 tot RVU	15	.24	.31	.46	16	.23	.31	.44
Total supp stf FTE/10,000 tot RVU	20	3.13	4.18	4.94	21	3.06	4.08	4.91
Tot empl supp stf/10,000 tot RVU	1	*	*	*	2	*	*	*
General administrative	2	*	*	*	3	*	*	*
Patient accounting	2	*	*	*	2	*	*	*
General accounting	0	*	*	*	0	*	*	*
Managed care administrative	0	*	*	*	0	*	*	*
Information technology	0	*	*	*	0	*	*	*
Housekeeping, maint, security	0	*	*	*	0	*	*	*
Medical receptionists	2	*	*	*	3	*	*	*
Med secretaries,transcribers	0	*	*	*	0	*	*	*
Medical records	0	*	*	*	0	*	*	*
Other admin support	1	*	*	*	1	*	*	*
*Total administrative supp staff	19	1.49	2.01	2.66	19	1.49	2.01	2.66
Registered Nurses	1	*	*	*	2	*	*	*
Licensed Practical Nurses	1	*	*	*	2	*	*	*
Med assistants, nurse aides	1	*	*	*	2	*	*	*
*Total clinical supp staff	19	1.40	1.84	2.32	20	1.43	1.80	2.29
Clinical laboratory	0	*	*	*	0	*	*	*
Radiology and imaging	0	*	*	*	0	*	*	*
Other medical support serv	0	*	*	*	0	*	*	*
*Total ancillary supp staff	3	*	*	*	3	*	*	*
Tot contracted supp staff	2	*	*	*	2	*	*	*
Physician work RVU/tot RVU	15	.48	.54	.94	16	.48	.54	.93
Patients/tot RVU	0	*	*	*	0	*	*	*
Tot procedures/tot RVU	2	*	*	*	3	*	*	*
Square feet/tot RVU	19	.10	.14	.19	20	.10	.13	.19
Total support staff FTE/phy	71	3.25	4.00	4.99	89	3.28	3.89	4.81

*See pages 260 and 261 for definition.

Table 11.8b: Charges, Revenue and Cost

	Pediatrics - Not Hospital Owned				Pediatrics - All			
	Count	25th %tile	Median	75th %tile	Count	25th %tile	Median	75th %tile
Total gross charges	20	$57.42	$67.11	$85.72	21	$57.74	$67.40	$84.14
Total medical revenue	20	$39.81	$47.36	$64.16	21	$38.87	$45.12	$64.11
Net fee-for-service revenue	2	*	*	*	3	*	*	*
Net capitation revenue	2	*	*	*	2	*	*	*
Net other medical revenue	1	*	*	*	1	*	*	*
Total supp staff cost/tot RVU	20	$11.37	$13.46	$17.03	21	$11.46	$13.34	$17.02
Total general operating cost	20	$14.14	$17.67	$19.76	21	$13.07	$17.18	$19.71
Total operating cost	20	$24.55	$30.00	$38.30	21	$23.95	$29.43	$38.26
Total med rev after oper cost	20	$14.57	$22.28	$25.72	21	$13.91	$22.12	$25.60
Total provider cost/tot RVU	20	$14.28	$16.46	$24.83	21	$14.45	$17.35	$24.57
Total NPP cost/tot RVU	15	$1.26	$2.31	$4.32	16	$1.39	$2.29	$4.00
Provider consultant cost	0	*	*	*	0	*	*	*
Total physician cost/tot RVU	20	$12.32	$15.34	$21.27	21	$12.32	$15.57	$21.37
Total phy compensation	1	*	*	*	2	*	*	*
Total phy benefit cost	1	*	*	*	2	*	*	*
Total cost	1	*	*	*	2	*	*	*
Net nonmedical revenue	12	$.01	$.12	$.73	12	$.01	$.12	$.73
Net inc, prac with fin sup	0	*	*	*	0	*	*	*
Net inc, prac w/o fin sup	18	$.00	$.58	$1.45	19	$.00	$.56	$1.15
Net inc, excl fin supp (all prac)	18	$.00	$.58	$1.45	19	$.00	$.56	$1.15
Total support staff FTE/phy	71	3.25	4.00	4.99	89	3.28	3.89	4.81

Primary Care Single Specialty Practices by Ownership — Pediatrics, Not Hospital or IDS Owned and All Owner Types (per Work RVU)

Table 11.9a: Staffing, Patients, Procedures and Square Footage

	Pediatrics - Not Hospital Owned				Pediatrics - All			
	Count	25th %tile	Median	75th %tile	Count	25th %tile	Median	75th %tile
Total prov FTE/10,000 work RVU	13	1.25	2.04	2.77	15	1.23	2.04	2.71
Tot phy FTE/10,000 work RVU	17	.99	1.72	2.10	19	.97	1.72	2.00
Prim care phy/10,000 work RVU	1	*	*	*	2	*	*	*
Nonsurg phy/10,000 work RVU	0	*	*	*	1	*	*	*
Surg spec phy/10,000 work RVU	0	*	*	*	0	*	*	*
Total NPP FTE/10,000 work RVU	13	.36	.53	.79	15	.35	.53	.84
Total supp stf FTE/10,000 wrk RVU	17	4.60	7.99	9.16	19	4.28	7.99	9.23
Tot empl supp stf/10,000 work RVU	1	*	*	*	3	*	*	*
General administrative	2	*	*	*	4	*	*	*
Patient accounting	2	*	*	*	2	*	*	*
General accounting	0	*	*	*	0	*	*	*
Managed care administrative	0	*	*	*	0	*	*	*
Information technology	0	*	*	*	0	*	*	*
Housekeeping, maint, security	0	*	*	*	0	*	*	*
Medical receptionists	2	*	*	*	4	*	*	*
Med secretaries,transcribers	0	*	*	*	0	*	*	*
Medical records	0	*	*	*	0	*	*	*
Other admin support	1	*	*	*	2	*	*	*
***Total administrative supp staff**	16	2.18	3.70	4.75	16	2.18	3.70	4.75
Registered Nurses	1	*	*	*	3	*	*	*
Licensed Practical Nurses	1	*	*	*	3	*	*	*
Med assistants, nurse aides	1	*	*	*	3	*	*	*
***Total clinical supp staff**	17	2.05	3.06	4.21	19	1.85	3.06	4.50
Clinical laboratory	0	*	*	*	0	*	*	*
Radiology and imaging	0	*	*	*	0	*	*	*
Other medical support serv	0	*	*	*	0	*	*	*
***Total ancillary supp staff**	2	*	*	*	2	*	*	*
Tot contracted supp staff	3	*	*	*	3	*	*	*
Tot RVU/work RVU	15	1.06	1.85	2.07	16	1.07	1.84	2.07
Patients/work RVU	0	*	*	*	0	*	*	*
Tot procedures/work RVU	2	*	*	*	4	*	*	*
Square feet/work RVU	16	.19	.22	.30	18	.18	.22	.31
Total support staff FTE/phy	71	3.25	4.00	4.99	89	3.28	3.89	4.81

*See pages 260 and 261 for definition.

Table 11.9b: Charges, Revenue and Cost

	Pediatrics - Not Hospital Owned				Pediatrics - All			
	Count	25th %tile	Median	75th %tile	Count	25th %tile	Median	75th %tile
Total gross charges	17	$76.34	$119.00	$151.85	19	$73.96	$119.00	$147.27
Total medical revenue	17	$53.45	$77.97	$105.74	19	$50.62	$77.97	$102.81
Net fee-for-service revenue	2	*	*	*	4	*	*	*
Net capitation revenue	2	*	*	*	3	*	*	*
Net other medical revenue	1	*	*	*	2	*	*	*
Total supp staff cost/work RVU	17	$14.30	$25.90	$30.23	19	$13.48	$25.90	$31.14
Total general operating cost	17	$19.80	$29.89	$38.74	19	$19.63	$29.89	$38.21
Total operating cost	17	$33.00	$51.82	$73.02	19	$30.79	$51.82	$70.41
Total med rev after oper cost	17	$19.36	$28.74	$48.67	19	$15.40	$28.74	$47.28
Total provider cost/work RVU	17	$19.00	$28.35	$47.35	19	$23.02	$28.35	$48.07
Total NPP cost/work RVU	13	$2.27	$4.32	$7.04	15	$1.94	$4.32	$6.20
Provider consultant cost	0	*	*	*	0	*	*	*
Total physician cost/work RVU	17	$16.74	$26.30	$43.02	19	$20.37	$26.30	$42.76
Total phy compensation	1	*	*	*	3	*	*	*
Total phy benefit cost	1	*	*	*	3	*	*	*
Total cost	17	$50.41	$83.38	$116.34	19	$50.81	$83.38	$115.99
Net nonmedical revenue	11	$.03	$.31	$1.36	12	$.04	$.43	$1.49
Net inc, prac with fin sup	0	*	*	*	1	*	*	*
Net inc, prac w/o fin sup	16	-$.18	$.71	$2.06	17	-$1.52	$.70	$1.79
Net inc, excl fin supp (all prac)	16	-$.18	$.71	$2.06	18	-$3.22	$.65	$1.52
Total support staff FTE/phy	71	3.25	4.00	4.99	89	3.28	3.89	4.81

Primary Care Single Specialty Practices by Ownership — Pediatrics, Not Hospital or IDS Owned and All Owner Types (per Patient)

Table 11.10a: Staffing, RVUs, Procedures and Square Footage

	Pediatrics - Not Hospital Owned				Pediatrics - All			
	Count	25th %tile	Median	75th %tile	Count	25th %tile	Median	75th %tile
Total prov FTE/10,000 patients	0	*	*	*	3	*	*	*
Total phy FTE/10,000 pat	1	*	*	*	9	*	*	*
Prim care phy/10,000 pat	1	*	*	*	9	*	*	*
Nonsurg phy/10,000 pat	0	*	*	*	0	*	*	*
Surg spec phy/10,000 pat	0	*	*	*	0	*	*	*
Total NPP FTE/10,000 pat	0	*	*	*	3	*	*	*
Total supp staff FTE/10,000 pat	1	*	*	*	9	*	*	*
Total empl supp staff/10,000 pat	1	*	*	*	9	*	*	*
General administrative	1	*	*	*	9	*	*	*
Patient accounting	1	*	*	*	2	*	*	*
General accounting	0	*	*	*	0	*	*	*
Managed care administrative	0	*	*	*	0	*	*	*
Information technology	0	*	*	*	0	*	*	*
Housekeeping, maint, security	0	*	*	*	0	*	*	*
Medical receptionists	1	*	*	*	8	*	*	*
Med secretaries,transcribers	0	*	*	*	3	*	*	*
Medical records	0	*	*	*	0	*	*	*
Other admin support	0	*	*	*	2	*	*	*
***Total administrative supp staff**	0	*	*	*	1	*	*	*
Registered Nurses	0	*	*	*	7	*	*	*
Licensed Practical Nurses	0	*	*	*	6	*	*	*
Med assistants, nurse aides	1	*	*	*	8	*	*	*
***Total clinical supp staff**	0	*	*	*	5	*	*	*
Clinical laboratory	0	*	*	*	3	*	*	*
Radiology and imaging	0	*	*	*	0	*	*	*
Other medical support serv	0	*	*	*	1	*	*	*
***Total ancillary supp staff**	0	*	*	*	0	*	*	*
Tot contracted supp staff	0	*	*	*	3	*	*	*
Tot RVU/patient	0	*	*	*	0	*	*	*
Physician work RVU/patient	0	*	*	*	0	*	*	*
Tot procedures/patient	1	*	*	*	9	*	*	*
Square feet/patient	1	*	*	*	9	*	*	*
Total support staff FTE/phy	71	3.25	4.00	4.99	89	3.28	3.89	4.81

*See pages 260 and 261 for definition.

Table 11.10b: Charges, Revenue and Cost

	Pediatrics - Not Hospital Owned				Pediatrics - All			
	Count	25th %tile	Median	75th %tile	Count	25th %tile	Median	75th %tile
Total gross charges	1	*	*	*	9	*	*	*
Total medical revenue	1	*	*	*	9	*	*	*
Net fee-for-service revenue	1	*	*	*	9	*	*	*
Net capitation revenue	0	*	*	*	1	*	*	*
Net other medical revenue	0	*	*	*	5	*	*	*
Total support staff cost/patient	1	*	*	*	9	*	*	*
Total general operating cost	1	*	*	*	9	*	*	*
Total operating cost	1	*	*	*	9	*	*	*
Total med rev after oper cost	1	*	*	*	9	*	*	*
Total provider cost/patient	1	*	*	*	9	*	*	*
Total NPP cost/patient	0	*	*	*	4	*	*	*
Provider consultant cost	0	*	*	*	0	*	*	*
Total physician cost/patient	1	*	*	*	9	*	*	*
Total phy compensation	1	*	*	*	9	*	*	*
Total phy benefit cost	1	*	*	*	9	*	*	*
Total cost	1	*	*	*	9	*	*	*
Net nonmedical revenue	0	*	*	*	2	*	*	*
Net inc, prac with fin sup	0	*	*	*	0	*	*	*
Net inc, prac w/o fin sup	1	*	*	*	5	*	*	*
Net inc, excl fin supp (all prac)	1	*	*	*	5	*	*	*
Total support staff FTE/phy	71	3.25	4.00	4.99	89	3.28	3.89	4.81

Primary Care Single Specialty Practices by Ownership — Pediatrics, Not Hospital or IDS Owned and All Owner Types (Procedure and Charge Data)

Table 11.11a: Activity Charges to Total Gross Charges Ratios

	Pediatrics - Not Hospital Owned				Pediatrics - All			
	Count	25th %tile	Median	75th %tile	Count	25th %tile	Median	75th %tile
Total proc gross charges	7	*	*	*	22	90.53%	99.30%	100.00%
Medical proc-inside practice	6	*	*	*	21	83.67%	87.17%	92.61%
Medical proc-outside practice	6	*	*	*	11	2.18%	3.55%	6.02%
Surg proc-inside practice	3	*	*	*	17	1.18%	1.97%	2.97%
Surg proc-outside practice	3	*	*	*	4	*	*	*
Laboratory procedures	7	*	*	*	21	1.91%	3.74%	5.83%
Radiology procedures	1	*	*	*	4	*	*	*
Tot nonproc gross charges	2	*	*	*	15	.22%	1.28%	11.58%
Total support staff FTE/phy	71	3.25	4.00	4.99	89	3.28	3.89	4.81

Table 11.11b: Medical Procedure Data (inside the practice)

	Pediatrics - Not Hospital Owned				Pediatrics - All			
	Count	25th %tile	Median	75th %tile	Count	25th %tile	Median	75th %tile
Gross charges/procedure	6	*	*	*	21	$57.15	$62.74	$90.19
Total cost/procedure	5	*	*	*	20	$39.88	$47.68	$73.50
Operating cost/procedure	5	*	*	*	15	$24.51	$29.01	$45.70
Provider cost/procedure	5	*	*	*	20	$16.41	$20.71	$35.37
Procedures/patient	1	*	*	*	9	*	*	*
Gross charges/patient	1	*	*	*	9	*	*	*
Procedures/physician	6	*	*	*	21	7,631	10,604	14,306
Gross charges/physician	6	*	*	*	21	$560,882	$686,175	$800,829
Procedures/provider	3	*	*	*	11	5,842	8,234	9,712
Gross charges/provider	3	*	*	*	11	$439,180	$495,505	$571,157
Gross charge to total cost ratio	5	*	*	*	20	1.15	1.29	1.40
Oper cost to total cost ratio	5	*	*	*	15	.54	.58	.61
Prov cost to total cost ratio	5	*	*	*	20	.39	.43	.47
Total support staff FTE/phy	71	3.25	4.00	4.99	89	3.28	3.89	4.81

Table 11.11c: Medical Procedure Data (outside the practice)

	Pediatrics - Not Hospital Owned				Pediatrics - All			
	Count	25th %tile	Median	75th %tile	Count	25th %tile	Median	75th %tile
Gross charges/procedure	6	*	*	*	11	$105.24	$122.62	$134.02
Total cost/procedure	5	*	*	*	10	$45.28	$55.25	$71.93
Operating cost/procedure	5	*	*	*	8	*	*	*
Provider cost/procedure	5	*	*	*	10	$29.65	$33.90	$48.10
Procedures/patient	1	*	*	*	4	*	*	*
Gross charges/patient	1	*	*	*	4	*	*	*
Procedures/physician	6	*	*	*	11	147	208	410
Gross charges/physician	6	*	*	*	11	$18,080	$24,974	$44,430
Procedures/provider	3	*	*	*	4	*	*	*
Gross charges/provider	3	*	*	*	4	*	*	*
Gross charge to total cost ratio	5	*	*	*	10	1.92	2.27	2.52
Oper cost to total cost ratio	5	*	*	*	8	*	*	*
Prov cost to total cost ratio	5	*	*	*	10	.58	.62	.73
Total support staff FTE/phy	71	3.25	4.00	4.99	89	3.28	3.89	4.81

Primary Care Single Specialty Practices by Ownership — Pediatrics, Not Hospital or IDS Owned and All Owner Types (Procedure and Charge Data)

Table 11.11d: Surgery/Anesthesia Procedure Data (inside the practice)

	Pediatrics - Not Hospital Owned				Pediatrics - All			
	Count	25th %tile	Median	75th %tile	Count	25th %tile	Median	75th %tile
Gross charges/procedure	3	*	*	*	17	$42.17	$97.08	$117.55
Total cost/procedure	2	*	*	*	16	$31.79	$70.64	$104.98
Operating cost/procedure	2	*	*	*	12	$15.21	$28.76	$55.04
Provider cost/procedure	2	*	*	*	16	$12.73	$31.05	$45.76
Procedures/patient	1	*	*	*	8	*	*	*
Gross charges/patient	1	*	*	*	8	*	*	*
Procedures/physician	3	*	*	*	17	100	217	462
Gross charges/physician	3	*	*	*	17	$8,039	$13,163	$25,592
Procedures/provider	1	*	*	*	9	*	*	*
Gross charges/provider	1	*	*	*	9	*	*	*
Gross charge to total cost ratio	2	*	*	*	16	1.14	1.19	1.37
Oper cost to total cost ratio	2	*	*	*	12	.53	.56	.60
Prov cost to total cost ratio	2	*	*	*	16	.41	.44	.48
Total support staff FTE/phy	71	3.25	4.00	4.99	89	3.28	3.89	4.81

Table 11.11e: Surgery/Anesthesia Procedure Data (outside the practice)

	Pediatrics - Not Hospital Owned				Pediatrics - All			
	Count	25th %tile	Median	75th %tile	Count	25th %tile	Median	75th %tile
Gross charges/procedure	3	*	*	*	4	*	*	*
Total cost/procedure	3	*	*	*	4	*	*	*
Operating cost/procedure	3	*	*	*	4	*	*	*
Provider cost/procedure	3	*	*	*	4	*	*	*
Procedures/patient	1	*	*	*	1	*	*	*
Gross charges/patient	1	*	*	*	1	*	*	*
Procedures/physician	3	*	*	*	4	*	*	*
Gross charges/physician	3	*	*	*	4	*	*	*
Procedures/provider	2	*	*	*	2	*	*	*
Gross charges/provider	2	*	*	*	2	*	*	*
Gross charge to total cost ratio	3	*	*	*	4	*	*	*
Oper cost to total cost ratio	3	*	*	*	4	*	*	*
Prov cost to total cost ratio	3	*	*	*	4	*	*	*
Total support staff FTE/phy	71	3.25	4.00	4.99	89	3.28	3.89	4.81

Primary Care Single Specialty Practices by Ownership — Pediatrics, Not Hospital or IDS Owned and All Owner Types (Procedure and Charge Data)

Table 11.11f: Clinical Laboratory/Pathology Procedure Data

	Pediatrics - Not Hospital Owned				Pediatrics - All			
	Count	25th %tile	Median	75th %tile	Count	25th %tile	Median	75th %tile
Gross charges/procedure	7	*	*	*	21	$8.11	$18.52	$25.10
Total cost/procedure	5	*	*	*	19	$6.78	$11.20	$19.40
Operating cost/procedure	5	*	*	*	15	$4.95	$9.09	$11.73
Provider cost/procedure	5	*	*	*	19	$2.17	$4.99	$8.28
Procedures/patient	1	*	*	*	8	*	*	*
Gross charges/patient	1	*	*	*	8	*	*	*
Procedures/physician	7	*	*	*	21	988	2,292	3,189
Gross charges/physician	7	*	*	*	21	$16,086	$24,136	$51,137
Procedures/provider	3	*	*	*	11	938	1,821	2,655
Gross charges/provider	3	*	*	*	11	$9,574	$27,696	$56,704
Gross charge to total cost ratio	5	*	*	*	19	1.17	1.53	1.60
Oper cost to total cost ratio	5	*	*	*	15	.50	.61	.70
Prov cost to total cost ratio	5	*	*	*	19	.32	.40	.50
Total support staff FTE/phy	71	3.25	4.00	4.99	89	3.28	3.89	4.81

Table 11.11g: Diagnostic Radiology and Imaging Procedure Data

	Pediatrics - Not Hospital Owned				Pediatrics - All			
	Count	25th %tile	Median	75th %tile	Count	25th %tile	Median	75th %tile
Gross charges/procedure	1	*	*	*	4	*	*	*
Total cost/procedure	1	*	*	*	4	*	*	*
Operating cost/procedure	1	*	*	*	3	*	*	*
Provider cost/procedure	1	*	*	*	4	*	*	*
Procedures/patient	1	*	*	*	3	*	*	*
Gross charges/patient	1	*	*	*	3	*	*	*
Procedures/physician	1	*	*	*	4	*	*	*
Gross charges/physician	1	*	*	*	4	*	*	*
Procedures/provider	0	*	*	*	1	*	*	*
Gross charges/provider	0	*	*	*	1	*	*	*
Gross charge to total cost ratio	1	*	*	*	4	*	*	*
Oper cost to total cost ratio	1	*	*	*	3	*	*	*
Prov cost to total cost ratio	1	*	*	*	4	*	*	*
Total support staff FTE/phy	71	3.25	4.00	4.99	89	3.28	3.89	4.81

Table 11.11h: Nonprocedural Gross Charge Data

	Pediatrics - Not Hospital Owned				Pediatrics - All			
	Count	25th %tile	Median	75th %tile	Count	25th %tile	Median	75th %tile
Gross charges/patient	0	*	*	*	7	*	*	*
Nonproc gross charges/physician	2	*	*	*	15	$2,127	$12,142	$84,079
Gross charges/provider	1	*	*	*	8	*	*	*
Total support staff FTE/phy	71	3.25	4.00	4.99	89	3.28	3.89	4.81

THIS PAGE INTENTIONALLY LEFT BLANK

Single Specialty Practices — Not Hospital or IDS Owned

Single Specialty Practices, Not Hospital or IDS Owned — Allergy/Immunology, Anesthesiology, Anesthesiology: Pain Management, Cardiology

Table 12.1: Staffing and Practice Data

	Allergy/Immunology		Anesthesiology		Anesthesiology: Pain Management		Cardiology	
	Count	Median	Count	Median	Count	Median	Count	Median
Total provider FTE	**5**	*****	**40**	**33.25**	**25**	**39.00**	**58**	**15.50**
Total physician FTE	11	4.00	58	17.45	32	20.13	85	11.50
Total nonphysician provider FTE	5	*	40	14.30	25	13.75	58	3.50
Total support staff FTE	**11**	**23.00**	**58**	**6.00**	**32**	**13.10**	**85**	**59.35**
Number of branch clinics	8	*	1	*	0	*	73	3
Square footage of all facilities	10	14,124	36	2,436	22	3,400	80	22,000

Table 12.2: Accounts Receivable Data, Collection Percentages and Financial Ratios

	Allergy/Immunology		Anesthesiology		Anesthesiology: Pain Management		Cardiology	
	Count	Median	Count	Median	Count	Median	Count	Median
Total AR/physician	**9**	*****	**54**	**$153,429**	**28**	**$188,318**	**79**	**$264,338**
Total AR/provider	**5**	*****	**37**	**$79,269**	**23**	**$85,510**	**54**	**$215,121**
0-30 days in AR	9	*	54	52.88%	29	44.18%	79	57.44%
31-60 days in AR	9	*	54	16.92%	29	17.17%	79	13.81%
61-90 days in AR	9	*	54	8.13%	29	9.22%	79	7.23%
91-120 days in AR	9	*	54	5.47%	29	5.86%	79	5.03%
120+ days in AR	9	*	54	11.27%	29	17.04%	79	15.71%
Re-aged: 0-30 days in AR	2	*	12	64.90%	8	*	28	49.95%
Re-aged: 31-60 days in AR	2	*	12	16.34%	8	*	28	15.33%
Re-aged: 61-90 days in AR	2	*	12	7.22%	8	*	28	6.82%
Re-aged: 91-120 days in AR	2	*	12	4.43%	8	*	28	5.07%
Re-aged: 120+ days in AR	2	*	12	7.56%	8	*	28	17.13%
Not re-aged: 0-30 days in AR	7	*	40	49.99%	21	44.18%	47	58.06%
Not re-aged: 31-60 days in AR	7	*	40	17.76%	21	17.17%	47	13.41%
Not re-aged: 61-90 days in AR	7	*	40	8.43%	21	9.22%	47	7.48%
Not re-aged: 91-120 days in AR	7	*	40	5.79%	21	6.05%	47	5.03%
Not re-aged: 120+ days in AR	7	*	40	14.39%	21	16.81%	47	16.26%
Months gross FFS charges in AR	9	*	5	*	1	*	76	1.52
Days gross FFS charges in AR	9	*	5	*	1	*	76	46.12
Gross FFS collection %	10	72.72%	5	*	1	*	82	44.60%
Adjusted FFS collection %	9	*	5	*	1	*	74	96.61%
Gross FFS + cap collection %	3	*	0	*	0	*	13	40.22%
Net cap rev % of gross cap chrg	3	*	0	*	0	*	11	39.63%
Current ratio	3	*	0	*	0	*	37	1.25
Tot asset turnover ratio	3	*	0	*	0	*	38	9.03
Debt to equity ratio	3	*	0	*	0	*	38	2.46
Debt ratio	3	*	0	*	0	*	38	71.07%
Return on total assets	3	*	6	*	4	*	38	9.02%
Return on equity	3	*	6	*	4	*	38	26.16%

Table 12.3: Breakout of Total Gross Charges by Type of Payer

	Allergy/Immunology		Anesthesiology		Anesthesiology: Pain Management		Cardiology	
	Count	Median	Count	Median	Count	Median	Count	Median
Medicare: fee-for-service	11	5.00%	58	26.52%	31	28.70%	79	45.00%
Medicare: managed care FFS	11	.00%	58	.00%	31	.00%	79	.00%
Medicare: capitation	11	.00%	58	.00%	31	.00%	79	.00%
Medicaid: fee-for-service	11	1.00%	58	8.10%	31	5.30%	79	2.50%
Medicaid: managed care FFS	11	.00%	58	.00%	31	.00%	79	.00%
Medicaid: capitation	11	.00%	58	.00%	31	.00%	79	.00%
Commercial: fee-for-service	11	14.50%	58	13.95%	31	13.28%	79	26.50%
Commercial: managed care FFS	11	70.50%	58	31.20%	31	35.30%	79	15.00%
Commercial: capitation	11	.00%	58	.00%	31	.00%	79	.00%
Workers' compensation	11	.00%	58	2.69%	31	3.00%	79	.00%
Charity care and prof courtesy	11	.02%	58	.00%	31	.00%	79	.02%
Self-pay	11	2.00%	58	3.00%	31	3.50%	79	3.00%
Other federal government payers	11	.04%	58	.15%	31	.20%	79	.00%

Single Specialty Practices, Not Hospital or IDS Owned — Allergy/Immunology, Anesthesiology, Anesthesiology: Pain Management, Cardiology (per FTE Physician)

Table 12.4a: Staffing, RVUs, Patients, Procedures and Square Footage

	Allergy/Immunology		Anesthesiology		Anesthesiology: Pain Management		Cardiology	
	Count	Median	Count	Median	Count	Median	Count	Median
Total provider FTE/physician	5	*	40	2.14	25	1.88	58	1.25
Prim care phy/physician	2	*	0	*	0	*	5	*
Nonsurg phy/physician	7	*	0	*	0	*	75	1.00
Surg spec phy/physician	0	*	3	*	0	*	12	.18
Total NPP FTE/physician	5	*	40	1.14	25	.88	58	.25
Total support staff FTE/phy	11	6.03	58	.45	32	.57	85	5.18
Total empl support staff FTE	10	6.84	3	*	1	*	83	5.01
General administrative	9	*	3	*	1	*	84	.28
Patient accounting	9	*	2	*	0	*	84	.76
General accounting	6	*	1	*	1	*	64	.10
Managed care administrative	2	*	0	*	0	*	21	.13
Information technology	2	*	0	*	0	*	41	.10
Housekeeping, maint, security	1	*	0	*	0	*	11	.06
Medical receptionists	9	*	0	*	0	*	83	.78
Med secretaries,transcribers	5	*	0	*	0	*	75	.31
Medical records	4	*	0	*	0	*	82	.42
Other admin support	6	*	0	*	1	*	35	.13
*Total administrative supp staff	4	*	49	.40	30	.52	43	2.98
Registered Nurses	8	*	2	*	0	*	77	.62
Licensed Practical Nurses	5	*	0	*	0	*	49	.16
Med assistants, nurse aides	6	*	0	*	0	*	81	.64
*Total clinical supp staff	6	*	17	.15	16	.14	64	1.40
Clinical laboratory	3	*	0	*	0	*	25	.18
Radiology and imaging	0	*	0	*	0	*	80	.53
Other medical support serv	4	*	0	*	0	*	50	.27
*Total ancillary supp staff	2	*	3	*	5	*	34	.81
Tot contracted supp staff	4	*	5	*	7	*	45	.11
Tot RVU/physician	5	*	45	12,703	24	13,880	37	19,947
Physician work RVU/physician	2	*	0	*	0	*	48	9,572
Patients/physician	4	*	3	*	0	*	48	1,532
Tot procedures/physician	6	*	4	*	1	*	76	10,664
Square feet/physician	10	3,327	36	121	22	150	80	1,860

*See pages 260 and 261 for definition.

Table 12.4b: Charges and Revenue

	Allergy/Immunology		Anesthesiology		Anesthesiology: Pain Management		Cardiology	
	Count	Median	Count	Median	Count	Median	Count	Median
Net fee-for-service revenue	10	$846,170	5	*	1	*	83	$963,821
Gross FFS charges	10	$1,104,520	5	*	1	*	82	$2,223,936
Adjustments to FFS charges	9	*	5	*	1	*	71	$1,157,065
Adjusted FFS charges	9	*	5	*	1	*	74	$1,015,064
Bad debts due to FFS activity	8	*	5	*	1	*	67	$33,706
Net capitation revenue	3	*	0	*	0	*	13	$59,213
Gross capitation charges	3	*	0	*	0	*	11	$215,843
Capitation revenue	3	*	0	*	0	*	11	$65,719
Purch serv for cap patients	0	*	0	*	0	*	0	*
Net other medical revenue	7	*	2	*	0	*	67	$20,409
Gross rev from other activity	6	*	2	*	0	*	64	$20,861
Other medical revenue	7	*	2	*	0	*	65	$11,189
Rev from sale of goods/services	1	*	0	*	0	*	18	$20,867
Cost of sales	1	*	0	*	0	*	2	*
Total gross charges	11	$1,156,693	56	$1,052,258	32	$1,262,964	84	$2,234,709
Total medical revenue	11	$922,286	58	$517,000	32	$616,709	85	$998,524

Single Specialty Practices, Not Hospital or IDS Owned — Allergy/Immunology, Anesthesiology, Anesthesiology: Pain Management, Cardiology (per FTE Physician)

Table 12.4c: Operating Cost

	Allergy/Immunology		Anesthesiology		Anesthesiology: Pain Management		Cardiology	
	Count	Median	Count	Median	Count	Median	Count	Median
Total support staff cost/phy	11	$271,716	58	$25,726	32	$33,688	85	$242,154
Total empl supp staff cost/phy	10	$226,963	3	*	1	*	82	$188,457
General administrative	9	*	3	*	1	*	81	$21,637
Patient accounting	9	*	2	*	0	*	81	$23,565
General accounting	6	*	1	*	1	*	62	$3,918
Managed care administrative	2	*	0	*	0	*	20	$3,886
Information technology	2	*	0	*	0	*	38	$4,746
Housekeeping, maint, security	1	*	0	*	0	*	13	$1,524
Medical receptionists	9	*	0	*	0	*	80	$20,066
Med secretaries,transcribers	6	*	0	*	0	*	72	$9,254
Medical records	4	*	0	*	0	*	79	$8,954
Other admin support	5	*	0	*	1	*	34	$4,541
***Total administrative supp staff**	4	*	48	$20,455	30	$24,952	40	$105,287
Registered Nurses	8	*	2	*	0	*	74	$28,726
Licensed Practical Nurses	5	*	0	*	0	*	46	$5,567
Med assistants, nurse aides	6	*	0	*	0	*	78	$16,509
***Total clinical supp staff**	6	*	17	$7,494	16	$6,754	60	$51,832
Clinical laboratory	3	*	0	*	0	*	24	$5,564
Radiology and imaging	0	*	0	*	0	*	77	$25,788
Other medical support serv	4	*	0	*	0	*	47	$9,794
***Total ancillary supp staff**	1	*	3	*	5	*	41	$36,877
Total empl supp staff benefits	9	*	33	$9,431	26	$9,559	81	$47,615
Tot contracted supp staff	5	*	4	*	8	*	54	$4,981
Total general operating cost	11	$242,752	58	$36,111	32	$43,915	85	$239,026
Information technology	9	*	2	*	1	*	84	$15,454
Medical and surgical supply	9	*	1	*	0	*	84	$14,415
Building and occupancy	9	*	3	*	1	*	85	$45,784
Furniture and equipment	8	*	2	*	1	*	76	$12,276
Admin supplies and services	9	*	3	*	1	*	85	$15,181
Prof liability insurance	10	$6,614	58	$16,073	31	$15,182	85	$14,825
Other insurance premiums	9	*	5	*	1	*	82	$1,885
Outside professional fees	9	*	5	*	1	*	85	$6,989
Promotion and marketing	9	*	2	*	1	*	85	$3,250
Clinical laboratory	3	*	0	*	0	*	31	$3,871
Radiology and imaging	1	*	0	*	0	*	73	$50,329
Other ancillary services	2	*	0	*	0	*	42	$6,905
Billing purchased services	6	*	4	*	1	*	39	$1,645
Management fees paid to MSO	0	*	1	*	0	*	5	*
Misc operating cost	9	*	5	*	1	*	81	$14,569
Cost allocated to prac from par	0	*	0	*	0	*	0	*
Total operating cost	11	$487,843	58	$66,866	32	$73,631	85	$484,754

*See pages 260 and 261 for definition.

Single Specialty Practices, Not Hospital or IDS Owned — Allergy/Immunology, Anesthesiology, Anesthesiology: Pain Management, Cardiology (per FTE Physician)

Table 12.4d: Provider Cost

	Allergy/Immunology		Anesthesiology		Anesthesiology: Pain Management		Cardiology	
	Count	Median	Count	Median	Count	Median	Count	Median
Total med rev after oper cost	11	$434,443	58	$447,913	32	$539,789	85	$492,434
Total provider cost/physician	11	$375,278	57	$462,721	32	$502,019	85	$485,857
Total NPP cost/physician	6	*	40	$150,374	25	$131,020	61	$22,672
Nonphysician provider comp	6	*	4	*	0	*	62	$18,086
Nonphysician prov benefit cost	5	*	2	*	0	*	59	$3,520
Provider consultant cost	0	*	4	*	2	*	10	$8,951
Total physician cost/physician	11	$375,278	58	$370,257	32	$412,525	85	$462,675
Total phy compensation	10	$351,319	3	*	0	*	84	$404,492
Total phy benefit cost	10	$47,740	3	*	0	*	83	$53,550

Table 12.4e: Net Income or Loss

	Allergy/Immunology		Anesthesiology		Anesthesiology: Pain Management		Cardiology	
	Count	Median	Count	Median	Count	Median	Count	Median
Total cost	11	$921,723	57	$542,619	32	$610,953	85	$978,949
Net nonmedical revenue	7	*	47	$4,315	24	$832	53	$2,433
Nonmedical revenue	4	*	3	*	0	*	51	$2,538
Fin support for oper costs	0	*	0	*	0	*	0	*
Goodwill amortization	1	*	0	*	0	*	4	*
Nonmedical cost	2	*	2	*	0	*	19	$1,083
Net inc, prac with fin sup	0	*	0	*	0	*	0	*
Net inc, prac w/o fin sup	11	$1,731	58	$8	31	$0	82	$4,156
Net inc, excl fin supp (all prac)	11	$1,731	58	$8	31	$0	82	$4,156

Table 12.4f: Assets and Liabilities

	Allergy/Immunology		Anesthesiology		Anesthesiology: Pain Management		Cardiology	
	Count	Median	Count	Median	Count	Median	Count	Median
Total assets	3	*	1	*	0	*	43	$97,875
Current assets	3	*	1	*	0	*	43	$32,191
Noncurrent assets	3	*	1	*	0	*	43	$51,186
Total liabilities	3	*	1	*	0	*	43	$66,686
Current liabilities	3	*	1	*	0	*	43	$33,610
Noncurrent liabilities	3	*	1	*	0	*	43	$28,696
Working capital	3	*	1	*	0	*	43	$6,125
Total net worth	3	*	1	*	0	*	43	$24,542
Total support staff FTE/phy	11	6.03	58	.45	32	.57	85	5.18

Single Specialty Practices, Not Hospital or IDS Owned — Allergy/Immunology, Anesthesiology, Anesthesiology: Pain Management, Cardiology (as a % of Total Medical Revenue)

Table 12.5a: Charges and Revenue

	Allergy/Immunology		Anesthesiology		Anesthesiology: Pain Management		Cardiology	
	Count	Median	Count	Median	Count	Median	Count	Median
Net fee-for-service revenue	10	95.90%	5	*	1	*	83	98.22%
Net capitation revenue	3	*	0	*	0	*	13	5.75%
Net other medical revenue	7	*	2	*	0	*	67	1.78%
Total gross charges	**11**	**124.01%**	**56**	**205.63%**	**32**	**205.86%**	**85**	**218.26%**

Table 12.5b: Operating Cost

	Allergy/Immunology		Anesthesiology		Anesthesiology: Pain Management		Cardiology	
	Count	Median	Count	Median	Count	Median	Count	Median
Total support staff cost	**11**	**30.29%**	**58**	**4.71%**	**32**	**5.72%**	**85**	**24.79%**
Total empl support staff cost	10	25.39%	3	*	1	*	82	19.42%
General administrative	9	*	3	*	1	*	81	2.23%
Patient accounting	9	*	2	*	0	*	81	2.35%
General accounting	6	*	1	*	1	*	62	.40%
Managed care administrative	2	*	0	*	0	*	20	.40%
Information technology	2	*	0	*	0	*	38	.42%
Housekeeping, maint, security	1	*	0	*	0	*	13	.20%
Medical receptionists	9	*	0	*	0	*	80	1.96%
Med secretaries,transcribers	6	*	0	*	0	*	72	1.03%
Medical records	4	*	0	*	0	*	79	1.02%
Other admin support	5	*	0	*	1	*	34	.43%
*Total administrative supp staff	4	*	48	4.03%	30	4.00%	40	10.20%
Registered Nurses	8	*	2	*	0	*	74	3.11%
Licensed Practical Nurses	5	*	0	*	0	*	46	.53%
Med assistants, nurse aides	6	*	0	*	0	*	78	1.53%
*Total clinical supp staff	6	*	17	1.04%	16	1.00%	60	5.44%
Clinical laboratory	3	*	0	*	0	*	24	.46%
Radiology and imaging	0	*	0	*	0	*	77	2.80%
Other medical support serv	4	*	0	*	0	*	47	1.05%
*Total ancillary supp staff	1	*	3	*	5	*	41	3.93%
Total empl supp staff benefits	9	*	33	1.61%	26	1.18%	81	4.76%
Tot contracted supp staff	5	*	4	*	8	*	54	.57%
Total general operating cost	**11**	**23.75%**	**58**	**7.53%**	**32**	**7.78%**	**85**	**24.02%**
Information technology	9	*	2	*	1	*	84	1.45%
Medical and surgical supply	9	*	1	*	0	*	84	1.36%
Building and occupancy	9	*	3	*	1	*	85	4.69%
Furniture and equipment	8	*	2	*	1	*	76	1.21%
Admin supplies and services	9	*	3	*	1	*	85	1.50%
Prof liability insurance	10	.59%	58	2.82%	31	2.56%	85	1.57%
Other insurance premiums	9	*	5	*	1	*	82	.20%
Outside professional fees	9	*	5	*	1	*	85	.72%
Promotion and marketing	9	*	2	*	1	*	85	.34%
Clinical laboratory	3	*	0	*	0	*	31	.38%
Radiology and imaging	1	*	0	*	0	*	73	5.52%
Other ancillary services	2	*	0	*	0	*	42	.80%
Billing purchased services	6	*	4	*	1	*	39	.17%
Management fees paid to MSO	0	*	1	*	0	*	5	*
Misc operating cost	9	*	5	*	1	*	81	1.39%
Cost allocated to prac from par	0	*	0	*	0	*	0	*
Total operating cost	**11**	**54.61%**	**58**	**12.43%**	**32**	**13.40%**	**85**	**48.75%**

*See pages 260 and 261 for definition.

Single Specialty Practices, Not Hospital or IDS Owned — Allergy/Immunology, Anesthesiology, Anesthesiology: Pain Management, Cardiology (as a % of Total Medical Revenue)

Table 12.5c: Provider Cost

	Allergy/Immunology		Anesthesiology		Anesthesiology: Pain Management		Cardiology	
	Count	Median	Count	Median	Count	Median	Count	Median
Total med rev after oper cost	11	44.97%	58	87.57%	32	87.12%	85	51.16%
Total provider cost	11	42.07%	57	89.84%	32	87.24%	85	49.93%
Total NPP cost	6	*	40	23.58%	25	20.57%	61	2.08%
Nonphysician provider comp	6	*	4	*	0	*	62	1.62%
Nonphysician prov benefit cost	5	*	2	*	0	*	59	.34%
Provider consultant cost	0	*	4	*	2	*	10	.88%
Total physician cost	11	40.60%	58	76.18%	32	66.55%	85	48.76%
Total phy compensation	10	33.68%	3	*	0	*	84	42.63%
Total phy benefit cost	10	5.08%	3	*	0	*	83	5.34%

Table 12.5d: Net Income or Loss

	Allergy/Immunology		Anesthesiology		Anesthesiology: Pain Management		Cardiology	
	Count	Median	Count	Median	Count	Median	Count	Median
Total cost	11	99.52%	57	100.71%	32	100.08%	85	99.88%
Net nonmedical revenue	7	*	47	.58%	24	.16%	53	.25%
Nonmedical revenue	4	*	3	*	0	*	51	.25%
Fin support for oper costs	0	*	0	*	0	*	0	*
Goodwill amortization	1	*	0	*	0	*	4	*
Nonmedical cost	2	*	2	*	0	*	19	.14%
Net inc, prac with fin sup	0	*	0	*	0	*	0	*
Net inc, prac w/o fin sup	11	.22%	58	.00%	31	.00%	82	.39%
Net inc, excl fin supp (all prac)	11	.22%	58	.00%	31	.00%	82	.39%

Table 12.5e: Assets and Liabilities

	Allergy/Immunology		Anesthesiology		Anesthesiology: Pain Management		Cardiology	
	Count	Median	Count	Median	Count	Median	Count	Median
Total assets	3	*	1	*	0	*	43	10.16%
Current assets	3	*	1	*	0	*	43	3.29%
Noncurrent assets	3	*	1	*	0	*	43	6.22%
Total liabilities	3	*	1	*	0	*	43	7.34%
Current liabilities	3	*	1	*	0	*	43	3.97%
Noncurrent liabilities	3	*	1	*	0	*	43	2.83%
Working capital	3	*	1	*	0	*	43	.59%
Total net worth	3	*	1	*	0	*	43	2.38%
Total support staff FTE/phy	11	6.03	58	.45	32	.57	85	5.18

Single Specialty Practices, Not Hospital or IDS Owned — Allergy/Immunology, Anesthesiology, Anesthesiology: Pain Management, Cardiology (per FTE Provider)

Table 12.6a: Staffing, RVUs, Patients, Procedures and Square Footage

	Allergy/Immunology		Anesthesiology		Anesthesiology: Pain Management		Cardiology	
	Count	Median	Count	Median	Count	Median	Count	Median
Total physician FTE/provider	5	*	40	.47	25	.53	58	.80
Prim care phy/provider	1	*	0	*	0	*	5	*
Nonsurg phy/provider	3	*	0	*	0	*	51	.79
Surg spec phy/provider	0	*	3	*	0	*	7	*
Total NPP FTE/provider	5	*	40	.53	25	.47	58	.20
Total support staff FTE/prov	5	*	40	.24	25	.31	58	4.29
Total empl supp staff FTE/prov	5	*	3	*	1	*	57	4.27
General administrative	5	*	3	*	1	*	57	.23
Patient accounting	5	*	2	*	0	*	57	.58
General accounting	4	*	1	*	1	*	47	.08
Managed care administrative	1	*	0	*	0	*	15	.11
Information technology	2	*	0	*	0	*	32	.07
Housekeeping, maint, security	1	*	0	*	0	*	9	*
Medical receptionists	5	*	0	*	0	*	57	.65
Med secretaries,transcribers	3	*	0	*	0	*	50	.26
Medical records	2	*	0	*	0	*	57	.38
Other admin support	2	*	0	*	1	*	26	.09
*Total administrative supp staff	0	*	35	.24	24	.29	28	2.55
Registered Nurses	5	*	2	*	0	*	52	.46
Licensed Practical Nurses	3	*	0	*	0	*	35	.13
Med assistants, nurse aides	3	*	0	*	0	*	57	.51
*Total clinical supp staff	2	*	14	.07	14	.08	44	1.12
Clinical laboratory	1	*	0	*	0	*	17	.13
Radiology and imaging	0	*	0	*	0	*	53	.47
Other medical support serv	3	*	0	*	0	*	35	.24
*Total ancillary supp staff	1	*	3	*	5	*	23	.68
Tot contracted supp staff	1	*	4	*	5	*	33	.09
Tot RVU/provider	1	*	29	8,707	17	7,852	25	15,289
Physician work RVU/provider	0	*	0	*	0	*	35	8,042
Patients/provider	1	*	3	*	0	*	35	1,288
Tot procedures/provider	2	*	4	*	1	*	53	8,332
Square feet/provider	4	*	24	76	19	75	56	1,547
Total support staff FTE/phy	11	6.03	58	.45	32	.57	85	5.18

*See pages 260 and 261 for definition.

Table 12.6b: Charges, Revenue and Cost

	Allergy/Immunology		Anesthesiology		Anesthesiology: Pain Management		Cardiology	
	Count	Median	Count	Median	Count	Median	Count	Median
Total gross charges	5	*	39	$593,523	25	$638,597	58	$1,785,252
Total medical revenue	5	*	40	$305,521	25	$322,364	58	$799,842
Net fee-for-service revenue	5	*	5	*	1	*	57	$770,404
Net capitation revenue	3	*	0	*	0	*	11	$58,801
Net other medical revenue	4	*	2	*	0	*	47	$16,135
Total support staff cost/prov	5	*	40	$14,975	25	$17,123	58	$192,562
Total general operating cost	5	*	40	$19,050	25	$28,658	58	$193,862
Total operating cost	5	*	40	$39,551	25	$52,762	58	$381,863
Total med rev after oper cost	5	*	40	$249,501	25	$288,547	58	$394,991
Total provider cost/provider	5	*	39	$272,139	25	$282,938	58	$388,585
Total NPP cost/provider	5	*	40	$70,299	25	$67,108	56	$17,995
Provider consultant cost	0	*	3	*	1	*	8	*
Total physician cost/provider	5	*	40	$182,531	25	$214,792	58	$371,257
Total phy compensation	5	*	3	*	0	*	58	$324,135
Total phy benefit cost	5	*	3	*	0	*	58	$43,954
Total cost	5	*	39	$321,727	25	$323,824	58	$778,932
Net nonmedical revenue	3	*	35	$1,388	19	$313	41	$1,998
Net inc, prac with fin sup	0	*	0	*	0	*	0	*
Net inc, prac w/o fin sup	5	*	40	$194	24	-$88	57	$1,534
Net inc, excl fin supp (all prac)	5	*	40	$194	24	-$88	57	$1,534
Total support staff FTE/phy	11	6.03	58	.45	32	.57	85	5.18

Single Specialty Practices, Not Hospital or IDS Owned — Allergy/Immunology, Anesthesiology, Anesthesiology: Pain Management, Cardiology (per Square Foot)

Table 12.7a: Staffing, RVUs, Patients and Procedures

	Allergy/Immunology		Anesthesiology		Anesthesiology: Pain Management		Cardiology	
	Count	Median	Count	Median	Count	Median	Count	Median
Total prov FTE/10,000 sq ft	4	*	24	131.91	19	134.19	56	6.46
Total phy FTE/10,000 sq ft	10	3.01	36	82.45	22	66.71	80	5.38
Prim care phy/10,000 sq ft	2	*	0	*	0	*	5	*
Nonsurg phy/10,000 sq ft	6	*	0	*	0	*	70	5.35
Surg spec phy/10,000 sq ft	0	*	1	*	0	*	11	1.99
Total NPP FTE/10,000 sq ft	4	*	24	63.42	19	40.91	56	1.14
Total supp stf FTE/10,000 sq ft	10	26.09	36	42.53	22	34.30	80	28.52
Total empl supp stf/10,000 sq ft	9	*	1	*	1	*	78	28.36
General administrative	8	*	1	*	1	*	79	1.50
Patient accounting	8	*	1	*	0	*	79	4.07
General accounting	5	*	0	*	1	*	60	.53
Managed care administrative	1	*	0	*	0	*	21	.47
Information technology	1	*	0	*	0	*	39	.50
Housekeeping, maint, security	0	*	0	*	0	*	10	.28
Medical receptionists	8	*	0	*	0	*	78	4.14
Med secretaries,transcribers	4	*	0	*	0	*	71	1.79
Medical records	4	*	0	*	0	*	78	2.20
Other admin support	5	*	0	*	1	*	31	.66
*Total administrative supp staff	4	*	33	40.00	21	32.64	42	16.04
Registered Nurses	7	*	1	*	0	*	73	3.16
Licensed Practical Nurses	4	*	0	*	0	*	46	.96
Med assistants, nurse aides	6	*	0	*	0	*	76	3.06
*Total clinical supp staff	6	*	12	12.55	14	4.55	61	7.42
Clinical laboratory	3	*	0	*	0	*	23	.94
Radiology and imaging	0	*	0	*	0	*	75	2.97
Other medical support serv	3	*	0	*	0	*	47	1.18
*Total ancillary supp staff	2	*	3	*	5	*	32	4.43
Tot contracted supp staff	4	*	4	*	7	*	43	.67
Tot RVU/sq ft	5	*	31	97.17	15	106.11	36	9.83
Physician work RVU/sq ft	2	*	0	*	0	*	48	4.82
Patients/sq ft	4	*	2	*	0	*	46	.78
Tot procedures/sq ft	5	*	1	*	1	*	72	5.70
Total support staff FTE/phy	11	6.03	58	.45	32	.57	85	5.18

*See pages 260 and 261 for definition.

Table 12.7b: Charges, Revenue and Cost

	Allergy/Immunology		Anesthesiology		Anesthesiology: Pain Management		Cardiology	
	Count	Median	Count	Median	Count	Median	Count	Median
Total gross charges	10	$369.37	34	$8,058.76	22	$7,706.07	80	$1,245.03
Total medical revenue	10	$285.56	36	$4,003.97	22	$3,920.14	80	$537.60
Net fee-for-service revenue	9	*	2	*	1	*	78	$535.51
Net capitation revenue	2	*	0	*	0	*	13	$24.19
Net other medical revenue	6	*	1	*	0	*	64	$9.49
Total support staff cost/sq ft	10	$88.58	36	$260.59	22	$247.88	80	$127.71
Total general operating cost	10	$68.02	36	$284.87	22	$236.19	80	$124.77
Total operating cost	10	$158.95	36	$539.12	22	$494.85	80	$256.15
Total med rev after oper cost	10	$131.30	36	$3,534.18	22	$3,187.98	80	$267.72
Total provider cost/sq ft	10	$133.94	36	$3,502.91	22	$3,511.62	80	$259.15
Total NPP cost/sq ft	5	*	24	$860.97	19	$635.56	59	$10.94
Provider consultant cost	0	*	4	*	2	*	10	$4.35
Total physician cost/sq ft	10	$129.53	36	$3,262.81	22	$2,956.32	80	$246.91
Total phy compensation	9	*	1	*	0	*	79	$218.10
Total phy benefit cost	9	*	1	*	0	*	78	$26.43
Total cost	10	$288.90	36	$4,035.17	22	$4,135.41	80	$532.88
Net nonmedical revenue/sq ft	6	*	29	$23.06	15	$8.89	53	$1.31
Net inc, prac with fin sup	0	*	0	*	0	*	0	*
Net inc, prac w/o fin sup	10	$.23	36	$.00	21	$.00	78	$1.55
Net inc, excl fin supp (all prac)	10	$.23	36	$.00	21	$.00	78	$1.55
Total support staff FTE/phy	11	6.03	58	.45	32	.57	85	5.18

Single Specialty Practices, Not Hospital or IDS Owned — Allergy/Immunology, Anesthesiology, Anesthesiology: Pain Management, Cardiology (per Total RVU)

Table 12.8a: Staffing, Patients, Procedures and Square Footage

	Allergy/Immunology		Anesthesiology		Anesthesiology: Pain Management		Cardiology	
	Count	Median	Count	Median	Count	Median	Count	Median
Total prov FTE/10,000 tot RVU	1	*	29	1.15	17	1.27	25	.65
Total phy FTE/10,000 tot RVU	5	*	45	.79	24	.72	37	.50
Prim care phy/10,000 tot RVU	0	*	0	*	0	*	2	*
Nonsurg phy/10,000 tot RVU	3	*	0	*	0	*	35	.50
Surg spec phy/10,000 tot RVU	0	*	2	*	0	*	5	*
Total NPP FTE/10,000 tot RVU	1	*	29	.55	17	.71	25	.11
Total supp stf FTE/10,000 tot RVU	5	*	45	.29	24	.33	37	2.60
Tot empl supp stf/10,000 tot RVU	4	*	3	*	0	*	37	2.57
General administrative	4	*	3	*	0	*	37	.15
Patient accounting	4	*	2	*	0	*	37	.39
General accounting	2	*	1	*	0	*	27	.06
Managed care administrative	1	*	0	*	0	*	11	.06
Information technology	0	*	0	*	0	*	20	.05
Housekeeping, maint, security	0	*	0	*	0	*	8	*
Medical receptionists	4	*	0	*	0	*	36	.35
Med secretaries,transcribers	2	*	0	*	0	*	33	.20
Medical records	3	*	0	*	0	*	35	.17
Other admin support	4	*	0	*	0	*	16	.06
*Total administrative supp staff	4	*	37	.29	23	.31	23	1.58
Registered Nurses	3	*	2	*	0	*	35	.33
Licensed Practical Nurses	2	*	0	*	0	*	23	.06
Med assistants, nurse aides	4	*	0	*	0	*	35	.32
*Total clinical supp staff	5	*	12	.11	12	.06	32	.60
Clinical laboratory	2	*	0	*	0	*	9	*
Radiology and imaging	0	*	0	*	0	*	36	.27
Other medical support serv	0	*	0	*	0	*	24	.19
*Total ancillary supp staff	1	*	2	*	3	*	17	.44
Tot contracted supp staff	3	*	5	*	6	*	23	.05
Physician work RVU/tot RVU	2	*	0	*	0	*	31	.42
Patients/tot RVU	2	*	3	*	0	*	26	.07
Tot procedures/tot RVU	3	*	3	*	0	*	36	.48
Square feet/tot RVU	5	*	31	.01	15	.01	36	.10
Total support staff FTE/phy	11	6.03	58	.45	32	.57	85	5.18

*See pages 260 and 261 for definition.

Table 12.8b: Charges, Revenue and Cost

	Allergy/Immunology		Anesthesiology		Anesthesiology: Pain Management		Cardiology	
	Count	Median	Count	Median	Count	Median	Count	Median
Total gross charges	5	*	44	$71.44	24	$78.96	37	$107.69
Total medical revenue	5	*	45	$34.14	24	$39.27	37	$45.62
Net fee-for-service revenue	4	*	4	*	0	*	37	$44.24
Net capitation revenue	0	*	0	*	0	*	6	*
Net other medical revenue	2	*	1	*	0	*	31	$.86
Total supp staff cost/tot RVU	5	*	45	$1.72	24	$2.04	37	$11.65
Total general operating cost	5	*	45	$2.58	24	$3.08	37	$11.46
Total operating cost	5	*	45	$4.33	24	$5.13	37	$22.96
Total med rev after oper cost	5	*	45	$30.54	24	$35.06	37	$22.90
Total provider cost/tot RVU	5	*	45	$29.84	24	$34.99	37	$22.25
Total NPP cost/tot RVU	2	*	29	$7.23	17	$8.87	25	$1.11
Provider consultant cost	0	*	4	*	1	*	4	*
Total physician cost/tot RVU	5	*	45	$27.48	24	$29.30	37	$21.13
Total phy compensation	4	*	2	*	0	*	37	$18.15
Total phy benefit cost	4	*	2	*	0	*	37	$2.69
Total cost	4	*	3	*	0	*	35	$85.68
Net nonmedical revenue	4	*	36	$.23	18	$.07	30	$.16
Net inc, prac with fin sup	0	*	0	*	0	*	0	*
Net inc, prac w/o fin sup	5	*	45	$.00	23	$.00	37	$.16
Net inc, excl fin supp (all prac)	5	*	45	$.00	23	$.00	37	$.16
Total support staff FTE/phy	11	6.03	58	.45	32	.57	85	5.18

Single Specialty Practices, Not Hospital or IDS Owned — Allergy/Immunology, Anesthesiology, Anesthesiology: Pain Management, Cardiology (per Work RVU)

Table 12.9a: Staffing, Patients, Procedures and Square Footage

	Allergy/Immunology		Anesthesiology		Anesthesiology: Pain Management		Cardiology	
	Count	Median	Count	Median	Count	Median	Count	Median
Total prov FTE/10,000 work RVU	0	*	0	*	0	*	35	**1.24**
Tot phy FTE/10,000 work RVU	2	*	0	*	0	*	48	1.04
Prim care phy/10,000 work RVU	0	*	0	*	0	*	2	*
Nonsurg phy/10,000 work RVU	1	*	0	*	0	*	46	1.04
Surg spec phy/10,000 work RVU	0	*	0	*	0	*	4	*
Total NPP FTE/10,000 work RVU	0	*	0	*	0	*	35	.22
Total supp stf FTE/10,000 wrk RVU	2	*	0	*	0	*	48	**5.66**
Tot empl supp stf/10,000 work RVU	1	*	0	*	0	*	48	5.60
General administrative	1	*	0	*	0	*	48	.28
Patient accounting	1	*	0	*	0	*	48	.88
General accounting	0	*	0	*	0	*	38	.12
Managed care administrative	0	*	0	*	0	*	14	.11
Information technology	0	*	0	*	0	*	27	.12
Housekeeping, maint, security	0	*	0	*	0	*	7	*
Medical receptionists	1	*	0	*	0	*	47	.85
Med secretaries,transcribers	0	*	0	*	0	*	42	.36
Medical records	0	*	0	*	0	*	47	.48
Other admin support	1	*	0	*	0	*	18	.17
*Total administrative supp staff	2	*	0	*	0	*	28	3.36
Registered Nurses	1	*	0	*	0	*	46	.72
Licensed Practical Nurses	0	*	0	*	0	*	30	.18
Med assistants, nurse aides	1	*	0	*	0	*	46	.65
*Total clinical supp staff	2	*	0	*	0	*	41	1.43
Clinical laboratory	0	*	0	*	0	*	13	.17
Radiology and imaging	0	*	0	*	0	*	46	.68
Other medical support serv	0	*	0	*	0	*	31	.37
*Total ancillary supp staff	0	*	0	*	0	*	20	.94
Tot contracted supp staff	1	*	0	*	0	*	28	.12
Tot RVU/work RVU	2	*	0	*	0	*	31	2.40
Patients/work RVU	1	*	0	*	0	*	31	.14
Tot procedures/work RVU	1	*	0	*	0	*	46	1.16
Square feet/work RVU	2	*	0	*	0	*	48	.21
Total support staff FTE/phy	11	6.03	58	.45	32	.57	85	5.18

*See pages 260 and 261 for definition.

Table 12.9b: Charges, Revenue and Cost

	Allergy/Immunology		Anesthesiology		Anesthesiology: Pain Management		Cardiology	
	Count	Median	Count	Median	Count	Median	Count	Median
Total gross charges	2	*	0	*	0	*	48	$238.62
Total medical revenue	2	*	0	*	0	*	48	$100.73
Net fee-for-service revenue	1	*	0	*	0	*	48	$96.10
Net capitation revenue	0	*	0	*	0	*	10	$6.92
Net other medical revenue	1	*	0	*	0	*	42	$2.10
Total supp staff cost/work RVU	2	*	0	*	0	*	48	$26.78
Total general operating cost	2	*	0	*	0	*	48	$23.03
Total operating cost	2	*	0	*	0	*	48	$50.46
Total med rev after oper cost	2	*	0	*	0	*	48	$50.13
Total provider cost/work RVU	2	*	0	*	0	*	48	$49.69
Total NPP cost/work RVU	1	*	0	*	0	*	37	$2.09
Provider consultant cost	0	*	0	*	0	*	8	*
Total physician cost/work RVU	2	*	0	*	0	*	48	$48.43
Total phy compensation	1	*	0	*	0	*	48	$42.44
Total phy benefit cost	1	*	0	*	0	*	48	$5.98
Total cost	2	*	0	*	0	*	48	$100.20
Net nonmedical revenue	2	*	0	*	0	*	36	$.27
Net inc, prac with fin sup	0	*	0	*	0	*	0	*
Net inc, prac w/o fin sup	2	*	0	*	0	*	47	$.29
Net inc, excl fin supp (all prac)	2	*	0	*	0	*	47	$.29
Total support staff FTE/phy	11	6.03	58	.45	32	.57	85	5.18

Single Specialty Practices, Not Hospital or IDS Owned — Allergy/Immunology, Anesthesiology, Anesthesiology: Pain Management, Cardiology (per Patient)

Table 12.10a: Staffing, RVUs, Procedures and Square Footage

	Allergy/Immunology		Anesthesiology		Anesthesiology: Pain Management		Cardiology	
	Count	Median	Count	Median	Count	Median	Count	Median
Total prov FTE/10,000 patients	1	*	3	*	0	*	35	7.76
Total phy FTE/10,000 pat	4	*	3	*	0	*	49	6.51
Prim care phy/10,000 pat	0	*	0	*	0	*	2	*
Nonsurg phy/10,000 pat	4	*	0	*	0	*	44	6.40
Surg spec phy/10,000 pat	0	*	2	*	0	*	8	*
Total NPP FTE/10,000 pat	1	*	3	*	0	*	35	1.48
Total supp staff FTE/10,000 pat	4	*	3	*	0	*	49	35.27
Total empl supp staff/10,000 pat	4	*	2	*	0	*	49	34.47
General administrative	4	*	2	*	0	*	49	1.82
Patient accounting	4	*	2	*	0	*	49	5.37
General accounting	2	*	1	*	0	*	37	.75
Managed care administrative	0	*	0	*	0	*	14	.82
Information technology	0	*	0	*	0	*	28	.72
Housekeeping, maint, security	0	*	0	*	0	*	6	*
Medical receptionists	4	*	0	*	0	*	48	4.31
Med secretaries,transcribers	2	*	0	*	0	*	42	1.90
Medical records	1	*	0	*	0	*	47	2.46
Other admin support	3	*	0	*	0	*	25	.50
*Total administrative supp staff	2	*	0	*	0	*	27	20.40
Registered Nurses	3	*	2	*	0	*	44	4.61
Licensed Practical Nurses	2	*	0	*	0	*	32	.90
Med assistants, nurse aides	3	*	0	*	0	*	47	3.71
*Total clinical supp staff	3	*	0	*	0	*	38	8.67
Clinical laboratory	2	*	0	*	0	*	16	.95
Radiology and imaging	0	*	0	*	0	*	48	3.47
Other medical support serv	2	*	0	*	0	*	34	1.57
*Total ancillary supp staff	1	*	0	*	0	*	24	5.55
Tot contracted supp staff	1	*	0	*	0	*	28	.67
Tot RVU/patient	2	*	3	*	0	*	26	14.92
Physician work RVU/patient	1	*	0	*	0	*	31	6.99
Tot procedures/patient	4	*	2	*	0	*	47	7.25
Square feet/patient	4	*	2	*	0	*	46	1.28
Total support staff FTE/phy	11	6.03	58	.45	32	.57	85	5.18

*See pages 260 and 261 for definition.

Table 12.10b: Charges, Revenue and Cost

	Allergy/Immunology		Anesthesiology		Anesthesiology: Pain Management		Cardiology	
	Count	Median	Count	Median	Count	Median	Count	Median
Total gross charges	4	*	3	*	0	*	49	$1,557.40
Total medical revenue	4	*	3	*	0	*	49	$663.01
Net fee-for-service revenue	4	*	3	*	0	*	49	$607.99
Net capitation revenue	1	*	0	*	0	*	7	*
Net other medical revenue	2	*	1	*	0	*	38	$8.77
Total support staff cost/patient	4	*	3	*	0	*	49	$159.89
Total general operating cost	4	*	3	*	0	*	49	$154.82
Total operating cost	4	*	3	*	0	*	49	$292.08
Total med rev after oper cost	4	*	3	*	0	*	49	$333.55
Total provider cost/patient	4	*	3	*	0	*	49	$327.43
Total NPP cost/patient	2	*	3	*	0	*	37	$11.38
Provider consultant cost	0	*	2	*	0	*	6	*
Total physician cost/patient	4	*	3	*	0	*	49	$313.51
Total phy compensation	4	*	2	*	0	*	49	$270.82
Total phy benefit cost	4	*	2	*	0	*	49	$32.60
Total cost	4	*	3	*	0	*	49	$685.33
Net nonmedical revenue	3	*	3	*	0	*	33	$1.51
Net inc, prac with fin sup	0	*	0	*	0	*	0	*
Net inc, prac w/o fin sup	4	*	3	*	0	*	47	$.54
Net inc, excl fin supp (all prac)	4	*	3	*	0	*	47	$.54
Total support staff FTE/phy	11	6.03	58	.45	32	.57	85	5.18

Single Specialty Practices, Not Hospital or IDS Owned — Allergy/Immunology, Anesthesiology, Anesthesiology: Pain Management, Cardiology (Procedure and Charge Data)

Table 12.11a: Activity Charges to Total Gross Charges Ratios

	Allergy/Immunology		Anesthesiology		Anesthesiology: Pain Management		Cardiology	
	Count	Median	Count	Median	Count	Median	Count	Median
Total proc gross charges	8	*	4	*	1	*	79	97.07%
Medical proc-inside practice	9	*	0	*	0	*	75	33.12%
Medical proc-outside practice	6	*	1	*	0	*	74	36.71%
Surg proc-inside practice	1	*	2	*	0	*	23	.04%
Surg proc-outside practice	0	*	2	*	0	*	57	3.74%
Laboratory procedures	5	*	0	*	1	*	59	.41%
Radiology procedures	1	*	1	*	0	*	75	17.52%
Tot nonproc gross charges	4	*	0	*	0	*	51	4.09%
Total support staff FTE/phy	11	6.03	58	.45	32	.57	85	5.18

Table 12.11b: Medical Procedure Data (inside the practice)

	Allergy/Immunology		Anesthesiology		Anesthesiology: Pain Management		Cardiology	
	Count	Median	Count	Median	Count	Median	Count	Median
Gross charges/procedure	7	*	0	*	0	*	74	$164.96
Total cost/procedure	6	*	0	*	0	*	69	$93.02
Operating cost/procedure	6	*	0	*	0	*	69	$52.19
Provider cost/procedure	6	*	0	*	0	*	69	$42.89
Procedures/patient	4	*	0	*	0	*	47	3.07
Gross charges/patient	4	*	0	*	0	*	47	$437.54
Procedures/physician	7	*	0	*	0	*	75	4,362
Gross charges/physician	9	*	0	*	0	*	75	$661,279
Procedures/provider	3	*	0	*	0	*	52	3,757
Gross charges/provider	5	*	0	*	0	*	53	$574,327
Gross charge to total cost ratio	6	*	0	*	0	*	69	1.75
Oper cost to total cost ratio	6	*	0	*	0	*	69	.54
Prov cost to total cost ratio	6	*	0	*	0	*	69	.46
Total support staff FTE/phy	11	6.03	58	.45	32	.57	85	5.18

Table 12.11c: Medical Procedure Data (outside the practice)

	Allergy/Immunology		Anesthesiology		Anesthesiology: Pain Management		Cardiology	
	Count	Median	Count	Median	Count	Median	Count	Median
Gross charges/procedure	4	*	1	*	0	*	73	$187.40
Total cost/procedure	4	*	1	*	0	*	68	$65.78
Operating cost/procedure	4	*	1	*	0	*	68	$21.59
Provider cost/procedure	4	*	1	*	0	*	68	$44.22
Procedures/patient	2	*	1	*	0	*	47	2.71
Gross charges/patient	2	*	1	*	0	*	47	$529.70
Procedures/physician	4	*	1	*	0	*	74	4,056
Gross charges/physician	6	*	1	*	0	*	74	$811,622
Procedures/provider	2	*	1	*	0	*	51	3,098
Gross charges/provider	4	*	1	*	0	*	52	$630,707
Gross charge to total cost ratio	4	*	1	*	0	*	68	2.89
Oper cost to total cost ratio	4	*	1	*	0	*	68	.32
Prov cost to total cost ratio	4	*	1	*	0	*	68	.68
Total support staff FTE/phy	11	6.03	58	.45	32	.57	85	5.18

Single Specialty Practices, Not Hospital or IDS Owned — Allergy/Immunology, Anesthesiology, Anesthesiology: Pain Management, Cardiology (Procedure and Charge Data)

Table 12.11d: Surgery/Anesthesia Procedure Data (inside the practice)

	Allergy/Immunology		Anesthesiology		Anesthesiology: Pain Management		Cardiology	
	Count	Median	Count	Median	Count	Median	Count	Median
Gross charges/procedure	1	*	2	*	0	*	23	**$78.89**
Total cost/procedure	1	*	1	*	0	*	22	**$50.43**
Operating cost/procedure	1	*	1	*	0	*	22	$28.33
Provider cost/procedure	1	*	2	*	0	*	22	$23.48
Procedures/patient	1	*	1	*	0	*	17	.00
Gross charges/patient	1	*	1	*	0	*	17	$.13
Procedures/physician	1	*	2	*	0	*	23	23
Gross charges/physician	1	*	2	*	0	*	23	$624
Procedures/provider	0	*	2	*	0	*	17	12
Gross charges/provider	0	*	2	*	0	*	17	$524
Gross charge to total cost ratio	1	*	1	*	0	*	22	1.64
Oper cost to total cost ratio	1	*	1	*	0	*	22	.54
Prov cost to total cost ratio	1	*	1	*	0	*	22	.46
Total support staff FTE/phy	11	6.03	58	.45	32	.57	85	5.18

Table 12.11e: Surgery/Anesthesia Procedure Data (outside the practice)

	Allergy/Immunology		Anesthesiology		Anesthesiology: Pain Management		Cardiology	
	Count	Median	Count	Median	Count	Median	Count	Median
Gross charges/procedure	0	*	2	*	0	*	57	**$1,060.92**
Total cost/procedure	0	*	1	*	0	*	52	**$381.33**
Operating cost/procedure	0	*	1	*	0	*	52	$111.79
Provider cost/procedure	0	*	2	*	0	*	52	$243.76
Procedures/patient	0	*	1	*	0	*	34	.04
Gross charges/patient	0	*	1	*	0	*	33	$53.12
Procedures/physician	0	*	2	*	0	*	58	72
Gross charges/physician	0	*	2	*	0	*	57	$90,698
Procedures/provider	0	*	2	*	0	*	40	64
Gross charges/provider	0	*	2	*	0	*	40	$70,634
Gross charge to total cost ratio	0	*	1	*	0	*	52	2.90
Oper cost to total cost ratio	0	*	1	*	0	*	52	.32
Prov cost to total cost ratio	0	*	1	*	0	*	52	.68
Total support staff FTE/phy	11	6.03	58	.45	32	.57	85	5.18

Single Specialty Practices, Not Hospital or IDS Owned — Allergy/Immunology, Anesthesiology, Anesthesiology: Pain Management, Cardiology (Procedure and Charge Data)

Table 12.11f: Clinical Laboratory/Pathology Procedure Data

	Allergy/Immunology		Anesthesiology		Anesthesiology: Pain Management		Cardiology	
	Count	Median	Count	Median	Count	Median	Count	Median
Gross charges/procedure	4	*	0	*	1	*	59	**$17.19**
Total cost/procedure	4	*	0	*	1	*	56	**$10.46**
Operating cost/procedure	4	*	0	*	1	*	56	$5.51
Provider cost/procedure	4	*	0	*	1	*	56	$4.32
Procedures/patient	2	*	0	*	0	*	39	.31
Gross charges/patient	2	*	0	*	0	*	39	$5.53
Procedures/physician	4	*	0	*	1	*	60	538
Gross charges/physician	5	*	0	*	1	*	59	$8,289
Procedures/provider	2	*	0	*	1	*	44	396
Gross charges/provider	3	*	0	*	1	*	43	$6,899
Gross charge to total cost ratio	4	*	0	*	1	*	56	2.00
Oper cost to total cost ratio	4	*	0	*	1	*	56	.53
Prov cost to total cost ratio	4	*	0	*	1	*	56	.47
Total support staff FTE/phy	11	6.03	58	.45	32	.57	85	5.18

Table 12.11g: Diagnostic Radiology and Imaging Procedure Data

	Allergy/Immunology		Anesthesiology		Anesthesiology: Pain Management		Cardiology	
	Count	Median	Count	Median	Count	Median	Count	Median
Gross charges/procedure	0	*	1	*	0	*	74	**$390.65**
Total cost/procedure	0	*	1	*	0	*	69	**$242.95**
Operating cost/procedure	0	*	1	*	0	*	69	$144.72
Provider cost/procedure	0	*	1	*	0	*	69	$91.17
Procedures/patient	0	*	1	*	0	*	48	.59
Gross charges/patient	0	*	1	*	0	*	47	$242.80
Procedures/physician	0	*	1	*	0	*	75	1,017
Gross charges/physician	1	*	1	*	0	*	75	$349,555
Procedures/provider	0	*	1	*	0	*	52	853
Gross charges/provider	1	*	1	*	0	*	53	$280,116
Gross charge to total cost ratio	0	*	1	*	0	*	69	1.59
Oper cost to total cost ratio	0	*	1	*	0	*	69	.61
Prov cost to total cost ratio	0	*	1	*	0	*	69	.39
Total support staff FTE/phy	11	6.03	58	.45	32	.57	85	5.18

Table 12.11h: Nonprocedural Gross Charge Data

	Allergy/Immunology		Anesthesiology		Anesthesiology: Pain Management		Cardiology	
	Count	Median	Count	Median	Count	Median	Count	Median
Gross charges/patient	3	*	0	*	0	*	33	$72.62
Nonproc gross charges/physician	4	*	0	*	0	*	51	$85,312
Gross charges/provider	1	*	0	*	0	*	36	$73,794
Total support staff FTE/phy	11	6.03	58	.45	32	.57	85	5.18

Single Specialty Practices, Not Hospital or IDS Owned — Gastroenterology, Hematology/Oncology, Neurology, Obstetrics/Gynecology

Table 13.1: Staffing and Practice Data

	Gastroenterology		Hematology/Oncology		Neurology		Ob/Gyn	
	Count	Median	Count	Median	Count	Median	Count	Median
Total provider FTE	**24**	**9.45**	**18**	**12.00**	**6**	*****	**38**	**7.75**
Total physician FTE	37	7.13	32	6.50	14	6.75	48	5.15
Total nonphysician provider FTE	24	2.00	18	2.13	6	*	38	2.50
Total support staff FTE	**37**	**31.02**	**32**	**46.55**	**14**	**27.63**	**48**	**28.90**
Number of branch clinics	22	2	1	*	7	*	23	1
Square footage of all facilities	36	10,401	28	13,631	14	13,000	46	10,175

Table 13.2: Accounts Receivable Data, Collection Percentages and Financial Ratios

	Gastroenterology		Hematology/Oncology		Neurology		Ob/Gyn	
	Count	Median	Count	Median	Count	Median	Count	Median
Total AR/physician	**31**	**$196,108**	**27**	**$517,583**	**12**	**$96,745**	**44**	**$125,325**
Total AR/provider	**20**	**$157,268**	**14**	**$542,366**	**4**	*****	**35**	**$90,609**
0-30 days in AR	31	57.16%	27	58.92%	12	53.52%	44	58.50%
31-60 days in AR	31	16.77%	27	16.34%	12	16.42%	44	15.62%
61-90 days in AR	31	7.50%	27	6.32%	12	8.03%	44	7.19%
91-120 days in AR	31	5.18%	27	3.88%	12	5.04%	44	4.18%
120+ days in AR	31	14.08%	27	12.77%	12	17.23%	44	10.83%
Re-aged: 0-30 days in AR	6	*	5	*	4	*	11	63.25%
Re-aged: 31-60 days in AR	6	*	5	*	4	*	11	17.87%
Re-aged: 61-90 days in AR	6	*	5	*	4	*	11	6.93%
Re-aged: 91-120 days in AR	6	*	5	*	4	*	11	3.49%
Re-aged: 120+ days in AR	6	*	5	*	4	*	11	7.42%
Not re-aged: 0-30 days in AR	23	57.16%	21	58.92%	6	*	32	58.35%
Not re-aged: 31-60 days in AR	23	16.77%	21	16.99%	6	*	32	14.10%
Not re-aged: 61-90 days in AR	23	7.84%	21	6.58%	6	*	32	7.33%
Not re-aged: 91-120 days in AR	23	5.18%	21	3.75%	6	*	32	4.25%
Not re-aged: 120+ days in AR	23	14.19%	21	12.77%	6	*	32	11.07%
Months gross FFS charges in AR	29	1.43	5	*	10	1.59	39	1.47
Days gross FFS charges in AR	29	43.40	5	*	10	48.45	39	44.71
Gross FFS collection %	35	48.59%	5	*	12	63.87%	43	65.05%
Adjusted FFS collection %	31	97.23%	5	*	11	98.01%	40	98.92%
Gross FFS + cap collection %	0	*	0	*	1	*	3	*
Net cap rev % of gross cap chrg	0	*	0	*	1	*	2	*
Current ratio	17	1.24	0	*	5	*	22	1.20
Tot asset turnover ratio	17	12.90	0	*	5	*	22	6.93
Debt to equity ratio	17	1.23	0	*	5	*	22	2.33
Debt ratio	17	55.06%	0	*	5	*	22	69.76%
Return on total assets	17	12.36%	0	*	5	*	22	7.85%
Return on equity	17	40.87%	0	*	5	*	22	36.16%

Table 13.3: Breakout of Total Gross Charges by Type of Payer

	Gastroenterology		Hematology/Oncology		Neurology		Ob/Gyn	
	Count	Median	Count	Median	Count	Median	Count	Median
Medicare: fee-for-service	36	33.50%	29	42.70%	13	25.00%	45	3.00%
Medicare: managed care FFS	36	.00%	29	.00%	13	3.00%	45	.00%
Medicare: capitation	36	.00%	29	.00%	13	.00%	45	.00%
Medicaid: fee-for-service	36	2.85%	29	1.50%	13	2.00%	45	4.00%
Medicaid: managed care FFS	36	.00%	29	.00%	13	.00%	45	.00%
Medicaid: capitation	36	.00%	29	.00%	13	.00%	45	.00%
Commercial: fee-for-service	36	33.50%	29	23.00%	13	18.71%	45	25.60%
Commercial: managed care FFS	36	12.00%	29	27.00%	13	35.00%	45	35.00%
Commercial: capitation	36	.00%	29	.00%	13	.00%	45	.00%
Workers' compensation	36	.00%	29	.00%	13	1.30%	45	.00%
Charity care and prof courtesy	36	.35%	29	.00%	13	.25%	45	.00%
Self-pay	36	2.70%	29	1.00%	13	3.00%	45	3.00%
Other federal government payers	36	.00%	29	.00%	13	.00%	45	.00%

Single Specialty Practices, Not Hospital or IDS Owned — Gastroenterology, Hematology/Oncology, Neurology, Obstetrics/Gynecology (per FTE Physician)

Table 13.4a: Staffing, RVUs, Patients, Procedures and Square Footage

	Gastroenterology		Hematology/Oncology		Neurology		Ob/Gyn	
	Count	Median	Count	Median	Count	Median	Count	Median
Total provider FTE/physician	**24**	**1.26**	**18**	**1.32**	**6**	*	**38**	**1.38**
Prim care phy/physician	2	*	0	*	0	*	3	*
Nonsurg phy/physician	27	1.00	1	*	12	1.00	3	*
Surg spec phy/physician	6	*	0	*	0	*	34	1.00
Total NPP FTE/physician	24	.26	18	.32	6	*	38	.38
Total support staff FTE/phy	**37**	**4.46**	**32**	**6.99**	**14**	**3.54**	**48**	**4.62**
Total empl support staff FTE	35	4.46	5	*	12	3.27	42	4.55
General administrative	33	.25	5	*	11	.29	42	.28
Patient accounting	33	.67	5	*	11	.63	41	.67
General accounting	22	.11	3	*	6	*	17	.08
Managed care administrative	5	*	0	*	1	*	7	*
Information technology	6	*	2	*	5	*	6	*
Housekeeping, maint, security	7	*	1	*	0	*	1	*
Medical receptionists	33	.80	4	*	11	.75	42	1.05
Med secretaries,transcribers	21	.25	4	*	8	*	18	.23
Medical records	29	.44	4	*	9	*	35	.38
Other admin support	13	.57	2	*	6	*	16	.17
*Total administrative supp staff	13	2.94	29	3.25	6	*	21	2.57
Registered Nurses	23	.59	5	*	6	*	32	.43
Licensed Practical Nurses	19	.40	3	*	3	*	28	.42
Med assistants, nurse aides	32	.68	4	*	5	*	36	.92
*Total clinical supp staff	22	1.51	30	2.58	6	*	34	1.70
Clinical laboratory	2	*	3	*	1	*	12	.20
Radiology and imaging	2	*	1	*	2	*	30	.22
Other medical support serv	7	*	1	*	8	*	2	*
*Total ancillary supp staff	0	*	23	.95	3	*	9	*
Tot contracted supp staff	13	.14	12	.42	6	*	18	.10
Tot RVU/physician	11	16,412	10	11,141	6	*	14	14,779
Physician work RVU/physician	9	*	8	*	7	*	8	*
Patients/physician	14	2,025	0	*	7	*	15	2,220
Tot procedures/physician	33	4,887	3	*	11	5,071	27	7,308
Square feet/physician	36	1,443	28	1,964	14	1,895	46	1,854

*See pages 260 and 261 for definition.

Table 13.4b: Charges and Revenue

	Gastroenterology		Hematology/Oncology		Neurology		Ob/Gyn	
	Count	Median	Count	Median	Count	Median	Count	Median
Net fee-for-service revenue	36	$762,131	5	*	12	$492,277	43	$663,067
Gross FFS charges	35	$1,612,819	5	*	12	$730,397	43	$1,027,629
Adjustments to FFS charges	30	$816,132	5	*	11	$242,871	39	$347,623
Adjusted FFS charges	31	$784,768	5	*	11	$514,099	40	$625,559
Bad debts due to FFS activity	29	$17,299	4	*	10	$12,296	36	$8,028
Net capitation revenue	0	*	0	*	1	*	3	*
Gross capitation charges	0	*	0	*	1	*	2	*
Capitation revenue	0	*	0	*	1	*	3	*
Purch serv for cap patients	0	*	0	*	0	*	0	*
Net other medical revenue	16	$14,283	0	*	9	*	18	$5,173
Gross rev from other activity	15	$18,791	0	*	9	*	15	$5,505
Other medical revenue	15	$18,791	0	*	8	*	13	$5,505
Rev from sale of goods/services	2	*	0	*	4	*	7	*
Cost of sales	3	*	0	*	2	*	1	*
Total gross charges	**37**	**$1,612,819**	**31**	**$4,245,902**	**14**	**$759,562**	**48**	**$1,032,250**
Total medical revenue	**37**	**$765,124**	**32**	**$2,722,930**	**14**	**$535,115**	**48**	**$686,222**

Single Specialty Practices, Not Hospital or IDS Owned — Gastroenterology, Hematology/Oncology, Neurology, Obstetrics/Gynecology (per FTE Physician)

Table 13.4c: Operating Cost

	Gastroenterology		Hematology/Oncology		Neurology		Ob/Gyn	
	Count	Median	Count	Median	Count	Median	Count	Median
Total support staff cost/phy	37	$167,333	32	$370,709	14	$152,183	48	$172,199
Total empl supp staff cost/phy	36	$138,971	5	*	12	$105,276	42	$140,858
General administrative	34	$19,070	5	*	11	$19,280	42	$16,553
Patient accounting	33	$17,943	5	*	11	$17,731	41	$19,432
General accounting	22	$3,757	3	*	6	*	17	$3,560
Managed care administrative	5	*	0	*	1	*	7	*
Information technology	6	*	2	*	5	*	6	*
Housekeeping, maint, security	7	*	1	*	0		1	*
Medical receptionists	34	$18,070	4	*	11	$18,853	41	$24,773
Med secretaries,transcribers	22	$7,182	4	*	8	*	17	$5,092
Medical records	30	$8,997	4	*	9	*	34	$7,286
Other admin support	13	$13,536	2	*	6	*	16	$4,931
*Total administrative supp staff	10	$89,230	28	$136,374	6	*	19	$71,942
Registered Nurses	24	$28,399	5	*	6	*	32	$17,320
Licensed Practical Nurses	19	$14,105	3	*	3	*	28	$11,935
Med assistants, nurse aides	32	$17,441	4	*	5	*	36	$23,650
*Total clinical supp staff	21	$48,887	29	$117,564	5	*	33	$53,609
Clinical laboratory	2	*	3	*	1	*	12	$7,339
Radiology and imaging	2	*	1	*	2	*	30	$12,064
Other medical support serv	7	*	2	*	8	*	3	*
*Total ancillary supp staff	0	*	22	$39,126	3	*	14	$20,717
Total empl supp staff benefits	36	$36,121	31	$68,325	14	$31,449	45	$37,492
Tot contracted supp staff	17	$2,715	14	$11,545	7	*	22	$2,289
Total general operating cost	37	$150,386	32	$1,536,601	14	$176,227	48	$177,896
Information technology	36	$11,920	4	*	11	$14,773	42	$10,074
Medical and surgical supply	35	$23,397	4	*	12	$10,735	42	$17,284
Building and occupancy	36	$37,106	4	*	12	$33,186	42	$42,052
Furniture and equipment	28	$4,522	4	*	12	$12,774	36	$4,695
Admin supplies and services	36	$16,857	4	*	12	$14,344	42	$13,417
Prof liability insurance	37	$13,523	31	$10,845	12	$8,350	47	$36,834
Other insurance premiums	34	$1,998	3	*	12	$2,630	39	$1,440
Outside professional fees	36	$6,304	4	*	12	$7,760	42	$5,872
Promotion and marketing	36	$1,343	4	*	11	$1,383	38	$3,823
Clinical laboratory	10	$2,801	4	*	1	*	22	$3,861
Radiology and imaging	1	*	2	*	3	*	26	$4,304
Other ancillary services	3	*	2	*	6	*	11	$5,819
Billing purchased services	19	$2,111	2	*	7	*	18	$1,367
Management fees paid to MSO	3	*	0	*	1	*	3	*
Misc operating cost	36	$7,326	4	*	12	$9,057	41	$9,790
Cost allocated to prac from par	0	*	0	*	0	*	1	*
Total operating cost	37	$326,677	32	$1,811,639	13	$356,896	48	$349,286

*See pages 260 and 261 for definition.

Single Specialty Practices, Not Hospital or IDS Owned — Gastroenterology, Hematology/Oncology, Neurology, Obstetrics/Gynecology (per FTE Physician)

Table 13.4d: Provider Cost

	Gastroenterology		Hematology/Oncology		Neurology		Ob/Gyn	
	Count	Median	Count	Median	Count	Median	Count	Median
Total med rev after oper cost	37	$451,132	32	$698,398	13	$241,832	48	$321,946
Total provider cost/physician	37	$442,739	32	$599,403	14	$230,363	48	$318,938
Total NPP cost/physician	28	$19,882	18	$23,695	7	*	40	$35,176
Nonphysician provider comp	27	$18,076	0	*	6	*	35	$28,713
Nonphysician prov benefit cost	25	$3,034	0	*	4	*	34	$6,492
Provider consultant cost	1	*	7	*	1	*	3	*
Total physician cost/physician	37	$422,157	32	$578,342	14	$205,252	48	$270,853
Total phy compensation	35	$372,237	1	*	12	$167,963	43	$220,210
Total phy benefit cost	34	$50,995	0	*	12	$33,687	42	$41,526

Table 13.4e: Net Income or Loss

	Gastroenterology		Hematology/Oncology		Neurology		Ob/Gyn	
	Count	Median	Count	Median	Count	Median	Count	Median
Total cost	37	$770,285	32	$2,588,581	14	$509,463	48	$650,252
Net nonmedical revenue	20	$858	19	$7,253	6	*	28	$529
Nonmedical revenue	18	$688	0	*	5	*	25	$1,218
Fin support for oper costs	1	*	0	*	0	*	1	*
Goodwill amortization	1	*	0	*	0	*	1	*
Nonmedical cost	9	*	0	*	2	*	11	$6,710
Net inc, prac with fin sup	1	*	0	*	0	*	1	*
Net inc, prac w/o fin sup	34	$5,756	29	$28,249	13	$14,227	47	$2,865
Net inc, excl fin supp (all prac)	35	$3,167	29	$28,249	13	$14,227	48	$2,778

Table 13.4f: Assets and Liabilities

	Gastroenterology		Hematology/Oncology		Neurology		Ob/Gyn	
	Count	Median	Count	Median	Count	Median	Count	Median
Total assets	19	$67,461	0	*	8	*	25	$83,911
Current assets	19	$31,965	0	*	8	*	25	$32,624
Noncurrent assets	19	$30,176	0	*	8	*	25	$20,795
Total liabilities	19	$42,555	0	*	8	*	25	$44,731
Current liabilities	19	$33,437	0	*	8	*	25	$19,119
Noncurrent liabilities	19	$0	0	*	8	*	25	$11,649
Working capital	19	$3,772	0	*	8	*	25	$5,310
Total net worth	19	$21,370	0	*	8	*	25	$17,255
Total support staff FTE/phy	37	4.46	32	6.99	14	3.54	48	4.62

Single Specialty Practices, Not Hospital or IDS Owned — Gastroenterology, Hematology/Oncology, Neurology, Obstetrics/Gynecology (as a % of Total Medical Revenue)

Table 13.5a: Charges and Revenue

	Gastroenterology		Hematology/Oncology		Neurology		Ob/Gyn	
	Count	Median	Count	Median	Count	Median	Count	Median
Net fee-for-service revenue	36	100.00%	5	*	12	96.36%	43	99.95%
Net capitation revenue	0	*	0	*	1	*	3	*
Net other medical revenue	16	1.76%	0	*	9	*	18	.76%
Total gross charges	37	203.04%	31	165.13%	14	151.04%	48	153.58%

Table 13.5b: Operating Cost

	Gastroenterology		Hematology/Oncology		Neurology		Ob/Gyn	
	Count	Median	Count	Median	Count	Median	Count	Median
Total support staff cost	37	23.31%	32	13.59%	14	26.51%	48	26.91%
Total empl support staff cost	36	18.82%	5	*	12	20.25%	42	21.29%
General administrative	34	2.33%	5	*	11	3.16%	42	2.30%
Patient accounting	33	2.57%	5	*	11	3.61%	41	3.11%
General accounting	22	.54%	3	*	6	*	17	.75%
Managed care administrative	5	*	0	*	1	*	7	*
Information technology	6	*	2	*	5	*	6	*
Housekeeping, maint, security	7	*	1	*	0	*	1	*
Medical receptionists	34	2.39%	4	*	11	2.26%	41	3.47%
Med secretaries,transcribers	22	.92%	4	*	8	*	17	.68%
Medical records	30	1.26%	4	*	9	*	34	.98%
Other admin support	13	1.33%	2	*	6	*	16	.71%
*Total administrative supp staff	10	12.09%	28	5.54%	6	*	19	11.98%
Registered Nurses	24	3.75%	5	*	6	*	32	2.49%
Licensed Practical Nurses	19	1.66%	3	*	3	*	28	1.32%
Med assistants, nurse aides	32	2.18%	4	*	5	*	36	3.41%
*Total clinical supp staff	21	6.39%	29	4.54%	5	*	33	7.63%
Clinical laboratory	2	*	3	*	1	*	12	.92%
Radiology and imaging	2	*	1	*	2	*	30	1.75%
Other medical support serv	7	*	2	*	8	*	3	*
*Total ancillary supp staff	0	*	22	1.61%	3	*	14	3.03%
Total empl supp staff benefits	36	4.64%	31	2.82%	14	5.13%	45	5.51%
Tot contracted supp staff	17	.39%	14	.40%	7	*	22	.35%
Total general operating cost	37	18.25%	32	59.81%	14	28.47%	48	25.27%
Information technology	36	1.42%	4	*	11	2.51%	42	1.60%
Medical and surgical supply	36	2.34%	4	*	12	2.04%	42	2.83%
Building and occupancy	36	4.70%	4	*	12	6.26%	42	7.01%
Furniture and equipment	28	.58%	4	*	12	1.95%	36	.59%
Admin supplies and services	36	1.93%	4	*	12	3.26%	42	1.85%
Prof liability insurance	37	1.89%	31	.37%	12	1.80%	47	5.54%
Other insurance premiums	34	.24%	3	*	12	.54%	39	.20%
Outside professional fees	36	.74%	4	*	12	1.11%	42	.81%
Promotion and marketing	36	.18%	4	*	11	.30%	38	.53%
Clinical laboratory	10	.33%	4	*	1	*	22	.55%
Radiology and imaging	1	*	2	*	3	*	26	.66%
Other ancillary services	3	*	2	*	6	*	11	1.16%
Billing purchased services	19	.21%	2	*	7	*	18	.20%
Management fees paid to MSO	3	*	0	*	1	*	3	*
Misc operating cost	36	.96%	4	*	12	1.35%	41	1.44%
Cost allocated to prac from par	0	*	0	*	0	*	1	*
Total operating cost	37	42.69%	32	75.09%	14	58.23%	48	52.81%

*See pages 260 and 261 for definition.

Single Specialty Practices, Not Hospital or IDS Owned — Gastroenterology, Hematology/Oncology, Neurology, Obstetrics/Gynecology (as a % of Total Medical Revenue)

Table 13.5c: Provider Cost

	Gastroenterology		Hematology/Oncology		Neurology		Ob/Gyn	
	Count	Median	Count	Median	Count	Median	Count	Median
Total med rev after oper cost	37	57.31%	32	25.08%	14	41.77%	48	47.19%
Total provider cost	37	55.23%	32	22.44%	14	40.04%	48	45.73%
Total NPP cost	28	2.52%	18	.78%	7	*	40	4.80%
Nonphysician provider comp	27	2.11%	0	*	6	*	35	3.68%
Nonphysician prov benefit cost	25	.36%	0	*	4	*	34	.80%
Provider consultant cost	1	*	7	*	1	*	3	*
Total physician cost	37	52.81%	32	21.57%	14	35.20%	48	41.90%
Total phy compensation	35	47.12%	1	*	12	29.33%	43	35.86%
Total phy benefit cost	34	5.79%	0	*	12	6.54%	42	6.35%

Table 13.5d: Net Income or Loss

	Gastroenterology		Hematology/Oncology		Neurology		Ob/Gyn	
	Count	Median	Count	Median	Count	Median	Count	Median
Total cost	37	99.60%	32	99.41%	14	97.34%	48	99.78%
Net nonmedical revenue	20	.09%	19	.26%	6	*	30	.07%
Nonmedical revenue	18	.07%	0	*	5	*	25	.28%
Fin support for oper costs	1	*	0	*	0	*	1	*
Goodwill amortization	1	*	0	*	0	*	1	*
Nonmedical cost	9	*	0	*	2	*	11	1.00%
Net inc, prac with fin sup	1	*	0	*	0	*	1	*
Net inc, prac w/o fin sup	34	.82%	29	1.54%	14	2.66%	47	.57%
Net inc, excl fin supp (all prac)	35	.44%	29	1.54%	14	2.66%	48	.55%

Table 13.5e: Assets and Liabilities

	Gastroenterology		Hematology/Oncology		Neurology		Ob/Gyn	
	Count	Median	Count	Median	Count	Median	Count	Median
Total assets	19	7.75%	0	*	8	*	25	14.32%
Current assets	19	3.76%	0	*	8	*	25	4.93%
Noncurrent assets	19	3.73%	0	*	8	*	25	2.93%
Total liabilities	19	5.24%	0	*	8	*	25	6.50%
Current liabilities	19	4.28%	0	*	8	*	25	2.42%
Noncurrent liabilities	19	.00%	0	*	8	*	25	1.68%
Working capital	19	.36%	0	*	8	*	25	.71%
Total net worth	19	2.72%	0	*	8	*	25	2.42%
Total support staff FTE/phy	37	4.46	32	6.99	14	3.54	48	4.62

Single Specialty Practices, Not Hospital or IDS Owned — Gastroenterology, Hematology/Oncology, Neurology, Obstetrics/Gynecology (per FTE Provider)

Table 13.6a: Staffing, RVUs, Patients, Procedures and Square Footage

	Gastroenterology		Hematology/Oncology		Neurology		Ob/Gyn	
	Count	Median	Count	Median	Count	Median	Count	Median
Total physician FTE/provider	24	.79	18	.76	6	*	38	.73
Prim care phy/provider	2	*	0	*	0	*	2	*
Nonsurg phy/provider	20	.80	0	*	5	*	3	*
Surg spec phy/provider	2	*	0	*	0	*	26	.74
Total NPP FTE/provider	24	.21	18	.24	6	*	38	.27
Total support staff FTE/prov	24	3.99	18	6.44	6	*	38	3.19
Total empl supp staff FTE/prov	23	3.97	1	*	5	*	32	3.11
General administrative	23	.25	1	*	5	*	32	.18
Patient accounting	23	.57	1	*	5	*	31	.42
General accounting	17	.10	1	*	2	*	14	.07
Managed care administrative	5	*	0	*	0	*	4	*
Information technology	6	*	1	*	2	*	4	*
Housekeeping, maint, security	4	*	0	*	0	*	1	*
Medical receptionists	23	.66	0	*	5	*	32	.75
Med secretaries,transcribers	13	.20	1	*	5	*	13	.11
Medical records	21	.33	1	*	4	*	27	.29
Other admin support	10	.44	0	*	1	*	13	.15
*Total administrative supp staff	9	*	17	3.26	3	*	15	1.60
Registered Nurses	18	.49	1	*	3	*	23	.32
Licensed Practical Nurses	16	.32	1	*	1	*	21	.33
Med assistants, nurse aides	23	.50	1	*	3	*	28	.57
*Total clinical supp staff	19	1.05	17	2.08	3	*	27	1.16
Clinical laboratory	1	*	1	*	0	*	9	*
Radiology and imaging	1	*	0	*	1	*	22	.18
Other medical support serv	4	*	1	*	5	*	2	*
*Total ancillary supp staff	0	*	15	.69	1	*	8	*
Tot contracted supp staff	8	*	7	*	3	*	17	.09
Tot RVU/provider	7	*	5	*	2	*	10	9,959
Physician work RVU/provider	7	*	3	*	3	*	6	*
Patients/provider	9	*	0	*	4	*	11	1,850
Tot procedures/provider	21	3,909	1	*	4	*	20	4,536
Square feet/provider	24	1,247	15	2,286	6	*	36	1,265
Total support staff FTE/phy	37	4.46	32	6.99	14	3.54	48	4.62

*See pages 260 and 261 for definition.

Table 13.6b: Charges, Revenue and Cost

	Gastroenterology		Hematology/Oncology		Neurology		Ob/Gyn	
	Count	Median	Count	Median	Count	Median	Count	Median
Total gross charges	24	$1,271,854	18	$3,635,827	6	*	38	$718,108
Total medical revenue	24	$625,000	18	$2,253,847	6	*	38	$479,409
Net fee-for-service revenue	23	$609,632	1	*	5	*	33	$466,111
Net capitation revenue	0	*	0	*	0	*	2	*
Net other medical revenue	13	$12,113	0	*	2	*	13	$4,161
Total support staff cost/prov	24	$136,814	18	$290,354	6	*	38	$120,603
Total general operating cost	24	$120,926	18	$1,215,791	6	*	38	$117,903
Total operating cost	24	$257,606	18	$1,570,783	6	*	38	$239,816
Total med rev after oper cost	24	$368,036	18	$563,487	6	*	38	$231,535
Total provider cost/provider	24	$366,603	18	$437,259	6	*	38	$214,273
Total NPP cost/provider	24	$15,502	18	$18,395	6	*	38	$24,376
Provider consultant cost	0	*	4	*	1	*	3	*
Total physician cost/provider	24	$356,680	18	$412,603	6	*	38	$189,931
Total phy compensation	23	$312,183	0	*	5	*	33	$173,056
Total phy benefit cost	23	$39,893	0	*	5	*	32	$29,686
Total cost	24	$617,777	18	$1,979,038	6	*	38	$461,695
Net nonmedical revenue	15	$217	10	$5,250	2	*	22	$173
Net inc, prac with fin sup	0	*	0	*	0	*	0	*
Net inc, prac w/o fin sup	23	$2,082	16	$33,447	6	*	38	$3,049
Net inc, excl fin supp (all prac)	23	$2,082	16	$33,447	6	*	38	$3,049
Total support staff FTE/phy	37	4.46	32	6.99	14	3.54	48	4.62

Single Specialty Practices, Not Hospital or IDS Owned — Gastroenterology, Hematology/Oncology, Neurology, Obstetrics/Gynecology (per Square Foot)

Table 13.7a: Staffing, RVUs, Patients and Procedures

	Gastroenterology		Hematology/Oncology		Neurology		Ob/Gyn	
	Count	Median	Count	Median	Count	Median	Count	Median
Total prov FTE/10,000 sq ft	24	8.03	15	4.37	6	*	36	7.90
Total phy FTE/10,000 sq ft	36	6.94	28	5.09	14	5.28	46	5.40
Prim care phy/10,000 sq ft	2	*	0	*	0	*	3	*
Nonsurg phy/10,000 sq ft	27	7.22	1	*	12	5.51	3	*
Surg spec phy/10,000 sq ft	6	*	0	*	0	*	33	5.66
Total NPP FTE/10,000 sq ft	24	1.60	15	1.05	6	*	36	2.23
Total supp stf FTE/10,000 sq ft	36	32.68	28	30.68	14	23.56	46	25.72
Total empl supp stf/10,000 sq ft	35	32.39	4	*	12	20.60	40	25.45
General administrative	33	1.89	4	*	11	2.15	40	1.42
Patient accounting	33	4.64	4	*	11	4.00	39	4.17
General accounting	22	.96	2	*	6	*	17	.49
Managed care administrative	5	*	0	*	1	*	6	*
Information technology	6	*	1	*	5	*	6	*
Housekeeping, maint, security	7	*	0	*	0	*	1	*
Medical receptionists	33	5.00	3	*	11	4.00	40	5.53
Med secretaries,transcribers	21	1.78	3	*	8	*	16	1.02
Medical records	29	3.13	3	*	9	*	34	2.14
Other admin support	13	3.18	1	*	6	*	15	.88
*Total administrative supp staff	13	18.09	26	15.28	6	*	20	14.40
Registered Nurses	23	3.15	4	*	6	*	30	2.35
Licensed Practical Nurses	19	2.10	2	*	3	*	27	1.89
Med assistants, nurse aides	32	4.74	4	*	5	*	34	5.42
*Total clinical supp staff	22	8.94	27	9.91	6	*	32	9.28
Clinical laboratory	2	*	3	*	1	*	11	1.43
Radiology and imaging	2	*	1	*	2	*	29	1.33
Other medical support serv	7	*	1	*	8	*	1	*
*Total ancillary supp staff	0	*	21	4.38	3	*	8	*
Tot contracted supp staff	13	1.43	11	1.30	6	*	18	.55
Tot RVU/sq ft	11	7.69	7	*	6	*	14	9.21
Physician work RVU/sq ft	9	*	5	*	7	*	8	*
Patients/sq ft	14	1.21	0	*	7	*	13	1.10
Tot procedures/sq ft	32	3.38	2	*	11	3.44	25	3.41
Total support staff FTE/phy	37	4.46	32	6.99	14	3.54	48	4.62

*See pages 260 and 261 for definition.

Table 13.7b: Charges, Revenue and Cost

	Gastroenterology		Hematology/Oncology		Neurology		Ob/Gyn	
	Count	Median	Count	Median	Count	Median	Count	Median
Total gross charges	36	$1,098.79	27	$1,725.55	14	$534.55	46	$572.71
Total medical revenue	36	$514.34	28	$1,126.11	14	$357.30	46	$363.10
Net fee-for-service revenue	35	$510.51	4	*	12	$340.47	41	$363.09
Net capitation revenue	0	*	0	*	1	*	3	*
Net other medical revenue	16	$12.10	0	*	9	*	16	$2.72
Total support staff cost/sq ft	36	$126.63	28	$139.74	14	$92.51	46	$88.64
Total general operating cost	36	$96.05	28	$666.28	14	$94.15	46	$97.03
Total operating cost	36	$216.61	28	$812.35	14	$184.89	46	$178.53
Total med rev after oper cost	36	$301.93	28	$287.11	14	$179.24	46	$179.78
Total provider cost/sq ft	36	$301.45	28	$270.10	14	$158.18	46	$173.19
Total NPP cost/sq ft	28	$12.60	15	$8.11	7	*	38	$18.99
Provider consultant cost	1	*	7	*	1	*	3	*
Total physician cost/sq ft	36	$290.27	28	$232.96	14	$134.72	46	$155.53
Total phy compensation	34	$266.65	1	*	12	$115.50	41	$138.85
Total phy benefit cost	33	$32.88	0	*	12	$22.28	40	$23.89
Total cost	36	$518.90	28	$1,080.36	14	$330.63	46	$358.54
Net nonmedical revenue/sq ft	19	$.31	16	$1.54	6	*	28	$.24
Net inc, prac with fin sup	1	*	0	*	0	*	1	*
Net inc, prac w/o fin sup	33	$5.17	25	$13.45	14	$12.83	45	$1.64
Net inc, excl fin supp (all prac)	34	$4.28	25	$13.45	14	$12.83	46	$1.30
Total support staff FTE/phy	37	4.46	32	6.99	14	3.54	48	4.62

Single Specialty Practices, Not Hospital or IDS Owned — Gastroenterology, Hematology/Oncology, Neurology, Obstetrics/Gynecology (per Total RVU)

Table 13.8a: Staffing, Patients, Procedures and Square Footage

	Gastroenterology		Hematology/Oncology		Neurology		Ob/Gyn	
	Count	Median	Count	Median	Count	Median	Count	Median
Total prov FTE/10,000 tot RVU	7	*	5	*	2	*	10	1.02
Total phy FTE/10,000 tot RVU	11	.61	10	.90	6	*	14	.68
Prim care phy/10,000 tot RVU	1	*	0	*	0	*	0	*
Nonsurg phy/10,000 tot RVU	9	*	0	*	6	*	0	*
Surg spec phy/10,000 tot RVU	2	*	0	*	0	*	13	.69
Total NPP FTE/10,000 tot RVU	7	*	5	*	2	*	10	.25
Total supp stf FTE/10,000 tot RVU	11	3.30	10	4.35	6	*	14	2.78
Tot empl supp stf/10,000 tot RVU	11	3.24	1	*	6	*	13	2.79
General administrative	11	.14	1	*	5	*	12	.14
Patient accounting	11	.36	1	*	5	*	12	.46
General accounting	8	*	1	*	3	*	6	*
Managed care administrative	2	*	0	*	1	*	3	*
Information technology	4	*	1	*	2	*	2	*
Housekeeping, maint, security	5	*	1	*	0	*	0	*
Medical receptionists	11	.65	1	*	5	*	12	.69
Med secretaries,transcribers	8	*	1	*	3	*	5	*
Medical records	10	.38	1	*	3	*	10	.29
Other admin support	5	*	1	*	3	*	4	*
*Total administrative supp staff	5	*	9	*	3	*	6	*
Registered Nurses	10	.32	1	*	2	*	9	*
Licensed Practical Nurses	8	*	1	*	1	*	7	*
Med assistants, nurse aides	11	.55	0	*	2	*	10	.55
*Total clinical supp staff	9	*	9	*	2	*	10	1.00
Clinical laboratory	0	*	0	*	0	*	6	*
Radiology and imaging	1	*	0	*	1	*	10	.13
Other medical support serv	4	*	0	*	4	*	1	*
*Total ancillary supp staff	0	*	5	*	1	*	2	*
Tot contracted supp staff	5	*	2	*	2	*	5	*
Physician work RVU/tot RVU	7	*	8	*	5	*	7	*
Patients/tot RVU	6	*	0	*	4	*	3	*
Tot procedures/tot RVU	10	.29	1	*	6	*	6	*
Square feet/tot RVU	11	.13	7	*	6	*	14	.11
Total support staff FTE/phy	37	4.46	32	6.99	14	3.54	48	4.62

*See pages 260 and 261 for definition.

Table 13.8b: Charges, Revenue and Cost

	Gastroenterology		Hematology/Oncology		Neurology		Ob/Gyn	
	Count	Median	Count	Median	Count	Median	Count	Median
Total gross charges	11	$103.60	10	$325.83	6	*	14	$71.54
Total medical revenue	11	$52.04	10	$205.56	6	*	14	$42.89
Net fee-for-service revenue	11	$50.96	1	*	6	*	13	$43.64
Net capitation revenue	0	*	0	*	0	*	1	*
Net other medical revenue	5	*	0	*	5	*	8	*
Total supp staff cost/tot RVU	11	$15.15	10	$21.89	6	*	14	$11.24
Total general operating cost	11	$11.67	10	$130.33	6	*	14	$10.82
Total operating cost	11	$26.81	10	$152.50	6	*	14	$22.36
Total med rev after oper cost	11	$27.78	10	$44.87	6	*	14	$21.97
Total provider cost/tot RVU	11	$32.33	10	$35.58	6	*	14	$22.05
Total NPP cost/tot RVU	8	*	5	*	2	*	10	$2.23
Provider consultant cost	1	*	2	*	0	*	1	*
Total physician cost/tot RVU	11	$28.70	10	$35.58	6	*	14	$18.54
Total phy compensation	11	$25.27	0	*	6	*	13	$14.78
Total phy benefit cost	11	$3.62	0	*	6	*	12	$3.47
Total cost	10	$98.41	1	*	6	*	9	*
Net nonmedical revenue	5	*	7	*	3	*	9	*
Net inc, prac with fin sup	1	*	0	*	0	*	1	*
Net inc, prac w/o fin sup	8	*	9	*	6	*	13	$.44
Net inc, excl fin supp (all prac)	9	*	9	*	6	*	14	$.43
Total support staff FTE/phy	37	4.46	32	6.99	14	3.54	48	4.62

Single Specialty Practices, Not Hospital or IDS Owned — Gastroenterology, Hematology/Oncology, Neurology, Obstetrics/Gynecology (per Work RVU)

Table 13.9a: Staffing, Patients, Procedures and Square Footage

	Gastroenterology		Hematology/Oncology		Neurology		Ob/Gyn	
	Count	Median	Count	Median	Count	Median	Count	Median
Total prov FTE/10,000 work RVU	7	*	3	*	3	*	6	*
Tot phy FTE/10,000 work RVU	9	*	8	*	7	*	8	*
Prim care phy/10,000 work RVU	1	*	0	*	0	*	0	*
Nonsurg phy/10,000 work RVU	7	*	0	*	7	*	0	*
Surg spec phy/10,000 work RVU	2	*	0	*	0	*	7	*
Total NPP FTE/10,000 work RVU	7	*	3	*	3	*	6	*
Total supp stf FTE/10,000 wrk RVU	9	*	8	*	7	*	8	*
Tot empl supp stf/10,000 work RVU	9	*	1	*	7	*	8	*
General administrative	9	*	1	*	7	*	7	*
Patient accounting	9	*	1	*	7	*	7	*
General accounting	6	*	1	*	4	*	3	*
Managed care administrative	0	*	0	*	1	*	2	*
Information technology	3	*	1	*	3	*	2	*
Housekeeping, maint, security	3	*	1	*	0	*	0	*
Medical receptionists	9	*	1	*	7	*	7	*
Med secretaries,transcribers	7	*	1	*	5	*	3	*
Medical records	8	*	1	*	5	*	7	*
Other admin support	4	*	1	*	4	*	2	*
*Total administrative supp staff	4	*	7	*	3	*	0	*
Registered Nurses	9	*	1	*	3	*	5	*
Licensed Practical Nurses	7	*	1	*	1	*	4	*
Med assistants, nurse aides	9	*	0	*	2	*	6	*
*Total clinical supp staff	8	*	7	*	2	*	3	*
Clinical laboratory	0	*	0	*	1	*	2	*
Radiology and imaging	0	*	0	*	1	*	6	*
Other medical support serv	4	*	0	*	5	*	0	*
*Total ancillary supp staff	0	*	4	*	1	*	0	*
Tot contracted supp staff	2	*	2	*	2	*	3	*
Tot RVU/work RVU	7	*	8	*	5	*	7	*
Patients/work RVU	6	*	0	*	6	*	2	*
Tot procedures/work RVU	8	*	1	*	7	*	4	*
Square feet/work RVU	9	*	5	*	7	*	8	*
Total support staff FTE/phy	37	4.46	32	6.99	14	3.54	48	4.62

*See pages 260 and 261 for definition.

Table 13.9b: Charges, Revenue and Cost

	Gastroenterology		Hematology/Oncology		Neurology		Ob/Gyn	
	Count	Median	Count	Median	Count	Median	Count	Median
Total gross charges	9	*	8	*	7	*	8	*
Total medical revenue	9	*	8	*	7	*	8	*
Net fee-for-service revenue	9	*	1	*	7	*	8	*
Net capitation revenue	0	*	0	*	0	*	1	*
Net other medical revenue	5	*	0	*	5	*	4	*
Total supp staff cost/work RVU	9	*	8	*	7	*	8	*
Total general operating cost	9	*	8	*	7	*	8	*
Total operating cost	9	*	8	*	7	*	8	*
Total med rev after oper cost	9	*	8	*	7	*	8	*
Total provider cost/work RVU	9	*	8	*	7	*	8	*
Total NPP cost/work RVU	8	*	3	*	3	*	6	*
Provider consultant cost	1	*	2	*	0	*	0	*
Total physician cost/work RVU	9	*	8	*	7	*	8	*
Total phy compensation	9	*	0	*	7	*	8	*
Total phy benefit cost	9	*	0	*	7	*	7	*
Total cost	9	*	8	*	7	*	8	*
Net nonmedical revenue	3	*	6	*	2	*	6	*
Net inc, prac with fin sup	1	*	0	*	0	*	0	*
Net inc, prac w/o fin sup	7	*	7	*	7	*	8	*
Net inc, excl fin supp (all prac)	8	*	7	*	7	*	8	*
Total support staff FTE/phy	37	4.46	32	6.99	14	3.54	48	4.62

Single Specialty Practices, Not Hospital or IDS Owned — Gastroenterology, Hematology/Oncology, Neurology, Obstetrics/Gynecology (per Patient)

Table 13.10a: Staffing, RVUs, Procedures and Square Footage

	Gastroenterology		Hematology/Oncology		Neurology		Ob/Gyn	
	Count	Median	Count	Median	Count	Median	Count	Median
Total prov FTE/10,000 patients	9	*	0	*	4	*	11	5.41
Total phy FTE/10,000 pat	14	4.94	0	*	7	*	15	4.50
Prim care phy/10,000 pat	1	*	0	*	0	*	1	*
Nonsurg phy/10,000 pat	12	5.37	0	*	7	*	1	*
Surg spec phy/10,000 pat	2	*	0	*	0	*	9	*
Total NPP FTE/10,000 pat	9	*	0	*	4	*	11	1.31
Total supp staff FTE/10,000 pat	14	24.44	0	*	7	*	15	20.33
Total empl supp staff/10,000 pat	14	24.44	0	*	7	*	15	19.40
General administrative	12	.87	0	*	7	*	15	.97
Patient accounting	12	3.12	0	*	7	*	15	1.98
General accounting	7	*	0	*	4	*	4	*
Managed care administrative	0	*	0	*	0	*	4	*
Information technology	3	*	0	*	3	*	3	*
Housekeeping, maint, security	1	*	0	*	0	*	0	*
Medical receptionists	12	3.40	0	*	7	*	15	4.53
Med secretaries,transcribers	8	*	0	*	6	*	7	*
Medical records	10	2.22	0	*	5	*	12	1.41
Other admin support	5	*	0	*	3	*	6	*
*Total administrative supp staff	4	*	0	*	3	*	6	*
Registered Nurses	9	*	0	*	4	*	12	2.41
Licensed Practical Nurses	7	*	0	*	2	*	8	*
Med assistants, nurse aides	11	6.14	0	*	2	*	14	2.81
*Total clinical supp staff	8	*	0	*	3	*	9	*
Clinical laboratory	0	*	0	*	1	*	5	*
Radiology and imaging	0	*	0	*	1	*	11	.79
Other medical support serv	3	*	0	*	5	*	2	*
*Total ancillary supp staff	0	*	0	*	1	*	2	*
Tot contracted supp staff	4	*	0	*	3	*	6	*
Tot RVU/patient	6	*	0	*	4	*	3	*
Physician work RVU/patient	6	*	0	*	6	*	2	*
Tot procedures/patient	12	1.85	0	*	7	*	11	3.53
Square feet/patient	14	.83	0	*	7	*	13	.91
Total support staff FTE/phy	37	4.46	32	6.99	14	3.54	48	4.62

*See pages 260 and 261 for definition.

Table 13.10b: Charges, Revenue and Cost

	Gastroenterology		Hematology/Oncology		Neurology		Ob/Gyn	
	Count	Median	Count	Median	Count	Median	Count	Median
Total gross charges	14	$743.55	0	*	7	*	15	$455.14
Total medical revenue	14	$369.66	0	*	7	*	15	$316.67
Net fee-for-service revenue	14	$369.66	0	*	7	*	15	$315.48
Net capitation revenue	0	*	0	*	0	*	0	*
Net other medical revenue	6	*	0	*	5	*	8	*
Total support staff cost/patient	14	$91.42	0	*	7	*	15	$87.56
Total general operating cost	14	$81.07	0	*	7	*	15	$87.96
Total operating cost	14	$166.69	0	*	7	*	15	$159.23
Total med rev after oper cost	14	$235.40	0	*	7	*	15	$140.77
Total provider cost/patient	14	$234.09	0	*	7	*	15	$135.09
Total NPP cost/patient	10	$10.45	0	*	4	*	13	$12.18
Provider consultant cost	1	*	0	*	0	*	1	*
Total physician cost/patient	14	$228.08	0	*	7	*	15	$122.91
Total phy compensation	14	$197.87	0	*	7	*	15	$99.92
Total phy benefit cost	13	$30.63	0	*	7	*	15	$20.26
Total cost	14	$370.88	0	*	7	*	15	$325.93
Net nonmedical revenue	6	*	0	*	2	*	12	$.07
Net inc, prac with fin sup	1	*	0	*	0	*	1	*
Net inc, prac w/o fin sup	11	$4.02	0	*	7	*	14	$.35
Net inc, excl fin supp (all prac)	12	$3.86	0	*	7	*	15	$.01
Total support staff FTE/phy	37	4.46	32	6.99	14	3.54	48	4.62

Single Specialty Practices, Not Hospital or IDS Owned — Gastroenterology, Hematology/ Oncology, Neurology, Obstetrics/Gynecology (Procedure and Charge Data)

Table 13.11a: Activity Charges to Total Gross Charges Ratios

	Gastroenterology		Hematology/Oncology		Neurology		Ob/Gyn	
	Count	Median	Count	Median	Count	Median	Count	Median
Total proc gross charges	33	100.00%	3	*	11	97.59%	36	99.13%
Medical proc-inside practice	31	11.90%	4	*	11	63.25%	35	24.27%
Medical proc-outside practice	31	8.41%	4	*	10	17.82%	32	.76%
Surg proc-inside practice	20	3.43%	1	*	7	*	32	5.58%
Surg proc-outside practice	29	67.87%	2	*	3	*	35	51.48%
Laboratory procedures	17	.22%	3	*	1	*	34	2.65%
Radiology procedures	8	*	2	*	3	*	34	9.12%
Tot nonproc gross charges	13	2.59%	3	*	9	*	29	1.00%
Total support staff FTE/phy	37	4.46	32	6.99	14	3.54	48	4.62

Table 13.11b: Medical Procedure Data (inside the practice)

	Gastroenterology		Hematology/Oncology		Neurology		Ob/Gyn	
	Count	Median	Count	Median	Count	Median	Count	Median
Gross charges/procedure	30	$124.11	4	*	11	$152.54	32	$87.71
Total cost/procedure	28	$109.62	3	*	10	$99.69	25	$74.35
Operating cost/procedure	28	$69.10	3	*	10	$50.53	24	$45.10
Provider cost/procedure	29	$43.07	3	*	11	$47.19	26	$28.19
Procedures/patient	12	.91	0	*	7	*	13	1.47
Gross charges/patient	12	$138.18	0	*	7	*	14	$117.53
Procedures/physician	32	1,672	4	*	11	3,667	32	2,748
Gross charges/physician	31	$220,187	4	*	11	$553,551	35	$247,159
Procedures/provider	21	1,404	1	*	4	*	23	1,973
Gross charges/provider	21	$178,528	1	*	4	*	25	$188,273
Gross charge to total cost ratio	28	1.05	3	*	10	1.43	25	1.01
Oper cost to total cost ratio	28	.64	3	*	10	.61	25	.60
Prov cost to total cost ratio	28	.36	3	*	10	.39	25	.40
Total support staff FTE/phy	37	4.46	32	6.99	14	3.54	48	4.62

Table 13.11c: Medical Procedure Data (outside the practice)

	Gastroenterology		Hematology/Oncology		Neurology		Ob/Gyn	
	Count	Median	Count	Median	Count	Median	Count	Median
Gross charges/procedure	30	$130.69	4	*	10	$127.70	31	$122.74
Total cost/procedure	28	$50.40	3	*	9	*	24	$51.54
Operating cost/procedure	28	$13.47	3	*	9	*	24	$20.61
Provider cost/procedure	29	$34.70	3	*	10	$42.91	25	$32.34
Procedures/patient	11	.41	0	*	6	*	14	.04
Gross charges/patient	12	$68.15	0	*	6	*	14	$5.60
Procedures/physician	30	1,056	4	*	10	533	31	66
Gross charges/physician	31	$159,270	4	*	10	$114,991	32	$9,334
Procedures/provider	20	821	1	*	3	*	22	48
Gross charges/provider	21	$115,832	1	*	3	*	23	$6,226
Gross charge to total cost ratio	28	2.55	3	*	9	*	24	2.23
Oper cost to total cost ratio	28	.28	3	*	9	*	24	.39
Prov cost to total cost ratio	28	.72	3	*	9	*	24	.61
Total support staff FTE/phy	37	4.46	32	6.99	14	3.54	48	4.62

Single Specialty Practices, Not Hospital or IDS Owned — Gastroenterology, Hematology/Oncology, Neurology, Obstetrics/Gynecology (Procedure and Charge Data)

Table 13.11d: Surgery/Anesthesia Procedure Data (inside the practice)

	Gastroenterology		Hematology/Oncology		Neurology		Ob/Gyn	
	Count	Median	Count	Median	Count	Median	Count	Median
Gross charges/procedure	20	$318.00	1	*	7	*	29	$209.45
Total cost/procedure	18	$296.96	0	*	7	*	22	$209.35
Operating cost/procedure	18	$140.64	0	*	7	*	22	$125.29
Provider cost/procedure	19	$97.41	0	*	7	*	23	$86.03
Procedures/patient	6	*	0	*	4	*	13	.09
Gross charges/patient	6	*	0	*	4	*	14	$25.11
Procedures/physician	20	421	1	*	7	*	29	271
Gross charges/physician	20	$54,019	1	*	7	*	32	$54,209
Procedures/provider	13	123	0	*	1	*	22	179
Gross charges/provider	13	$25,478	0	*	1	*	24	$39,038
Gross charge to total cost ratio	18	1.25	0	*	7	*	22	1.03
Oper cost to total cost ratio	18	.62	0	*	7	*	22	.60
Prov cost to total cost ratio	18	.38	0	*	7	*	22	.40
Total support staff FTE/phy	37	4.46	32	6.99	14	3.54	48	4.62

Table 13.11e: Surgery/Anesthesia Procedure Data (outside the practice)

	Gastroenterology		Hematology/Oncology		Neurology		Ob/Gyn	
	Count	Median	Count	Median	Count	Median	Count	Median
Gross charges/procedure	28	$729.15	2	*	3	*	33	$1,393.35
Total cost/procedure	26	$244.82	1	*	3	*	26	$557.33
Operating cost/procedure	26	$68.88	1	*	3	*	26	$202.42
Provider cost/procedure	27	$193.68	1	*	3	*	27	$354.47
Procedures/patient	11	.75	0	*	3	*	14	.13
Gross charges/patient	11	$582.39	0	*	3	*	14	$213.25
Procedures/physician	29	1,527	2	*	3	*	33	369
Gross charges/physician	29	$1,009,575	2	*	3	*	35	$517,349
Procedures/provider	19	1,241	0	*	1	*	24	252
Gross charges/provider	20	$825,912	0	*	1	*	25	$354,405
Gross charge to total cost ratio	26	2.55	1	*	3	*	26	2.25
Oper cost to total cost ratio	26	.28	1	*	3	*	26	.39
Prov cost to total cost ratio	26	.72	1	*	3	*	26	.61
Total support staff FTE/phy	37	4.46	32	6.99	14	3.54	48	4.62

Single Specialty Practices, Not Hospital or IDS Owned — Gastroenterology, Hematology/Oncology, Neurology, Obstetrics/Gynecology (Procedure and Charge Data)

Table 13.11f: Clinical Laboratory/Pathology Procedure Data

	Gastroenterology		Hematology/Oncology		Neurology		Ob/Gyn	
	Count	Median	Count	Median	Count	Median	Count	Median
Gross charges/procedure	17	$18.39	3	*	1	*	32	$18.29
Total cost/procedure	15	$9.63	3	*	1	*	25	$12.99
Operating cost/procedure	15	$5.86	3	*	1	*	25	$6.93
Provider cost/procedure	16	$4.14	3	*	1	*	26	$4.68
Procedures/patient	5	*	0	*	0	*	14	.49
Gross charges/patient	5	*	0	*	0	*	14	$7.68
Procedures/physician	17	163	3	*	1	*	32	1,621
Gross charges/physician	17	$4,410	3	*	1	*	34	$21,932
Procedures/provider	12	160	1	*	0	*	24	1,230
Gross charges/provider	12	$2,165	1	*	0	*	25	$14,254
Gross charge to total cost ratio	15	1.44	3	*	1	*	25	1.42
Oper cost to total cost ratio	15	.62	3	*	1	*	25	.63
Prov cost to total cost ratio	15	.38	3	*	1	*	25	.37
Total support staff FTE/phy	37	4.46	32	6.99	14	3.54	48	4.62

Table 13.11g: Diagnostic Radiology and Imaging Procedure Data

	Gastroenterology		Hematology/Oncology		Neurology		Ob/Gyn	
	Count	Median	Count	Median	Count	Median	Count	Median
Gross charges/procedure	7	*	2	*	3	*	32	$195.85
Total cost/procedure	6	*	2	*	3	*	25	$134.54
Operating cost/procedure	6	*	2	*	3	*	25	$90.49
Provider cost/procedure	7	*	2	*	3	*	26	$52.93
Procedures/patient	4	*	0	*	2	*	14	.24
Gross charges/patient	4	*	0	*	2	*	14	$40.24
Procedures/physician	7	*	2	*	3	*	32	499
Gross charges/physician	8	*	2	*	3	*	34	$90,144
Procedures/provider	6	*	1	*	2	*	24	308
Gross charges/provider	7	*	1	*	2	*	25	$66,279
Gross charge to total cost ratio	6	*	2	*	3	*	25	1.35
Oper cost to total cost ratio	6	*	2	*	3	*	25	.63
Prov cost to total cost ratio	6	*	2	*	3	*	25	.37
Total support staff FTE/phy	37	4.46	32	6.99	14	3.54	48	4.62

Table 13.11h: Nonprocedural Gross Charge Data

	Gastroenterology		Hematology/Oncology		Neurology		Ob/Gyn	
	Count	Median	Count	Median	Count	Median	Count	Median
Gross charges/patient	4	*	0	*	6	*	12	$2.99
Nonproc gross charges/physician	13	$48,396	3	*	9	*	29	$9,964
Gross charges/provider	11	$38,432	1	*	4	*	20	$5,762
Total support staff FTE/phy	37	4.46	32	6.99	14	3.54	48	4.62

Single Specialty Practices, Not Hospital or IDS Owned — Opthalmology, Orthopedic Surgery, Otorhinolaryngology

Table 14.1: Staffing and Practice Data

	Ophthalmology		Orthopedic Surgery		Otorhinolaryngology	
	Count	Median	Count	Median	Count	Median
Total provider FTE	16	11.30	78	13.30	9	*
Total physician FTE	21	8.00	100	8.40	14	5.00
Total nonphysician provider FTE	16	2.65	78	4.00	9	*
Total support staff FTE	21	51.67	100	48.15	14	30.05
Number of branch clinics	15	4	72	2	12	2
Square footage of all facilities	19	23,000	98	20,450	14	10,000

Table 14.2: Accounts Receivable Data, Collection Percentages and Financial Ratios

	Ophthalmology		Orthopedic Surgery		Otorhinolaryngology	
	Count	Median	Count	Median	Count	Median
Total AR/physician	16	$158,243	95	$323,596	11	$195,933
Total AR/provider	12	$108,251	74	$213,252	8	*
0-30 days in AR	16	50.50%	95	45.54%	11	53.11%
31-60 days in AR	16	13.93%	95	17.40%	11	16.00%
61-90 days in AR	16	7.61%	95	8.91%	11	8.02%
91-120 days in AR	16	4.04%	95	5.96%	11	4.20%
120+ days in AR	16	16.72%	95	19.73%	11	15.27%
Re-aged: 0-30 days in AR	6	*	22	51.59%	3	*
Re-aged: 31-60 days in AR	6	*	22	16.29%	3	*
Re-aged: 61-90 days in AR	6	*	22	8.34%	3	*
Re-aged: 91-120 days in AR	6	*	22	4.98%	3	*
Re-aged: 120+ days in AR	6	*	22	16.45%	3	*
Not re-aged: 0-30 days in AR	9	*	68	44.39%	8	*
Not re-aged: 31-60 days in AR	9	*	68	17.70%	8	*
Not re-aged: 61-90 days in AR	9	*	68	9.18%	8	*
Not re-aged: 91-120 days in AR	9	*	68	6.13%	8	*
Not re-aged: 120+ days in AR	9	*	68	21.09%	8	*
Months gross FFS charges in AR	14	1.45	90	1.87	11	1.42
Days gross FFS charges in AR	14	43.99	90	56.80	11	43.30
Gross FFS collection %	18	63.04%	94	47.77%	14	57.26%
Adjusted FFS collection %	15	98.82%	89	96.82%	13	97.49%
Gross FFS + cap collection %	0	*	4	*	1	*
Net cap rev % of gross cap chrg	0	*	3	*	1	*
Current ratio	11	1.13	51	1.05	8	*
Tot asset turnover ratio	11	5.51	51	6.66	9	*
Debt to equity ratio	11	1.17	51	3.00	9	*
Debt ratio	11	53.98%	51	75.01%	9	*
Return on total assets	11	1.53%	48	3.30%	8	*
Return on equity	11	3.20%	48	11.98%	8	*

Table 14.3: Breakout of Total Gross Charges by Type of Payer

	Ophthalmology		Orthopedic Surgery		Otorhinolaryngology	
	Count	Median	Count	Median	Count	Median
Medicare: fee-for-service	19	43.00%	91	24.00%	12	13.49%
Medicare: managed care FFS	19	.00%	91	.00%	12	.00%
Medicare: capitation	19	.00%	91	.00%	12	.00%
Medicaid: fee-for-service	19	3.00%	91	2.00%	12	9.38%
Medicaid: managed care FFS	19	.00%	91	.00%	12	.00%
Medicaid: capitation	19	.00%	91	.00%	12	.00%
Commercial: fee-for-service	19	30.00%	91	25.00%	12	5.15%
Commercial: managed care FFS	19	10.00%	91	20.00%	12	51.50%
Commercial: capitation	19	.00%	91	.00%	12	.00%
Workers' compensation	19	.50%	91	10.00%	12	.50%
Charity care and prof courtesy	19	.00%	91	.13%	12	1.00%
Self-pay	19	6.00%	91	2.40%	12	3.75%
Other federal government payers	19	.00%	91	.00%	12	.00%

Single Specialty Practices, Not Hospital or IDS Owned — Opthalmology, Orthopedic Surgery, Otorhinolaryngology (per FTE Physician)

Table 14.4a: Staffing, RVUs, Patients, Procedures and Square Footage

	Ophthalmology		Orthopedic Surgery		Otorhinolaryngology	
	Count	Median	Count	Median	Count	Median
Total provider FTE/physician	16	**1.38**	78	**1.40**	9	*
Prim care phy/physician	2	*	6	*	0	*
Nonsurg phy/physician	1	*	54	.10	1	*
Surg spec phy/physician	15	1.00	95	.95	12	1.00
Total NPP FTE/physician	16	.38	78	.40	9	*
Total support staff FTE/phy	21	**8.25**	100	**5.42**	14	**5.19**
Total empl support staff FTE	17	9.31	93	5.44	14	5.10
General administrative	18	.43	97	.29	14	.24
Patient accounting	18	.87	96	.88	14	.92
General accounting	13	.14	69	.12	10	.20
Managed care administrative	3	*	26	.10	2	*
Information technology	6	*	41	.09	3	*
Housekeeping, maint, security	6	*	26	.09	2	*
Medical receptionists	18	1.77	96	.99	14	1.02
Med secretaries,transcribers	13	.20	87	.50	10	.32
Medical records	14	.37	89	.39	11	.38
Other admin support	12	.19	48	.23	8	*
***Total administrative supp staff**	4	*	34	**3.64**	5	*
Registered Nurses	4	*	55	.30	10	.27
Licensed Practical Nurses	2	*	36	.25	11	.63
Med assistants, nurse aides	14	3.46	81	.80	12	1.11
***Total clinical supp staff**	4	*	44	**1.26**	10	**1.88**
Clinical laboratory	2	*	3	*	1	*
Radiology and imaging	1	*	96	.50	2	*
Other medical support serv	11	1.52	53	.50	8	*
***Total ancillary supp staff**	1	*	26	**1.02**	2	*
Tot contracted supp staff	7	*	33	.18	7	*
Tot RVU/physician	4	*	34	17,956	4	*
Physician work RVU/physician	2	*	25	8,465	2	*
Patients/physician	9	*	38	1,391	5	*
Tot procedures/physician	16	10,914	71	7,635	10	10,539
Square feet/physician	19	3,167	98	2,414	14	1,982

*See pages 260 and 261 for definition.

Table 14.4b: Charges and Revenue

	Ophthalmology		Orthopedic Surgery		Otorhinolaryngology	
	Count	Median	Count	Median	Count	Median
Net fee-for-service revenue	18	$1,006,346	96	$973,330	14	$809,826
Gross FFS charges	18	$1,463,395	95	$2,120,547	14	$1,436,559
Adjustments to FFS charges	16	$543,493	89	$1,025,763	13	$578,701
Adjusted FFS charges	15	$961,643	90	$1,031,525	13	$826,901
Bad debts due to FFS activity	16	$10,057	84	$26,424	13	$13,142
Net capitation revenue	0	*	4	*	1	*
Gross capitation charges	0	*	3	*	1	*
Capitation revenue	0	*	3	*	1	*
Purch serv for cap patients	0	*	0	*	0	*
Net other medical revenue	14	$110,041	55	$9,628	12	$65,949
Gross rev from other activity	12	$182,609	54	$16,002	12	$111,958
Other medical revenue	4	*	30	$3,983	3	*
Rev from sale of goods/services	12	$168,865	38	$22,031	11	$94,162
Cost of sales	12	$65,469	27	$11,171	11	$42,547
Total gross charges	20	**$1,463,395**	99	**$2,138,471**	14	**$1,483,382**
Total medical revenue	21	**$1,031,408**	100	**$998,827**	14	**$862,697**

Single Specialty Practices, Not Hospital or IDS Owned — Opthalmology, Orthopedic Surgery, Otorhinolaryngology (per FTE Physician)

Table 14.4c: Operating Cost

	Ophthalmology		Orthopedic Surgery		Otorhinolaryngology	
	Count	Median	Count	Median	Count	Median
Total support staff cost/phy	**21**	**$299,739**	**100**	**$231,041**	**14**	**$217,126**
Total empl supp staff cost/phy	18	$242,448	95	$180,682	13	$173,585
General administrative	18	$23,435	94	$21,432	13	$15,655
Patient accounting	18	$23,340	93	$25,399	13	$26,256
General accounting	12	$4,288	69	$4,788	9	*
Managed care administrative	3	*	25	$3,446	2	*
Information technology	6	*	39	$4,303	3	*
Housekeeping, maint, security	6	*	24	$2,780	2	*
Medical receptionists	18	$39,519	94	$24,282	13	$25,694
Med secretaries,transcribers	13	$5,543	84	$14,529	9	*
Medical records	14	$6,340	87	$8,386	10	$7,219
Other admin support	12	$6,243	46	$6,227	7	*
*Total administrative supp staff	4	*	31	$112,500	4	*
Registered Nurses	4	*	54	$15,435	9	*
Licensed Practical Nurses	2	*	36	$8,474	10	$22,799
Med assistants, nurse aides	14	$97,529	78	$23,579	11	$24,810
*Total clinical supp staff	4	*	40	$46,452	9	*
Clinical laboratory	2	*	3	*	1	*
Radiology and imaging	1	*	93	$19,162	2	*
Other medical support serv	11	$54,571	53	$16,661	7	*
*Total ancillary supp staff	1	*	29	$31,329	1	*
Total empl supp staff benefits	20	$64,976	97	$46,611	13	$43,694
Tot contracted supp staff	9	*	42	$5,466	8	*
Total general operating cost	**21**	**$253,112**	**100**	**$221,759**	**14**	**$196,645**
Information technology	18	$11,633	96	$14,206	13	$16,070
Medical and surgical supply	18	$19,146	94	$29,084	13	$14,831
Building and occupancy	18	$77,243	96	$59,610	13	$54,602
Furniture and equipment	16	$31,788	83	$6,821	11	$6,345
Admin supplies and services	18	$22,710	95	$18,929	13	$18,697
Prof liability insurance	20	$10,473	99	$26,138	13	$18,248
Other insurance premiums	18	$3,143	91	$2,005	13	$2,484
Outside professional fees	17	$9,041	96	$6,971	13	$6,785
Promotion and marketing	18	$13,559	95	$5,705	12	$6,088
Clinical laboratory	0	*	5	*	2	*
Radiology and imaging	0	*	94	$10,159	4	*
Other ancillary services	2	*	35	$17,445	6	*
Billing purchased services	5	*	51	$3,182	9	*
Management fees paid to MSO	1	*	2	*	1	*
Misc operating cost	17	$15,174	93	$11,089	12	$13,112
Cost allocated to prac from par	0	*	0	*	0	*
Total operating cost	**21**	**$512,682**	**100**	**$450,406**	**14**	**$415,391**

*See pages 260 and 261 for definition.

Single Specialty Practices, Not Hospital or IDS Owned — Opthalmology, Orthopedic Surgery, Otorhinolaryngology (per FTE Physician)

Table 14.4d: Provider Cost

	Ophthalmology		Orthopedic Surgery		Otorhinolaryngology	
	Count	Median	Count	Median	Count	Median
Total med rev after oper cost	21	$504,232	100	$514,861	14	$449,736
Total provider cost/physician	21	$448,959	100	$497,979	14	$411,047
Total NPP cost/physician	16	$52,224	84	$38,568	10	$48,121
Nonphysician provider comp	15	$44,546	79	$30,625	10	$40,363
Nonphysician prov benefit cost	13	$6,834	77	$5,883	10	$8,227
Provider consultant cost	2	*	3	*	1	*
Total physician cost/physician	21	$397,328	100	$475,333	14	$374,399
Total phy compensation	18	$350,840	95	$406,421	14	$324,282
Total phy benefit cost	18	$51,721	93	$62,406	14	$57,563

Table 14.4e: Net Income or Loss

	Ophthalmology		Orthopedic Surgery		Otorhinolaryngology	
	Count	Median	Count	Median	Count	Median
Total cost	21	$1,022,283	100	$997,279	14	$812,632
Net nonmedical revenue	9	*	70	$3,992	7	*
Nonmedical revenue	8	*	63	$5,950	7	*
Fin support for oper costs	0	*	1	*	0	*
Goodwill amortization	3	*	1	*	1	*
Nonmedical cost	9	*	33	$1,153	5	*
Net inc, prac with fin sup	0	*	1	*	0	*
Net inc, prac w/o fin sup	19	$401	94	$2,628	13	$6,117
Net inc, excl fin supp (all prac)	19	$401	95	$2,541	13	$6,117

Table 14.4f: Assets and Liabilities

	Ophthalmology		Orthopedic Surgery		Otorhinolaryngology	
	Count	Median	Count	Median	Count	Median
Total assets	11	$177,002	56	$113,089	9	*
Current assets	11	$34,524	56	$41,067	9	*
Noncurrent assets	11	$142,477	56	$56,566	9	*
Total liabilities	11	$60,808	56	$60,702	9	*
Current liabilities	11	$24,036	56	$35,821	9	*
Noncurrent liabilities	11	$33,502	56	$20,253	9	*
Working capital	11	$1,970	56	$2,839	9	*
Total net worth	11	$66,669	56	$41,021	9	*
Total support staff FTE/phy	21	8.25	100	5.42	14	5.19

Single Specialty Practices, Not Hospital or IDS Owned — Opthalmology, Orthopedic Surgery, Otorhinolaryngology (as a % of Total Medical Revenue)

Table 14.5a: Charges and Revenue

	Ophthalmology		Orthopedic Surgery		Otorhinolaryngology	
	Count	Median	Count	Median	Count	Median
Net fee-for-service revenue	18	95.67%	96	99.78%	14	92.29%
Net capitation revenue	0	*	4	*	1	*
Net other medical revenue	14	9.88%	55	1.05%	12	8.03%
Total gross charges	**20**	**161.75%**	**99**	**208.12%**	**14**	**168.80%**

Table 14.5b: Operating Cost

	Ophthalmology		Orthopedic Surgery		Otorhinolaryngology	
	Count	Median	Count	Median	Count	Median
Total support staff cost	**21**	**29.28%**	**100**	**23.33%**	**14**	**24.39%**
Total empl support staff cost	18	22.88%	95	18.28%	13	18.64%
General administrative	18	2.51%	94	1.94%	13	2.01%
Patient accounting	18	2.00%	93	2.47%	13	2.54%
General accounting	12	.43%	69	.42%	9	*
Managed care administrative	3	*	25	.37%	2	*
Information technology	6	*	39	.47%	3	*
Housekeeping, maint, security	6	*	24	.29%	2	*
Medical receptionists	18	4.18%	94	2.36%	13	2.96%
Med secretaries,transcribers	13	.51%	84	1.44%	9	*
Medical records	14	.53%	87	.80%	10	.63%
Other admin support	12	.53%	46	.70%	7	*
*Total administrative supp staff	4	*	31	11.35%	4	*
Registered Nurses	4	*	54	1.69%	9	*
Licensed Practical Nurses	2	*	36	.81%	10	2.88%
Med assistants, nurse aides	14	9.98%	78	2.27%	11	2.84%
*Total clinical supp staff	4	*	40	4.94%	9	*
Clinical laboratory	2	*	3	*	1	*
Radiology and imaging	1	*	93	1.86%	2	*
Other medical support serv	11	5.24%	53	1.62%	7	*
*Total ancillary supp staff	1	*	29	3.37%	1	*
Total empl supp staff benefits	20	6.06%	97	4.68%	13	5.09%
Tot contracted supp staff	9	*	42	.51%	8	*
Total general operating cost	**21**	**22.23%**	**100**	**23.51%**	**14**	**25.30%**
Information technology	18	1.20%	96	1.43%	13	1.85%
Medical and surgical supply	18	1.64%	94	2.96%	13	1.69%
Building and occupancy	18	7.81%	96	5.78%	13	6.07%
Furniture and equipment	16	2.78%	83	.71%	11	.67%
Admin supplies and services	18	2.11%	95	1.87%	13	1.78%
Prof liability insurance	20	1.11%	99	2.69%	13	1.74%
Other insurance premiums	18	.32%	91	.20%	13	.31%
Outside professional fees	17	.84%	96	.74%	13	.93%
Promotion and marketing	18	1.34%	95	.52%	12	.62%
Clinical laboratory	0	*	5	*	2	*
Radiology and imaging	0	*	94	1.09%	4	*
Other ancillary services	2	*	35	1.87%	6	*
Billing purchased services	5	*	51	.32%	9	*
Management fees paid to MSO	1	*	2	*	1	*
Misc operating cost	17	1.66%	93	1.31%	12	1.40%
Cost allocated to prac from par	0	*	0	*	0	*
Total operating cost	**21**	**55.70%**	**100**	**47.04%**	**14**	**47.83%**

*See pages 260 and 261 for definition.

Single Specialty Practices, Not Hospital or IDS Owned — Opthalmology, Orthopedic Surgery, Otorhinolaryngology (as a % of Total Medical Revenue)

Table 14.5c: Provider Cost

	Ophthalmology		Orthopedic Surgery		Otorhinolaryngology	
	Count	Median	Count	Median	Count	Median
Total med rev after oper cost	21	44.30%	100	53.04%	14	52.17%
Total provider cost	21	43.45%	100	52.73%	14	47.49%
Total NPP cost	16	4.61%	84	3.97%	10	5.66%
Nonphysician provider comp	15	3.93%	79	3.28%	10	4.83%
Nonphysician prov benefit cost	13	.77%	77	.60%	10	1.00%
Provider consultant cost	2	*	3	*	1	*
Total physician cost	21	37.05%	100	48.60%	14	42.98%
Total phy compensation	18	32.08%	95	43.65%	14	38.38%
Total phy benefit cost	18	5.15%	93	6.05%	14	6.06%

Table 14.5d: Net Income or Loss

	Ophthalmology		Orthopedic Surgery		Otorhinolaryngology	
	Count	Median	Count	Median	Count	Median
Total cost	21	99.72%	100	100.00%	14	99.66%
Net nonmedical revenue	15	.03%	70	.35%	7	*
Nonmedical revenue	11	.25%	63	.63%	7	*
Fin support for oper costs	0	*	1	*	0	*
Goodwill amortization	3	*	1	*	1	*
Nonmedical cost	9	*	33	.13%	5	*
Net inc, prac with fin sup	0	*	1	*	0	*
Net inc, prac w/o fin sup	19	.04%	94	.29%	13	.73%
Net inc, excl fin supp (all prac)	19	.04%	95	.22%	13	.73%

Table 14.5e: Assets and Liabilities

	Ophthalmology		Orthopedic Surgery		Otorhinolaryngology	
	Count	Median	Count	Median	Count	Median
Total assets	11	18.15%	56	11.34%	9	*
Current assets	11	4.11%	56	4.16%	9	*
Noncurrent assets	11	15.46%	56	6.22%	9	*
Total liabilities	11	6.84%	56	6.37%	9	*
Current liabilities	11	2.34%	56	3.54%	9	*
Noncurrent liabilities	11	3.52%	56	2.05%	9	*
Working capital	11	.24%	56	.35%	9	*
Total net worth	11	5.73%	56	3.92%	9	*

Single Specialty Practices, Not Hospital or IDS Owned — Opthalmology, Orthopedic Surgery, Otorhinolaryngology (per FTE Provider)

Table 14.6a: Staffing, RVUs, Patients, Procedures and Square Footage

	Ophthalmology		Orthopedic Surgery		Otorhinolaryngology	
	Count	Median	Count	Median	Count	Median
Total physician FTE/provider	16	.73	78	.71	9	*
Prim care phy/provider	2	*	6	*	0	*
Nonsurg phy/provider	0	*	42	.06	1	*
Surg spec phy/provider	12	.72	74	.66	7	*
Total NPP FTE/provider	16	.27	78	.29	9	*
Total support staff FTE/prov	16	**6.42**	78	**3.77**	9	*
Total empl supp staff FTE/prov	14	7.25	72	3.77	9	*
General administrative	15	.36	75	.20	9	*
Patient accounting	15	.78	74	.61	9	*
General accounting	10	.12	58	.08	6	*
Managed care administrative	2	*	23	.07	2	*
Information technology	5	*	34	.07	3	*
Housekeeping, maint, security	5	*	21	.07	1	*
Medical receptionists	15	1.46	74	.68	9	*
Med secretaries,transcribers	11	.16	68	.33	7	*
Medical records	12	.33	70	.28	7	*
Other admin support	11	.17	36	.17	5	*
*Total administrative supp staff	1	*	29	2.51	3	*
Registered Nurses	3	*	44	.19	6	*
Licensed Practical Nurses	1	*	31	.19	7	*
Med assistants, nurse aides	11	2.87	63	.50	8	*
*Total clinical supp staff	1	*	39	.90	6	*
Clinical laboratory	2	*	2	*	0	*
Radiology and imaging	1	*	74	.36	1	*
Other medical support serv	10	1.19	44	.32	3	*
*Total ancillary supp staff	1	*	22	.67	1	*
Tot contracted supp staff	6	*	28	.17	6	*
Tot RVU/provider	3	*	28	12,319	2	*
Physician work RVU/provider	2	*	21	6,298	1	*
Patients/provider	8	*	32	991	4	*
Tot procedures/provider	13	7,932	56	5,293	7	*
Square feet/provider	16	2,626	77	1,721	9	*
Total support staff FTE/phy	21	8.25	100	5.42	14	5.19

*See pages 260 and 261 for definition.

Table 14.6b: Charges, Revenue and Cost

	Ophthalmology		Orthopedic Surgery		Otorhinolaryngology	
	Count	Median	Count	Median	Count	Median
Total gross charges	16	$1,202,672	77	$1,369,988	9	*
Total medical revenue	16	$744,053	78	$663,868	9	*
Net fee-for-service revenue	15	$697,927	74	$659,579	9	*
Net capitation revenue	0	*	3	*	1	*
Net other medical revenue	13	$95,915	48	$6,541	7	*
Total support staff cost/prov	16	$209,827	78	$159,383	9	*
Total general operating cost	16	$161,597	78	$144,829	9	*
Total operating cost	16	$389,274	78	$303,973	9	*
Total med rev after oper cost	16	$321,350	78	$340,465	9	*
Total provider cost/provider	16	$316,511	78	$323,394	9	*
Total NPP cost/provider	16	$38,211	78	$26,487	9	*
Provider consultant cost	1	*	2	*	0	*
Total physician cost/provider	16	$272,483	78	$303,752	9	*
Total phy compensation	15	$233,549	73	$263,266	9	*
Total phy benefit cost	15	$37,222	73	$40,509	9	*
Total cost	16	$704,890	78	$652,200	9	*
Net nonmedical revenue	12	$471	55	$2,668	5	*
Net inc, prac with fin sup	0	*	1	*	0	*
Net inc, prac w/o fin sup	16	$119	72	$1,599	8	*
Net inc, excl fin supp (all prac)	16	$119	73	$1,513	8	*
Total support staff FTE/phy	21	8.25	100	5.42	14	5.19

Single Specialty Practices, Not Hospital or IDS Owned — Opthalmology, Orthopedic Surgery, Otorhinolaryngology (per Square Foot)

Table 14.7a: Staffing, RVUs, Patients and Procedures

	Ophthalmology		Orthopedic Surgery		Otorhinolaryngology	
	Count	Median	Count	Median	Count	Median
Total prov FTE/10,000 sq ft	**16**	**3.81**	**77**	**5.81**	**9**	*
Total phy FTE/10,000 sq ft	19	3.16	98	4.14	14	5.05
Prim care phy/10,000 sq ft	2	*	6	*	0	*
Nonsurg phy/10,000 sq ft	1	*	52	.43	1	*
Surg spec phy/10,000 sq ft	14	2.84	93	3.68	12	5.00
Total NPP FTE/10,000 sq ft	16	1.06	77	1.67	9	*
Total supp stf FTE/10,000 sq ft	**19**	**26.10**	**98**	**21.99**	**14**	**27.20**
Total empl supp stf/10,000 sq ft	16	26.50	91	22.29	14	27.20
General administrative	17	1.38	95	1.08	14	1.12
Patient accounting	17	2.76	94	3.52	14	4.12
General accounting	12	.48	67	.52	10	.81
Managed care administrative	3	*	25	.41	2	*
Information technology	5	*	40	.41	3	*
Housekeeping, maint, security	6	*	25	.41	2	*
Medical receptionists	17	5.44	94	4.13	14	4.90
Med secretaries,transcribers	12	.60	85	2.08	10	1.59
Medical records	13	.96	87	1.67	11	1.43
Other admin support	12	.56	46	.89	8	*
*Total administrative supp staff	3	*	33	14.14	5	*
Registered Nurses	3	*	54	1.36	10	1.16
Licensed Practical Nurses	1	*	35	1.07	11	3.12
Med assistants, nurse aides	13	10.73	79	3.13	12	3.99
*Total clinical supp staff	3	*	43	5.33	10	9.01
Clinical laboratory	2	*	2	*	1	*
Radiology and imaging	1	*	94	2.06	2	*
Other medical support serv	11	3.90	52	1.93	8	*
*Total ancillary supp staff	1	*	25	3.56	2	*
Tot contracted supp staff	6	*	33	.75	7	*
Tot RVU/sq ft	4	*	34	8.16	4	*
Physician work RVU/sq ft	2	*	25	3.86	2	*
Patients/sq ft	9	*	39	.59	5	*
Tot procedures/sq ft	15	3.07	69	3.51	10	5.18
Total support staff FTE/phy	**21**	**8.25**	**100**	**5.42**	**14**	**5.19**

*See pages 260 and 261 for definition.

Table 14.7b: Charges, Revenue and Cost

	Ophthalmology		Orthopedic Surgery		Otorhinolaryngology	
	Count	Median	Count	Median	Count	Median
Total gross charges	19	$442.02	97	$879.09	14	$712.40
Total medical revenue	19	$325.65	98	$431.42	14	$423.66
Net fee-for-service revenue	17	$295.36	94	$423.59	14	$409.05
Net capitation revenue	0	*	4	*	1	*
Net other medical revenue	13	$33.45	54	$4.13	12	$30.73
Total support staff cost/sq ft	19	$95.23	98	$93.28	14	$96.19
Total general operating cost	19	$70.42	98	$94.20	14	$107.44
Total operating cost	19	$157.96	98	$189.95	14	$204.95
Total med rev after oper cost	19	$167.99	98	$222.49	14	$226.96
Total provider cost/sq ft	19	$128.02	98	$220.35	14	$233.58
Total NPP cost/sq ft	16	$16.11	82	$16.99	10	$22.82
Provider consultant cost	1	*	3	*	1	*
Total physician cost/sq ft	19	$99.82	98	$201.74	14	$207.44
Total phy compensation	17	$87.58	93	$176.27	14	$176.09
Total phy benefit cost	17	$13.62	91	$21.50	14	$25.03
Total cost	19	$260.94	98	$419.19	14	$414.68
Net nonmedical revenue/sq ft	15	$.12	68	$1.17	7	*
Net inc, prac with fin sup	0	*	1	*	0	*
Net inc, prac w/o fin sup	19	$.12	92	$1.07	13	$1.87
Net inc, excl fin supp (all prac)	19	$.12	93	$.98	13	$1.87
Total support staff FTE/phy	**21**	**8.25**	**100**	**5.42**	**14**	**5.19**

Single Specialty Practices, Not Hospital or IDS Owned — Opthalmology, Orthopedic Surgery, Otorhinolaryngology (per Total RVU)

Table 14.8a: Staffing, Patients, Procedures and Square Footage

	Ophthalmology		Orthopedic Surgery		Otorhinolaryngology	
	Count	Median	Count	Median	Count	Median
Total prov FTE/10,000 tot RVU	3	*	28	.81	2	*
Total phy FTE/10,000 tot RVU	4	*	34	.56	4	*
Prim care phy/10,000 tot RVU	1	*	2	*	0	*
Nonsurg phy/10,000 tot RVU	1	*	20	.05	1	*
Surg spec phy/10,000 tot RVU	3	*	33	.50	4	*
Total NPP FTE/10,000 tot RVU	3	*	28	.22	2	*
Total supp stf FTE/10,000 tot RVU	4	*	34	2.77	4	*
Tot empl supp stf/10,000 tot RVU	4	*	34	2.75	4	*
General administrative	4	*	34	.17	4	*
Patient accounting	4	*	34	.43	4	*
General accounting	3	*	30	.06	4	*
Managed care administrative	0	*	13	.07	1	*
Information technology	2	*	20	.07	0	*
Housekeeping, maint, security	3	*	13	.04	1	*
Medical receptionists	4	*	33	.51	4	*
Med secretaries, transcribers	4	*	31	.29	3	*
Medical records	4	*	33	.21	4	*
Other admin support	3	*	17	.11	4	*
*Total administrative supp staff	1	*	15	1.91	0	*
Registered Nurses	0	*	19	.25	4	*
Licensed Practical Nurses	0	*	12	.15	3	*
Med assistants, nurse aides	3	*	29	.40	4	*
*Total clinical supp staff	1	*	16	.67	3	*
Clinical laboratory	0	*	1	*	0	*
Radiology and imaging	0	*	33	.25	1	*
Other medical support serv	4	*	18	.18	2	*
*Total ancillary supp staff	0	*	8	*	1	*
Tot contracted supp staff	0	*	13	.10	2	*
Physician work RVU/tot RVU	2	*	23	.45	2	*
Patients/tot RVU	4	*	21	.07	1	*
Tot procedures/tot RVU	3	*	29	.38	3	*
Square feet/tot RVU	4	*	34	.12	4	*
Total support staff FTE/phy	21	8.25	100	5.42	14	5.19

*See pages 260 and 261 for definition.

Table 14.8b: Charges, Revenue and Cost

	Ophthalmology		Orthopedic Surgery		Otorhinolaryngology	
	Count	Median	Count	Median	Count	Median
Total gross charges	4	*	34	$100.39	4	*
Total medical revenue	4	*	34	$48.12	4	*
Net fee-for-service revenue	4	*	34	$47.87	4	*
Net capitation revenue	0	*	1	*	0	*
Net other medical revenue	3	*	22	$.65	3	*
Total supp staff cost/tot RVU	4	*	34	$11.54	4	*
Total general operating cost	4	*	34	$11.05	4	*
Total operating cost	4	*	34	$23.70	4	*
Total med rev after oper cost	4	*	34	$23.90	4	*
Total provider cost/tot RVU	4	*	34	$24.86	4	*
Total NPP cost/tot RVU	3	*	29	$2.05	2	*
Provider consultant cost	0	*	2	*	0	*
Total physician cost/tot RVU	4	*	34	$22.38	4	*
Total phy compensation	4	*	33	$18.68	4	*
Total phy benefit cost	4	*	33	$2.91	4	*
Total cost	4	*	30	$83.45	3	*
Net nonmedical revenue	3	*	25	$.13	1	*
Net inc, prac with fin sup	0	*	1	*	0	*
Net inc, prac w/o fin sup	4	*	30	$.00	4	*
Net inc, excl fin supp (all prac)	4	*	31	$.00	4	*
Total support staff FTE/phy	21	8.25	100	5.42	14	5.19

Single Specialty Practices, Not Hospital or IDS Owned — Opthalmology, Orthopedic Surgery, Otorhinolaryngology (per Work RVU)

Table 14.9a: Staffing, Patients, Procedures and Square Footage

	Ophthalmology		Orthopedic Surgery		Otorhinolaryngology	
	Count	Median	Count	Median	Count	Median
Total prov FTE/10,000 work RVU	2	*	21	1.59	1	*
Tot phy FTE/10,000 work RVU	2	*	25	1.18	2	*
Prim care phy/10,000 work RVU	1	*	2	*	0	*
Nonsurg phy/10,000 work RVU	0	*	17	.11	0	*
Surg spec phy/10,000 work RVU	1	*	25	1.09	2	*
Total NPP FTE/10,000 work RVU	2	*	21	.37	1	*
Total supp stf FTE/10,000 wrk RVU	2	*	25	6.26	2	*
Tot empl supp stf/10,000 work RVU	2	*	25	6.24	2	*
General administrative	2	*	25	.35	2	*
Patient accounting	2	*	25	.98	2	*
General accounting	2	*	23	.12	2	*
Managed care administrative	0	*	10	.14	1	*
Information technology	2	*	17	.11	0	*
Housekeeping, maint, security	2	*	8	*	1	*
Medical receptionists	2	*	25	1.22	2	*
Med secretaries,transcribers	2	*	24	.55	1	*
Medical records	2	*	25	.44	2	*
Other admin support	2	*	13	.20	2	*
*Total administrative supp staff	0	*	11	4.58	0	*
Registered Nurses	0	*	16	.46	2	*
Licensed Practical Nurses	0	*	12	.26	1	*
Med assistants, nurse aides	2	*	21	.77	2	*
*Total clinical supp staff	0	*	14	1.38	1	*
Clinical laboratory	0	*	1	*	0	*
Radiology and imaging	0	*	24	.52	1	*
Other medical support serv	2	*	14	.38	1	*
*Total ancillary supp staff	0	*	6	*	0	*
Tot contracted supp staff	0	*	12	.15	1	*
Tot RVU/work RVU	2	*	23	2.20	2	*
Patients/work RVU	2	*	14	.16	0	*
Tot procedures/work RVU	1	*	21	.84	2	*
Square feet/work RVU	2	*	25	.26	2	*
Total support staff FTE/phy	21	8.25	100	5.42	14	5.19

*See pages 260 and 261 for definition.

Table 14.9b: Charges, Revenue and Cost

	Ophthalmology		Orthopedic Surgery		Otorhinolaryngology	
	Count	Median	Count	Median	Count	Median
Total gross charges	2	*	25	$219.42	2	*
Total medical revenue	2	*	25	$115.38	2	*
Net fee-for-service revenue	2	*	25	$108.82	2	*
Net capitation revenue	0	*	1	*	0	*
Net other medical revenue	2	*	17	$1.14	1	*
Total supp staff cost/work RVU	2	*	25	$27.21	2	*
Total general operating cost	2	*	25	$23.84	2	*
Total operating cost	2	*	25	$50.40	2	*
Total med rev after oper cost	2	*	25	$53.10	2	*
Total provider cost/work RVU	2	*	25	$52.27	2	*
Total NPP cost/work RVU	2	*	22	$4.12	1	*
Provider consultant cost	0	*	1	*	0	*
Total physician cost/work RVU	2	*	25	$48.14	2	*
Total phy compensation	2	*	25	$42.68	2	*
Total phy benefit cost	2	*	25	$6.65	2	*
Total cost	2	*	25	$102.98	2	*
Net nonmedical revenue	2	*	21	$.27	1	*
Net inc, prac with fin sup	0	*	0	*	0	*
Net inc, prac w/o fin sup	2	*	24	-$.08	2	*
Net inc, excl fin supp (all prac)	2	*	24	-$.08	2	*
Total support staff FTE/phy	21	8.25	100	5.42	14	5.19

Single Specialty Practices, Not Hospital or IDS Owned — Opthalmology, Orthopedic Surgery, Otorhinolaryngology (per Patient)

Table 14.10a: Staffing, RVUs, Procedures and Square Footage

	Ophthalmology		Orthopedic Surgery		Otorhinolaryngology	
	Count	Median	Count	Median	Count	Median
Total prov FTE/10,000 patients	8	*	32	10.09	4	*
Total phy FTE/10,000 pat	9	*	39	7.16	5	*
Prim care phy/10,000 pat	1	*	4	*	0	*
Nonsurg phy/10,000 pat	1	*	19	.67	1	*
Surg spec phy/10,000 pat	8	*	39	6.17	5	*
Total NPP FTE/10,000 pat	8	*	32	3.07	4	*
Total supp staff FTE/10,000 pat	9	*	39	41.29	5	*
Total empl supp staff/10,000 pat	8	*	39	41.29	5	*
General administrative	9	*	39	2.02	5	*
Patient accounting	9	*	38	6.45	5	*
General accounting	8	*	31	.60	4	*
Managed care administrative	1	*	13	1.23	1	*
Information technology	4	*	18	1.07	1	*
Housekeeping, maint, security	6	*	11	1.23	1	*
Medical receptionists	9	*	39	7.48	5	*
Med secretaries,transcribers	9	*	34	3.52	4	*
Medical records	7	*	36	2.37	4	*
Other admin support	5	*	20	1.71	3	*
*Total administrative supp staff	1	*	12	31.35	2	*
Registered Nurses	3	*	21	1.45	4	*
Licensed Practical Nurses	1	*	13	1.30	5	*
Med assistants, nurse aides	8	*	32	4.73	5	*
*Total clinical supp staff	2	*	15	8.82	4	*
Clinical laboratory	0	*	1	*	1	*
Radiology and imaging	0	*	38	3.64	1	*
Other medical support serv	7	*	26	2.74	2	*
*Total ancillary supp staff	0	*	9	*	1	*
Tot contracted supp staff	1	*	15	.90	3	*
Tot RVU/patient	4	*	21	14.65	1	*
Physician work RVU/patient	2	*	14	6.24	0	*
Tot procedures/patient	8	*	31	5.36	5	*
Square feet/patient	9	*	39	1.70	5	*
Total support staff FTE/phy	21	8.25	100	5.42	14	5.19

*See pages 260 and 261 for definition.

Table 14.10b: Charges, Revenue and Cost

	Ophthalmology		Orthopedic Surgery		Otorhinolaryngology	
	Count	Median	Count	Median	Count	Median
Total gross charges	9	*	39	$1,492.54	5	*
Total medical revenue	9	*	39	$697.10	5	*
Net fee-for-service revenue	9	*	38	$700.45	5	*
Net capitation revenue	0	*	0	*	0	*
Net other medical revenue	7	*	24	$8.76	4	*
Total support staff cost/patient	9	*	39	$161.78	5	*
Total general operating cost	9	*	39	$148.56	5	*
Total operating cost	9	*	39	$333.69	5	*
Total med rev after oper cost	9	*	39	$365.28	5	*
Total provider cost/patient	9	*	39	$379.75	5	*
Total NPP cost/patient	8	*	33	$26.14	4	*
Provider consultant cost	0	*	2	*	0	*
Total physician cost/patient	9	*	39	$349.41	5	*
Total phy compensation	9	*	38	$287.46	5	*
Total phy benefit cost	9	*	36	$45.74	5	*
Total cost	9	*	39	$730.14	5	*
Net nonmedical revenue	7	*	28	$.68	3	*
Net inc, prac with fin sup	0	*	1	*	0	*
Net inc, prac w/o fin sup	9	*	34	$.01	4	*
Net inc, excl fin supp (all prac)	9	*	35	$.00	4	*
Total support staff FTE/phy	21	8.25	100	5.42	14	5.19

Single Specialty Practices, Not Hospital or IDS Owned — Opthalmology, Orthopedic Surgery, Otorhinolaryngology (Procedure and Charge Data)

Table 14.11a: Activity Charges to Total Gross Charges Ratios

	Ophthalmology		Orthopedic Surgery		Otorhinolaryngology	
	Count	Median	Count	Median	Count	Median
Total proc gross charges	16	99.91%	78	98.31%	10	98.59%
Medical proc-inside practice	16	44.96%	79	16.50%	10	31.98%
Medical proc-outside practice	13	.15%	67	.72%	10	.90%
Surg proc-inside practice	14	11.46%	58	8.36%	10	8.25%
Surg proc-outside practice	15	35.99%	76	60.93%	10	46.08%
Laboratory procedures	1	*	9	*	4	*
Radiology procedures	12	1.75%	79	9.25%	5	*
Tot nonproc gross charges	9	*	53	2.71%	8	*
Total support staff FTE/phy	21	8.25	100	5.42	14	5.19

Table 14.11b: Medical Procedure Data (inside the practice)

	Ophthalmology		Orthopedic Surgery		Otorhinolaryngology	
	Count	Median	Count	Median	Count	Median
Gross charges/procedure	15	$65.44	75	$75.58	10	$51.51
Total cost/procedure	14	$61.45	66	$57.62	8	*
Operating cost/procedure	13	$38.22	66	$30.90	8	*
Provider cost/procedure	14	$22.19	68	$22.35	8	*
Procedures/patient	8	*	32	2.87	5	*
Gross charges/patient	9	*	34	$221.99	5	*
Procedures/physician	16	9,595	75	4,372	10	8,293
Gross charges/physician	16	$620,782	79	$336,666	10	$482,870
Procedures/provider	13	6,784	59	3,181	7	*
Gross charges/provider	13	$443,996	62	$235,977	7	*
Gross charge to total cost ratio	14	1.17	66	1.37	8	*
Oper cost to total cost ratio	13	.61	66	.57	8	*
Prov cost to total cost ratio	14	.40	66	.43	8	*
Total support staff FTE/phy	21	8.25	100	5.42	14	5.19

Table 14.11c: Medical Procedure Data (outside the practice)

	Ophthalmology		Orthopedic Surgery		Otorhinolaryngology	
	Count	Median	Count	Median	Count	Median
Gross charges/procedure	13	$111.96	63	$156.36	10	$143.43
Total cost/procedure	12	$52.35	54	$56.13	8	*
Operating cost/procedure	12	$19.13	54	$18.61	8	*
Provider cost/procedure	12	$32.34	56	$38.09	8	*
Procedures/patient	7	*	29	.07	5	*
Gross charges/patient	7	*	31	$10.42	5	*
Procedures/physician	13	18	63	83	10	84
Gross charges/physician	13	$1,938	67	$13,619	10	$12,609
Procedures/provider	11	15	50	57	7	*
Gross charges/provider	11	$1,947	53	$9,341	7	*
Gross charge to total cost ratio	12	2.36	54	2.78	8	*
Oper cost to total cost ratio	12	.38	54	.32	8	*
Prov cost to total cost ratio	12	.62	54	.68	8	*
Total support staff FTE/phy	21	8.25	100	5.42	14	5.19

Single Specialty Practices, Not Hospital or IDS Owned — Opthalmology, Orthopedic Surgery, Otorhinolaryngology (Procedure and Charge Data)

Table 14.11d: Surgery/Anesthesia Procedure Data (inside the practice)

	Ophthalmology		Orthopedic Surgery		Otorhinolaryngology	
	Count	Median	Count	Median	Count	Median
Gross charges/procedure	14	$440.79	54	$218.55	10	$224.51
Total cost/procedure	13	$407.76	47	$170.12	8	*
Operating cost/procedure	13	$276.84	47	$102.64	8	*
Provider cost/procedure	13	$141.72	48	$68.42	8	*
Procedures/patient	7	*	27	.38	5	*
Gross charges/patient	7	*	28	$126.01	5	*
Procedures/physician	14	347	54	654	10	797
Gross charges/physician	14	$170,175	58	$155,907	10	$131,414
Procedures/provider	11	263	42	462	7	*
Gross charges/provider	11	$82,418	45	$110,658	7	*
Gross charge to total cost ratio	13	1.16	47	1.44	8	*
Oper cost to total cost ratio	13	.61	47	.58	8	*
Prov cost to total cost ratio	13	.39	47	.42	8	*
Total support staff FTE/phy	21	8.25	100	5.42	14	5.19

Table 14.11e: Surgery/Anesthesia Procedure Data (outside the practice)

	Ophthalmology		Orthopedic Surgery		Otorhinolaryngology	
	Count	Median	Count	Median	Count	Median
Gross charges/procedure	14	$1,179.82	72	$1,714.73	10	$760.43
Total cost/procedure	13	$504.24	65	$649.57	8	*
Operating cost/procedure	12	$174.13	65	$208.12	8	*
Provider cost/procedure	13	$342.62	65	$428.14	8	*
Procedures/patient	8	*	31	.43	5	*
Gross charges/patient	9	*	33	$793.26	5	*
Procedures/physician	15	384	72	701	10	869
Gross charges/physician	15	$558,069	76	$1,182,961	10	$697,380
Procedures/provider	13	248	57	486	7	*
Gross charges/provider	13	$379,526	60	$790,004	7	*
Gross charge to total cost ratio	13	2.37	65	2.80	8	*
Oper cost to total cost ratio	12	.38	65	.32	8	*
Prov cost to total cost ratio	13	.62	65	.68	8	*
Total support staff FTE/phy	21	8.25	100	5.42	14	5.19

Single Specialty Practices, Not Hospital or IDS Owned — Opthalmology, Orthopedic Surgery, Otorhinolaryngology (Procedure and Charge Data)

Table 14.11f: Clinical Laboratory/Pathology Procedure Data

	Ophthalmology		Orthopedic Surgery		Otorhinolaryngology	
	Count	Median	Count	Median	Count	Median
Gross charges/procedure	1	*	8	*	4	*
Total cost/procedure	1	*	8	*	4	*
Operating cost/procedure	1	*	8	*	4	*
Provider cost/procedure	1	*	8	*	4	*
Procedures/patient	0	*	2	*	3	*
Gross charges/patient	0	*	2	*	3	*
Procedures/physician	1	*	8	*	4	*
Gross charges/physician	1	*	9	*	4	*
Procedures/provider	1	*	7	*	2	*
Gross charges/provider	1	*	8	*	2	*
Gross charge to total cost ratio	1	*	8	*	4	*
Oper cost to total cost ratio	1	*	8	*	4	*
Prov cost to total cost ratio	1	*	8	*	4	*
Total support staff FTE/phy	21	8.25	100	5.42	14	5.19

Table 14.11g: Diagnostic Radiology and Imaging Procedure Data

	Ophthalmology		Orthopedic Surgery		Otorhinolaryngology	
	Count	Median	Count	Median	Count	Median
Gross charges/procedure	12	$100.31	76	$107.61	5	*
Total cost/procedure	12	$58.93	66	$82.17	5	*
Operating cost/procedure	12	$36.06	66	$51.10	5	*
Provider cost/procedure	12	$25.73	68	$28.06	5	*
Procedures/patient	7	*	33	1.15	4	*
Gross charges/patient	7	*	34	$126.94	4	*
Procedures/physician	12	267	76	1,744	5	*
Gross charges/physician	12	$27,500	79	$184,817	5	*
Procedures/provider	9	*	60	1,248	3	*
Gross charges/provider	9	*	62	$130,460	3	*
Gross charge to total cost ratio	12	1.60	66	1.49	5	*
Oper cost to total cost ratio	12	.58	66	.65	5	*
Prov cost to total cost ratio	12	.42	66	.35	5	*
Total support staff FTE/phy	21	8.25	100	5.42	14	5.19

Table 14.11h: Nonprocedural Gross Charge Data

	Ophthalmology		Orthopedic Surgery		Otorhinolaryngology	
	Count	Median	Count	Median	Count	Median
Gross charges/patient	6	*	21	$47.43	4	*
Nonproc gross charges/physician	9	*	53	$51,533	8	*
Gross charges/provider	7	*	42	$34,996	5	*
Total support staff FTE/phy	21	8.25	100	5.42	14	5.19

Single Specialty Practices, Not Hospital or IDS Owned — Radiology, Surgery: Cardiovascular, Surgery: General

Table 15.1: Staffing and Practice Data

	Radiology		Surg: Cardiovascular		Surgery: General	
	Count	Median	Count	Median	Count	Median
Total provider FTE	2	*	11	12.00	5	*
Total physician FTE	12	11.50	14	7.00	22	5.50
Total nonphysician provider FTE	2	*	11	2.00	5	*
Total support staff FTE	12	46.92	14	13.75	22	15.08
Number of branch clinics	4	*	8	*	9	*
Square footage of all facilities	11	8,334	14	7,167	21	6,437

Table 15.2: Accounts Receivable Data, Collection Percentages and Financial Ratios

	Radiology		Surg: Cardiovascular		Surgery: General	
	Count	Median	Count	Median	Count	Median
Total AR/physician	11	$179,943	14	$220,074	20	$152,137
Total AR/provider	1	*	11	$171,738	4	*
0-30 days in AR	11	55.93%	14	54.02%	20	52.27%
31-60 days in AR	11	14.03%	14	13.83%	20	15.47%
61-90 days in AR	11	9.20%	14	6.76%	20	8.27%
91-120 days in AR	11	5.88%	14	6.00%	20	5.26%
120+ days in AR	11	13.09%	14	19.75%	20	14.77%
Re-aged: 0-30 days in AR	4	*	3	*	8	*
Re-aged: 31-60 days in AR	4	*	3	*	8	*
Re-aged: 61-90 days in AR	4	*	3	*	8	*
Re-aged: 91-120 days in AR	4	*	3	*	8	*
Re-aged: 120+ days in AR	4	*	3	*	8	*
Not re-aged: 0-30 days in AR	7	*	10	51.64%	12	49.99%
Not re-aged: 31-60 days in AR	7	*	10	15.65%	12	16.06%
Not re-aged: 61-90 days in AR	7	*	10	7.77%	12	8.62%
Not re-aged: 91-120 days in AR	7	*	10	6.16%	12	6.72%
Not re-aged: 120+ days in AR	7	*	10	20.40%	12	14.77%
Months gross FFS charges in AR	11	1.56	12	1.45	17	1.71
Days gross FFS charges in AR	11	47.33	12	44.02	17	51.88
Gross FFS collection %	11	43.99%	12	36.63%	19	45.84%
Adjusted FFS collection %	10	90.98%	11	93.23%	17	96.48%
Gross FFS + cap collection %	2	*	1	*	1	*
Net cap rev % of gross cap chrg	1	*	1	*	1	*
Current ratio	4	*	2	*	7	*
Tot asset turnover ratio	4	*	4	*	7	*
Debt to equity ratio	4	*	4	*	7	*
Debt ratio	4	*	4	*	7	*
Return on total assets	4	*	4	*	7	*
Return on equity	4	*	4	*	7	*

Table 15.3: Breakout of Total Gross Charges by Type of Payer

	Radiology		Surg: Cardiovascular		Surgery: General	
	Count	Median	Count	Median	Count	Median
Medicare: fee-for-service	11	21.20%	14	50.80%	22	31.50%
Medicare: managed care FFS	11	.00%	14	.50%	22	.00%
Medicare: capitation	11	.00%	14	.00%	22	.00%
Medicaid: fee-for-service	11	5.90%	14	2.55%	22	4.00%
Medicaid: managed care FFS	11	.00%	14	.00%	22	.00%
Medicaid: capitation	11	.00%	14	.00%	22	.00%
Commercial: fee-for-service	11	2.00%	14	10.00%	22	30.00%
Commercial: managed care FFS	11	34.80%	14	18.00%	22	23.05%
Commercial: capitation	11	.00%	14	.00%	22	.00%
Workers' compensation	11	2.00%	14	.11%	22	.80%
Charity care and prof courtesy	11	.00%	14	.33%	22	.28%
Self-pay	11	6.00%	14	2.55%	22	4.76%
Other federal government payers	11	.00%	14	.00%	22	.00%

Single Specialty Practices, Not Hospital or IDS Owned — Radiology, Surgery: Cardiovascular, Surgery: General (per FTE Physician)

Table 15.4a: Staffing, RVUs, Patients, Procedures and Square Footage

	Radiology		Surg: Cardiovascular		Surgery: General	
	Count	Median	Count	Median	Count	Median
Total provider FTE/physician	2	*	11	1.56	5	*
Prim care phy/physician	1	*	0	*	0	*
Nonsurg phy/physician	6	*	0	*	0	*
Surg spec phy/physician	3	*	12	1.00	19	1.00
Total NPP FTE/physician	2	*	11	.56	5	*
Total support staff FTE/phy	12	2.27	14	1.86	22	2.92
Total empl support staff FTE	12	2.23	13	1.78	20	3.04
General administrative	12	.16	11	.29	20	.20
Patient accounting	11	1.13	11	.44	20	.60
General accounting	8	*	4	*	8	*
Managed care administrative	2	*	2	*	3	*
Information technology	7	*	2	*	3	*
Housekeeping, maint, security	1	*	1	*	2	*
Medical receptionists	5	*	11	.33	20	.60
Med secretaries,transcribers	6	*	10	.30	7	*
Medical records	4	*	8	*	13	.14
Other admin support	3	*	6	*	8	*
*Total administrative supp staff	2	*	7	*	5	*
Registered Nurses	0	*	9	*	14	.27
Licensed Practical Nurses	0	*	2	*	12	.30
Med assistants, nurse aides	2	*	7	*	17	.50
*Total clinical supp staff	1	*	6	*	13	.72
Clinical laboratory	0	*	0	*	1	*
Radiology and imaging	8	*	1	*	7	*
Other medical support serv	2	*	2	*	4	*
*Total ancillary supp staff	1	*	2	*	2	*
Tot contracted supp staff	4	*	3	*	4	*
Tot RVU/physician	5	*	6	*	9	*
Physician work RVU/physician	6	*	5	*	10	7,299
Patients/physician	3	*	5	*	8	*
Tot procedures/physician	10	18,309	8	*	16	3,608
Square feet/physician	11	705	14	941	21	1,189

*See pages 260 and 261 for definition.

Table 15.4b: Charges and Revenue

	Radiology		Surg: Cardiovascular		Surgery: General	
	Count	Median	Count	Median	Count	Median
Net fee-for-service revenue	11	$671,574	13	$647,909	19	$529,755
Gross FFS charges	11	$1,728,232	12	$1,957,999	19	$1,155,731
Adjustments to FFS charges	10	$811,796	11	$1,078,525	17	$609,452
Adjusted FFS charges	10	$836,166	11	$698,321	17	$537,059
Bad debts due to FFS activity	10	$65,907	11	$48,733	17	$24,578
Net capitation revenue	2	*	2	*	1	*
Gross capitation charges	1	*	1	*	1	*
Capitation revenue	2	*	1	*	1	*
Purch serv for cap patients	0	*	0	*	0	*
Net other medical revenue	8	*	9	*	12	$30,963
Gross rev from other activity	7	*	8	*	11	$29,072
Other medical revenue	5	*	9	*	8	*
Rev from sale of goods/services	4	*	1	*	8	*
Cost of sales	0	*	0	*	3	*
Total gross charges	11	$1,728,232	13	$2,134,878	22	$1,159,733
Total medical revenue	12	$763,551	14	$704,227	22	$529,797

Single Specialty Practices, Not Hospital or IDS Owned — Radiology, Surgery: Cardiovascular, Surgery: General (per FTE Physician)

Table 15.4c: Operating Cost

	Radiology		Surg: Cardiovascular		Surgery: General	
	Count	Median	Count	Median	Count	Median
Total support staff cost/phy	**12**	**$101,557**	**14**	**$104,027**	**22**	**$112,371**
Total empl supp staff cost/phy	12	$75,498	13	$76,911	20	$89,363
General administrative	12	$11,654	10	$18,570	20	$13,989
Patient accounting	11	$34,673	10	$13,482	20	$16,518
General accounting	8	*	3	*	8	*
Managed care administrative	2	*	1	*	3	*
Information technology	7	*	2	*	3	*
Housekeeping, maint, security	1	*	0	*	2	*
Medical receptionists	5	*	9	*	19	$14,610
Med secretaries,transcribers	6	*	9	*	7	*
Medical records	4	*	7	*	13	$3,454
Other admin support	3	*	4	*	8	*
*Total administrative supp staff	0	*	5	*	4	*
Registered Nurses	0	*	8	*	14	$10,607
Licensed Practical Nurses	0	*	2	*	12	$8,926
Med assistants, nurse aides	2	*	6	*	17	$13,363
*Total clinical supp staff	0	*	5	*	12	$25,303
Clinical laboratory	0	*	0	*	1	*
Radiology and imaging	8	*	1	*	7	*
Other medical support serv	2	*	2	*	5	*
*Total ancillary supp staff	0	*	2	*	2	*
Total empl supp staff benefits	11	$23,246	14	$23,762	22	$23,132
Tot contracted supp staff	4	*	4	*	6	*
Total general operating cost	**12**	**$86,357**	**14**	**$113,931**	**22**	**$103,527**
Information technology	11	$6,736	12	$11,742	20	$9,689
Medical and surgical supply	3	*	12	$1,107	20	$3,794
Building and occupancy	11	$6,274	12	$21,289	20	$27,011
Furniture and equipment	9	*	11	$2,146	19	$2,313
Admin supplies and services	12	$7,739	12	$5,971	20	$9,358
Prof liability insurance	12	$19,231	13	$28,752	22	$29,271
Other insurance premiums	10	$1,603	10	$2,089	18	$747
Outside professional fees	12	$8,760	12	$4,986	20	$4,743
Promotion and marketing	11	$1,977	12	$1,578	20	$2,130
Clinical laboratory	0	*	0	*	2	*
Radiology and imaging	8	*	2	*	6	*
Other ancillary services	2	*	0	*	1	*
Billing purchased services	5	*	7	*	10	$1,000
Management fees paid to MSO	0	*	0	*	2	*
Misc operating cost	11	$6,240	12	$8,662	20	$4,027
Cost allocated to prac from par	0	*	0	*	0	*
Total operating cost	**10**	**$217,503**	**14**	**$220,018**	**22**	**$222,272**

*See pages 260 and 261 for definition.

Single Specialty Practices, Not Hospital or IDS Owned — Radiology, Surgery: Cardiovascular, Surgery: General (per FTE Physician)

Table 15.4d: Provider Cost

	Radiology		Surg: Cardiovascular		Surgery: General	
	Count	Median	Count	Median	Count	Median
Total med rev after oper cost	11	$469,748	14	$518,089	22	$312,675
Total provider cost/physician	12	$471,552	14	$538,227	22	$299,327
Total NPP cost/physician	2	*	11	$57,110	5	*
Nonphysician provider comp	2	*	10	$52,506	5	*
Nonphysician prov benefit cost	1	*	10	$12,141	5	*
Provider consultant cost	0	*	1	*	1	*
Total physician cost/physician	12	$468,697	14	$505,580	22	$295,513
Total phy compensation	12	$405,933	12	$410,403	20	$243,642
Total phy benefit cost	11	$63,050	11	$61,590	20	$50,907

Table 15.4e: Net Income or Loss

	Radiology		Surg: Cardiovascular		Surgery: General	
	Count	Median	Count	Median	Count	Median
Total cost	12	$804,146	14	$738,171	22	$531,758
Net nonmedical revenue	12	$2,397	6	*	17	$382
Nonmedical revenue	11	$3,578	6	*	15	$382
Fin support for oper costs	0	*	0	*	1	*
Goodwill amortization	0	*	0	*	0	*
Nonmedical cost	6	*	1	*	6	*
Net inc, prac with fin sup	0	*	0	*	1	*
Net inc, prac w/o fin sup	12	$1,197	13	$3,163	17	$6,766
Net inc, excl fin supp (all prac)	12	$1,197	13	$3,163	18	$7,016

Table 15.4f: Assets and Liabilities

	Radiology		Surg: Cardiovascular		Surgery: General	
	Count	Median	Count	Median	Count	Median
Total assets	7	*	9	*	11	$34,181
Current assets	7	*	9	*	11	$15,597
Noncurrent assets	7	*	9	*	11	$15,660
Total liabilities	7	*	9	*	11	$12,834
Current liabilities	7	*	9	*	11	$11,194
Noncurrent liabilities	7	*	9	*	11	$0
Working capital	7	*	9	*	11	$4,422
Total net worth	7	*	9	*	11	$23,051
Total support staff FTE/phy	12	2.27	14	1.86	22	2.92

Single Specialty Practices, Not Hospital or IDS Owned — Radiology, Surgery: Cardiovascular, Surgery: General (as a % of Total Medical Revenue)

Table 15.5a: Charges and Revenue

	Radiology		Surg: Cardiovascular		Surgery: General	
	Count	Median	Count	Median	Count	Median
Net fee-for-service revenue	11	98.90%	13	99.03%	19	99.66%
Net capitation revenue	2	*	2	*	1	*
Net other medical revenue	8	*	9	*	12	5.36%
Total gross charges	**11**	**204.53%**	**13**	**261.50%**	**22**	**214.53%**

Table 15.5b: Operating Cost

	Radiology		Surg: Cardiovascular		Surgery: General	
	Count	Median	Count	Median	Count	Median
Total support staff cost	**12**	**14.62%**	**14**	**14.70%**	**22**	**22.19%**
Total empl support staff cost	12	10.77%	13	11.92%	20	16.48%
General administrative	12	1.76%	10	2.02%	20	2.71%
Patient accounting	11	4.32%	10	1.66%	20	2.91%
General accounting	8	*	3	*	8	*
Managed care administrative	2	*	1	*	3	*
Information technology	7	*	2	*	3	*
Housekeeping, maint, security	1	*	0	*	2	*
Medical receptionists	5	*	9	*	19	2.62%
Med secretaries,transcribers	6	*	9	*	7	*
Medical records	4	*	7	*	13	.53%
Other admin support	3	*	4	*	8	*
*Total administrative supp staff	0	*	5	*	4	*
Registered Nurses	0	*	8	*	14	2.20%
Licensed Practical Nurses	0	*	2	*	12	1.34%
Med assistants, nurse aides	2	*	6	*	17	2.29%
*Total clinical supp staff	0	*	5	*	12	4.80%
Clinical laboratory	0	*	0	*	1	*
Radiology and imaging	8	*	1	*	7	*
Other medical support serv	2	*	2	*	5	*
*Total ancillary supp staff	0	*	2	*	2	*
Total empl supp staff benefits	11	3.24%	14	3.32%	22	4.37%
Tot contracted supp staff	4	*	4	*	6	*
Total general operating cost	**12**	**12.63%**	**14**	**15.48%**	**22**	**19.92%**
Information technology	12	1.12%	12	1.50%	20	1.57%
Medical and surgical supply	3	*	11	.15%	20	.73%
Building and occupancy	12	1.05%	12	3.21%	20	4.97%
Furniture and equipment	10	1.02%	11	.29%	19	.45%
Admin supplies and services	12	1.12%	12	.70%	20	1.62%
Prof liability insurance	12	2.10%	13	4.18%	22	5.99%
Other insurance premiums	10	.26%	10	.24%	18	.14%
Outside professional fees	12	.94%	12	.86%	20	.93%
Promotion and marketing	11	.26%	12	.21%	20	.36%
Clinical laboratory	0	*	0	*	2	*
Radiology and imaging	8	*	2	*	6	*
Other ancillary services	2	*	0	*	1	*
Billing purchased services	5	*	7	*	10	.19%
Management fees paid to MSO	0	*	0	*	2	*
Misc operating cost	11	.76%	12	1.31%	20	.69%
Cost allocated to prac from par	0	*	0	*	0	*
Total operating cost	**12**	**25.75%**	**14**	**27.01%**	**22**	**41.76%**

*See pages 260 and 261 for definition.

Single Specialty Practices, Not Hospital or IDS Owned — Radiology, Surgery: Cardiovascular, Surgery: General (as a % of Total Medical Revenue)

Table 15.5c: Provider Cost

	Radiology		Surg: Cardiovascular		Surgery: General	
	Count	Median	Count	Median	Count	Median
Total med rev after oper cost	**12**	**74.25%**	**14**	**72.99%**	**22**	**59.59%**
Total provider cost	**12**	**76.15%**	**14**	**72.26%**	**22**	**58.56%**
Total NPP cost	2	*	11	7.65%	5	*
Nonphysician provider comp	2	*	10	6.26%	5	*
Nonphysician prov benefit cost	1	*	10	1.95%	5	*
Provider consultant cost	0	*	1	*	1	*
Total physician cost	12	76.12%	14	64.55%	22	57.85%
Total phy compensation	12	65.16%	12	57.20%	20	48.59%
Total phy benefit cost	11	10.00%	11	8.06%	20	9.18%

Table 15.5d: Net Income or Loss

	Radiology		Surg: Cardiovascular		Surgery: General	
	Count	Median	Count	Median	Count	Median
Total cost	**12**	**100.13%**	**14**	**100.00%**	**22**	**98.62%**
Net nonmedical revenue	12	.33%	6	*	17	.06%
Nonmedical revenue	11	.43%	6	*	15	.07%
Fin support for oper costs	0	*	0	*	1	*
Goodwill amortization	0	*	0	*	0	*
Nonmedical cost	6	*	1	*	6	*
Net inc, prac with fin sup	0	*	0	*	1	*
Net inc, prac w/o fin sup	12	.18%	13	.51%	17	1.41%
Net inc, excl fin supp (all prac)	12	.18%	13	.51%	18	1.49%

Table 15.5e: Assets and Liabilities

	Radiology		Surg: Cardiovascular		Surgery: General	
	Count	Median	Count	Median	Count	Median
Total assets	**7**	*	**9**	*	**11**	**5.62%**
Current assets	7	*	9	*	11	2.75%
Noncurrent assets	7	*	9	*	11	2.94%
Total liabilities	**7**	*	**9**	*	**11**	**2.52%**
Current liabilities	7	*	9	*	11	1.92%
Noncurrent liabilities	7	*	9	*	11	.00%
Working capital	7	*	9	*	11	.88%
Total net worth	**7**	*	**9**	*	**11**	**4.24%**

Single Specialty Practices, Not Hospital or IDS Owned — Radiology, Surgery: Cardiovascular, Surgery: General (per FTE Provider)

Table 15.6a: Staffing, RVUs, Patients, Procedures and Square Footage

	Radiology		Surg: Cardiovascular		Surgery: General	
	Count	Median	Count	Median	Count	Median
Total physician FTE/provider	2	*	11	.64	5	*
Prim care phy/provider	0	*	0	*	0	*
Nonsurg phy/provider	1	*	0	*	0	*
Surg spec phy/provider	0	*	9	*	5	*
Total NPP FTE/provider	2	*	11	.36	5	*
Total support staff FTE/prov	2	*	11	1.25	5	*
Total empl supp staff FTE/prov	2	*	10	1.25	5	*
General administrative	2	*	9	*	5	*
Patient accounting	2	*	9	*	5	*
General accounting	2	*	3	*	2	*
Managed care administrative	1	*	2	*	2	*
Information technology	2	*	1	*	1	*
Housekeeping, maint, security	0	*	1	*	0	*
Medical receptionists	1	*	9	*	5	*
Med secretaries,transcribers	1	*	8	*	4	*
Medical records	1	*	6	*	4	*
Other admin support	0	*	5	*	3	*
*Total administrative supp staff	0	*	5	*	1	*
Registered Nurses	0	*	7	*	4	*
Licensed Practical Nurses	0	*	2	*	2	*
Med assistants, nurse aides	0	*	5	*	4	*
*Total clinical supp staff	0	*	4	*	3	*
Clinical laboratory	0	*	0	*	0	*
Radiology and imaging	1	*	1	*	4	*
Other medical support serv	0	*	2	*	2	*
*Total ancillary supp staff	0	*	2	*	1	*
Tot contracted supp staff	0	*	3	*	1	*
Tot RVU/provider	0	*	4	*	4	*
Physician work RVU/provider	1	*	3	*	4	*
Patients/provider	0	*	3	*	4	*
Tot procedures/provider	1	*	6	*	4	*
Square feet/provider	2	*	11	631	5	*
Total support staff FTE/phy	12	2.27	14	1.86	22	2.92

*See pages 260 and 261 for definition.

Table 15.6b: Charges, Revenue and Cost

	Radiology		Surg: Cardiovascular		Surgery: General	
	Count	Median	Count	Median	Count	Median
Total gross charges	1	*	10	$1,264,583	5	*
Total medical revenue	2	*	11	$509,314	5	*
Net fee-for-service revenue	1	*	10	$453,944	5	*
Net capitation revenue	1	*	1	*	0	*
Net other medical revenue	1	*	6	*	4	*
Total support staff cost/prov	2	*	11	$66,099	5	*
Total general operating cost	2	*	11	$73,644	5	*
Total operating cost	2	*	11	$157,851	5	*
Total med rev after oper cost	2	*	11	$314,637	5	*
Total provider cost/provider	2	*	11	$311,886	5	*
Total NPP cost/provider	2	*	11	$36,714	5	*
Provider consultant cost	0	*	1	*	0	*
Total physician cost/provider	2	*	11	$274,063	5	*
Total phy compensation	2	*	9	*	5	*
Total phy benefit cost	2	*	8	*	5	*
Total cost	2	*	11	$420,680	5	*
Net nonmedical revenue	2	*	5	*	4	*
Net inc, prac with fin sup	0	*	0	*	1	*
Net inc, prac w/o fin sup	2	*	11	$2,008	3	*
Net inc, excl fin supp (all prac)	2	*	11	$2,008	4	*
Total support staff FTE/phy	12	2.27	14	1.86	22	2.92

Single Specialty Practices, Not Hospital or IDS Owned — Radiology, Surgery: Cardiovascular, Surgery: General (per Square Foot)

Table 15.7a: Staffing, RVUs, Patients and Procedures

	Radiology		Surg: Cardiovascular		Surgery: General	
	Count	Median	Count	Median	Count	Median
Total prov FTE/10,000 sq ft	2	*	11	15.84	5	*
Total phy FTE/10,000 sq ft	11	14.18	14	10.63	21	8.41
Prim care phy/10,000 sq ft	1	*	0	*	0	*
Nonsurg phy/10,000 sq ft	6	*	0	*	0	*
Surg spec phy/10,000 sq ft	3	*	12	10.63	18	7.83
Total NPP FTE/10,000 sq ft	2	*	11	5.84	5	*
Total supp stf FTE/10,000 sq ft	11	49.70	14	20.98	21	22.28
Total empl supp stf/10,000 sq ft	11	48.82	13	20.67	19	23.29
General administrative	11	3.35	11	2.21	19	1.58
Patient accounting	11	22.55	11	4.67	19	4.68
General accounting	8	*	4	*	8	*
Managed care administrative	2	*	2	*	3	*
Information technology	7	*	2	*	3	*
Housekeeping, maint, security	1	*	1	*	2	*
Medical receptionists	5	*	11	3.43	19	4.34
Med secretaries,transcribers	6	*	10	2.50	7	*
Medical records	4	*	8	*	13	1.54
Other admin support	3	*	6	*	8	*
*Total administrative supp staff	2	*	7	*	5	*
Registered Nurses	0	*	9	*	14	1.96
Licensed Practical Nurses	0	*	2	*	12	1.87
Med assistants, nurse aides	2	*	7	*	16	3.44
*Total clinical supp staff	1	*	6	*	13	5.92
Clinical laboratory	0	*	0	*	1	*
Radiology and imaging	7	*	1	*	7	*
Other medical support serv	1	*	2	*	4	*
*Total ancillary supp staff	1	*	2	*	2	*
Tot contracted supp staff	4	*	3	*	4	*
Tot RVU/sq ft	5	*	6	*	9	*
Physician work RVU/sq ft	5	*	5	*	10	4.81
Patients/sq ft	3	*	5	*	8	*
Tot procedures/sq ft	9	*	8	*	15	2.93
Total support staff FTE/phy	12	2.27	14	1.86	22	2.92

*See pages 260 and 261 for definition.

Table 15.7b: Charges, Revenue and Cost

	Radiology		Surg: Cardiovascular		Surgery: General	
	Count	Median	Count	Median	Count	Median
Total gross charges	10	$2,347.28	13	$1,733.48	21	$938.49
Total medical revenue	11	$1,257.90	14	$713.94	21	$419.16
Net fee-for-service revenue	10	$902.06	13	$658.76	18	$389.66
Net capitation revenue	2	*	2	*	1	*
Net other medical revenue	7	*	9	*	12	$20.28
Total support staff cost/sq ft	11	$236.43	14	$110.29	21	$90.30
Total general operating cost	11	$187.29	14	$107.58	21	$83.48
Total operating cost	11	$421.75	14	$207.36	21	$178.41
Total med rev after oper cost	11	$881.88	14	$495.13	21	$254.02
Total provider cost/sq ft	11	$832.73	14	$502.69	21	$259.11
Total NPP cost/sq ft	2	*	11	$60.00	5	*
Provider consultant cost	0	*	1	*	1	*
Total physician cost/sq ft	11	$832.73	14	$436.30	21	$253.56
Total phy compensation	11	$648.76	12	$391.44	19	$195.26
Total phy benefit cost	11	$183.97	11	$47.63	19	$43.86
Total cost	11	$1,208.74	14	$712.04	21	$439.99
Net nonmedical revenue/sq ft	11	$7.30	6	*	17	$.47
Net inc, prac with fin sup	0	*	0	*	1	*
Net inc, prac w/o fin sup	11	$4.32	13	$6.15	17	$6.24
Net inc, excl fin supp (all prac)	11	$4.32	13	$6.15	18	$6.77
Total support staff FTE/phy	12	2.27	14	1.86	22	2.92

Single Specialty Practices, Not Hospital or IDS Owned — Radiology, Surgery: Cardiovascular, Surgery: General (per Total RVU)

Table 15.8a: Staffing, Patients, Procedures and Square Footage

	Radiology		Surg: Cardiovascular		Surgery: General	
	Count	Median	Count	Median	Count	Median
Total prov FTE/10,000 tot RVU	0	*	4	*	4	*
Total phy FTE/10,000 tot RVU	5	*	6	*	9	*
Prim care phy/10,000 tot RVU	1	*	0	*	0	*
Nonsurg phy/10,000 tot RVU	2	*	0	*	0	*
Surg spec phy/10,000 tot RVU	2	*	5	*	7	*
Total NPP FTE/10,000 tot RVU	0	*	4	*	4	*
Total supp stf FTE/10,000 tot RVU	5	*	6	*	9	*
Tot empl supp stf/10,000 tot RVU	5	*	6	*	8	*
General administrative	5	*	6	*	8	*
Patient accounting	5	*	6	*	8	*
General accounting	3	*	2	*	6	*
Managed care administrative	1	*	0	*	2	*
Information technology	2	*	2	*	2	*
Housekeeping, maint, security	1	*	0	*	1	*
Medical receptionists	2	*	5	*	8	*
Med secretaries,transcribers	3	*	5	*	4	*
Medical records	2	*	4	*	7	*
Other admin support	2	*	4	*	3	*
*Total administrative supp staff	1	*	4	*	1	*
Registered Nurses	0	*	6	*	6	*
Licensed Practical Nurses	0	*	1	*	3	*
Med assistants, nurse aides	1	*	4	*	7	*
*Total clinical supp staff	0	*	5	*	4	*
Clinical laboratory	0	*	0	*	1	*
Radiology and imaging	4	*	0	*	4	*
Other medical support serv	0	*	1	*	2	*
*Total ancillary supp staff	1	*	0	*	0	*
Tot contracted supp staff	1	*	1	*	2	*
Physician work RVU/tot RVU	2	*	5	*	8	*
Patients/tot RVU	3	*	4	*	6	*
Tot procedures/tot RVU	4	*	6	*	6	*
Square feet/tot RVU	5	*	6	*	9	*
Total support staff FTE/phy	12	2.27	14	1.86	22	2.92

*See pages 260 and 261 for definition.

Table 15.8b: Charges, Revenue and Cost

	Radiology		Surg: Cardiovascular		Surgery: General	
	Count	Median	Count	Median	Count	Median
Total gross charges	5	*	6	*	9	*
Total medical revenue	5	*	6	*	9	*
Net fee-for-service revenue	5	*	6	*	8	*
Net capitation revenue	1	*	1	*	0	*
Net other medical revenue	2	*	4	*	5	*
Total supp staff cost/tot RVU	5	*	6	*	9	*
Total general operating cost	5	*	6	*	9	*
Total operating cost	5	*	6	*	9	*
Total med rev after oper cost	5	*	6	*	9	*
Total provider cost/tot RVU	5	*	6	*	9	*
Total NPP cost/tot RVU	0	*	4	*	4	*
Provider consultant cost	0	*	0	*	0	*
Total physician cost/tot RVU	5	*	6	*	9	*
Total phy compensation	5	*	5	*	8	*
Total phy benefit cost	5	*	5	*	8	*
Total cost	2	*	6	*	6	*
Net nonmedical revenue	5	*	2	*	7	*
Net inc, prac with fin sup	0	*	0	*	1	*
Net inc, prac w/o fin sup	5	*	5	*	7	*
Net inc, excl fin supp (all prac)	5	*	5	*	8	*
Total support staff FTE/phy	12	2.27	14	1.86	22	2.92

Single Specialty Practices, Not Hospital or IDS Owned — Radiology, Surgery: Cardiovascular, Surgery: General (per Work RVU)

Table 15.9a: Staffing, Patients, Procedures and Square Footage

	Radiology		Surg: Cardiovascular		Surgery: General	
	Count	Median	Count	Median	Count	Median
Total prov FTE/10,000 work RVU	1	*	3	*	4	*
Tot phy FTE/10,000 work RVU	6	*	5	*	10	1.37
Prim care phy/10,000 work RVU	0	*	0	*	0	*
Nonsurg phy/10,000 work RVU	4	*	0	*	0	*
Surg spec phy/10,000 work RVU	1	*	4	*	8	*
Total NPP FTE/10,000 work RVU	1	*	3	*	4	*
Total supp stf FTE/10,000 wrk RVU	6	*	5	*	10	5.16
Tot empl supp stf/10,000 work RVU	6	*	5	*	9	*
General administrative	6	*	5	*	9	*
Patient accounting	5	*	5	*	9	*
General accounting	3	*	2	*	6	*
Managed care administrative	1	*	0	*	3	*
Information technology	3	*	2	*	2	*
Housekeeping, maint, security	0	*	0	*	1	*
Medical receptionists	0	*	5	*	9	*
Med secretaries,transcribers	0	*	5	*	5	*
Medical records	0	*	4	*	8	*
Other admin support	1	*	3	*	3	*
*Total administrative supp stf	1	*	4	*	2	*
Registered Nurses	0	*	5	*	8	*
Licensed Practical Nurses	0	*	1	*	5	*
Med assistants, nurse aides	0	*	3	*	7	*
*Total clinical supp stf	0	*	5	*	5	*
Clinical laboratory	0	*	0	*	1	*
Radiology and imaging	3	*	0	*	5	*
Other medical support serv	2	*	1	*	4	*
*Total ancillary supp stf	1	*	0	*	1	*
Tot contracted supp staff	2	*	1	*	2	*
Tot RVU/work RVU	2	*	5	*	8	*
Patients/work RVU	2	*	3	*	6	*
Tot procedures/work RVU	5	*	5	*	8	*
Square feet/work RVU	5	*	5	*	10	.21
Total support staff FTE/phy	12	2.27	14	1.86	22	2.92

*See pages 260 and 261 for definition.

Table 15.9b: Charges, Revenue and Cost

	Radiology		Surg: Cardiovascular		Surgery: General	
	Count	Median	Count	Median	Count	Median
Total gross charges	5	*	5	*	10	$173.82
Total medical revenue	6	*	5	*	10	$80.70
Net fee-for-service revenue	5	*	5	*	9	*
Net capitation revenue	1	*	1	*	0	*
Net other medical revenue	4	*	4	*	5	*
Total supp staff cost/work RVU	6	*	5	*	10	$19.11
Total general operating cost	6	*	5	*	10	$15.90
Total operating cost	6	*	5	*	10	$35.57
Total med rev after oper cost	6	*	5	*	10	$46.87
Total provider cost/work RVU	6	*	5	*	10	$45.98
Total NPP cost/work RVU	1	*	3	*	4	*
Provider consultant cost	0	*	0	*	0	*
Total physician cost/work RVU	6	*	5	*	10	$44.69
Total phy compensation	6	*	4	*	9	*
Total phy benefit cost	5	*	4	*	9	*
Total cost	6	*	5	*	10	$79.80
Net nonmedical revenue	6	*	2	*	8	*
Net inc, prac with fin sup	0	*	0	*	1	*
Net inc, prac w/o fin sup	6	*	4	*	7	*
Net inc, excl fin supp (all prac)	6	*	4	*	8	*
Total support staff FTE/phy	12	2.27	14	1.86	22	2.92

Single Specialty Practices, Not Hospital or IDS Owned — Radiology, Surgery: Cardiovascular, Surgery: General (per Patient)

Table 15.10a: Staffing, RVUs, Procedures and Square Footage

	Radiology		Surg: Cardiovascular		Surgery: General	
	Count	Median	Count	Median	Count	Median
Total prov FTE/10,000 patients	0	*	3	*	4	*
Total phy FTE/10,000 pat	3	*	5	*	8	*
Prim care phy/10,000 pat	1	*	0	*	0	*
Nonsurg phy/10,000 pat	2	*	0	*	0	*
Surg spec phy/10,000 pat	0	*	4	*	8	*
Total NPP FTE/10,000 pat	0	*	3	*	4	*
Total supp staff FTE/10,000 pat	3	*	5	*	8	*
Total empl supp staff/10,000 pat	3	*	5	*	8	*
General administrative	3	*	4	*	8	*
Patient accounting	3	*	4	*	8	*
General accounting	2	*	3	*	5	*
Managed care administrative	1	*	1	*	2	*
Information technology	1	*	2	*	2	*
Housekeeping, maint, security	0	*	1	*	0	*
Medical receptionists	1	*	4	*	8	*
Med secretaries,transcribers	1	*	3	*	3	*
Medical records	1	*	2	*	6	*
Other admin support	2	*	3	*	5	*
*Total administrative supp staff	1	*	3	*	0	*
Registered Nurses	0	*	4	*	6	*
Licensed Practical Nurses	0	*	0	*	2	*
Med assistants, nurse aides	0	*	3	*	7	*
*Total clinical supp staff	0	*	3	*	3	*
Clinical laboratory	0	*	0	*	0	*
Radiology and imaging	3	*	0	*	4	*
Other medical support serv	0	*	0	*	3	*
*Total ancillary supp staff	1	*	0	*	0	*
Tot contracted supp staff	1	*	0	*	2	*
Tot RVU/patient	3	*	4	*	6	*
Physician work RVU/patient	2	*	3	*	6	*
Tot procedures/patient	2	*	5	*	7	*
Square feet/patient	3	*	5	*	8	*
Total support staff FTE/phy	12	2.27	14	1.86	22	2.92

*See pages 260 and 261 for definition.

Table 15.10b: Charges, Revenue and Cost

	Radiology		Surg: Cardiovascular		Surgery: General	
	Count	Median	Count	Median	Count	Median
Total gross charges	3	*	4	*	8	*
Total medical revenue	3	*	5	*	8	*
Net fee-for-service revenue	3	*	5	*	8	*
Net capitation revenue	1	*	2	*	0	*
Net other medical revenue	1	*	3	*	5	*
Total support staff cost/patient	3	*	5	*	8	*
Total general operating cost	3	*	5	*	8	*
Total operating cost	3	*	5	*	8	*
Total med rev after oper cost	3	*	5	*	8	*
Total provider cost/patient	3	*	5	*	8	*
Total NPP cost/patient	0	*	3	*	4	*
Provider consultant cost	0	*	0	*	0	*
Total physician cost/patient	3	*	5	*	8	*
Total phy compensation	3	*	4	*	8	*
Total phy benefit cost	3	*	3	*	8	*
Total cost	3	*	5	*	8	*
Net nonmedical revenue	3	*	1	*	7	*
Net inc, prac with fin sup	0	*	0	*	1	*
Net inc, prac w/o fin sup	3	*	4	*	6	*
Net inc, excl fin supp (all prac)	3	*	4	*	7	*
Total support staff FTE/phy	12	2.27	14	1.86	22	2.92

Single Specialty Practices, Not Hospital or IDS Owned — Radiology, Surgery: Cardiovascular, Surgery: General (Procedure and Charge Data)

Table 15.11a: Activity Charges to Total Gross Charges Ratios

	Radiology		Surg: Cardiovascular		Surgery: General	
	Count	Median	Count	Median	Count	Median
Total proc gross charges	**11**	**100.00%**	**9**	*	**16**	**100.00%**
Medical proc-inside practice	4	*	8	*	16	10.48%
Medical proc-outside practice	4	*	7	*	13	5.81%
Surg proc-inside practice	2	*	4	*	13	4.09%
Surg proc-outside practice	5	*	8	*	16	76.79%
Laboratory procedures	1	*	0	*	3	*
Radiology procedures	10	95.75%	4	*	15	2.71%
Tot nonproc gross charges	3	*	1	*	5	*
Total support staff FTE/phy	**12**	**2.27**	**14**	**1.86**	**22**	**2.92**

Table 15.11b: Medical Procedure Data (inside the practice)

	Radiology		Surg: Cardiovascular		Surgery: General	
	Count	Median	Count	Median	Count	Median
Gross charges/procedure	**4**	*	**8**	*	**16**	**$77.69**
Total cost/procedure	**4**	*	**7**	*	**15**	**$65.69**
Operating cost/procedure	4	*	7	*	15	$40.95
Provider cost/procedure	4	*	8	*	15	$21.56
Procedures/patient	1	*	5	*	7	*
Gross charges/patient	1	*	4	*	7	*
Procedures/physician	4	*	9	*	16	1,822
Gross charges/physician	4	*	8	*	16	$150,114
Procedures/provider	0	*	7	*	4	*
Gross charges/provider	0	*	6	*	4	*
Gross charge to total cost ratio	4	*	7	*	15	1.31
Oper cost to total cost ratio	4	*	7	*	15	.67
Prov cost to total cost ratio	4	*	7	*	15	.33
Total support staff FTE/phy	**12**	**2.27**	**14**	**1.86**	**22**	**2.92**

Table 15.11c: Medical Procedure Data (outside the practice)

	Radiology		Surg: Cardiovascular		Surgery: General	
	Count	Median	Count	Median	Count	Median
Gross charges/procedure	**4**	*	**7**	*	**13**	**$129.69**
Total cost/procedure	**4**	*	**6**	*	**12**	**$47.11**
Operating cost/procedure	4	*	6	*	12	$15.48
Provider cost/procedure	4	*	7	*	12	$30.54
Procedures/patient	1	*	4	*	7	*
Gross charges/patient	1	*	3	*	7	*
Procedures/physician	4	*	8	*	13	575
Gross charges/physician	4	*	7	*	13	$71,502
Procedures/provider	0	*	6	*	4	*
Gross charges/provider	0	*	5	*	4	*
Gross charge to total cost ratio	4	*	6	*	12	2.71
Oper cost to total cost ratio	4	*	6	*	12	.32
Prov cost to total cost ratio	4	*	6	*	12	.68
Total support staff FTE/phy	**12**	**2.27**	**14**	**1.86**	**22**	**2.92**

Single Specialty Practices, Not Hospital or IDS Owned — Radiology, Surgery: Cardiovascular, Surgery: General (Procedure and Charge Data)

Table 15.11d: Surgery/Anesthesia Procedure Data (inside the practice)

	Radiology		Surg: Cardiovascular		Surgery: General	
	Count	Median	Count	Median	Count	Median
Gross charges/procedure	2	*	4	*	13	$285.71
Total cost/procedure	2	*	3	*	12	$261.81
Operating cost/procedure	2	*	3	*	12	$179.90
Provider cost/procedure	2	*	4	*	12	$78.95
Procedures/patient	1	*	1	*	7	*
Gross charges/patient	1	*	1	*	13	221
Procedures/physician	2	*	4	*	13	$47,150
Gross charges/physician	2	*	4	*	13	$47,150
Procedures/provider	0	*	3	*	4	*
Gross charges/provider	0	*	3	*	4	*
Gross charge to total cost ratio	2	*	3	*	12	1.25
Oper cost to total cost ratio	2	*	3	*	12	.68
Prov cost to total cost ratio	2	*	3	*	12	.32
Total support staff FTE/phy	**12**	**2.27**	**14**	**1.86**	**22**	**2.92**

Table 15.11e: Surgery/Anesthesia Procedure Data (outside the practice)

	Radiology		Surg: Cardiovascular		Surgery: General	
	Count	Median	Count	Median	Count	Median
Gross charges/procedure	5	*	8	*	16	$1,087.65
Total cost/procedure	5	*	7	*	15	$410.79
Operating cost/procedure	5	*	7	*	15	$126.52
Provider cost/procedure	5	*	8	*	15	$291.24
Procedures/patient	1	*	5	*	7	*
Gross charges/patient	1	*	4	*	7	*
Procedures/physician	5	*	9	*	16	788
Gross charges/physician	5	*	8	*	16	$872,358
Procedures/provider	0	*	7	*	4	*
Gross charges/provider	0	*	6	*	4	*
Gross charge to total cost ratio	5	*	7	*	15	2.60
Oper cost to total cost ratio	5	*	7	*	15	.31
Prov cost to total cost ratio	5	*	7	*	15	.69
Total support staff FTE/phy	**12**	**2.27**	**14**	**1.86**	**22**	**2.92**

Single Specialty Practices, Not Hospital or IDS Owned — Radiology, Surgery: Cardiovascular, Surgery: General (Procedure and Charge Data)

Table 15.11f: Clinical Laboratory/Pathology Procedure Data

	Radiology		Surg: Cardiovascular		Surgery: General	
	Count	Median	Count	Median	Count	Median
Gross charges/procedure	1	*	0	*	3	*
Total cost/procedure	1	*	0	*	3	*
Operating cost/procedure	1	*	0	*	3	*
Provider cost/procedure	1	*	0	*	3	*
Procedures/patient	1	*	0	*	1	*
Gross charges/patient	1	*	0	*	1	*
Procedures/physician	1	*	0	*	3	*
Gross charges/physician	1	*	0	*	3	*
Procedures/provider	0	*	0	*	0	*
Gross charges/provider	0	*	0	*	0	*
Gross charge to total cost ratio	1	*	0	*	3	*
Oper cost to total cost ratio	1	*	0	*	3	*
Prov cost to total cost ratio	1	*	0	*	3	*
Total support staff FTE/phy	12	2.27	14	1.86	22	2.92

Table 15.11g: Diagnostic Radiology and Imaging Procedure Data

	Radiology		Surg: Cardiovascular		Surgery: General	
	Count	Median	Count	Median	Count	Median
Gross charges/procedure	10	$85.11	4	*	15	$222.63
Total cost/procedure	10	$37.32	4	*	14	$138.23
Operating cost/procedure	10	$8.10	4	*	14	$88.50
Provider cost/procedure	10	$24.92	4	*	14	$61.59
Procedures/patient	3	*	2	*	7	*
Gross charges/patient	3	*	2	*	7	*
Procedures/physician	10	18,524	4	*	15	128
Gross charges/physician	10	$1,532,392	4	*	13	$20,274
Procedures/provider	1	*	2	*	4	*
Gross charges/provider	1	*	2	*	4	*
Gross charge to total cost ratio	10	2.21	4	*	14	1.54
Oper cost to total cost ratio	10	.25	4	*	14	.61
Prov cost to total cost ratio	10	.75	4	*	14	.39
Total support staff FTE/phy	12	2.27	14	1.86	22	2.92

Table 15.11h: Nonprocedural Gross Charge Data

	Radiology		Surg: Cardiovascular		Surgery: General	
	Count	Median	Count	Median	Count	Median
Gross charges/patient	1	*	1	*	2	*
Nonproc gross charges/physician	3	*	1	*	5	*
Gross charges/provider	0	*	0	*	1	*
Total support staff FTE/phy	12	2.27	14	1.86	22	2.92

Single Specialty Practices, Not Hospital or IDS Owned — Surgery: Neurological, Surgery: Oral, Urology

Table 16.1: Staffing and Practice Data

	Surg: Neurological		Surg: Oral		Urology	
	Count	Median	Count	Median	Count	Median
Total provider FTE	5	*	2	*	27	9.00
Total physician FTE	10	5.40	11	4.50	84	5.00
Total nonphysician provider FTE	5	*	2	*	27	1.60
Total support staff FTE	10	20.00	11	32.00	84	22.50
Number of branch clinics	4	*	4	*	2	*
Square footage of all facilities	10	10,556	11	13,000	78	9,148

Table 16.2: Accounts Receivable Data, Collection Percentages and Financial Ratios

	Surg: Neurological		Surg: Oral		Urology	
	Count	Median	Count	Median	Count	Median
Total AR/physician	8	*	11	$144,619	69	$177,071
Total AR/provider	4	*	2	*	22	$149,668
0-30 days in AR	8	*	11	46.34%	69	56.82%
31-60 days in AR	8	*	11	21.98%	69	15.76%
61-90 days in AR	8	*	11	9.71%	69	7.40%
91-120 days in AR	8	*	11	7.51%	69	3.99%
120+ days in AR	8	*	11	16.24%	69	12.93%
Re-aged: 0-30 days in AR	2	*	2	*	17	56.82%
Re-aged: 31-60 days in AR	2	*	2	*	17	17.25%
Re-aged: 61-90 days in AR	2	*	2	*	17	6.14%
Re-aged: 91-120 days in AR	2	*	2	*	17	3.50%
Re-aged: 120+ days in AR	2	*	2	*	17	11.71%
Not re-aged: 0-30 days in AR	6	*	9	*	50	58.49%
Not re-aged: 31-60 days in AR	6	*	9	*	50	14.57%
Not re-aged: 61-90 days in AR	6	*	9	*	50	7.49%
Not re-aged: 91-120 days in AR	6	*	9	*	50	4.14%
Not re-aged: 120+ days in AR	6	*	9	*	50	13.56%
Months gross FFS charges in AR	8	*	6	*	5	*
Days gross FFS charges in AR	8	*	6	*	5	*
Gross FFS collection %	10	36.66%	6	*	6	*
Adjusted FFS collection %	9	*	6	*	6	*
Gross FFS + cap collection %	1	*	0	*	1	*
Net cap rev % of gross cap chrg	1	*	0	*	1	*
Current ratio	4	*	3	*	2	*
Tot asset turnover ratio	4	*	3	*	2	*
Debt to equity ratio	4	*	3	*	2	*
Debt ratio	4	*	3	*	2	*
Return on total assets	4	*	4	*	5	*
Return on equity	4	*	4	*	5	*

Table 16.3: Breakout of Total Gross Charges by Type of Payer

	Surg: Neurological		Surg: Oral		Urology	
	Count	Median	Count	Median	Count	Median
Medicare: fee-for-service	10	25.50%	10	2.00%	77	41.00%
Medicare: managed care FFS	10	.00%	10	.00%	77	.00%
Medicare: capitation	10	.00%	10	.00%	77	.00%
Medicaid: fee-for-service	10	2.00%	10	.32%	77	2.00%
Medicaid: managed care FFS	10	.00%	10	.00%	77	.00%
Medicaid: capitation	10	.00%	10	.00%	77	.00%
Commercial: fee-for-service	10	8.20%	10	37.50%	77	21.00%
Commercial: managed care FFS	10	43.00%	10	13.50%	77	19.00%
Commercial: capitation	10	.00%	10	.00%	77	.00%
Workers' compensation	10	5.50%	10	.03%	77	.02%
Charity care and prof courtesy	10	1.35%	10	.75%	77	.50%
Self-pay	10	1.00%	10	23.50%	77	3.00%
Other federal government payers	10	.00%	10	.00%	77	.00%

Single Specialty Practices, Not Hospital or IDS Owned — Surgery: Neurological, Surgery: Oral, Urology (per FTE Physician)

Table 16.4a: Staffing, RVUs, Patients, Procedures and Square Footage

	Surg: Neurological		Surg: Oral		Urology	
	Count	Median	Count	Median	Count	Median
Total provider FTE/physician	5	*	2	*	27	1.25
Prim care phy/physician	0	*	0	*	1	*
Nonsurg phy/physician	1	*	0	*	1	*
Surg spec phy/physician	9	*	6	*	0	*
Total NPP FTE/physician	5	*	2	*	27	.25
Total support staff FTE/phy	10	3.42	11	6.24	84	4.21
Total empl support staff FTE	10	3.24	6	*	6	*
General administrative	9	*	5	*	6	*
Patient accounting	9	*	5	*	6	*
General accounting	3	*	1	*	5	*
Managed care administrative	2	*	1	*	0	*
Information technology	2	*	0	*	4	*
Housekeeping, maint, security	0	*	0	*	0	*
Medical receptionists	8	*	5	*	6	*
Med secretaries,transcribers	8	*	3	*	4	*
Medical records	8	*	1	*	5	*
Other admin support	3	*	2	*	3	*
*Total administrative supp staff	2	*	6	*	80	2.67
Registered Nurses	2	*	5	*	6	*
Licensed Practical Nurses	4	*	3	*	5	*
Med assistants, nurse aides	5	*	3	*	6	*
*Total clinical supp staff	2	*	7	*	79	1.50
Clinical laboratory	0	*	0	*	5	*
Radiology and imaging	2	*	0	*	5	*
Other medical support serv	2	*	3	*	3	*
*Total ancillary supp staff	1	*	0	*	45	.25
Tot contracted supp staff	3	*	3	*	25	.27
Tot RVU/physician	4	*	1	*	15	17,605
Physician work RVU/physician	2	*	1	*	16	7,933
Patients/physician	6	*	5	*	1	*
Tot procedures/physician	8	*	5	*	5	*
Square feet/physician	10	1,623	11	2,333	78	1,800

*See pages 260 and 261 for definition.

Table 16.4b: Charges and Revenue

	Surg: Neurological		Surg: Oral		Urology	
	Count	Median	Count	Median	Count	Median
Net fee-for-service revenue	10	$1,049,663	6	*	6	*
Gross FFS charges	10	$2,622,333	6	*	6	*
Adjustments to FFS charges	9	*	6	*	6	*
Adjusted FFS charges	9	*	6	*	6	*
Bad debts due to FFS activity	9	*	5	*	6	*
Net capitation revenue	1	*	0	*	1	*
Gross capitation charges	1	*	0	*	1	*
Capitation revenue	1	*	0	*	0	*
Purch serv for cap patients	0	*	0	*	0	*
Net other medical revenue	5	*	1	*	0	*
Gross rev from other activity	5	*	1	*	0	*
Other medical revenue	2	*	1	*	0	*
Rev from sale of goods/services	3	*	0	*	0	*
Cost of sales	0	*	0	*	0	*
Total gross charges	10	$2,622,333	10	$1,195,257	81	$1,665,256
Total medical revenue	10	$1,049,659	11	$943,941	84	$853,312

Single Specialty Practices, Not Hospital or IDS Owned — Surgery: Neurological, Surgery: Oral, Urology (per FTE Physician)

Table 16.4c: Operating Cost

	Surg: Neurological		Surg: Oral		Urology	
	Count	Median	Count	Median	Count	Median
Total support staff cost/phy	10	$166,780	11	$232,561	84	$155,644
Total empl supp staff cost/phy	10	$128,882	6	*	6	*
General administrative	9	*	5	*	6	*
Patient accounting	9	*	5	*	6	*
General accounting	3	*	1	*	5	*
Managed care administrative	2	*	1	*	0	*
Information technology	2	*	0	*	4	*
Housekeeping, maint, security	0	*	0	*	0	*
Medical receptionists	8	*	5	*	6	*
Med secretaries,transcribers	8	*	3	*	4	*
Medical records	8	*	1	*	5	*
Other admin support	3	*	2	*	3	*
***Total administrative supp staff**	2	*	5	*	78	$83,174
Registered Nurses	2	*	5	*	6	*
Licensed Practical Nurses	4	*	3	*	5	*
Med assistants, nurse aides	5	*	3	*	6	*
***Total clinical supp staff**	2	*	6	*	77	$42,323
Clinical laboratory	0	*	0	*	5	*
Radiology and imaging	2	*	0	*	5	*
Other medical support serv	2	*	3	*	3	*
***Total ancillary supp staff**	1	*	0	*	43	$8,825
Total empl supp staff benefits	10	$35,412	9	*	69	$33,045
Tot contracted supp staff	3	*	3	*	27	$6,267
Total general operating cost	10	$159,132	11	$287,559	84	$270,280
Information technology	10	$14,624	6	*	6	*
Medical and surgical supply	10	$1,739	6	*	6	*
Building and occupancy	10	$33,395	6	*	6	*
Furniture and equipment	8	*	3	*	4	*
Admin supplies and services	10	$21,720	6	*	6	*
Prof liability insurance	8	*	10	$11,031	84	$15,404
Other insurance premiums	10	$981	6	*	6	*
Outside professional fees	9	*	6	*	6	*
Promotion and marketing	10	$1,753	6	*	6	*
Clinical laboratory	0	*	1	*	6	*
Radiology and imaging	3	*	4	*	4	*
Other ancillary services	1	*	0	*	2	*
Billing purchased services	5	*	5	*	1	*
Management fees paid to MSO	3	*	0	*	0	*
Misc operating cost	9	*	5	*	5	*
Cost allocated to prac from par	0	*	0	*	0	*
Total operating cost	10	$333,113	11	$485,306	84	$423,699

*See pages 260 and 261 for definition.

Single Specialty Practices, Not Hospital or IDS Owned — Surgery: Neurological, Surgery: Oral, Urology (per FTE Physician)

Table 16.4d: Provider Cost

	Surg: Neurological		Surg: Oral		Urology	
	Count	Median	Count	Median	Count	Median
Total med rev after oper cost	10	$708,986	11	$471,859	84	$414,926
Total provider cost/physician	10	$716,457	11	$418,666	84	$387,222
Total NPP cost/physician	5	*	2	*	27	$19,946
Nonphysician provider comp	5	*	1	*	1	*
Nonphysician prov benefit cost	5	*	1	*	1	*
Provider consultant cost	0	*	0	*	9	*
Total physician cost/physician	10	$687,866	11	$402,397	84	$373,438
Total phy compensation	9	*	6	*	2	*
Total phy benefit cost	8	*	6	*	2	*

Table 16.4e: Net Income or Loss

	Surg: Neurological		Surg: Oral		Urology	
	Count	Median	Count	Median	Count	Median
Total cost	10	$1,057,130	11	$942,504	84	$846,736
Net nonmedical revenue	4	*	1	*	37	$1,440
Nonmedical revenue	4	*	1	*	1	*
Fin support for oper costs	1	*	0	*	0	*
Goodwill amortization	0	*	0	*	0	*
Nonmedical cost	3	*	1	*	0	*
Net inc, prac with fin sup	1	*	0	*	0	*
Net inc, prac w/o fin sup	8	*	11	$19,830	80	$13,592
Net inc, excl fin supp (all prac)	9	*	11	$19,830	80	$13,592

Table 16.4f: Assets and Liabilities

	Surg: Neurological		Surg: Oral		Urology	
	Count	Median	Count	Median	Count	Median
Total assets	5	*	3	*	2	*
Current assets	5	*	3	*	2	*
Noncurrent assets	5	*	3	*	2	*
Total liabilities	5	*	3	*	2	*
Current liabilities	5	*	3	*	2	*
Noncurrent liabilities	5	*	3	*	2	*
Working capital	5	*	3	*	2	*
Total net worth	5	*	3	*	2	*
Total support staff FTE/phy	10	3.42	11	6.24	84	4.21

Single Specialty Practices, Not Hospital or IDS Owned — Surgery: Neurological, Surgery: Oral, Urology (as a % of Total Medical Revenue)

Table 16.5a: Charges and Revenue

	Surg: Neurological		Surg: Oral		Urology	
	Count	Median	Count	Median	Count	Median
Net fee-for-service revenue	10	99.72%	6	*	6	*
Net capitation revenue	1	*	0	*	1	*
Net other medical revenue	5	*	1	*	0	*
Total gross charges	**10**	**272.01%**	**10**	**120.16%**	**81**	**175.42%**

Table 16.5b: Operating Cost

	Surg: Neurological		Surg: Oral		Urology	
	Count	Median	Count	Median	Count	Median
Total support staff cost	**10**	**15.50%**	**11**	**22.08%**	**84**	**18.53%**
Total empl support staff cost	10	11.61%	6	*	6	*
General administrative	9	*	5	*	6	*
Patient accounting	9	*	5	*	6	*
General accounting	3	*	1	*	5	*
Managed care administrative	2	*	1	*	0	*
Information technology	2	*	0	*	4	*
Housekeeping, maint, security	0	*	0	*	0	*
Medical receptionists	8	*	5	*	6	*
Med secretaries,transcribers	8	*	3	*	4	*
Medical records	8	*	1	*	5	*
Other admin support	3	*	2	*	3	*
*Total administrative supp staff	2	*	5	*	78	9.68%
Registered Nurses	2	*	5	*	6	*
Licensed Practical Nurses	4	*	3	*	5	*
Med assistants, nurse aides	5	*	3	*	6	*
*Total clinical supp staff	2	*	6	*	77	4.89%
Clinical laboratory	0	*	0	*	5	*
Radiology and imaging	2	*	0	*	5	*
Other medical support serv	2	*	3	*	3	*
*Total ancillary supp staff	1	*	0	*	43	1.13%
Total empl supp staff benefits	10	3.57%	9	*	69	3.66%
Tot contracted supp staff	3	*	3	*	27	.70%
Total general operating cost	**10**	**16.29%**	**11**	**28.25%**	**84**	**30.13%**
Information technology	10	1.66%	6	*	6	*
Medical and surgical supply	10	.18%	6	*	6	*
Building and occupancy	10	3.43%	6	*	6	*
Furniture and equipment	8	*	3	*	4	*
Admin supplies and services	10	2.10%	6	*	6	*
Prof liability insurance	8	*	10	.96%	84	1.74%
Other insurance premiums	10	.09%	6	*	6	*
Outside professional fees	9	*	6	*	6	*
Promotion and marketing	10	.19%	6	*	6	*
Clinical laboratory	0	*	1	*	6	*
Radiology and imaging	3	*	4	*	4	*
Other ancillary services	1	*	0	*	2	*
Billing purchased services	5	*	5	*	1	*
Management fees paid to MSO	3	*	0	*	0	*
Misc operating cost	9	*	5	*	5	*
Cost allocated to prac from par	0	*	0	*	0	*
Total operating cost	**10**	**31.98%**	**11**	**51.88%**	**84**	**50.67%**

*See pages 260 and 261 for definition.

Single Specialty Practices, Not Hospital or IDS Owned — Surgery: Neurological, Surgery: Oral, Urology (as a % of Total Medical Revenue)

Table 16.5c: Provider Cost

	Surg: Neurological		Surg: Oral		Urology	
	Count	Median	Count	Median	Count	Median
Total med rev after oper cost	10	68.02%	11	48.12%	84	49.20%
Total provider cost	10	67.14%	11	47.24%	84	45.84%
Total NPP cost	5	*	2	*	27	1.99%
Nonphysician provider comp	5	*	1	*	1	*
Nonphysician prov benefit cost	5	*	1	*	1	*
Provider consultant cost	0	*	0	*	9	*
Total physician cost	10	62.94%	11	47.24%	84	44.91%
Total phy compensation	9	*	6	*	2	*
Total phy benefit cost	8	*	6	*	2	*

Table 16.5d: Net Income or Loss

	Surg: Neurological		Surg: Oral		Urology	
	Count	Median	Count	Median	Count	Median
Total cost	10	99.57%	11	97.89%	84	98.67%
Net nonmedical revenue	4	*	1	*	37	.18%
Nonmedical revenue	4	*	1	*	1	*
Fin support for oper costs	1	*	0	*	0	*
Goodwill amortization	0	*	0	*	0	*
Nonmedical cost	3	*	1	*	0	*
Net inc, prac with fin sup	1	*	0	*	0	*
Net inc, prac w/o fin sup	8	*	11	2.11%	81	1.63%
Net inc, excl fin supp (all prac)	9	*	11	2.11%	81	1.63%

Table 16.5e: Assets and Liabilities

	Surg: Neurological		Surg: Oral		Urology	
	Count	Median	Count	Median	Count	Median
Total assets	5	*	3	*	2	*
Current assets	5	*	3	*	2	*
Noncurrent assets	5	*	3	*	2	*
Total liabilities	5	*	3	*	2	*
Current liabilities	5	*	3	*	2	*
Noncurrent liabilities	5	*	3	*	2	*
Working capital	5	*	3	*	2	*
Total net worth	5	*	3	*	2	*

Single Specialty Practices, Not Hospital or IDS Owned — Surgery: Neurological, Surgery: Oral, Urology (per FTE Provider)

Table 16.6a: Staffing, RVUs, Patients, Procedures and Square Footage

	Surg: Neurological		Surg: Oral		Urology	
	Count	Median	Count	Median	Count	Median
Total physician FTE/provider	5	*	2	*	27	.80
Prim care phy/provider	0	*	0	*	1	*
Nonsurg phy/provider	1	*	0	*	1	*
Surg spec phy/provider	5	*	1	*	0	*
Total NPP FTE/provider	5	*	2	*	27	.20
Total support staff FTE/prov	5	*	2	*	27	4.00
Total empl supp staff FTE/prov	5	*	1	*	2	*
General administrative	4	*	0	*	2	*
Patient accounting	4	*	0	*	2	*
General accounting	2	*	0	*	1	*
Managed care administrative	0	*	0	*	0	*
Information technology	1	*	0	*	2	*
Housekeeping, maint, security	0	*	0	*	0	*
Medical receptionists	4	*	0	*	2	*
Med secretaries,transcribers	4	*	0	*	2	*
Medical records	4	*	0	*	2	*
Other admin support	0	*	0	*	0	*
*Total administrative supp staff	0	*	1	*	26	2.15
Registered Nurses	1	*	0	*	2	*
Licensed Practical Nurses	2	*	0	*	2	*
Med assistants, nurse aides	3	*	0	*	2	*
*Total clinical supp staff	1	*	1	*	26	1.28
Clinical laboratory	0	*	0	*	2	*
Radiology and imaging	1	*	0	*	1	*
Other medical support serv	1	*	0	*	1	*
*Total ancillary supp staff	0	*	0	*	18	.29
Tot contracted supp staff	2	*	1	*	10	.13
Tot RVU/provider	2	*	0	*	8	*
Physician work RVU/provider	0	*	0	*	11	6,343
Patients/provider	3	*	0	*	1	*
Tot procedures/provider	3	*	0	*	2	*
Square feet/provider	5	*	2	*	24	1,523
Total support staff FTE/phy	10	3.42	11	6.24	84	4.21

*See pages 260 and 261 for definition.

Table 16.6b: Charges, Revenue and Cost

	Surg: Neurological		Surg: Oral		Urology	
	Count	Median	Count	Median	Count	Median
Total gross charges	5	*	2	*	27	$1,323,665
Total medical revenue	5	*	2	*	27	$750,980
Net fee-for-service revenue	5	*	1	*	2	*
Net capitation revenue	0	*	0	*	1	*
Net other medical revenue	3	*	1	*	0	*
Total support staff cost/prov	5	*	2	*	27	$140,399
Total general operating cost	5	*	2	*	27	$221,918
Total operating cost	5	*	2	*	27	$375,343
Total med rev after oper cost	5	*	2	*	27	$329,438
Total provider cost/provider	5	*	2	*	27	$329,266
Total NPP cost/provider	5	*	2	*	27	$15,225
Provider consultant cost	0	*	0	*	4	*
Total physician cost/provider	5	*	2	*	27	$316,463
Total phy compensation	5	*	1	*	1	*
Total phy benefit cost	5	*	1	*	1	*
Total cost	5	*	2	*	27	$743,748
Net nonmedical revenue	2	*	0	*	17	$1,333
Net inc, prac with fin sup	0	*	0	*	0	*
Net inc, prac w/o fin sup	4	*	2	*	26	$3,662
Net inc, excl fin supp (all prac)	4	*	2	*	26	$3,662
Total support staff FTE/phy	10	3.42	11	6.24	84	4.21

Single Specialty Practices, Not Hospital or IDS Owned — Surgery: Neurological, Surgery: Oral, Urology (per Square Foot)

Table 16.7a: Staffing, RVUs, Patients and Procedures

	Surg: Neurological		Surg: Oral		Urology	
	Count	Median	Count	Median	Count	Median
Total prov FTE/10,000 sq ft	5	*	2	*	24	6.57
Total phy FTE/10,000 sq ft	10	6.16	11	4.29	78	5.56
Prim care phy/10,000 sq ft	0	*	0	*	1	*
Nonsurg phy/10,000 sq ft	1	*	0	*	1	*
Surg spec phy/10,000 sq ft	9	*	6	*	0	*
Total NPP FTE/10,000 sq ft	5	*	2	*	24	1.50
Total supp stf FTE/10,000 sq ft	10	20.77	11	28.41	78	22.89
Total empl supp stf/10,000 sq ft	10	20.36	6	*	5	*
General administrative	9	*	5	*	5	*
Patient accounting	9	*	5	*	5	*
General accounting	3	*	1	*	4	*
Managed care administrative	2	*	1	*	0	*
Information technology	2	*	0	*	4	*
Housekeeping, maint, security	0	*	0	*	0	*
Medical receptionists	8	*	5	*	5	*
Med secretaries,transcribers	8	*	3	*	4	*
Medical records	8	*	1	*	4	*
Other admin support	3	*	2	*	3	*
*Total administrative supp staff	2	*	6	*	75	14.02
Registered Nurses	2	*	5	*	5	*
Licensed Practical Nurses	4	*	3	*	5	*
Med assistants, nurse aides	5	*	3	*	5	*
*Total clinical supp staff	2	*	7	*	74	7.52
Clinical laboratory	0	*	0	*	5	*
Radiology and imaging	2	*	0	*	4	*
Other medical support serv	2	*	3	*	3	*
*Total ancillary supp staff	1	*	0	*	43	1.40
Tot contracted supp staff	3	*	3	*	24	1.39
Tot RVU/sq ft	4	*	1	*	13	10.79
Physician work RVU/sq ft	2	*	1	*	16	3.83
Patients/sq ft	6	*	5	*	1	*
Tot procedures/sq ft	8	*	5	*	4	*
Total support staff FTE/phy	10	3.42	11	6.24	84	4.21

*See pages 260 and 261 for definition.

Table 16.7b: Charges, Revenue and Cost

	Surg: Neurological		Surg: Oral		Urology	
	Count	Median	Count	Median	Count	Median
Total gross charges	10	$1,638.69	10	$531.49	75	$814.63
Total medical revenue	10	$697.14	11	$423.53	78	$476.72
Net fee-for-service revenue	10	$694.31	6	*	5	*
Net capitation revenue	1	*	0	*	1	*
Net other medical revenue	5	*	1	*	0	*
Total support staff cost/sq ft	10	$93.03	11	$107.34	78	$87.92
Total general operating cost	10	$99.63	11	$121.49	78	$144.52
Total operating cost	10	$217.56	11	$223.99	78	$238.01
Total med rev after oper cost	10	$476.68	11	$199.78	78	$212.81
Total provider cost/sq ft	10	$476.63	11	$199.73	78	$203.36
Total NPP cost/sq ft	5	*	2	*	24	$10.04
Provider consultant cost	0	*	0	*	8	*
Total physician cost/sq ft	10	$448.83	11	$199.73	78	$201.64
Total phy compensation	9	*	6	*	1	*
Total phy benefit cost	8	*	6	*	1	*
Total cost	10	$697.08	11	$422.73	78	$471.19
Net nonmedical revenue/sq ft	4	*	1	*	33	$.80
Net inc, prac with fin sup	1	*	0	*	0	*
Net inc, prac w/o fin sup	8	*	11	$8.50	75	$7.59
Net inc, excl fin supp (all prac)	9	*	11	$8.50	75	$7.59
Total support staff FTE/phy	10	3.42	11	6.24	84	4.21

Single Specialty Practices, Not Hospital or IDS Owned — Surgery: Neurological, Surgery: Oral, Urology (per Total RVU)

Table 16.8a: Staffing, Patients, Procedures and Square Footage

	Surg: Neurological		Surg: Oral		Urology	
	Count	Median	Count	Median	Count	Median
Total prov FTE/10,000 tot RVU	2	*	0	*	8	*
Total phy FTE/10,000 tot RVU	4	*	1	*	15	.57
Prim care phy/10,000 tot RVU	0	*	0	*	1	*
Nonsurg phy/10,000 tot RVU	0	*	0	*	1	*
Surg spec phy/10,000 tot RVU	4	*	1	*	0	*
Total NPP FTE/10,000 tot RVU	2	*	0	*	8	*
Total supp stf FTE/10,000 tot RVU	4	*	1	*	15	2.96
Tot empl supp stf/10,000 tot RVU	4	*	1	*	3	*
General administrative	3	*	1	*	3	*
Patient accounting	3	*	1	*	3	*
General accounting	2	*	0	*	2	*
Managed care administrative	1	*	1	*	0	*
Information technology	1	*	0	*	3	*
Housekeeping, maint, security	0	*	0	*	0	*
Medical receptionists	3	*	1	*	3	*
Med secretaries,transcribers	3	*	1	*	2	*
Medical records	3	*	0	*	3	*
Other admin support	2	*	1	*	1	*
*Total administrative supp staff	1	*	1	*	14	2.02
Registered Nurses	0	*	1	*	3	*
Licensed Practical Nurses	0	*	0	*	3	*
Med assistants, nurse aides	1	*	1	*	3	*
*Total clinical supp staff	0	*	1	*	13	.86
Clinical laboratory	0	*	0	*	3	*
Radiology and imaging	1	*	0	*	2	*
Other medical support serv	0	*	0	*	1	*
*Total ancillary supp staff	1	*	0	*	10	.18
Tot contracted supp staff	0	*	1	*	8	.40
Physician work RVU/tot RVU	2	*	1	*	10	.40
Patients/tot RVU	3	*	1	*	1	*
Tot procedures/tot RVU	3	*	1	*	3	*
Square feet/tot RVU	4	*	1	*	13	.09
Total support staff FTE/phy	10	3.42	11	6.24	84	4.21

*See pages 260 and 261 for definition.

Table 16.8b: Charges, Revenue and Cost

	Surg: Neurological		Surg: Oral		Urology	
	Count	Median	Count	Median	Count	Median
Total gross charges	4	*	1	*	15	$99.08
Total medical revenue	4	*	1	*	15	$53.62
Net fee-for-service revenue	4	*	1	*	3	*
Net capitation revenue	0	*	0	*	1	*
Net other medical revenue	2	*	0	*	0	*
Total supp staff cost/tot RVU	4	*	1	*	15	$11.69
Total general operating cost	4	*	1	*	15	$16.11
Total operating cost	4	*	1	*	15	$28.70
Total med rev after oper cost	4	*	1	*	15	$23.17
Total provider cost/tot RVU	4	*	1	*	15	$23.31
Total NPP cost/tot RVU	2	*	0	*	8	*
Provider consultant cost	0	*	0	*	3	*
Total physician cost/tot RVU	4	*	1	*	15	$22.69
Total phy compensation	4	*	1	*	1	*
Total phy benefit cost	4	*	1	*	1	*
Total cost	3	*	1	*	3	*
Net nonmedical revenue	1	*	0	*	9	*
Net inc, prac with fin sup	0	*	0	*	0	*
Net inc, prac w/o fin sup	3	*	1	*	15	$.22
Net inc, excl fin supp (all prac)	3	*	1	*	15	$.22
Total support staff FTE/phy	10	3.42	11	6.24	84	4.21

Single Specialty Practices, Not Hospital or IDS Owned — Surgery: Neurological, Surgery: Oral, Urology (per Work RVU)

Table 16.9a: Staffing, Patients, Procedures and Square Footage

	Surg: Neurological		Surg: Oral		Urology	
	Count	Median	Count	Median	Count	Median
Total prov FTE/10,000 work RVU	0	*	0	*	11	1.58
Tot phy FTE/10,000 work RVU	2	*	1	*	16	1.26
Prim care phy/10,000 work RVU	0	*	0	*	1	*
Nonsurg phy/10,000 work RVU	0	*	0	*	1	*
Surg spec phy/10,000 work RVU	2	*	1	*	0	*
Total NPP FTE/10,000 work RVU	0	*	0	*	11	.30
Total supp stf FTE/10,000 wrk RVU	2	*	1	*	16	7.05
Tot empl supp stf/10,000 work RVU	2	*	1	*	3	*
General administrative	2	*	1	*	3	*
Patient accounting	2	*	1	*	3	*
General accounting	1	*	0	*	2	*
Managed care administrative	1	*	1	*	0	*
Information technology	1	*	0	*	3	*
Housekeeping, maint, security	0	*	0	*	0	*
Medical receptionists	2	*	1	*	3	*
Med secretaries,transcribers	2	*	1	*	2	*
Medical records	2	*	0	*	3	*
Other admin support	2	*	1	*	1	*
*Total administrative supp staff	1	*	1	*	15	4.73
Registered Nurses	0	*	1	*	3	*
Licensed Practical Nurses	0	*	0	*	3	*
Med assistants, nurse aides	1	*	1	*	3	*
*Total clinical supp staff	0	*	1	*	15	2.31
Clinical laboratory	0	*	0	*	3	*
Radiology and imaging	1	*	0	*	2	*
Other medical support serv	0	*	0	*	1	*
*Total ancillary supp staff	1	*	0	*	11	.48
Tot contracted supp staff	0	*	1	*	6	*
Tot RVU/work RVU	2	*	1	*	10	2.51
Patients/work RVU	2	*	1	*	1	*
Tot procedures/work RVU	2	*	1	*	3	*
Square feet/work RVU	2	*	1	*	16	.26
Total support staff FTE/phy	10	3.42	11	6.24	84	4.21

*See pages 260 and 261 for definition.

Table 16.9b: Charges, Revenue and Cost

	Surg: Neurological		Surg: Oral		Urology	
	Count	Median	Count	Median	Count	Median
Total gross charges	2	*	1	*	16	$264.74
Total medical revenue	2	*	1	*	16	$126.75
Net fee-for-service revenue	2	*	1	*	3	*
Net capitation revenue	0	*	0	*	1	*
Net other medical revenue	1	*	0	*	0	*
Total supp staff cost/work RVU	2	*	1	*	16	$27.99
Total general operating cost	2	*	1	*	16	$35.72
Total operating cost	2	*	1	*	16	$67.09
Total med rev after oper cost	2	*	1	*	16	$58.80
Total provider cost/work RVU	2	*	1	*	16	$59.53
Total NPP cost/work RVU	0	*	0	*	11	$2.59
Provider consultant cost	0	*	0	*	2	*
Total physician cost/work RVU	2	*	1	*	16	$56.76
Total phy compensation	2	*	1	*	1	*
Total phy benefit cost	2	*	1	*	1	*
Total cost	2	*	1	*	16	$132.71
Net nonmedical revenue	0	*	0	*	10	$.22
Net inc, prac with fin sup	0	*	0	*	0	*
Net inc, prac w/o fin sup	2	*	1	*	16	$.26
Net inc, excl fin supp (all prac)	2	*	1	*	16	$.26
Total support staff FTE/phy	10	3.42	11	6.24	84	4.21

Single Specialty Practices, Not Hospital or IDS Owned — Surgery: Neurological, Surgery: Oral, Urology (per Patient)

Table 16.10a: Staffing, RVUs, Procedures and Square Footage

	Surg: Neurological		Surg: Oral		Urology	
	Count	Median	Count	Median	Count	Median
Total prov FTE/10,000 patients	3	*	0	*	1	*
Total phy FTE/10,000 pat	6	*	5	*	1	*
Prim care phy/10,000 pat	0	*	0	*	1	*
Nonsurg phy/10,000 pat	1	*	0	*	1	*
Surg spec phy/10,000 pat	6	*	5	*	0	*
Total NPP FTE/10,000 pat	3	*	0	*	1	*
Total supp staff FTE/10,000 pat	6	*	5	*	1	*
Total empl supp staff/10,000 pat	6	*	5	*	1	*
General administrative	6	*	5	*	1	*
Patient accounting	6	*	5	*	1	*
General accounting	3	*	1	*	0	*
Managed care administrative	1	*	1	*	0	*
Information technology	2	*	0	*	1	*
Housekeeping, maint, security	0	*	0	*	0	*
Medical receptionists	5	*	5	*	1	*
Med secretaries,transcribers	5	*	3	*	1	*
Medical records	5	*	1	*	1	*
Other admin support	2	*	2	*	0	*
*Total administrative supp staff	1	*	2	*	0	*
Registered Nurses	1	*	5	*	1	*
Licensed Practical Nurses	3	*	3	*	1	*
Med assistants, nurse aides	3	*	3	*	1	*
*Total clinical supp staff	1	*	3	*	0	*
Clinical laboratory	0	*	0	*	1	*
Radiology and imaging	2	*	0	*	0	*
Other medical support serv	2	*	3	*	1	*
*Total ancillary supp staff	1	*	0	*	0	*
Tot contracted supp staff	2	*	1	*	1	*
Tot RVU/patient	3	*	1	*	1	*
Physician work RVU/patient	2	*	1	*	1	*
Tot procedures/patient	6	*	5	*	1	*
Square feet/patient	6	*	5	*	1	*
Total support staff FTE/phy	10	3.42	11	6.24	84	4.21

*See pages 260 and 261 for definition.

Table 16.10b: Charges, Revenue and Cost

	Surg: Neurological		Surg: Oral		Urology	
	Count	Median	Count	Median	Count	Median
Total gross charges	6	*	5	*	1	*
Total medical revenue	6	*	5	*	1	*
Net fee-for-service revenue	6	*	5	*	1	*
Net capitation revenue	0	*	0	*	1	*
Net other medical revenue	3	*	0	*	0	*
Total support staff cost/patient	6	*	5	*	1	*
Total general operating cost	6	*	5	*	1	*
Total operating cost	6	*	5	*	1	*
Total med rev after oper cost	6	*	5	*	1	*
Total provider cost/patient	6	*	5	*	1	*
Total NPP cost/patient	3	*	0	*	1	*
Provider consultant cost	0	*	0	*	0	*
Total physician cost/patient	6	*	5	*	1	*
Total phy compensation	6	*	5	*	1	*
Total phy benefit cost	5	*	5	*	1	*
Total cost	6	*	5	*	1	*
Net nonmedical revenue	3	*	1	*	1	*
Net inc, prac with fin sup	1	*	0	*	0	*
Net inc, prac w/o fin sup	5	*	5	*	1	*
Net inc, excl fin supp (all prac)	6	*	5	*	1	*
Total support staff FTE/phy	10	3.42	11	6.24	84	4.21

Single Specialty Practices, Not Hospital or IDS Owned — Surgery: Neurological, Surgery: Oral, Urology (Procedure and Charge Data)

Table 16.11a: Activity Charges to Total Gross Charges Ratios

	Surg: Neurological		Surg: Oral		Urology	
	Count	Median	Count	Median	Count	Median
Total proc gross charges	8	*	4	*	5	*
Medical proc-inside practice	8	*	4	*	5	*
Medical proc-outside practice	8	*	2	*	5	*
Surg proc-inside practice	3	*	5	*	5	*
Surg proc-outside practice	8	*	3	*	5	*
Laboratory procedures	0	*	0	*	5	*
Radiology procedures	5	*	5	*	5	*
Tot nonproc gross charges	4	*	1	*	5	*
Total support staff FTE/phy	10	3.42	11	6.24	84	4.21

Table 16.11b: Medical Procedure Data (inside the practice)

	Surg: Neurological		Surg: Oral		Urology	
	Count	Median	Count	Median	Count	Median
Gross charges/procedure	8	*	4	*	5	*
Total cost/procedure	8	*	4	*	4	*
Operating cost/procedure	7	*	4	*	4	*
Provider cost/procedure	8	*	4	*	4	*
Procedures/patient	6	*	4	*	1	*
Gross charges/patient	6	*	4	*	1	*
Procedures/physician	8	*	4	*	5	*
Gross charges/physician	8	*	4	*	5	*
Procedures/provider	3	*	0	*	2	*
Gross charges/provider	3	*	0	*	2	*
Gross charge to total cost ratio	8	*	4	*	4	*
Oper cost to total cost ratio	7	*	4	*	4	*
Prov cost to total cost ratio	8	*	4	*	4	*
Total support staff FTE/phy	10	3.42	11	6.24	84	4.21

Table 16.11c: Medical Procedure Data (outside the practice)

	Surg: Neurological		Surg: Oral		Urology	
	Count	Median	Count	Median	Count	Median
Gross charges/procedure	8	*	2	*	5	*
Total cost/procedure	8	*	2	*	4	*
Operating cost/procedure	7	*	2	*	4	*
Provider cost/procedure	8	*	2	*	4	*
Procedures/patient	6	*	2	*	1	*
Gross charges/patient	6	*	2	*	1	*
Procedures/physician	8	*	2	*	5	*
Gross charges/physician	8	*	2	*	5	*
Procedures/provider	3	*	0	*	2	*
Gross charges/provider	3	*	0	*	2	*
Gross charge to total cost ratio	8	*	2	*	4	*
Oper cost to total cost ratio	7	*	2	*	4	*
Prov cost to total cost ratio	8	*	2	*	4	*
Total support staff FTE/phy	10	3.42	11	6.24	84	4.21

Single Specialty Practices, Not Hospital or IDS Owned — Surgery: Neurological, Surgery: Oral, Urology (Procedure and Charge Data)

Table 16.11d: Surgery/Anesthesia Procedure Data (inside the practice)

	Surg: Neurological		Surg: Oral		Urology	
	Count	Median	Count	Median	Count	Median
Gross charges/procedure	3	*	5	*	5	*
Total cost/procedure	3	*	5	*	4	*
Operating cost/procedure	2	*	5	*	4	*
Provider cost/procedure	3	*	5	*	4	*
Procedures/patient	2	*	5	*	1	*
Gross charges/patient	2	*	5	*	1	*
Procedures/physician	3	*	5	*	5	*
Gross charges/physician	3	*	5	*	5	*
Procedures/provider	0	*	0	*	2	*
Gross charges/provider	0	*	0	*	2	*
Gross charge to total cost ratio	3	*	5	*	4	*
Oper cost to total cost ratio	2	*	5	*	4	*
Prov cost to total cost ratio	3	*	5	*	4	*
Total support staff FTE/phy	10	3.42	11	6.24	84	4.21

Table 16.11e: Surgery/Anesthesia Procedure Data (outside the practice)

	Surg: Neurological		Surg: Oral		Urology	
	Count	Median	Count	Median	Count	Median
Gross charges/procedure	8	*	3	*	5	*
Total cost/procedure	8	*	3	*	4	*
Operating cost/procedure	7	*	3	*	4	*
Provider cost/procedure	8	*	3	*	4	*
Procedures/patient	6	*	3	*	1	*
Gross charges/patient	6	*	3	*	1	*
Procedures/physician	8	*	3	*	5	*
Gross charges/physician	8	*	3	*	5	*
Procedures/provider	3	*	0	*	2	*
Gross charges/provider	3	*	0	*	2	*
Gross charge to total cost ratio	8	*	3	*	4	*
Oper cost to total cost ratio	7	*	3	*	4	*
Prov cost to total cost ratio	8	*	3	*	4	*
Total support staff FTE/phy	10	3.42	11	6.24	84	4.21

Single Specialty Practices, Not Hospital or IDS Owned — Surgery: Neurological, Surgery: Oral, Urology (Procedure and Charge Data)

Table 16.11f: Clinical Laboratory/Pathology Procedure Data

	Surg: Neurological		Surg: Oral		Urology	
	Count	Median	Count	Median	Count	Median
Gross charges/procedure	0	*	0	*	5	*
Total cost/procedure	0	*	0	*	4	*
Operating cost/procedure	0	*	0	*	4	*
Provider cost/procedure	0	*	0	*	4	*
Procedures/patient	0	*	0	*	1	*
Gross charges/patient	0	*	0	*	1	*
Procedures/physician	0	*	0	*	5	*
Gross charges/physician	0	*	0	*	5	*
Procedures/provider	0	*	0	*	2	*
Gross charges/provider	0	*	0	*	2	*
Gross charge to total cost ratio	0	*	0	*	4	*
Oper cost to total cost ratio	0	*	0	*	4	*
Prov cost to total cost ratio	0	*	0	*	4	*
Total support staff FTE/phy	10	3.42	11	6.24	84	4.21

Table 16.11g: Diagnostic Radiology and Imaging Procedure Data

	Surg: Neurological		Surg: Oral		Urology	
	Count	Median	Count	Median	Count	Median
Gross charges/procedure	5	*	5	*	5	*
Total cost/procedure	5	*	5	*	4	*
Operating cost/procedure	5	*	5	*	4	*
Provider cost/procedure	5	*	5	*	4	*
Procedures/patient	5	*	5	*	1	*
Gross charges/patient	5	*	5	*	1	*
Procedures/physician	5	*	5	*	5	*
Gross charges/physician	5	*	5	*	5	*
Procedures/provider	3	*	0	*	2	*
Gross charges/provider	3	*	0	*	2	*
Gross charge to total cost ratio	5	*	5	*	4	*
Oper cost to total cost ratio	5	*	5	*	4	*
Prov cost to total cost ratio	5	*	5	*	4	*
Total support staff FTE/phy	10	3.42	11	6.24	84	4.21

Table 16.11h: Nonprocedural Gross Charge Data

	Surg: Neurological		Surg: Oral		Urology	
	Count	Median	Count	Median	Count	Median
Gross charges/patient	3	*	1	*	1	*
Nonproc gross charges/physician	4	*	1	*	5	*
Gross charges/provider	2	*	0	*	2	*
Total support staff FTE/phy	10	3.42	11	6.24	84	4.21

THIS PAGE INTENTIONALLY LEFT BLANK

Appendices

Appendices

Appendix A: Abbreviations, Acronyms & Geographic Section

admin	administrative	oper	operating
AR	accounts receivable	otorhinolaryng	otorhinolaryngology
ASA	American Society of Anesthesiologists	par	parent
		pat	patients
cap	capitation	phy	physician(s)
cardiovasc	cardiovascular	PPMC	Physician Practice Management Company
chrg	charges		
empl	employed	prac	practice(s)
excl	excluding	prim	primary
FFS	fee-for-service	proc	procedural
fin	financial	proc	procedure(s)
ft	foot or feet	prof	professional
FTE	full-time-equivalent	prov	provider
gyn	gynecology	purch	purchased
HMO	Health Maintenance Organization	RBRVS	Resource Based Relative Value Scale
IBNR	incurred but not reported	rev	revenue
IDS	integrated delivery system	RVU	relative value unit(s)
immun	immunology	serv	service(s)
inc	income	sf	staff
maint	maintenance	spec	specialist
med	medical	spec	specialty
med	medicine	sp	support
MGMA	Medical Group Management Association	sq	square
		std dev	standard deviation
misc	miscellaneous	stf	staff
MSO	Management Services Organization	sup/supp	support
		surg	surgery
nonproc	nonprocedural	surg	surgical
NPP	Nonphysician provider	tot	total
ob	obstetrics	w/o	without
onc	oncology	wrk	work

Geographic Sections

Eastern Section:	Midwest Section:	Southern Section:	Western Section:
Connecticut	Illinois	Alabama	Alaska
Delaware	Indiana	Arkansas	Arizona
District of Columbia	Iowa	Florida	California
Maine	Michigan	Georgia	Colorado
Maryland	Minnesota	Kansas	Hawaii
Massachusetts	Nebraska	Kentucky	Idaho
New Hampshire	North Dakota	Louisiana	Montana
New Jersey	Ohio	Mississippi	Nevada
New York	South Dakota	Missouri	New Mexico
North Carolina	Wisconsin	Oklahoma	Oregon
Pennsylvania		South Carolina	Utah
Rhode Island		Tennessee	Washington
Vermont		Texas	Wyoming
Virginia			
West Virginia			

Appendix B: Terms Used in Report

A

Accrual accounting
A system of accounting where revenues are recorded as earned and when services are performed, rather than when cash is exchanged. Cost is recorded in the period during which it is incurred, that is, when the asset or service is used, regardless of when cash is paid. Costs for goods and services that will be used to produce revenues in the future are reported as assets and recorded as costs in future periods.

Adjustments to fee-for-service charges
The difference between "Gross fee-for-service charges" and the amount expected to be paid by patients or third-party payers. This represents the value of services performed for which payment is not expected.
See page 292 for additional information.

Administrative supplies and services cost
Cost of printing, postage, books, subscriptions, administrative and medical forms, stationery, bank processing fees and other administrative supplies and services.
See page 299 for additional information.

Administrative support staff
Administrative support staff includes general administrative, patient accounting, general accounting, managed care administrative, information technology, housekeeping, maintenance, security, medical receptionists, medical secretaries, transcribers, medical records and other administrative support.
See terms in this appendix for additional information.

Ancillary support staff
Ancillary support staff equals Clinical laboratory plus Radiology and imaging plus Other medical support services.

B

Bad debts due to fee-for-service activity
The difference between "Adjusted fee-for-service charges" and the amount actually collected.
See page 292 for additional information.

Billing and collections purchased services
When a medical practice decides to purchase billing and collections services from an outside organization as opposed to hiring and developing its own employed staff to conduct billing and collections activities.

Branch or satellite clinic
A smaller clinical facility for which the practice incurs occupancy costs (lease, depreciation, utilities, etc.). A branch is in a separate location from the practice's principal facility. Merely having physicians practice in another location does not qualify that location as a branch or satellite clinic.

Building and occupancy cost
Cost of general operation of buildings and grounds.
See page 299 for additional information.

Business corporation
A for-profit organization recognized by law as a business entity separate and distinct from its shareholders. Shareholders need not be licensed in the profession practiced by the corporation.

C

Capitation contract
A contract in which the practice agrees to provide medical services to a defined population for a fixed price per beneficiary per month, regardless of actual services provided. Capitation contracts, which always contain an element of risk, include HMO, Medicare and Medicaid capitation contracts.

Capitation: prepaid Medicare, Medicaid, and commercial
Fee-for-service equivalent gross charges, at the practice's undiscounted rates, for all services provided to patients under a commercial HMO capitated contract, or under a Medicare/TEFRA, Medicaid or similar state health care capitated contract.
See page 312 for additional information.

Cash accounting
A system of accounting where revenues are recorded when cash is received and costs are recorded when cash is paid out.

Charity care and professional courtesy
Fee-for-service gross charges, at the practice's undiscounted rates, for all services provided to charity patients. Charity patients are patients who do not have the resources to pay for services.

Clinical laboratory cost
Cost of clinical laboratory and pathology procedures defined by CPT codes 80048-89399.
See page 300 for additional information.

Appendix B: Terms Used in Report

Clinical laboratory support staff
The clinical laboratory and pathology department staff which conducts procedures for clinical laboratory and pathology CPT codes 80048-89399.

Clinical science department
A unit of organization in a medical school with an independent chair and a single budget. The department's mission is to conduct teaching, research and/or clinical activities related to the entire spectrum of health care delivery to humans, from prevention through treatment. Residents in training or fellows may be present.

Clinical support staff
Clinical support staff includes Registered Nurses, Licensed Practical Nurses, medical assistants and nurse's aides.
See terms in this appendix for additional information.

Commercial: fee-for-service
Fee-for-service gross charges, at the practice's undiscounted rates, for all services provided to fee-for-service patients who were covered by commercial contracts. A commercial contract is any contract that is not Medicare, Medicaid, or workers' compensation.
See page 313 for additional information.

Cost allocated to medical practice from parent organization
When a medical practice is owned by a hospital or integrated delivery system, the parent organization often allocates indirect costs to the medical practice. These indirect costs may vary, depending on the situation. Examples of alternative names are "shared services costs" or "uncontrollable costs." These costs may be arbitrarily assigned to the medical practice, may be the result of negotiations between the practice and the parent organization, or the result of some sort of cost accounting system.
See page 301 for additional information.

Current assets
Cash and other assets expected to be converted to cash, sold or consumed in the normal course of operations within one year.

E

Encounters
A documented, face-to-face contact between a patient and a provider who exercises independent judgment in the provision of services to the individual in an ambulatory or hospital setting.
See page 311 for additional information.

F

Faculty practice plan
A formal organizational framework that structures the clinical practice activities of the medical school faculty. The plan performs a range of services including billing, collections, contract negotiations and the distribution of income. Plans may form a separate legal organization or may be affiliated with the medical school through a clinical science department or teaching hospital. Faculty associated with the plan must provide patient care as part of a teaching or research program.

Fee-for-service: Medicare, Medicaid, and commercial
Fee-for-service equivalent gross charges, at the practice's established undiscounted rates, for all services provided to patients under a commercial contract, or under a Medicare/TEFRA, Medicaid or similar state healthcare contract.

Financial support for operating costs
Medical practice may receives operational support from a parent organization within a hospital or other integrated delivery system.
See page 305 for additional information.

Freestanding Ambulatory Surgery Center (ASC)
A freestanding entity that is specifically licensed to provide surgery services that are performed on a same-day outpatient basis. A freestanding ambulatory surgery center does not employ physicians.

Furniture and equipment cost
Cost of furniture and equipment in general use in the practice.
See page 299 for additional information.

G

General accounting support staff
General accounting office staff includes controller, financial accounting manager, accounts payable, payroll, bookkeeping and financial accounting input staff.

General administrative support staff
Administrative and practice management staff and supporting secretaries, administrative assistants, etc.
See page 295 for additional information.

Goodwill amortization
Goodwill is the premium paid in excess of the value of the tangible assets. Goodwill may be amortized over a period of time.
See page 305 for additional information.

Appendix B: Terms Used in Report

Government (ownership)
A governmental organization at the federal, state or local level. Government funding is not a sufficient criterion. Government ownership is the key factor. An example would be a medical clinic at a federal, state or county correctional facility.

Gross capitation revenue
Revenue received in a fixed per member payment, usually on a prospective and monthly basis, to pay for all covered goods and services due to capitation patients.
See page 293 for additional information.

Gross charges for patients covered by capitation contracts
Also known as fee-for-service equivalent gross charges. The full value, at a practice's undiscounted rates, of all covered services provided to patients covered by all capitation contracts, regardless of payer.
See page 292 for additional information.

Gross fee-for-service charges
The full value, at the practice's undiscounted rates, of all services provided to fee-for-service, discounted fee-for-service and non-capitated patients for all payers.
See page 291 for additional information.

Gross square footage
The total number of finished and occupied square feet within outside walls for all facilities (both administrative and clinical) that comprise the practice. Hallways, closets, elevators, stairways and other such spaces are included.

H

Health Maintenance Organization (HMO)
An HMO is an insurance company that accepts responsibility for providing and delivering a predetermined set of comprehensive health maintenance and treatment services to a voluntarily enrolled population for a negotiated and fixed periodic premium.

Hospital
A hospital is an inpatient facility that admits patients for overnight stays, incurs nursing care costs and generates bed-day revenues.

Housekeeping, maintenance, security support staff
Includes housekeeping, maintenance and security staff.

I

Incurred but not reported (IBNR) liability account
"Incurred but not reported" (IBNR) liability accounts are special liability accounts used by medical practices with capitation contracts to keep track of amounts owed to providers outside the practice for services provided to the practice's capitated patients.

Independent Practice Associations (IPA)
An IPA is an association or network of licensed providers and/or medical practices. An IPA is usually a unique legal entity, most often operating on a for-profit basis. Typically, the primary purpose of the IPA is to secure and maintain contractual relationships between providers and health plans.

Information technology cost
Cost of practice-wide data processing, computer, telephone and telecommunications services.
See page 298 for additional information.

Information technology support staff
Data processing, computer programming and telecommunications staff.

Insurance company
An insurance company is an organization that indemnifies an insured party against a specified loss in return for premiums paid, as stipulated by a contract.

Integrated delivery systems (IDS)
An IDS is a network of organizations that provide or coordinate and arrange for the provision of a continuum of health care services to consumers and are willing to be held clinically and fiscally responsible for the outcomes and the health status of the populations served. Generally consisting of hospitals, physician groups, health plans, home health agencies, hospices, skilled nursing facilities, or other provider entities, these networks may be built through "virtual" integration processes encompassing contractual arrangements and strategic alliances as well as through direct ownership.

L

Licensed Practical Nurse
Includes only Licensed Practical Nurses.

Limited liability company
A legal entity that is a hybrid between a corporation and a partnership, because it provides limited liability to owners like a corporation while passing profits and losses through to owners like a partnership.

Appendix B: Terms Used in Report

M

Managed care

Managed health care is a system in which the provider of care is incentivized to establish mechanisms to contain costs, control utilization, and deliver services in the most appropriate settings. There are three key factors: 1) controlling the utilization of medical services; 2) shifting financial risk to the provider; and 3) reducing the use of resources in rendering treatments to patients.

Managed care administrative support staff

Managed care administrative staff and supporting secretaries, administrative assistants.

Managed care fee-for-service: Medicare, Medicaid, and commercial

Fee-for-service equivalent gross charges, at the practice's established undiscounted rates, for all services provided to patients through a managed care plan under a commercial contract, or under a Medicare/TEFRA, Medicaid or similar state healthcare contract.

Management fees paid to an MSO or PPMC

Medical practices may receive management or other services from an MSO, PPMC, hospital or other parent organization in return for a fee. The fee could be a contracted fixed amount, a percentage of collections, or any other mutually agreed upon arrangement.
See page 300 for additional information.

Management Services Organizations (MSO)

An MSO is an entity organized to provide various forms of practice management and administrative support services to health care providers. These services may include centralized billing and collections services, management information services and other components of the managed care infrastructure. MSOs do not actually deliver health care services. MSOs may be jointly or solely owned and sponsored by physicians, hospitals or other parties. Some MSOs also purchase assets of affiliated physicians and enter into long-term management service arrangements with a provider network. Some expand their ownership base by involving outside investors to help capitalize the development of such practice infrastructure.

Medical and surgical supply cost

Cost of supplies purchased for general practice use.
See page 298 for additional information.

Medical group practice

A single legal entity or collection of legal entities consisting of at least three physicians who deliver health care services.

Medical assistants, nurse's aides

Includes medical assistants and nurse's aides.

Medical records

Include medical records clerks.

Medical receptionists support staff

Medical receptionists, switchboard operators, schedulers and appointment staff.

Medical secretaries, transcribers

Include medical secretaries and transcribers.

Medical school

A medical school is an institution that trains physicians and awards medical and osteopathic degrees.

Metropolitan (50,000 to 250,000)

The community in which the practice is located is a "metropolitan statistical area" (MSA) or Census Bureau defined urbanized area of 50,000 to 250,000 population.

Metropolitan (250,001 to 1,000,000)

The community in which the practice is located is a "metropolitan statistical area" (MSA) or Census Bureau defined urbanized area of 250,001 to 1,000,000 population.

Metropolitan (over 1,000,000):

The community in which the practice is located is a "primary metropolitan statistical area" (PMSA) having over 1,000,000 population.

Miscellaneous operating cost

Operating cost such as charitable contributions, employee relations dinners, picnics, entertainment, practice uniforms, business transportation, interest on loans, health, business and property taxes, recruiting cost, job position classified advertising, moving cost, payouts to retired physicians from accounts receivable, etc.
See page 301 for additional information.

Modified cash accounting

A system of accounting that is primarily a cash basis system, but allows the cost of long-lived (fixed) assets to be expensed through depreciation. The modified cash system recognizes inventories of goods intended for resale as assets. Under a modified cash system, purchases of buildings and equipment, leasehold improvements

Appendix B: Terms Used in Report

and payments of insurance premiums applicable to more than one accounting period are normally recorded as assets. Costs for these assets are allocated to accounting periods in a systematic manner over the length of time the practice benefits from the assets.

Multispecialty with primary and specialty care
A medical practice which consists of physicians practicing in different specialties, including at least one primary care specialty listed below.
Family practice: general
Family practice: sports medicine
Family practice: urgent care
Family practice: with obstetrics
Family practice: without obstetrics
Geriatrics
Internal medicine: general
Internal medicine: urgent care
Pediatrics: adolescent medicine
Pediatrics: general
Pediatrics: sports medicine

Multispecialty with primary care only
A medical practice, which consists of physicians practicing in more than one of the following prmary care specialties listed above or the surgical specialties of obstetrics/gynecology, gynecology (only), obstetrics (only).

Multispecialty with specialty care only
A medical practice, which consists of physicians practicing in different specialties, none of which are the primary care specialties listed above.

N

Net fee-for-service collections/revenue
Revenue collected from patients and third-party payers for services provided to fee-for-service, discounted fee-for-service, and non-capitated Medicare/Medicaid patients. This is the revenue remaining after patient refunds and checks returned to patients.
See page 292 for additional information.

Noncurrent and all other liabilities
Long-term liabilities that mature and require payment at some time beyond one year.

Nonphysician provider
Nonphysician providers are specially trained and licensed providers who can provide medical care and billable services. Examples of nonphysician providers include audiologists, Certified Registered Nurse Anesthetists (CRNAs), dieticians/nutritionists, midwives, nurse practitioners, occupational therapists, optometrists, physical therapists, physician assistants, psychologists, social workers, speech therapists and surgeon's assistants.

Not-for-profit corporation/foundation
An organization that has obtained special exemption under Section 501(c) of the Internal Revenue Service code that qualifies the organization to be exempt from federal income taxes. To qualify as a tax-exempt organization, a practice or faculty practice plan would have to provide evidence of a charitable, educational or research purpose.

Non-metropolitan (under 50,000)
The community in which the practice is located is generally referred to as "rural." It is located outside of a "metropolitan statistical area" (MSA), as defined by the United States Office of Management and Budget, and has a population under 50,000.

O

Other administrative support staff
Other administrative staff including shipping and receiving, cafeteria, mailroom and laundry staff.

Other ancillary services costs
Operating costs for all ancillary services departments except clinical laboratory and radiology and imaging.
See page 300 for additional information.

Other medical revenue
Grants, honoraria, research contract revenues, government support payments and educational subsidies.
See page 293 for additional information.

Other medical support services
Support staff in any ancillary services department other than clinical laboratory and radiology and imaging.
See page 297 for additional information.

Other insurance premiums
Cost of other policies such as fire, flood, theft, casualty, general liability, officers' and directors' liability, reinsurance, etc.

Outside professional fees
Fees for professional services performed on a onetime or sporadic basis.
See page 299 for additional information.

Appendix B: Terms Used in Report

P

Partnership
An organization where two or more individuals have agreed that they will share profits, losses, assets and liabilities, although not necessarily on an equal basis. The partnership agreement may or may not be formalized in writing.

Patient accounting support staff
Patient accounting (billing and collections) staff, such as billing/accounts receivable manager, coding, charge entry, insurance, billing, collections, payment posting, refund, adjustment, and cashiering staff.

Performance-based incentive
Some fee-for-service contracts stipulate that the payer will reward the provider with additional payments beyond those guaranteed in the fee-for-service contract if the provider meets certain performance specifications. Since no funds are withheld by the payer up front, this type of contract is not typically viewed as an "at-risk" contract.

Physician
Any doctor of medicine (MD) or doctor of osteopathy (DO) who is duly licensed and qualified under the law of jurisdiction in which treatment is received.

Physician Practice Management Companies (PPMC)
PPMCs are usually publicly held or entrepreneurial directed enterprises that acquire total or partial ownership interests in physician organizations. PPMCs are a type of MSO, however, the motivations, goals, strategies, and structures arising from their unequivocal ownership character – development of growth and profits for their investors, not for the participating providers – differentiate them from other MSO models.

Physician Work RVUs
Physician Work RVUs refer the physician work component of the total RVU.
See also "Relative Value Units"

Primary clinic location
The clinic with the most FTE physicians out of all the practice branches.

Professional corporation/association
A for-profit organization recognized by law as a business entity separate and distinct from its shareholders. Shareholders must be licensed in the profession practiced by the organization.

Professional liability insurance premiums
Premiums paid or self-insurance cost for malpractice and professional liability insurance for practice physicians, nonphysician providers and employees.

Promotion and marketing cost
Cost of promotion, advertising and marketing activities, including patient newsletters, information booklets, fliers, brochures, yellow page listings and public relations consultants.

Purchased services for capitation patients
Fees paid to health care providers and organizations external to the practice for services provided to capitation patients under the terms of capitation contracts.
See page 293 for additional information.

R

Radiology and imaging
Film library staff and the diagnostic radiology and imaging department staff who conduct procedures for diagnostic radiology CPT codes 70010-76499, diagnostic ultrasound CPT codes 76506-76999 and diagnostic nuclear medicine CPT codes 78000-78999, echocardiography CPT codes are 93303-93350, noninvasive vascular diagnostic studies CPT codes 93875-93990 and electrocardiograph CPT codes 93000-93350.

Registered Nurses support staff
Registered Nurse staff and Registered Nurses working as frontline managers or lead nurses.

Relative Value Units (RVUs)
Relative value units are nonmonetary, relative units of measure that indicate the value of health care services and relative difference in resources consumed when providing different procedures and services. RVUs assign relative values or weights to medical procedures primarily for the purpose of the reimbursement of services performed. They are used as a standardized method of analyzing resources involved in the provision of services or procedures.

Appendix B: Terms Used in Report

S

Self-pay
Fee-for-service gross charges, at the practice's undiscounted rates, for all services provided to patients who pay the medical practice directly. Note that these patients may or may not have insurance.

Single-specialty practice
Classifying the type of specialty is the focus of clinical work and not necessarily the specialties of the physicians in the practice. For example, a single-specialty neurosurgery practice may include a neurologist and a radiologist.

Sole proprietorship
An organization with a single owner who is responsible for all profit, losses, assets and liabilities.

T

Total contracted support staff
"Contracted support staff" represents all the staff hired on a contract basis that are not employed by any of the legal entities that comprise the medical practice. The utilization of contracted support staff occurs when the medical practice (including all the associated legal entities that comprise the medical practice) decides not to hire support staff as employees to conduct the ongoing support staff activities. Instead, the practice contracts to have these full-time and/or ongoing activities conducted by contracted staff.

U

University
An institution of higher learning with teaching and research facilities comprising undergraduate, graduate and professional schools.

W

Withhold
Some fee-for-service contracts specify a withholding of payments to the provider by the payer as a means for funding a risk pool. This withholding of payments is often called a "withhold." The funds in the risk pool (the withhold) may be returned to the provider by the payer, in whole or in part, based on goals related to financial performance and/or utilization of outpatient and/or inpatient services. When a contract involves a "withhold," the provider is "at-risk" for losing the withhold if certain performance standards are not met. Hence, contracts involving "withholds" are often referred to as "at-risk" contracts. "At-risk" contracts are not limited to fee-for-service contracts with a withhold. By definition, all capitation contracts are also referred to as "at-risk" contracts since the practice is at-risk of losing money if utilization of services is higher than anticipated when the capitation contract was initially analyzed and signed.

Workers' compensation
Fee-for-service gross charges, at the practice's undiscounted rates, for all services provided to patients covered by workers' compensation insurance.

Appendix C: Calculations and Formulas

Formulas for Created Variables

Adjusted fee-for-service collection percentage =
$$\frac{(\text{Net FFS revenue, \#22}) \times 100}{(\text{Adjusted FFS charges, \#20})}$$

Current ratio =
$$\frac{(\text{Current assets, \#90})}{(\text{Current liabilities, \#93})}$$

Days of gross fee-for-service charges in accounts receivable =
$$\frac{(\text{Total accounts receivable, \#102})}{(\text{Gross FFS charges, \#18}) \times (1/365)}$$

Debt ratio =
$$\frac{(\text{Total liabilities, \#95}) \times 100}{(\text{Total assets, \#92})}$$

Debt to equity ratio =
$$\frac{(\text{Total liabilities, \#95})}{(\text{Total net worth, \#96})}$$

Gross fee-for-service collection percentage =
$$\frac{(\text{Net FFS revenue, \#22}) \times 100}{(\text{Gross FFS charges, \#18})}$$

Gross fee-for-service plus capitation collection percentage =
$$\frac{((\text{Net FFS revenue, \#22}) + (\text{Net capitation revenue, \#26})) \times 100}{(\text{Total gross charges, \#32})}$$

Months of gross fee-for-service charges in accounts receivable =
$$\frac{(\text{Total accounts receivable, \#102})}{(\text{Gross FFS charges, \#18}) \times (1/12)}$$

Net capitation revenue percentage of gross capitation charges =
$$\frac{(\text{Net capitation revenue, \#26}) \times 100}{(\text{Gross capitation charges, \#23})}$$

Return on equity =
$$\frac{(\text{Net practice income or loss, \#89}) \times 100}{(\text{Total net worth, \#96})}$$

Return on total assets =
$$\frac{(\text{Net practice income or loss, \#89}) \times 100}{(\text{Total assets, \#92})}$$

Total asset turnover ratio =
$$\frac{(\text{Total medical revenue, \#33})}{(\text{Total assets, \#92})}$$

Total cost =
(Total operating cost, #70) + (Total provider cost, #83b)

Working capital =
(Current assets, #90) – (Current liabilities, #93)

Data Normalization Calculations

Per FTE physician =
$$\frac{<\text{performance measure}>}{(\text{Total physician FTE, \#82a})}$$

As a percent of total medical revenue =
$$\frac{<\text{performance measure}>}{(\text{Total medical revenue, \#33})}$$

Per FTE provider =
$$\frac{<\text{performance measure}>}{(\text{Total provider FTE, \#83a})}$$

Per square foot =
$$\frac{<\text{performance measure}>}{(\text{Square feet, \#15})}$$

Per total RVU =
$$\frac{<\text{performance measure}>}{(\text{Total RVUs, \#113a})}$$

Per work RVU =
$$\frac{<\text{performance measure}>}{(\text{Physician work RVUs, \#113b})}$$

Per patient =
$$\frac{<\text{performance measure}>}{(\text{Number of patients, \#114a})}$$

Per encounter =
$$\frac{<\text{performance measure}>}{(\text{Patient encounters, \#114b}) \times 10{,}000}$$

Note: Numbers preceded by # symbol refer to question numbers on the questionnaire.

Appendix D: Activity Based Cost Allocation Model

In a prospective pay and managed care environment, identifying and controlling costs per covered life is crucial for medical practices. To control costs per covered life, a practice must understand the costs of its health care services.

The first step in achieving this objective is for practices to understand what activities they perform (outputs) and what resources (inputs) go into performing these activities. Examples of outputs include surgical or radiology procedures. Inputs include support staff labor, physician labor, supplies, rent, insurance, etc. Costs for inputs can be allocated to one or more activities to determine cost per activity or procedure. Evaluation at this level helps practices benchmark cost performance, do budgeting, and analyze payer contracts.

MGMA has developed an activity based cost allocation model that allocates medical practice input costs to medical practice activities (outputs). The model calculates operating cost, provider cost and total cost per procedure. To develop the model, the cost (input) and activity (output) data collected in the survey were used. Procedure and charge data were collected for the six types of medical practice activities listed in Table 1: Outputs, Procedures, and Charges.

Cost data fell into two categories: operating cost and provider cost, as shown in Table 2: Inputs, Costs, and Allocation Patterns. These data provided the framework for the model.

Due to the complexity of the model, a case study example is used to illustrate how the model is structured, how costs are allocated to activities and how cost per procedure is determined. The medical practice in the example is a multispecialty practice with 40 FTE physicians. The case study data are shown in Tables 1 and 2. This case study only calculates total cost per procedure. The same logic was used to generate the operating cost per procedure and provider cost per procedure data that appear in the Cost Survey tables.

Step 1: Identify the procedure(s) to receive cost allocations: Each cost in Table 2 was analyzed individually to determine which procedure or procedures should receive an allocation of the cost. The type of procedure and whether the procedure took place

inside or outside the practice were considered. Depending on the costs' characteristics, costs were allocated to one type of procedure or to multiple procedures. For instance, general administrative support staff cost (question 34b) and total physician cost (question 82b) were allocated to all six types of procedures (A through F), while Registered Nurses' support staff costs (question 44b) were allocated only to medical and surgical procedures that took place within the practice (A and C). Clinical laboratory costs (questions 47b and 63) were allocated only to laboratory procedures (E). The allocation pattern for each cost is shown in Table 2, Cost Allocation Pattern column.

The cost allocation patterns in Table 2 can be summarized as follows, where the letters refer to the procedure types described in Table 1:

ABCDEF	All procedures
ACEF	Medical and surgical procedures that occur inside the practice's facilities and the ancillary procedures of laboratory and radiology
AC	Medical and surgical procedures that occur inside the practice's facilities but not ancillary procedures
E	Laboratory procedures only
F	Radiology procedures only

Step 2: Determine the total cost associated with each cost allocation pattern: Using the last column in Table 2 to identify the cost allocation pattern, sum the associated costs for each pattern. For example, the first five cost rows listed in Table 2 (questions 34b, 35b, 36b, 37b and 38b) would all be added to the total for pattern ABCDEF, and so on. The total costs for each pattern are listed in the second column of Table 8: Total Cost per Procedure Worksheet. This column sums to $21,805,000, which is equal to total cost listed on the bottom row of Table 2.

Step 3: Use procedural gross charges data to calculate ratios of specific procedure charges to total charges: The proportion of cost allocated to each procedure type is based on the amount of gross charges generated by each procedure compared to total gross charges for all procedures. In this case study, the

Table 1: Outputs, Procedures and Charges

Procedure Type	Procedure (Activity) Name	Cost Survey Question Number	Number of Procedures	Total Gross Charges
A	Medical procedures inside the practice	104	200,000	$11,000,000
B	Medical Procedures outside the practice	105	30,000	$6,300,000
C	Surgery and anesthesia procedures inside the practice	106	10,000	$1,300,000
D	Surgery and anesthesia procedures outside the practice	107	10.000	$13,000,000
E	Clinical laboratory and pathology procedures	108	135,000	$4,000,000
F	Diagnostic radiology and imaging procedures	109	25,000	$3,000,000
	Totals		410,000	$40,600,000

Appendix D: Activity Based Cost Allocation Model

Table 2: Inputs, Costs and Allocation Patterns

Cost Survey Question Number	Inputs (Type of Cost)	Cost	Cost Allocation Pattern
34b	General administrative	$400,000	ABCDEF
35b	Patient accounting	$400,000	ABCDEF
36b	General accounting	$100,000	ABCDEF
37b	Managed care administrative	$200,000	ABCDEF
38b	Information technology	$100,000	ABCDEF
39b	Housekeeping, maintenance, security	$20,000	ACEF
40b	Medical receptionists	$500,000	ACEF
41b	Medical secretaries, transcribers	$200,000	ABCDEF
42b	Medical records	$200,000	ABCDEF
43b	Other administrative support	$30,000	ACEF
44b	Registered Nurses	$100,000	AC
45b	Licensed Practical Nurses	$500,000	AC
46b	Medical assistants, nurse's aides	$600,000	AC
47b	Clinical laboratory	$300,000	E
48b	Radiology and imaging	$200,000	F
49b	Other medical support services	$250,000	ACEF
51b	Total employed support staff benefits	$800,000	ABCDEF
52b	Total contracted support staff	$300,000	ABCDEF
53b	**Total operating cost, support staff**	$5,200,000	
54	Information technology	$225,000	ABCDEF
55	Medical and surgical supply	$775,000	AC
56	Building and occupancy	$1,350,000	ACEF
57	Furniture and equipment	$475,000	AC
58	Administrative supplies and services	$300,000	ABCDEF
59	Professional liability insurance	$450,000	ABCDEF
60	Other insurance premiums	$10,000	ABCDEF
61	Outside professional fees	$85,000	ABCDEF
62	Promotion and marketing	$35,000	ABCDEF
63	Clinical laboratory	$700,000	E
64	Radiology and imaging	$300,000	F
65	Other ancillary services	$150,000	ACEF
66	Billing purchased services	$0	ABCDEF
67	Management fees paid to MSO	$100,000	ABCDEF
68	Miscellaneous operating cost	$1,375,000	ABCDEF
69	Cost allocated to practice from parent	$0	ABCDEF
70	**Total operating cost, general**	$6,330,000	
71	**Total operating cost**	$11,530,000	
75b	Total nonphysician provider cost	$250,000	AC
76b	Provider consultant cost	$25,000	ABCDEF
82b	Total physician cost	$10,000,000	ABCDEF
83b	**Total provider cost**	$10,275,000	
	Total cost	$21,805,000	

Appendix D: Activity Based Cost Allocation Model

charges generated by each type of procedure are shown in Table 1. For example, surgical procedures performed outside the practice generated 33.68% of the total gross charges for cost allocation pattern ABCDEF (see row D in Table 3). For costs that are allocated to all procedures (the ABCDEF pattern costs), surgical procedures performed outside the practice would be allocated 33.68% of the ABCDEF total costs. In the model, the ratios of procedure gross charges to total gross charges determine the proportion of total cost allocated to each procedure type.

For each cost allocation pattern, the gross charges for each procedure type are summed. (See the bottom row of Tables 3 through 7 for these sums.) Then, the ratios of procedure charges to total charges (the allocation ratios) are calculated by dividing the individual procedure charge amount by the total gross charges. Tables 3 through 7: Ratio of Procedure Charges to Total Charges for Cost Allocation Patterns present the complete set of ratios for all cost allocation patterns.

Step 4: Calculate the total cost allocated to each procedure type: The structure of the cost allocation model is now in place. Table 8: Total Cost per Procedure Worksheet illustrates the final step in this process. The total cost allocated to each procedure type is determined by multiplying the total cost for each pattern (column 2 of Table 8) by the appropriate ratio of procedure charges to total charges for each cost allocation pattern to get a cost for each cost allocation

Table 3: Ratio of Procedure Charges to Total Charges for Cost Allocation Pattern ABCDEF

Procedure Type	Procedure Name	Total Gross Charges	Ratio of Procedure Charges to Total Charges
A	Medical procedures inside the practice (#102)	$11,000,000	0.2850
B	Medical procedures outside the practice (#103)	$6,300,000	0.1632
C	Surgery and anesthesia procedures inside the practice (#104)	$1,300,000	0.0337
D	Surgery and anesthesia procedures outside the practice (#105)	$13,000,000	0.3368
E	Clinical laboratory and pathology procedures (#106)	$4,000,000	0.1036
F	Diagnostic radiology and imaging procedures (#107)	$3,000,000	0.0777
	Totals	$38,600,000	1.0000

Table 4: Ratio of Procedure Charges to Total Charges for Cost Allocation Pattern ACEF

Procedure Type	Procedure Name	Total Gross Charges	Ratio of Procedure Charges to Total Charges
A	Medical procedures inside the practice (#102)	$11,000,000	0.5699
C	Surgery and anesthesia procedures inside the practice (#104)	$1,300,000	0.0674
E	Clinical laboratory and pathology procedures (#106)	$4,000,000	0.2073
F	Diagnostic radiology and imaging procedures (#107)	$3,000,000	0.1554
	Totals	$19,300,000	1.0000

Table 5: Ratio of Procedure Charges to Total Charges for Cost Allocation Pattern AC

Procedure Type	Procedure Name	Total Gross Charges	Ratio of Procedure Charges to Total Charges
A	Medical procedures inside the practice (#102)	$11,000,000	0.8943
C	Surgery and anesthesia procedures inside the practice (#104)	$1,300,000	0.1057
	Totals	$12,300,000	1.0000

Table 6: Ratio of Procedure Charges to Total Charges for Cost Allocation Pattern E

Procedure Type	Procedure Name	Total Gross Charges	Ratio of Procedure Charges to Total Charges
E	Clinical laboratory and pathology procedures (#106)	$4,000,000	1.0000
	Totals	$38,600,000	1.0000

Table 7: Ratio of Procedure Charges to Total Charges for Cost Allocation Pattern F

Procedure Type	Procedure Name	Total Gross Charges	Ratio of Procedure Charges to Total Charges
F	Diagnostic radiology and imaging procedures (#107)	$3,000,000	1.0000
	Totals	$38,600,000	1.0000

Appendix D: Activity Based Cost Allocation Model

pattern – procedure type combination. Then, the costs for each combination are summed. These costs are not shown in Table 8, but the sums of these costs (the total cost allocated to each procedure type) are shown in columns A through F of Table 8.

For example, the total cost allocated to "medical procedures inside the practice" is calculated as follows:

$15,305,000 x 0.2850	=	$ 4,361,925
$ 2,300,000 x 0.5699	=	$ 1,310,770
$ 2,700,000 x 0.8943	=	$ 2,414,610
Total	=	$ 8,087,305

The figure of $8,087,305 is shown in column A of Table 8. Total costs allocated to the other five procedures are calculated in a similar manner.

Step 5: Calculate total cost per procedure: Divide the total cost allocated to each procedure type by the total number of procedures for each procedure type to get the total cost per procedure. The final results for this case study are shown on the last row of Table 8.

The data can now be analyzed at the procedure level. This information can help assess a practice's fee schedule and the impact of managed care discounts. It is also useful in evaluating capitation contracts. As a baseline measure, it can be compared to national medians. These national standards can be found in tables *.11b through *.11g of each data section in the report.

Table 8: Total Cost per Procedure Worksheet

Cost allocation pattern	Total cost for each pattern	A — Medical procedures inside the practice (#102)	B — Medical procedures outside the practice (#103)	C — Surgery and anesthesia procedures inside the practice (#104)	D — Surgery and amesthesia procedures outside the practice (#105)	E — Clinical laboratory and pathology procedures (#106)	F — Diagnostic radiology and imaging procedures (#107)
		Ratio of procedure charges to total charges by cost allocation pattern					
All procedures (ABCDEF)	$15,305,000	0.2850	0.1632	0.0337	0.3368	0.1036	0.0777
Medical/ surgical inside and lab/ radiology (ACEF)	$2,300,000	0.5699		0.0674		0,2073	0.1554
Medical/ surgical inside (AC)	$2,700,000	0.8943		0.1057			
Laboratory (E)	$1,000,000					1.0000	
Radiology (F)	$500,000						1.0000
Total	$21,805,000						
		Total cost allocated to each procedure type					
		$8,087,305	$2,497,776	$956,189	$5,154,724	$3,062,388	$2,046,619
		Total number of procedures					
		200,000	30,000	10,000	10,000	135,000	25,000
		Total cost per procedure					
		$40.44	$83.26	$95.62	$515.47	$22.68	$81.86

Appendix E: Cost Survey: 2004 Questionnaire Based on 2003 Data

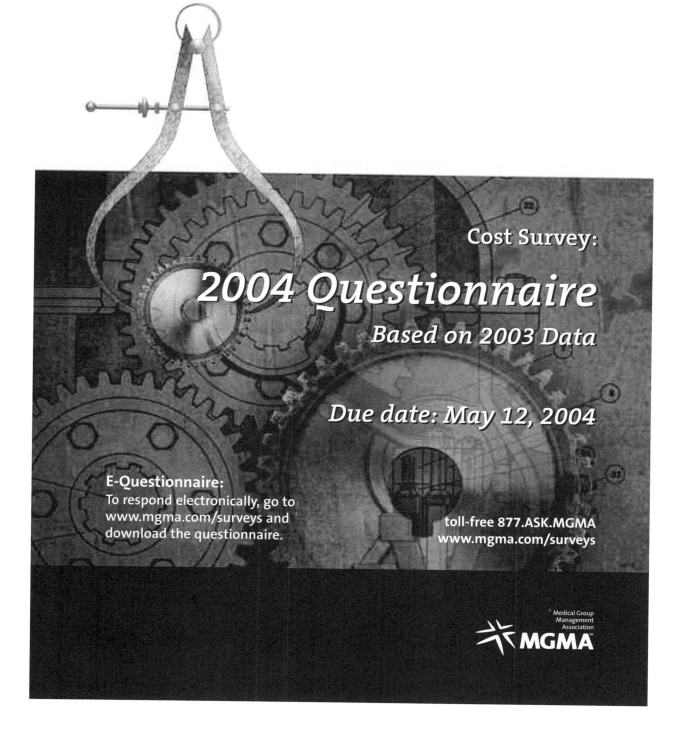

Appendix E: Cost Survey: 2004 Questionnaire Based on 2003 Data

Medical Group Management Association
Cost Survey: 2004 Questionnaire Based on 2003 Data

Instructions

The unit of observation for this survey is the medical group practice. For the purpose of this survey, a medical group practice is defined as a single legal entity or collection of legal entities consisting of one or more physicians who deliver health care services.

A survey response should represent one complete medical practice. If your organization is an Integrated Delivery System (IDS), hospital, Management Services Organization (MSO), Physician Practice Management Company (PPMC), Independent Practice Association (IPA), or other type of organization that owns, manages, or provides services to medical practices, one questionnaire should be completed for each practice.

Freestanding ambulatory surgery centers, medical school faculty practice plans and medical school clinical science departments should not participate in this survey.

Please refer to the *Cost Survey: 2004 Guide to the Questionnaire Based on 2003 Data* (Guide) for definitions and instructions for completing the questionnaire. If you need help in filling out this questionnaire, please contact the MGMA Survey Operations Department, toll-free, 877.ASK.MGMA (275.6462), ext. 895, or e-mail surveys@mgma.com.

2003 Fiscal Year Definition

All the questions on this questionnaire refer to the 2003 fiscal year. This is typically January 2003 through December 2003. If your practice uses an alternative fiscal year, you are encouraged to use it in your responses.

† 1. For the purposes of reporting the information in this questionnaire, what fiscal year was used?

Beginning month $_a$ [   ]   Beginning year $_b$ [   ]   *through* Ending month $_c$ [   ]   Ending year $_d$ [   ]

Medical Practice Information

Please answer the following questions in the way that best describes your practice at the end of the 2003 fiscal year. Pages 6 to 9 in the Guide contain additional information for answering questions in this section.

† 2. What was your practice type? (check only one)

Single-specialty .... $_1$ [   ]

Multispecialty with primary and
specialty care .... $_2$ [   ]

Multispecialty with primary care only .... $_3$ [   ]

Multispecialty with specialty care only .... $_4$ [   ]

† 3. If you answered "Single-specialty" for question 2, what specialty was your practice?

[   ]

† 4. Was your organization a freestanding ambulatory surgery center only? Answer "No" if the ambulatory surgery center was a unit of the medical practice.

Yes .... $_1$ [   ]

No .... $_2$ [   ]

† 5. Was your practice a medical school faculty practice plan and/or clinical science department?

Yes .... $_1$ [   ]

No .... $_2$ [   ]

6. Was your practice affiliated with a medical school?

Yes .... $_1$ [   ]

No .... $_2$ [   ]

7. Did an MSO or a PPMC provide services to your practice?

Yes .... $_1$ [   ]

No .... $_2$ [   ]

†Denotes required questions for data inclusion.

Need Help? Call Survey Operations at 877.275.6462, ext. 895.

MEDICAL GROUP MANAGEMENT ASSOCIATION™   2   ©2004 Medical Group Management Association. All rights reserved.

Appendix E: Cost Survey: 2004 Questionnaire Based on 2003 Data

Medical Group Management Association
Cost Survey: 2004 Questionnaire Based on 2003 Data

Medical Practice Information (continued)

8. **What was the legal organization of your practice? (check only one)**

   Business corporation .... ₁ ☐

   Limited liability company .... ₂ ☐

   Not-for-profit corporation/foundation .... ₃ ☐

   Partnership .... ₄ ☐

   Professional corporation/association .... ₅ ☐

   Sole proprietorship .... ₆ ☐

   Other [   ] ₇ ☐

†9. **Who was the majority owner of your practice? (check only one)**

   Government .... ₁ ☐

   *Hospital/integrated delivery system .... ₂ ☐

   Insurance company or health
   maintenance organization (HMO) .... ₃ ☐

   *MSO or PPMC .... ₄ ☐

   Physicians .... ₅ ☐

   *University or medical school .... ₆ ☐

   *Other [   ] ₇ ☐

10. **If you are a hospital/integrated delivery system, MSO or PPMC, and/or a medical practice with more than one legal entity, do you have a centralized administrative department?**

    Yes .... ₁ ☐

    No .... ₂ ☐

11. **Which population designation best describes the area surrounding the primary location of your practice? If your practice had multiple sites, choose the option that represents the location with the largest number of FTE physicians. (check only one)**

    Non-metropolitan (under 50,000) .... ₁ ☐

    Metropolitan (50,000 to 250,000) .... ₂ ☐

    Metropolitan (250,001 to 1,000,000) .... ₃ ☐

    Metropolitan (over 1,000,000) .... ₄ ☐

12. **Did your practice derive revenue from capitation contracts?**

    Yes .... ₁ ☐

    No .... ₂ ☐

13. **If you answered "Yes" to question 12, did your practice maintain a liability account for "incurred but not reported" (IBNR) amounts owed to providers outside the practice for services provided to the practice's capitated patients?**

    Yes .... ₁ ☐

    No .... ₂ ☐

14. **How many branch or satellite clinics did your practice have, not counting the primary clinic location? (if none, enter 0)**

    [   ] branch clinics

15. **What was the gross square footage of all practice facilities? (include hallways, closets, stairways and elevators)**

    [   ] square feet

16. **What accounting method was used for tax reporting purposes?**

    Cash .... ₁ ☐

    Accrual .... ₂ ☐

17. **What accounting method was used for internal management purposes?**

    Cash or modified cash .... ₁ ☐

    Accrual .... ₂ ☐

*Please indicate the name and location of your parent organization (owner) on lines 151 through 154 on page 12.
†Denotes required questions for data inclusion.

Appendix E: Cost Survey: 2004 Questionnaire Based on 2003 Data

Medical Group Management Association
Cost Survey: 2004 Questionnaire Based on 2003 Data

Medical Charges and Revenue

The questions below request information on your practice's medical charges and revenue (to the nearest whole dollar). Please provide this information for the fiscal year reported in question 1. Pages 9 to 12 in the Guide contain additional information for answering questions in this section.

Fee-for-Service Activity

Amount

18. Gross fee-for-service charges .... $ _____

19. Adjustments to fee-for-service charges (value of services performed for which payment is not expected) .... $ _____

20. Adjusted fee-for-service charges (subtract line 19 from line 18) .... $ _____

21. Bad debts due to fee-for-service activity (accounts assigned to collection agencies) .... $ _____

22. Net fee-for-service collections/revenue .... $ _____

Capitation Activity

Amount

23. Gross charges for patients covered by capitation contracts .... $ _____

24. Gross capitation revenue (per member per month capitation payments, capitation patient co-payments) .... $ _____

25. Purchased services for capitation patients .... $ _____

26. Net capitation revenue (subtract line 25 from line 24) .... $ _____

Other Medical Activity

Amount

27. Other medical revenue (research contract revenue, honoraria, teaching income) .... $ _____

28. Revenue from the sale of medical goods and services .... $ _____

29. Gross revenue from other medical activities (add lines 27 and 28) .... $ _____

30. Cost of sales and/or cost of other medical activities .... $ _____

31. Net other medical revenue (subtract line 30 from line 29) .... $ _____

Summary of Medical Charges and Revenue

Please provide the following totals even if you are unable to provide all the values requested on lines 18 through 31.

Amount

32. Total gross charges (add lines 18 and 23) .... $ _____

† 33. Total medical revenue (add lines 22, 26 and 31) .... $ _____

†Denotes required questions for data inclusion.

Need Help? Call Survey Operations at 877.275.6462, ext. 895.

MEDICAL GROUP MANAGEMENT ASSOCIATION™   4   ©2004 Medical Group Management Association. All rights reserved.

Appendix E: Cost Survey: 2004 Questionnaire Based on 2003 Data

Medical Group Management Association
Cost Survey: 2004 Questionnaire Based on 2003 Data

Support Staffing and Cost

Please provide the total full-time equivalent (FTE) support staff (to the nearest tenth FTE) in the FTE column and the associated cost (to the nearest whole dollar) in the Cost column for each category below. Pages 12 to 16 in the Guide contain additional information for answering questions in this section.

	FTE $_a$	Cost $_b$
34. General administrative (administrators, chief financial officer, medical director, human resources, marketing, purchasing, site/branch/office managers)		$
35. Patient accounting (billing manager, charge entry, billing, collection, payment and posting)		$
36. General accounting (controller, accounting manager, accounts payable, payroll accounting, budget, bookkeeping)		$
37. Managed care administrative (HMO/PPO contract administrators, quality assurance, utilization review, case management, referral coordinators)		$
38. Information technology (data processing, programming, telecommunications)		$
39. Housekeeping, maintenance, security		$
40. Medical receptionists		$
41. Medical secretaries, transcribers		$
42. Medical records		$
43. Other administrative support		$
44. Registered Nurses		$
45. Licensed Practical Nurses		$
46. Medical assistants, nurse's aides		$
47. Clinical laboratory (laboratory manager, nurses, secretaries, technicians)		$
48. Radiology and imaging (radiology manager, nurses, secretaries, technicians)		$
49. Other medical support services (services in all ancillary departments other than those listed above such as optical, physical therapy, etc.)		$
50. Total employed support staff FTE and cost (add lines 34 through 49)		$
51. Total employed support staff benefit cost (FICA, payroll taxes, employee health and life insurance, retirement)	■	$
52. Total contracted support staff (temporary)		$
† 53. Total support staff		$

(for Total support staff FTE add lines 50 and 52, FTE column)
(for Total support staff cost add lines 50, 51 and 52, Cost column)

†Denotes required questions for data inclusion.

　　　5　　　MEDICAL GROUP MANAGEMENT ASSOCIATION™

Appendix E: Cost Survey: 2004 Questionnaire Based on 2003 Data

Medical Group Management Association
Cost Survey: 2004 Questionnaire Based on 2003 Data

General Operating Cost

Please provide the operating cost (to the nearest whole dollar) for each item requested below. Pages 16 to 19 in the Guide contain additional information for answering questions in this section.

Amount

54. Information technology (data processing, computer, telecommunication services, telephone) .... $_____

55. Medical and surgical supply .... $_____

56. Building and occupancy (rental/lease, depreciation, interest on real estate loans, utilities, maintenance, security) .... $_____

57. Furniture and equipment (exclude cost for furniture and equipment used in departments described on lines 54, 63, 64 and 65) .... $_____

58. Administrative supplies and services (printing, postage, books, subscriptions, forms, stationery, purchased medical transcription services) .... $_____

59. Professional liability insurance premiums (malpractice and professional liability insurance for physicians, employees) .... $_____

60. Other insurance premiums (other policies such as fire, flood, theft, casualty, general liability, officers' and directors' liability, reinsurance) .... $_____

61. Outside professional fees (infrequent services such as legal and accounting services; management, financial and actuarial consultants) .... $_____

62. Promotion and marketing (promotion, advertising and marketing activities; fliers, brochures, yellow page listings) .... $_____

63. Clinical laboratory .... $_____

64. Radiology and imaging .... $_____

65. Other ancillary services (all ancillary services except clinical laboratory and radiology/imaging) .... $_____

66. Billing and collections purchased services .... $_____

67. Management fees paid to an MSO or PPMC .... $_____

68. Miscellaneous operating cost (recruiting; health, business and property taxes; other interest; charitable contributions; entertainment; business transportation) .... $_____

69. Cost allocated to medical practice from parent organization (indirect cost allocations or shared services) .... $_____

†70. Total general operating cost (add lines 54 through 69) .... $_____

†Denotes required questions for data inclusion.

Need Help? Call Survey Operations at 877.275.6462, ext. 895.

MEDICAL GROUP MANAGEMENT ASSOCIATION™   6

Appendix E: Cost Survey: 2004 Questionnaire Based on 2003 Data

Medical Group Management Association
Cost Survey: 2004 Questionnaire Based on 2003 Data

Total Operating Cost and Total Medical Revenue after Operating Cost

Page 19 in the Guide contains additional information for answering questions in this section.

Amount

† 71. Total operating cost (add line 53, Cost column, and line 70) .... $ [   ]

† 72. Total medical revenue after operating cost (subtract line 71 from line 33) .... $ [   ]

Provider Staffing and Cost

Please provide staffing FTE (to the nearest tenth FTE) in the FTE column and the associated cost (to the nearest whole dollar) in the Cost column. Pages 19 to 22 in the Guide contain additional information for answering questions in this section.

	FTE $_a$	Cost $_b$
Nonphysician Providers		
73. Nonphysician provider compensation	■	$
74. Nonphysician provider benefit cost	■	$
75. Total nonphysician provider (for Total nonphysician provider cost add lines 73 and 74, Cost column)	[ ]	$
Provider Consultants		
76. Provider consultant cost	■	$
Physicians		
77. Primary care physicians	[ ]	■
78. Nonsurgical specialty physicians	[ ]	■
79. Surgical specialty physicians	[ ]	■
80. Total physician compensation	■	$
81. Total physician benefit cost	■	$
† 82. Total physician	[ ]	$

(for Total physician FTE add lines 77, 78 and 79, FTE column)
(for Total physician cost add lines 80 and 81, Cost column)

83. Total provider	[ ]	$

(for Total provider FTE add lines 75 and 82, FTE column)
(for Total provider cost add lines 75, 76 and 82, Cost column)

†Denotes required questions for data inclusion.

7

MEDICAL GROUP MANAGEMENT ASSOCIATION™

Appendix E: Cost Survey: 2004 Questionnaire Based on 2003 Data

Medical Group Management Association
Cost Survey: 2004 Questionnaire Based on 2003 Data

Nonmedical Revenue and Cost

Please provide the nonmedical revenue and nonmedical cost (to the nearest whole dollar). Page 23 in the Guide contain additional information for answering questions in this section.

Amount

84. Nonmedical revenue (investment and rental revenue) .... $

85. Financial support for operating costs (from parent organization)........................ $

86. Goodwill amortization .... $

87. Nonmedical cost (income taxes).. $

88. Net nonmedical revenue (add lines 84 and 85 and subtract lines 86 and 87) .... $

Net Practice Income or Loss

Amount

89. Net practice income or loss (subtract line 83, Cost column, from line 72 and add line 88) .... $

Balance Sheet Data

Please provide the following balance sheet data (to the nearest whole dollar) at the end of your fiscal year. Page 24 in the Guide contains additional information for answering questions in this section.

Amount

90. Current assets .... $

91. Noncurrent and all other assets .... $

92. Total assets (add lines 90 and 91).. $

93. Current liabilities .... $

94. Noncurrent and all other liabilities .... $

95. Total liabilities (add lines 93 and 94) .... $

96. Total net worth (subtract line 95 from line 92) .... $

Need Help? Call Survey Operations at 877.275.6462, ext. 895.

Appendix E: Cost Survey: 2004 Questionnaire Based on 2003 Data

Medical Group Management Association
Cost Survey: 2004 Questionnaire Based on 2003 Data

Accounts Receivable

Please provide the information regarding the age of your practice's accounts receivable at the end of your fiscal year. Do not include accounts that have been assigned to collection agencies. Pages 24 and 25 in the Guide contain additional information for answering questions in this section.

Amount

97. Current to 30 days .... $ ☐

98. 31 to 60 days .... $ ☐

99. 61 to 90 days .... $ ☐

100. 91 to 120 days .... $ ☐

101. Over 120 days .... $ ☐

102. Total accounts receivable (add lines 97 through 101) .... $ ☐

103. Did your practice re-age accounts receivable when a balance was transferred to a secondary carrier or the patient's private account? .... Yes ☐₁ No ☐₂

Output Measures

Please provide the following practice output measures. For lines 104 to 112, report the number of procedures and the associated gross charges. Pages 25 to 29 in the Guide contain additional information for answering questions in this section.

	Number of Procedures$_a$	Gross Charges$_b$
104. Medical procedures conducted inside the practice's facilities (CPT codes 90281-99091, 99170-99199, 99201-99499, 77261-77799, 79000-79999)		$
105. Medical procedures conducted outside the practice's facilities (CPT codes 90281-99091, 99170-99199, 99201-99600, 77261-77799, 79000-79999)		$
106. Surgery and anesthesia procedures conducted inside the practice's facilities (CPT codes 00100-01999, 10021-69990, 99100-99142)		$
107. Surgery and anesthesia procedures conducted outside the practice's facilities (CPT codes 00100-01999, 10021-69990, 99100-99142)		$
108. Clinical laboratory and pathology procedures (CPT codes 80048-89399)		$
109. Diagnostic radiology and imaging procedures (CPT codes 70010-76499, 76506-76999, 78000-78999)		$
110. Total procedures and procedural gross charges (add lines 104 through 109)		$
111. Nonprocedural gross charges (include chemotherapy drug charges)	■	$
112. Total gross charges (add lines 110 and 111, Gross Charges column)	■	$

✔**Computation Check**: Note that the "Total gross charges" on line 112 should equal the "Total gross charges" on line 32. If these totals are not the same, an error has been made. Compare lines 32 and 112 and reconcile any discrepancy in the numbers.

9
MEDICAL GROUP MANAGEMENT ASSOCIATION™

Appendix E: Cost Survey: 2004 Questionnaire Based on 2003 Data

Medical Group Management Association
Cost Survey: 2004 Questionnaire Based on 2003 Data

Output Measures (continued)

113. How many Resource Based Relative Value Scale (RBRVS) total and physician work relative value units (RVUs) and/or American Society of Anesthesiology (ASA) units did your practice produce?

[   ] total RVUs$_a$

[   ] physician work RVUs$_b$

[   ] ASA units$_c$

114. How many patients did your practice serve?

[   ] individual patients$_a$

[   ] patient encounters$_b$

Breakout of Charges By Payer

Please estimate the percentage of your practice's "Total gross charges" (lines 32 and 112, Gross Charges column) by type of payer. The sum of the percentages on lines 115 to 127 must add to 100%. Pages 29 to 31 in the Guide contain additional information for answering questions in this section.

	Percentage
115. Medicare: fee-for-service	[ ] %
116. Medicare: managed care fee-for-service	[ ] %
117. Medicare: capitation	[ ] %
118. Medicaid: fee-for-service	[ ] %
119. Medicaid: managed care fee-for-service	[ ] %
120. Medicaid: capitation	[ ] %
121. Commercial: fee-for-service	[ ] %
122. Commercial: managed care fee-for-service	[ ] %
123. Commerical: capitation	[ ] %
124. Workers' compensation	[ ] %
125. Charity care and professional courtesy	[ ] %
126. Self-pay	[ ] %
127. Other federal government payers	[ ] %
Total	100 %

Need Help? Call Survey Operations at 877.275.6462, ext. 895.

Appendix E: Cost Survey: 2004 Questionnaire Based on 2003 Data

Medical Group Management Association
Cost Survey: 2004 Questionnaire Based on 2003 Data

Public Recognition Agreement

128. The *Performance and Practices of Successful Medical Groups: 2004 Report Based on 2003 Data* **will be based upon observed medical practices that meet established "better performer" criteria. MGMA would like to publicly recognize the exceptional performance of the practices that have earned the "better performer" distinction. In the event your practice meets or exceeds the "better performer" criteria, does your practice agree to this public recognition?**

Yes... $_1$ ☐

No... $_2$ ☐

Comments

We are very interested in your suggestions for improving this survey and other comments.

Appendix E: Cost Survey: 2004 Questionnaire Based on 2003 Data

Medical Group Management Association
Cost Survey: 2004 Questionnaire Based on 2003 Data

Questionnaire Contact

Please provide contact information for the individual who completed this questionnaire, as well as the name of the observed practice for which data is reported.

129. Name _____

130. Title _____

131. Telephone number (____) _____

132. Fax number (____) _____

133. E-mail address _____

134. Observed Practice Name _____

135. Address _____

136. City _____ 137. State _____

138. Please provide the Federal Tax ID# for the observed practice _____

139. Please report the total number of hours required to complete all parts of this survey questionnaire _____

Organizations will be mailed a Respondent Ranking Report and a complimentary copy of the survey report as a benefit of participation. To ensure this confidential information reaches the appropriate individual, please indicate below the recipient's name, organization, and mailing address in the spaces provided, if different from the information appearing on the mailing label. Please provide complete information.

140. Name _____

141. Title _____

142. Organization _____

143. Address _____

144. City _____

145. State _____

146. Zip _____

147. Telephone number (____) _____

148. E-mail address _____

149. MGMA member # _____

150. MGMA Use Only – _____

Parent Organization Information

The observed medical practice is the medical practice for which data has been reported on this questionnaire. If you indicated in question 9 on page 3, ownership of the observed practice by a 'hospital/integrated delivery system', 'MSO', 'PPMC', 'University' or 'Other' type of organization, please provide the name of the parent organization (owner) and their location in the spaces provided below.

151. Parent Name _____

152. Address _____

153. City _____

154. State _____

Comments

_____

_____

_____

_____

_____

_____

Thank you for participating and remember to keep a copy of this questionnaire for your records.

12

Appendix F: Cost Survey: 2004 Guide to the Questionnaire Based on 2003 Data

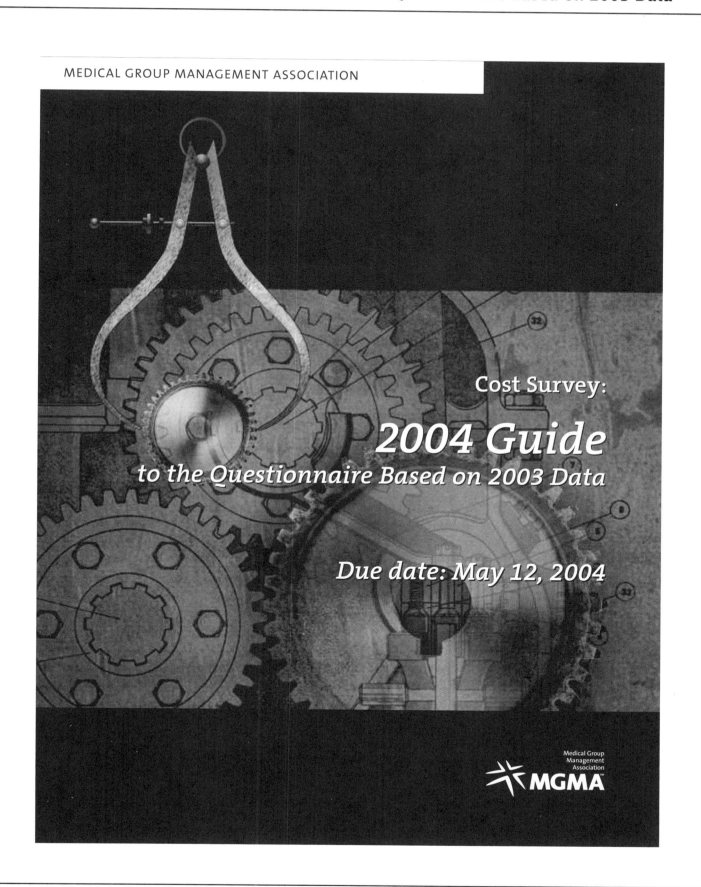

MEDICAL GROUP MANAGEMENT ASSOCIATION

Cost Survey:

2004 Guide

to the Questionnaire Based on 2003 Data

Due date: May 12, 2004

Medical Group
Management
Association

※ **MGMA**

Appendix F: Cost Survey: 2004 Guide to the Questionnaire Based on 2003 Data

Frequently Asked Questions

What is the purpose of this survey?
This survey questionnaire collects data for the *Cost Survey: 2004 Report Based on 2003 Data*. This report provides information to evaluate different aspects of medical practice performance and to help make policy decisions about medical practice operations. This questionnaire is also the principal data source for identification and evaluation of medical practices for inclusion in the Medical Group Management Association *Performance and Practices of Successful Medical Groups: 2004 Report Based on 2003 Data.*

Who is conducting this survey?
The Medical Group Management Association (MGMA) Survey Operations Department.

Who should complete this survey?
One questionnaire should be completed by the medical practice. Medical group practices comprised of at least three FTE physicians will be included in tables published in the *Cost Survey: 2004 Report Based on 2003 Data.*

If your practice consists of fewer than three physicians, you may participate in the survey, though your data may not be used in the compilation of the final report. Data from practices of fewer than three physicians in the following specialties, along with those in integrated delivery systems, will be used in the compilation of their respective specialty reports, including: cardiology, cardiovascular/thoracic surgery, anesthesia, pediatrics, pathology, orthopedics and urology.

If your organization is an Integrated Delivery System (IDS), hospital, Management Services Organization (MSO), Physician Practice Management Company (PPMC), Independent Practice Association (IPA), or other entity that owns, manages, or provides services to medical practices, one questionnaire should be completed for each medical practice that you own, manage, or service. See the Instructions on pages 4 and 5 for definitions.

Academic practices, faculty practice plans, and clinical science departments associated with medical schools should not participate in this survey. Freestanding ambulatory surgery centers should not participate in this survey. See questions 4, 5 and 6 on pages 6 and 7 for definitions. Instead, they should participate respectively in the *Academic Practice Compensation and Production Survey Questionnaire* or the *Ambulatory Surgery Center Performance Survey Questionnaire.*

Questionnaires should not be submitted for departments within multispecialty practices. A questionnaire must represent a complete medical practice.

Why should I participate?
Please see the enclosed postcard for information.

What should I do if my practice has branch or satellite clinics?
Practices with branch or satellite clinics should combine data for all sites onto one questionnaire.

Do I need to answer all of the questions on the survey?
We would appreciate receiving the requested information on your organization to the extent you can provide it. The quality of our reported results depends upon the completeness and accuracy of every response.

Survey questions with a (=) sign next to the number are required. Therefore, if any of the following questions are omitted the respondent's questionnaire will be considered incomplete and ineligible for data inclusion:
  Fiscal year (Line 1)
  Practice type (Line 2)
  Single-specialty (if applicable, Line 3)
  Freestanding ambulatory surgery center (Line 4)
  Medical school faculty practice plan/clinical science department (Line 5)
  Majority owner (Line 9)
  Total medical revenue (Line 33)
  Total support staff FTE and cost (Line 53)
  Total general operating cost (Line 70)
  Total operating cost (Line 71)
  Total medical revenue after operating cost (Line 72)
  Total physician FTE and cost (Line 82)

Appendix F: Cost Survey: 2004 Guide to the Questionnaire Based on 2003 Data

What if I am unsure about how to answer a question properly?
Please refer to the Definitions section of this Guide. For any questions about the survey questionnaire, please contact the MGMA Survey Operations Department toll-free 877.ASK.MGMA, (275.6462), extension 895, or e-mail surveys@mgma.com.

Are all survey data confidential?
Yes. The MGMA and the MGMA Center for Research Policy on Data Confidentiality states: All data submitted to the Medical Group Management Association or to the MGMA Center for Research will be kept confidential. All submitted data and related materials that identify a specific organization or individual will be safeguarded and will not be published or voluntarily released within the public domain without written permission.

Only summary statistics will be published. A summary statistic will be reported only if there are sufficient responses and if the anonymity of those submitting data is protected.

When is my response due?
The due date is May 12, 2004. The survey results will be much more useful to you if we can report the results on a timely basis. We have a very tight schedule for obtaining responses, processing the data and publishing the *Cost Survey: 2004 Report Based on 2003 Data*. Therefore, we would sincerely appreciate your giving this survey a high priority and returning your completed questionnaire as soon as you can.

What if my practice uses the *Chart of Accounts for Health Care Organizations*?
The *2004 Cost Survey Questionnaire* uses the *Chart of Accounts for Health Care Organizations* (Center for Research in Ambulatory Health Care Administration, 1999) to provide guidance in completing this questionnaire. The numbers in parentheses in the Definitions section of this booklet represent the Chart of Accounts' numbers. In some cases, the Chart of Accounts may be incomplete or over inclusive. When inconsistencies exist between the survey definitions and the Chart of Accounts, the survey definition will take precedence. The survey can be completed if the practice utilizes either cash or accrual basis accounting.

Can the data be submitted electronically?
Yes. Please go to www.mgma.com/surveys and follow the directions on the screen.

Where do I send a completed questionnaire?
Use the enclosed reply envelope and mail the completed questionnaire to the MGMA Survey Operations Department, 104 Inverness Terrace East, Englewood, CO 80112-5306. Or you may fax your response to 303.643.9567, Attention: Survey Operations. If you used the electronic version of the questionnaire, you may e-mail your response to surveys@mgma.com. **Be sure to keep a photocopy of the completed questionnaire for your reference.**

Appendix F: Cost Survey: 2004 Guide to the Questionnaire Based on 2003 Data

Instructions

The unit of observation for this survey is the medical group practice. For the purpose of this survey, a medical group practice is defined as a single legal entity or collection of legal entities consisting of three or more physicians who deliver health care services.

If your practice consists of fewer than three physicians, you may participate in the survey, though your data may not be used in the compilation of the final report. Data from practices of fewer than three physicians in the following specialties, along with those in integrated delivery systems, will be used in the compilation of their respective specialty reports, including: cardiology, cardiovascular/thoracic surgery, anesthesia, pediatrics, pathology, orthopedics and urology.

Integrated delivery systems (IDS) /Hospitals
An IDS is a network of organizations that provide or coordinate and arrange for the provision of a continuum of health care services to consumers and are willing to be held clinically and fiscally responsible for the outcomes and the health status of the populations served. Generally consisting of hospitals, physician groups, health plans, home health agencies, hospices, skilled nursing facilities, or other provider entities, these networks may be built through "virtual" integration processes encompassing contractual arrangements and strategic alliances as well as through direct ownership.

A hospital is an inpatient facility that admits patients for overnight stays, incurs nursing care costs and generates bed-day revenues.

If your organization is an IDS or hospital, that owns and/or manages medical practices, you should complete one questionnaire for each practice that you own or manage. Be sure to report the appropriate "Cost allocated to medical practice from parent organization" on line 69. A properly completed questionnaire in such a case will represent a consolidation of a portion of the information on the integrated delivery system's or hospital's income statement and balance sheet with the information from the medical practice's income statement and balance sheet. Also, complete the supplement pages found in

the *Cost Survey for Integrated Delivery System Practices: 2004 Questionnaire Based on 2003 Data.*

When completing a paper questionnaire on behalf of an owned practice, please identify the parent organization (owner) by completing the Parent Organization Information section on page 12 of the questionnaire.

Management Services Organizations (MSO), Physician Practice Management Companies (PPMC), Independent Practice Associations (IPA), etc.
If your organization is an MSO, PPMC or other type of management organization, you may also participate in the *Management Services Organization Performance Survey: 2004 Questionnaire Based on 2003 Data*, available in June 2004.

If you would like to receive a copy of the *2004 Management Services Organization Performance Survey Questionnaire*, you can call the MGMA Survey Operations Department toll-free, 877.275.6462, ext. 895, or e-mail surveys@mgma.com.

An MSO is an entity organized to provide various forms of practice management and administrative support services to health care providers. These services may include centralized billing and collections services, management information services and other components of the managed care infrastructure. MSOs do not actually deliver health care services. MSOs may be jointly or solely owned and sponsored by physicians, hospitals or other parties. Some MSOs also purchase assets of affiliated physicians and enter into long-term management service arrangements with a provider network. Some expand their ownership base by involving outside investors to help capitalize the development of such practice infrastructure.

PPMCs are usually publicly held or entrepreneurial directed enterprises that acquire total or partial ownership interests in physician organizations. PPMCs are a type of MSO, however, the motivations, goals, strategies, and structures arising from their unequivocal ownership character – development of growth and profits for their

Appendix F: Cost Survey: 2004 Guide to the Questionnaire Based on 2003 Data

investors, not for the participating providers – differentiate them from other MSO models.

An IPA is an association or network of licensed providers and/or medical practices. An IPA is usually a unique legal entity, most often operating on a for-profit basis. Typically, the primary purpose of the IPA is to secure and maintain contractual relationships between providers and health plans.

If your organization is an MSO, PPMC, IPA or other type of management organization, you should complete one questionnaire for each medical practice that you manage or service. You may make as many photocopies of this questionnaire as necessary or call MGMA to receive additional copies.

If some of the support staff functions for the medical practice are conducted by employees of an MSO, PPMC, or IPA, your responses to lines 34 through 49 should include the appropriate allocation of FTE and cost of the MSO/PPMC/IPA employees. For example, an MSO has one staff member working on managed care contracting issues on behalf of five practices. That 1.0 FTE should be disaggregated into five components and reported on five separate questionnaires. If this

MSO employee devotes an equal level of effort to each of the five managed practices, then 0.2 FTE would be included in "Managed care administrative" on line 37, FTE column, and 20% of the given MSO employee's salary would be included in "Managed care administrative" on line 37, Cost column, on each of the five questionnaires submitted by the MSO.

When completing a questionnaire on behalf of a managed practice, please identify the parent organization (owner) by completing the Parent Organization Information section on page 12 of the questionnaire.

Medical practice consisting of multiple legal entities

If your organization is a medical practice that consists of multiple legal entities, such as a professional corporation consisting of physicians, a limited liability company that provides management services and another limited liability company that owns the real estate and capital equipment, a properly completed questionnaire will represent a consolidation of the balance sheets and income statements for the three distinct legal entities.

Appendix F: Cost Survey: 2004 Guide to the Questionnaire Based on 2003 Data

Definitions

2003 Fiscal Year Definition

1. **For the purposes of reporting the information in this questionnaire, what fiscal year was used?**
   For many practices, this is January 2003 through December 2003. If your practice uses an alternative fiscal year, you are encouraged to use it in your responses. Do not report data for periods less than 12 months.

   If your medical practice was involved in a merger or acquisition during 2003 and you cannot assemble 12 months of practice data, you may not be able to participate this year. Please call the MGMA Survey Operations Department if you are uncertain about your eligibility to participate.

Medical Practice Information

2. **What was your practice type? (check only one)**
   Single-specialty: A medical practice that focuses its clinical work in one specialty. The determining factor for classifying the type of specialty is the focus of clinical work and not necessarily the specialties of the physicians in the practice. For example, a single-specialty neurosurgery practice may include a neurologist and a radiologist.

   Practices that include only the subspecialties of internal medicine should be classified as a single-specialty internal medicine practice. Internal medicine subspecialties include:
   > Allergy and immunology
   > Cardiology
   > Endocrinology/metabolism
   > Gastroenterology
   > Hematology/oncology
   > Infectious disease
   > Nephrology
   > Pulmonary disease
   > Rheumatology

   Multispecialty with primary and specialty care: A medical practice that consists of physicians practicing in different specialties, including at least one primary care specialty listed below.
   > Family practice: general
   > Family practice: sports medicine
   > Family practice: urgent care
   > Family practice: with obstetrics
   > Family practice: without obstetrics
   > Geriatrics
   > Internal medicine: general
   > Internal medicine: urgent care
   > Pediatrics: adolescent medicine
   > Pediatrics: general
   > Pediatrics: sports medicine

   Multispecialty with primary care only: A medical practice that consists of physicians practicing in more than one of the primary care specialties listed above or the surgical specialties of:
   > Obstetrics/gynecology
   > Gynecology (only)
   > Obstetrics (only)

   Multispecialty with specialty care only: A medical practice that consists of physicians practicing in different specialties, none of which are the primary care specialties listed above.

3. **If you answered "Single-specialty" for question 2, what specialty was your practice?**
   State the name of the single-specialty that most closely describes your practice.

4. **Was your organization a freestanding ambulatory surgery center only? Answer "No" if the ambulatory surgery center was a unit of the medical practice.**
   An ambulatory surgery center is a freestanding entity that is specifically licensed to provide surgery services that are performed on a same-day outpatient basis. A freestanding ambulatory surgery center does not employ physicians.

5. **Was your practice a medical school faculty practice plan and/or clinical science department?**
   A faculty practice plan is a formal framework that structures the clinical practice activities of the medical school faculty. The plan performs a range of services including billing, collections, contract negotiations and the distribution of income. Plans may form a separate legal organization or may be affiliated with the medical school through a clinical science department or teaching hospital. Faculty

Appendix F: Cost Survey: 2004 Guide to the Questionnaire Based on 2003 Data

associated with the plan must provide patient care as part of a teaching or research program.

A clinical science department is a unit of organization in a medical school with an independent chair and a single budget. The department's mission is to conduct teaching, research and/or clinical activities related to the entire spectrum of health care delivery to humans, from prevention through treatment.

6. **Was your practice affiliated with a medical school?** Answer "Yes" if your practice had a relationship in which:
   - clinicians from the medical group practice hold non-tenure appointments on a medical school faculty and/or are part of a health system that is associated with a medical school that grants a doctor of medicine (MD) degree.
   - practices having a legal standing with a medical school, faculty practice plan, or clinical science department.

   Answer "No" if your medical practice:
   - provides residency rotations, but does not meet the above criteria.

7. **Did an MSO or a PPMC provide services to your practice?**
   Answer "Yes" if your practice had a contract with an MSO or a PPMC to provide services to your practice. See pages 4 and 5 for a definition of MSO and/or PPMC.

8. **What was the legal organization of your practice? (check only one)**
   Business corporation: A for-profit organization recognized by law as a business entity separate and distinct from its shareholders. Shareholders need not be licensed in the profession practiced by the corporation.
   Limited liability company: A legal entity that is a hybrid between a corporation and a partnership, because it provides limited liability to owners like a corporation while passing profits and losses through to owners like a partnership.
   Not-for-profit corporation/foundation: An organization that has obtained special exemption under Section 501(c) of the Internal Revenue Service code that qualifies the organization to be exempt from federal income taxes. To qualify as a tax-exempt organization, a practice or faculty practice plan would have to

provide evidence of a charitable, educational or research purpose.
Partnership: An unincorporated organization where two or more individuals have agreed that they will share profits, losses, assets and liabilities, although not necessarily on an equal basis. The partnership agreement may or may not be formalized in writing.
Professional corporation/association: A for-profit organization recognized by law as a business entity separate and distinct from its shareholders. Shareholders must be licensed in the profession practiced by the organization.
Sole proprietorship: An organization with a single owner who is responsible for all profit, losses, assets and liabilities.

9. Who was the majority owner of your practice? (check only one)
   Government: A governmental organization at the federal, state or local level. Government funding is not a sufficient criterion. Government ownership is the key factor. An example would be a medical clinic at a federal, state or county correctional facility.
   Hospital/integrated delivery system (IDS): See page 3 for a definition of a hospital and IDS. If your practice is owned by a hospital/IDS, please indicate the name of your parent organization (owner) on lines 151-154, on page 12 of the questionnaire.
   Insurance company or health maintenance organization (HMO): An insurance company is an organization that indemnifies an insured party against a specified loss in return for premiums paid, as stipulated by a contract. An HMO is an insurance company that accepts responsibility for providing and delivering a predetermined set of comprehensive health maintenance and treatment services to a voluntarily enrolled population for a negotiated and fixed periodic premium.
   MSO or PPMC: See page 4 for a definition of an MSO or a PPMC. If your practice is owned by an MSO or PPMC, please indicate the name and location of your parent organization (owner) on lines 151-154, on page 12 of the questionnaire.
   Physicians: Any doctor of medicine (MD) or doctor of osteopathy (DO) who is duly licensed and qualified under the law of jurisdiction in which treatment is received.

Appendix F: Cost Survey: 2004 Guide to the Questionnaire Based on 2003 Data

University or medical school: A university is an institution of higher learning with teaching and research facilities comprising undergraduate, graduate and professional schools.
A medical school is an institution that trains physicians and awards medical and osteopathic degrees. If your practice is owned by a university or medical school, please indicate the name and location of your parent organization (owner) on lines 151-154, on page 12 of the questionnaire.
Other: If your practice is owned by an entity other than the options provided, please indicate the type of entity and location of your parent organization (owner) on lines 151-154, on page 12.

10. If you are a hospital/integrated delivery system, MSO or PPMC, and/or a medical practice with more than one legal entity, do you have a centralized administrative department?
Answer "Yes" if you have a centralized administrative department that provides leadership and has the authority/responsibility for the operations of the various physician practices within the entity. This department would provide oversight and encompass many or all of the following types of activities: establishing policies, negotiating managed care agreements, strategic planning, physician contracting, approving expenditures, as well as affording any other resources required to manage the physician practices.

11. Which population designation best describes the area surrounding the primary location of your practice? If your practice had multiple sites, choose the option that represents the location with the largest number of FTE physicians. (check only one)
Non-metropolitan (under 50,000): The community in which the practice is located is generally referred to as "rural". It is located outside of a "metropolitan statistical area" (MSA), as defined by the United States Office of Management and Budget, and has a population under 50,000.
Metropolitan (50,000 to 250,000): The community in which the practice is located is an MSA or Census Bureau defined urbanized area with a population of 50,000 to 250,000.
Metropolitan (250,001 to 1,000,000): The community in which the practice is located is an MSA or Census Bureau defined urbanized area with a population of 250,001 to 1,000,000.
Metropolitan (over 1,000,000): The community in which the practice is located is a "primary metropolitan statistical area" (PMSA) with a population over 1,000,000.

12. Did your practice derive revenue from capitation contracts?
A capitation contract is a contract in which the practice agrees to provide medical services to a defined population for a fixed price per beneficiary per month, regardless of actual services provided. Capitation contracts, which always contain an element of risk, include HMO, Medicare and Medicaid capitation contracts.

13. If you answered "Yes" to question 12, did your practice maintain a liability account for "incurred but not reported" (IBNR) amounts owed to providers outside the practice for services provided to the practice's capitated patients?
"Incurred but not reported" (IBNR) liability accounts are special liability accounts used by medical practices with capitation contracts to keep track of amounts owed to providers outside the practice for services provided to the practice's capitated patients.

14. How many branch or satellite clinics did your practice have, not counting the primary clinic location? (if none, enter 0)
The primary clinic location is the clinic with the most FTE physicians out of all the practice branches. A branch or satellite clinic is a smaller clinical facility for which the practice incurs occupancy costs (lease, depreciation, utilities, etc.). A branch is in a separate location from the practice's principal facility. Merely having physicians practice in another location does not qualify that location as a branch or satellite clinic. For example, if a physician sees patients in a hospital, this would not normally be counted as a branch or satellite clinic unless the practice pays rent for the space.

15. What was the gross square footage of all practice facilities? (include hallways, closets, stairways and elevators)
The total number of finished and occupied square feet within outside walls for all the facilities (both administrative and clinical) that

Appendix F: Cost Survey: 2004 Guide to the Questionnaire Based on 2003 Data

comprise the practice. Hallways, closets, elevators, stairways and other such spaces are included.

16. **What accounting method was used for tax reporting purposes?**
Cash: An accounting system where revenues are recorded when cash is received and costs are recorded when cash is paid out. Receivables, payables, accruals and deferrals arising from operations are ignored. On a pure cash basis, long-lived (fixed) assets are expensed when acquired, leaving cash and investments as the only assets, and borrowings and payroll withholds as the only liabilities.
Accrual: An accounting system where revenues are recorded as earned when services are performed rather than when cash is received. Cost is recorded in the period during which it is incurred, that is, when the asset or service is used, regardless of when cash is paid. Costs for goods and services that will be used to produce revenues in the future are reported as assets and recorded as costs in future periods. The accrual system balance sheet includes not only the assets and liabilities from the cash basis balance sheet but also includes the receivables from patients, prepayments and deferrals of costs, accruals of costs and revenues, and payables to suppliers.

17. **What accounting method was used for internal management purposes?**
Cash or modified cash: For "Cash," refer to the definition in question 16 above. Modified cash is an accounting system that is primarily a cash basis system, but allows the cost of long-lived (fixed) assets to be expensed through depreciation. The modified cash system recognizes inventories of goods intended for resale as assets. Under a modified cash system, purchases of buildings and equipment, leasehold improvements and payments of insurance premiums applicable to more than one accounting period are normally recorded as assets. Costs for these assets are allocated to accounting periods in a systematic manner over the length of time the practice benefits from the assets.
Accrual: Refer to the definition in question 16.

Medical Charges and Revenue

18. **Gross fee-for-service charges** (4110, 4120)
The full value, at the practice's undiscounted rates, of all services provided to fee-for-service, discounted fee-for-service and non-capitated patients for all payers.
Include:
1. professional services provided by physicians, nonphysician providers and other physician extenders such as nurses and medical assistants.
2. both the professional and technical components (TC) of laboratory, radiology, medical diagnostic and surgical procedures.
3. contractual adjustments such as Medicare charge restrictions, third-party payer contractual adjustments, charitable adjustments, and professional courtesy adjustments.
4. drug charges, including vaccinations, allergy injections, immunizations, and chemotherapy and antinausea drugs.
5. charges for supplies consumed during a patient encounter inside the practice's facilities. Charges for supplies sold to patients for consumption outside the practice's facilities are reported as a subset of "Revenue from the sale of medical goods and services" on line 28.
6. facility fees. Examples of facility fees include fees for the operation of an ambulatory surgery unit or fees for the operation of a medical practice owned by a hospital where split billing for professional and facility services is utilized.
7. charges for fee-for-service services allowed under the terms of capitation contracts.
8. charges for professional services provided on a case-rate reimbursement basis.
9. charges for purchased services for fee-for-service patients. Purchased services for fee-for-service patients are defined as services that are purchased by the practice from external providers and facilities on behalf of the practice's fee-for-service patients. For purchased services, please note the following:
   a. the revenue for such services should be included in "Net fee-for-service collections/revenue" on line 22.
   b. the cost for such services should be included, as appropriate, in "Clinical laboratory" on line 63, "Radiology and imaging" on line 64, "Other ancillary services" on line 65 and/or "Provider consultant cost" on line 76.

Appendix F: Cost Survey: 2004 Guide to the Questionnaire Based on 2003 Data

c. the count of the number of purchased procedures for fee-for-service patients should be included on lines 104 through 109, Number of Procedures column.

Do not include:

1. charges for services provided to capitation patients. Such charges are included in "Gross charges for patients covered by capitation contracts" on line 23.
2. charges for pharmaceuticals, medical supplies and equipment sold to patients primarily for use outside the practice. Examples include prescription drugs, hearing aids, optical goods, orthopedic supplies, etc. The revenue generated by such charges is included in "Revenue from the sale of medical goods and services" on line 28.
3. charges for any other activities that generate the revenue reported in "Revenue from the sale of medical goods and services" on line 28.

19. **Adjustments to fee-for-service charges** (4510, 4520, 4600-4700)
    The difference between "Gross fee-for-service charges" on line 18 and the amount expected to be paid by patients or third-party payers. This represents the value of services performed for which payment is not expected.
    Include:
    1. Medicare/Medicaid charge restrictions (the difference between the practice's full, undiscounted charge and the Medicare limiting charge).
    2. third-party payer contractual adjustments (commercial insurance and/or managed care organization).
    3. charitable, professional courtesy or employee adjustments.
    4. the difference between a gross charge and the Federally Qualified Health Center (FQHC) payment. This could be a positive or negative adjustment.

20. **Adjusted fee-for-service charges**
    Subtract line 19 from line 18.

21. **Bad debts due to fee-for-service activity** (6710, 6720)
    The difference between "Adjusted fee-for-service charges" (line 20) and the amount actually collected.
    Include:
    1. losses on settlements for less than the billed amount.

2. accounts written off as not collectible.
3. accounts assigned to collection agencies.
4. in the case of accrual accounting, the provision for bad debts.

22. **Net fee-for-service collections/revenue** (4210, 4220, 4292, 4300)
    Revenue collected from patients and third-party payers for services provided to fee-for-service, discounted fee-for-service, and non-capitated Medicare/Medicaid patients. This is the revenue remaining after patient refunds and checks returned to patients. If the practice used accrual basis accounting, "Net fee-for-service collections/revenue" on line 22 should equal "Gross fee-for-service charges" on line 18 minus "Adjustments to fee-for-service charges" on line 19, minus "Bad debts due to fee-for-service activity" on line 21.
    Include:
    1. portions of the withholds returned to a practice as part of a risk-sharing arrangement.
    2. bonuses and incentive payments paid to a practice for good performance.
    3. patient copayments.
    4. payments received due to a coordination of benefits and/or reinsurance recovery situation.
    5. revenue due to purchased services (services that are purchased by the practice from external providers and facilities on behalf of the practice's patients) for fee-for-service patients.

23. **Gross charges for patients covered by capitation contracts** (4130)
    Also known as fee-for-service equivalent gross charges. The full value, at a practice's undiscounted rates, of all covered services provided to patients covered by all capitation contracts, regardless of payer.
    Include:
    Fee-for-service equivalent gross charges for all services covered under the terms of the practice's capitation contracts, such as:
    1. professional services provided by physicians, nonphysician providers and other physician extenders such as nurses and medical assistants.
    2. both the professional and technical components (TC) of laboratory, radiology, medical diagnostic and surgical procedures.
    3. drug charges, including vaccinations, allergy injections, immunizations, and chemotherapy and antinausea drugs.

Appendix F: Cost Survey: 2004 Guide to the Questionnaire Based on 2003 Data

4. charges for supplies consumed during a patient encounter inside the practice's facilities. Charges for supplies sold to patients for consumption outside the practice's facilities are reported as a subset of "Revenue from the sale of medical goods and services" on line 28.

5. facility fees. Examples of facility fees include fees for the operation of an ambulatory surgery unit or fees for the operation of a medical practice owned by a hospital where split billing for professional and facility services is utilized.

Do not include:

1. pharmaceuticals, medical supplies and equipment sold to patients primarily for use outside the practice. Examples include prescription drugs, hearing aids, optical goods, orthopedic supplies, etc. If such goods are not covered under the capitation contract, the revenue from these charges is included in "Revenue from the sale of medical goods and services" on line 28.

2. the value of purchased services from external providers and facilities on behalf of the practice's capitation patients. The cost of these purchased services is included in "Purchased services for capitation patients" on line 25.

3. charges for fee-for-service activity allowed under the terms of capitation contracts. Such charges are reported as "Gross fee-for-service charges" on line 18.

24. **Gross capitation revenue** (4230-4283, 4530, 4291)
Revenue received in a fixed per member payment, usually on a prospective and monthly basis, to pay for all covered goods and services due to capitation patients.
Include:

1. per member per month capitation payments including those received from an HMO, Medicare AAPCC (average annual per capita cost) payments, state capitation payments for Medicaid beneficiaries and capitation payments from other medical groups.

2. portions of the capitation withholds returned to a practice as part of a risk-sharing arrangement.

3. bonuses and incentive payments paid to a practice for good capitation contract performance.

4. patient copayments or other direct payments made by capitation patients.

5. payments received due to a coordination of benefits and/or reinsurance recovery situation for capitation patients.

6. payments made by other payers for care provided to capitation patients.

Do not include:

1. payments paid to a practice by an HMO under the terms of a discounted fee-for-service managed care contract. Such payments are included in "Net fee-for-service collections/revenue," line 22.

25. **Purchased services for capitation patients** (7800)
Fees paid to health care providers and organizations external to the practice for services provided to capitation patients under the terms of capitation contracts.
Include:

1. payments to providers outside the practice for physician professional, nonphysician professional, clinical laboratory, radiology and imaging, hospital inpatient and emergency, ambulance, out of area emergency and pharmacy services, etc.

2. accrued expenses for "incurred but not reported" (IBNR) claims for purchased services for capitation patients for which invoices have not been received.

26. **Net capitation revenue**
Subtract line 25 from line 24.

27. **Other medical revenue** (4140, 4150, 4421, 4430-4480, 4540, 4550)
Grants, honoraria, research contract revenues, government support payments and educational subsidies.
Include:

1. federal, state or local government or private foundation grants to provide indigent patient care or for case management of the frail and elderly.

2. honoraria income for practice participation in educational programs.

3. research contract revenues for activities such as pharmaceutical studies.

4. educational subsidies used to train residents.

Do not include:

1. charges for the delivery of services made possible by subsidies or grants. Such charges are included in "Gross fee-for-service charges" on line 18 and/or "Gross charges

Appendix F: Cost Survey: 2004 Guide to the Questionnaire Based on 2003 Data

for patients covered by capitation contracts" on line 23.

2. the value of operating subsidies from parent organizations such as hospitals or integrated systems. Such subsidies should be included in "Financial support for operating costs" on line 85.

28. **Revenue from the sale of medical goods and services** (4140, 4410, 4420, 4540)
    Include:
    1. revenue from pharmaceuticals, medical supplies and equipment sold to patients primarily for use outside the practice. This amount should be net of write-offs and discounts. Examples include prescription drugs, hearing aids, optical goods, orthopedic supplies, etc.
    2. compensation paid by a hospital to a practice physician for services as a medical director.
    3. the hourly wages of physicians working in a hospital emergency room.
    4. contract revenue from a hospital for physician services in staffing a hospital indigent care clinic or emergency room.
    5. contract revenue from a school district for physician services in conducting physical exams for high school athletes.
    6. revenue from the preparation of court depositions, expert testimony, postmortem reports and other special reports.
    7. fees received from patients for the photocopying of patient medical records.
    Do not include:
    1. capitation revenue used to pay for covered goods and services for capitation patients. Such revenue is included in "Gross capitation revenue," line 24.

29. **Gross revenue from other medical activities**
    Add lines 27 and 28.
    Do not include:
    1. interest income, which is reported as "Nonmedical revenue" on line 84.
    2. income from practice nonmedical property such as parking areas or commercial real estate, which is reported as "Nonmedical revenue" on line 84.
    3. income from business ventures such as a billing service or parking lot, which is reported as "Nonmedical revenue" on line 84.

4. onetime gains from the sale of equipment or property, which is reported as "Nonmedical revenue" on line 84.
5. cash received from loans, which is not reported anywhere on this survey.

30. **Cost of sales and/or cost of other medical activities** (7600)
    Cost of activities that generate revenue included in "Revenue from the sale of medical goods and services" on line 28, as long as this cost is not also included in "Total operating cost" on line 71 or "Nonmedical cost" on line 87.
    Include:
    1. cost of pharmaceuticals, medical supplies and equipment sold to patients primarily for use outside the practice. Examples include prescription drugs, hearing aids, optical goods, orthopedic supplies, etc.
    Do not include:
    1. cost of drugs used in providing services including vaccinations, allergy injections, immunizations, and chemotherapy and antinausea drugs. Such cost is included in "Medical and surgical supply," on line 55.
    2. cost of medical/surgical supplies and instruments used in providing medical/surgical services. Such cost is included in "Medical and surgical supply" on line 55.

31. **Net other medical revenue**
    Subtract line 30 from line 29.

Summary of Medical Charges and Revenue
32. **Total gross charges**
    Add lines 18 and 23.

33. **Total medical revenue**
    Add lines 22, 26 and 31.

Support Staffing and Cost
Include on lines 34 through 49, FTE column:
1. the full-time equivalency (FTE) for all support staff employed by all the legal entities working in support of the medical practice represented on this questionnaire.
2. the FTE for both full-time and part-time support staff. To compute FTE, add the number of full-time (1.0 FTE) support staff to the FTE count for the part-time support staff. A full-time support staff employee works whatever number of hours the practice considers to be the minimum for a normal

Appendix F: Cost Survey: 2004 Guide to the Questionnaire Based on 2003 Data

workweek, which could be 37.5, 40, 50 hours or some other standard. To compute the FTE of a part-time support staff employee, divide the total hours worked in an average week by the number of hours that your practice considered to be a normal workweek. An employee working 30 hours compared to a normal workweek of 40 hours would be 0.75 FTE (30 divided by 40 hours). An employee working full-time for three months during a year would be 0.25 FTE (3 divided by 12 months). A support staff employee cannot be counted as more than 1.0 FTE regardless of the number of hours worked.

3. the allocated FTE where the practice consists of multiple legal entities. For example, an MSO managing two medical practices and employing one billing clerk who devotes an equal amount of time to each practice would add 0.5 FTE to the total FTE count in "Patient accounting" on line 33, FTE column, for each managed practice.

Do not include:

1. the FTE of contracted support staff, which should be reported as "Total contracted support staff" on line 52, FTE column.

Include on lines 34 through 49, Cost column:

1. salaries, bonuses, incentive payments, honoraria and profit distributions.
2. voluntary employee salary deductions used as contributions to 401(k), 403(b), or Section 125 plans.
3. compensation paid to the total FTE count reported in the FTE column.
4. compensation for all support staff employed by all of the legal entities working in support of the medical practice represented on this questionnaire.
5. the allocated support staff cost where the practice consists of multiple legal entities. For example, an MSO managing two medical practices and employing one billing clerk who devotes an equal amount of time to each practice would add 50% of the one billing clerk's compensation to the total cost of "Patient accounting" on line 35, Cost column, for each managed practice.
6. compensation for both full-time and part-time employed support staff.

Do not include:

1. nonphysician provider cost, which is reported on lines 73, 74 and 75, Cost column.

2. any benefits for employed support staff, which should be reported as "Total employed support staff benefit cost" on line 51, Cost column.
3. expense reimbursements.
4. any benefits or the cost of contracted support staff who do not work for any of the legal entities that comprise the medical practice. These costs should be reported as "Total contracted support staff" on line 52, Cost column.

34. **General administrative** (5710, 8170, 8370)
FTE and cost of general administrative and practice management staff and supporting secretaries, administrative assistants, etc.
Include:
1. FTE and cost of executive staff such as administrator, assistant administrator, chief financial officer, medical director, site/branch/office managers, human resources, marketing, credentialing and purchasing department staff.
Do not include:
1. FTE and cost of directors of departments listed separately on this questionnaire. Examples include information technology director (line 38), medical records director (line 42), laboratory director (line 47), and radiology director (line 48). Such FTE and cost should be reported on lines 38, 42, 47, or 48, as appropriate.
2. Credentialing staff as they pertain to managed care departments, such FTE and cost should be reported on line 37 "Managed care administrative."

35. **Patient accounting** (5715)
FTE and cost of patient accounting (billing and collections) staff, such as billing/accounts receivable manager, coding, charge entry, insurance, billing, collections, payment posting, refund, adjustment, and cashiering staff.

36. **General accounting** (5715)
FTE and cost of general accounting office staff such as controller, financial accounting manager, accounts payable, payroll, bookkeeping and financial accounting input staff.

Appendix F: Cost Survey: 2004 Guide to the Questionnaire Based on 2003 Data

37. **Managed care administrative** (5720)
    FTE and cost of managed care administrative staff and supporting secretaries, administrative assistants.
    Include:
    1. HMO/PPO contract administrators, case management staff, actuaries, managed care medical directors and managed care marketing, quality assurance, referral coordinators, utilization review and credentialing staff.

38. **Information technology** (5725)
    FTE and cost of data processing, computer programming and telecommunications staff.
    Include:
    1. FTE and cost of department director or manager.

39. **Housekeeping, maintenance, security** (5730)
    FTE and cost of housekeeping, maintenance and security staff.
    Do not include:
    1. FTE and cost of parking attendants if parking generates revenue, which is reported as "Nonmedical revenue" on line 84. The cost of parking attendants should be included as "Nonmedical cost" on line 87.

40. **Medical receptionists** (5735)
    FTE and cost of medical receptionists, switch-board operators, schedulers and appointment staff.
    Do not include:
    1. FTE and cost of medical receptionists, etc. who worked exclusively in the departments of clinical laboratory, radiology and imaging or other ancillary departments. Such FTE and cost is included on lines 47, 48 and 49.

41. **Medical secretaries, transcribers** (5740)
    FTE and cost of medical secretaries and transcribers.
    Do not include:
    1. FTE and cost of medical secretaries and transcribers who worked exclusively in the departments of clinical laboratory, radiology and imaging or other ancillary departments. Such FTE and cost is included on lines 47, 48 and 49.

42. **Medical records** (5745)
    FTE and cost of medical records clerks.

Include:
1. FTE and cost of department director or manager.
Do not include:
1. FTE and cost of medical records and coding staff who worked exclusively in the departments of clinical laboratory, radiology and imaging or other ancillary departments. Such FTE and cost is included on lines 47, 48 and 49.

43. **Other administrative support** (5750)
    FTE and cost of other administrative staff such as shipping and receiving, cafeteria, mailroom and laundry staff.

44. **Registered Nurses** (5755)
    FTE and cost of Registered Nurse staff and Registered Nurses working as frontline managers or lead nurses.
    Do not include:
    1. FTE and cost of nonphysician providers such as nurse practitioners, Certified Registered Nurse Anesthetists (CRNAs), or nurse midwives, which are included in "Total nonphysician provider" FTE and cost on line 75.
    2. FTE and cost of Registered Nurses who worked exclusively in the departments of clinical laboratory, radiology and imaging or other ancillary departments. Such FTE and cost is included on lines 47, 48 and 49.

45. **Licensed Practical Nurses** (5760)
    FTE and cost of Licensed Practical Nurses.
    Do not include:
    1. FTE and cost of Licensed Practical Nurses who worked exclusively in the departments of clinical laboratory, radiology and imaging or other ancillary departments. Such FTE and cost is included on lines 47, 48 and 49.

46. **Medical assistants, nurse's aides** (5765)
    FTE and cost of medical assistants and nurse's aides.
    Do not include:
    1. FTE and cost of medical assistants and nurse's aides who worked exclusively in the departments of clinical laboratory, radiology and imaging or other ancillary departments. Such FTE and cost is included on lines 47, 48 and 49.

Appendix F: Cost Survey: 2004 Guide to the Questionnaire Based on 2003 Data

47. **Clinical laboratory** (5520)
    The clinical laboratory and pathology department conducts procedures for clinical laboratory and pathology CPT codes 80048-89399.
    Include:
    1. FTE and cost of support staff such as nurses, secretaries and technicians.
    2. FTE and cost of department director or manager.

48. **Radiology and imaging** (5510)
    Film library staff and the diagnostic radiology and imaging department conducts procedures for diagnostic radiology CPT codes 70010-76499, diagnostic ultrasound CPT codes 76506-76999 and diagnostic nuclear medicine CPT codes 78000-78999, echocardiography CPT codes are 93303-93350, noninvasive vascular diagnostic studies CPT codes 93875-93990 and electrocardiograph CPT codes 93000-93350.
    Include:
    1. FTE and cost of support staff such as nurses, secretaries and technicians.
    2. FTE and cost of department director or manager.
    Do not include:
    1. FTE and staff cost for radiation oncology CPT codes 77261-77799 or therapeutic nuclear medicine CPT codes 79000-79999. Such FTE and cost is included as "Other medical support services" on line 49.

49. **Other medical support services** (5530-5550)
    FTE and cost of support staff in any ancillary services department other than clinical laboratory and radiology and imaging.
    Include:
    1. FTE and cost of support staff who provide assistance to patients, such as patient relations staff or lay counselors.
    2. FTE and cost of support staff such as nurses, secretaries and technicians in ancillary services departments such as physical therapy, optical, ambulatory surgery, radiation oncology, therapeutic nuclear medicine, clinical research, pharmacists and pharmacy support staff.
    3. FTE and cost of the department directors and managers in these ancillary services departments.

50. **Total employed support staff FTE and cost**
    Add lines 34 through 49.

51. **Total employed support staff benefit cost**
    (5610-5695, 5810-5895)
    The answer for "Total employed support staff benefit cost" on line 51, Cost column, should represent the total benefits for the FTE count of all employed support staff reported on line 50, FTE column.
    Include:
    1. employer's share of FICA (Federal Insurance Contributions Act), payroll and unemployment insurance taxes.
    2. employer's share of health, disability, life and workers' compensation insurance.
    3. employer payments to defined benefit and contribution, 401(k), 403(b) and nonqualified retirement plans.
    4. deferred compensation paid or expensed during the year.
    5. dues and memberships in professional organizations, state and local license fees, etc.
    6. allowances for education, professional meetings, travel, automobile, etc.
    7. entertainment, country/athletic club membership, travel for spouse, etc.
    Do not include:
    1. voluntary employee salary deductions used as contributions to 401(k) and 403(b) plans.
    2. expense reimbursements.

52. **Total contracted support staff (temporary)**
    (5903, 5904, 5913, 5914, 7710)
    Contracted support staff represents all the staff hired on a contract basis that are not employed by any of the legal entities that comprise the medical practice. The utilization of contracted support staff occurs when the medical practice (including all the associated legal entities that comprise the medical practice) decides not to hire support staff as employees to conduct the ongoing support staff activities described on lines 34 through 49. Instead, the practice contracts to have these full-time and/or ongoing activities conducted by contracted staff.

    A defining characteristic of contracted support staff is that the hours worked (hence the FTE) by the contracted support staff are easily identified and reported. If the hours worked are not easily identified and reported, then the FTE

Appendix F: Cost Survey: 2004 Guide to the Questionnaire Based on 2003 Data

count cannot be accurately reported and the cost for such services should be reported on one of the lines 54 through 69, as appropriate. One example of this type of cost would be purchased services for billing and collections activities. When a practice decides to hire a billing company to conduct billing activities that the practice decides not to fulfill with practice employees, it is often not possible to track the hours that the billing company devotes to the given practice. Such cost should be reported as "Billing and collections purchased services" on line 66.

Include:
1. temporary staff working for temporary agencies.

Do not include:
1. the FTE and cost of support staff employed directly by the practice or any of the legal entities comprising the medical practice. Such FTE counts and related costs are included on lines 34 through 49, FTE and Cost columns.
2. the FTE and cost for legal, accounting, management, and/or other consultants for services performed on a one time or sporadic basis. The FTE counts for these types of consultants are not reported on this questionnaire. The costs for these types of consultants are reported as "Outside professional fees" on line 61.

In the case where the exact FTE count is unknown, use your best judgment to estimate the FTE counts for "Total contracted support staff" on line 52. One method is to estimate the annual total hours worked by all the "contracted support staff" and divide that estimate by the total number of hours that the practice expects one full-time support staff employee to work during the course of one year.

53. **Total support staff**
For "Total support staff" FTE add lines 50 and 52 in the FTE column. For "Total support staff" cost add lines 50, 51 and 52 in the Cost column.

General Operating Cost
Do not include:
1. cost of sales and/or cost of other medical activities which is reported on line 30.
2. support staff cost, which is included on lines 34 through 53.

3. nonphysician provider cost, which is included on lines 73, 74 and 75.
4. cost included in "Purchased services for capitation patients" on line 25.
5. nonmedical cost which is reported on line 87.

54. **Information technology** (6120, 6220, 6304, 6420, 6430, 6530, 7120)
Cost of practice-wide data processing, computer, telephone and telecommunications services.
Include:
1. cost of local and long-distance telephone, radio paging, answering services, etc.
2. rental and/or depreciation cost of major data processing, computer and telecommunications furniture, equipment, hardware and software subject to capitalization.
3. hardware and software repair and maintenance contract cost.
4. cost of data processing services purchased from an outside service bureau.
5. cost of data processing supplies and minor software and equipment not subject to capitalization.

Do not include:
1. cost of specialized information services equipment dedicated for exclusive use in the departments of clinical laboratory, radiology and imaging or other ancillary services departments. Such cost is included on lines 63, 64 and 65.
2. cost of contract programmers, which is included in "Total contracted support staff" on line 52, Cost column.

55. **Medical and surgical supply** (7010, 7020, 7030, 7040, 7060)
Cost of supplies purchased for general practice use.
Include:
1. cost of chemotherapy drugs, allergy drugs, vaccines, etc. used in providing medical/surgical services.
2. cost of medical/surgical supplies and instruments used in providing medical/surgical services.
3. cost of laundry and linens.

Do not include:
1. cost of specialized supplies dedicated for exclusive use in the departments of clinical laboratory, radiology and imaging or other

Appendix F: Cost Survey: 2004 Guide to the Questionnaire Based on 2003 Data

ancillary services departments. Such cost is included on lines 63, 64 and 65.

2. cost of pharmaceuticals, medical supplies and equipment sold to patients primarily for use outside the practice and not used in providing medical/surgical services. Examples include prescription drugs, hearing aids, optical goods, orthopedic supplies, etc. Such cost is included in "Cost of sales and/or cost of other medical activities" on line 30.

3. the cost of any equipment subject to depreciation. Such cost is reported as a subset of lines 54, 57, 63, 64 and 65.

56. **Building and occupancy** (6150, 7070, 7510-7544, 7560, 7570, 7590, 7595)
Cost of general operation of buildings and grounds.
Include:
1. rental, operating lease and leasehold improvements for buildings and grounds
2. depreciation cost for buildings and grounds.
3. interest paid on loans for real estate used in practice operations.
4. cost of utilities such as water, electric power, space heating fuels, etc.
5. cost of supplies and materials used in housekeeping and maintenance.
6. other costs such as building repairs and security systems.
Do not include:
1. interest paid on short-term loans, which is included in "Miscellaneous operating cost" on line 68.
2. interest paid on loans for real estate not used in practice operations, such as nonmedical office space in practice-owned properties. Such interest is included in "Nonmedical cost" on line 87.
3. cost of producing revenue from sources such as parking lots or leased office space from practice-owned properties. Such cost is included in "Nonmedical cost" on line 87.

57. **Furniture and equipment** (6110, 6115, 6301-6303, 6305-6307, 6510, 6515, 6580, 7100, 7110, 7161)
Cost of furniture and equipment in general use in the practice.
Include:
1. rental and/or depreciation cost of furniture and equipment used in reception areas, patient treatment/exam rooms, physician offices, administrative areas, etc.

2. other costs related to clinic furniture and equipment, such as maintenance cost.
Do not include:
1. cost of specialized furniture and equipment dedicated for exclusive use in the information technology, clinical laboratory, radiology and imaging or other ancillary services departments. Such cost is included on lines 54, 63, 64 and 65.

58. **Administrative supplies and services** (6130, 6140, 6160, 6190-6210, 6370, 6380, 6400, 6540-6570, 6600, 6650, 6730, 7130, 7140, 7720)
Cost of printing, postage, books, subscriptions, administrative and medical forms, stationery, bank processing fees and other administrative supplies and services.
Include:
1. purchased medical transcription services.

59. **Professional liability insurance premiums** (6185-6189)
Premiums paid or self-insurance cost for malpractice and professional liability insurance for practice physicians, nonphysician providers and employees.

60. **Other insurance premiums** (6180-6184, 7580)
Cost of other policies such as fire, flood, theft, casualty, general liability, officers' and directors' liability, reinsurance, etc.

61. **Outside professional fees** (6310-6360)
Fees for professional services performed on a one time or sporadic basis.
Include:
1. fees for legal and accounting services.
2. fees for management, financial and actuarial consultants.
Do not include:
1. information services, architectural and public relations consultant fees. Such costs are included in "Information technology" on line 54, "Building and occupancy" on line 56 and "Promotion and marketing" on line 62.
2. cost for contracted support staff, which is reported as "Total contracted support staff" on line 52, Cost column.

62. **Promotion and marketing** (6170, 7050)
Cost of promotion, advertising and marketing activities, including patient newsletters,

Appendix F: Cost Survey: 2004 Guide to the Questionnaire Based on 2003 Data

information booklets, fliers, brochures, yellow page listings and public relations consultants.

63. **Clinical laboratory** (7022, 7163)
    Cost of clinical laboratory and pathology procedures defined by CPT codes 80048-89399.
    Include:
    1. rental and/or depreciation cost of major furniture and equipment subject to capitalization.
    2. repair and maintenance contract cost.
    3. cost of supplies and minor equipment not subject to capitalization.
    4. other costs unique to the clinical laboratory.
    5. cost of purchased laboratory technical services for fee-for-service patients.
    Do not include:
    1. cost of purchased laboratory technical services for capitation patients. Such cost should be reported as "Purchased services for capitation patients" on line 25.

64. **Radiology and imaging** (7021, 7162)
    Cost of diagnostic radiology and imaging procedures defined by diagnostic radiology CPT codes 70010-76499, diagnostic ultrasound CPT codes 76506-76999, diagnostic nuclear medicine CPT codes 78000-78999, echocardio-graphy CPT codes 93303-93350, noninvasive vascular diagnostic studies CPT codes 93825-93990 and electrocardiograph CPT Codes 93300-93350.
    Include:
    1. rental and/or depreciation cost of major furniture and equipment subject to capitalization.
    2. repair and maintenance contract cost.
    3. cost of supplies and minor equipment not subject to capitalization. This amount is the net after subtracting the revenue from silver recovery from X-ray film and processing fixer.
    4. other costs unique to the radiology and imaging department.
    5. cost of purchased radiology technical services for fee-for-service patients.
    Do not include:
    1. cost of purchased radiology technical services for capitation patients. Such cost should be reported as "Purchased services for capitation patients" on line 25.
    2. cost of procedures for radiation oncology CPT codes 77261-77799 or therapeutic nuclear medicine CPT codes 79000-79999.

Such costs are included in "Other ancillary services," on line 65.

65. **Other ancillary services** (7023)
    Operating costs for all ancillary services departments except clinical laboratory and radiology and imaging.
    Include:
    1. operating costs for departments such as physical therapy, optical, ambulatory surgery, radiation oncology, therapeutic nuclear medicine, etc.
    2. rental and/or depreciation cost of major furniture and equipment subject to capitalization.
    3. repair and maintenance cost.
    4. cost of supplies and minor equipment not subject to capitalization.
    5. other costs unique to the ancillary services departments.
    6. cost of purchased "other ancillary" technical services for fee-for-service patients.
    Do not include:
    1. cost of purchased "other ancillary" technical services for capitation patients. Such cost should be reported as "Purchased services for capitation patients" on line 25.
    2. cost of physical therapy and orthopedic items such as crutches, braces, etc. sold to patients. Such cost is included in "Cost of sales and/or cost of other medical activities" on line 30.
    3. cost of optical items such as eyeglasses, contact lenses, etc. sold to patients. Such cost is included in "Cost of sales and/or cost of other medical activities" on line 30.

66. **Billing and collections purchased services** (6520)
    When a medical practice decides to purchase billing and collections services from an outside organization as opposed to hiring and developing its own employed staff to conduct billing and collections activities, the cost for such purchased services should be considered "Billing and collections purchased services" and reported on line 66.

67. **Management fees paid to an MSO or PPMC** (7730-7740)
    Medical practices may receive management or other services from an MSO, PPMC, hospital or other parent organization in return for a fee.

Appendix F: Cost Survey: 2004 Guide to the Questionnaire Based on 2003 Data

The fee could be a contracted fixed amount, a percentage of collections, or any other mutually agreed upon arrangement. Whatever the methodology, report the amount here.
Include:
1. fees paid to an MSO/PPMC, hospital or parent organization for management services including management, administrative, and/or related support services.
2. the cost of support staff employed by the MSO/PPMC, etc., if these costs were not reported separately on lines 34 through 50. The decision of whether to report these support staff costs on lines 34 through 50, or on line 67 depends on the quality of the FTE data. If FTE data for the MSO/PPMC support staff is accurate and easily obtainable, it is preferable to report the MSO/PPMC support staff FTE and cost on lines 34 through 53. If the FTE counts are not known, it is suggested that the support staff cost be treated as a purchased service and be reported on line 67.

Do not include:
1. the cost of support staff employed by the MSO/PPMC, etc., if these costs were reported on lines 34 through 50.

68. **Miscellaneous operating cost** (6230-6270, 6390, 6410, 6440, 7150, 7550)
Operating cost not stated above, such as charitable contributions, employee relations dinners, picnics, entertainment, practice uniforms, business transportation, interest on loans, health, business and property taxes, recruiting cost, job position classified advertising, moving cost, payouts to retired physicians from accounts receivable, etc.
Do not include:
1. federal or state income taxes, which are included in "Nonmedical cost" on line 87.
2. principal paid on loans, which is not reported anywhere on this survey.

69. **Cost allocated to medical practice from parent organization**
When a medical practice is owned by a hospital or integrated delivery system, the parent organization often allocates indirect costs to the medical practice. These indirect costs may have different names depending on the situation. Examples of alternative names are "shared services costs" or "uncontrollable

costs." These costs may be arbitrarily assigned to the medical practice, may be the result of negotiations between the practice and the parent organization, or the result of some sort of cost accounting system. Often, these indirect costs include a portion of the salaries of the senior management team of the parent organization, a portion of corporate human resources costs, a portion of corporate marketing costs, etc.

Depending on the type of cost, the cost may be allocated to the medical practice as a function of the ratio of medical practice FTE to total system FTE, the ratio of medical practice square footage to total system square footage, or the ratio of medical practice gross charges to total system gross charges. Depending on the culture of the integrated system, these indirect costs may or may not even show up on the financial statements of the medical practice.

Regardless of what these costs are called in your system, how the costs are allocated, or what the reporting culture may be, please try to identify these costs and report them on line 69.
Do not include:
1. cash loans made to subsidiaries. Cash for loans does not appear anywhere on this survey.

70. **Total general operating cost**
Add lines 54 through 69.

Total Operating Cost and Total Medical Revenue after Operating Cost
71. **Total operating cost**
Add line 53 in the Cost column and line 70.

72. **Total medical revenue after operating cost**
Subtract line 71 from line 33.

Provider Staffing and Cost
Nonphysician Providers
73. **Nonphysician provider compensation** (8310-8360, 8380)
Nonphysician providers are specially trained and licensed providers who can provide medical care and billable services. Examples of nonphysician providers include audiologists, Certified Registered Nurse Anesthetists (CRNAs), dieticians/nutritionists, midwives, nurse practitioners, occupational therapists,

Appendix F: Cost Survey: 2004 Guide to the Questionnaire Based on 2003 Data

optometrists, physical therapists, physician assistants, psychologists, social workers, speech therapists and surgeon's assistants. Report the total compensation paid to nonphysician providers who comprise the count of "Total nonphysician provider" on line 73, FTE column.

Include:
1. compensation for both employed and contracted nonphysician providers.
2. compensation for full-time and part-time nonphysician providers.
3. salaries, bonuses, incentive payments, research contract revenue, honoraria and profit distributions.
4. voluntary employee salary deductions used as contributions to 401(k), 403(b), or Section 125 plans.

Do not include:
1. amounts included in "Nonphysician provider benefit cost" on line 74, Cost column.
2. expense reimbursements.

74. **Nonphysician provider benefit cost** (8410-8495)
    Include:
    1. employer's share of FICA, payroll and unemployment insurance taxes.
    2. employer's share of health, disability, life and workers' compensation insurance.
    3. employer payments to defined benefit and contribution, 401(k), 403(b) and nonqualified retirement plans.
    4. deferred compensation paid or expensed during the year.
    5. dues and memberships in professional organizations and state and local license fees, etc.
    6. allowances for education, professional meetings, travel, automobile, etc.
    7. entertainment, country/athletic club membership, travel for spouse, etc.

    Do not include:
    1. voluntary employee salary deductions used as contributions to 401(k) and 403(b) plans.
    2. expense reimbursements.

75. **Total nonphysician provider**
    To compute "Total nonphysician provider," FTE column, add the number of full-time (1.0 FTE) nonphysician providers to the FTE count for part-time nonphysician providers. A full-time

nonphysician provider works whatever number of hours the practice considers to be the minimum for a normal workweek, which could be 37.5, 40, 50 hours, or some other standard. To compute the FTE of a part-time nonphysician provider, divide the total hours worked by the number of hours that your practice considered to be a normal workweek. A nonphysician provider working 30 hours compared to a normal workweek of 40 hours would be 0.75 FTE (30 hours divided by 40 hours). A nonphysician provider working full-time for three months during a year would be 0.25 FTE (3 months divided by 12 months). A nonphysician provider cannot be counted as more than 1.0 FTE regardless of the number of hours worked.

To compute "Total nonphysician provider," Cost column, add lines 73 and 74 in the Cost column.

Provider Consultants
76. **Provider consultant cost** (5901, 5902, 5911, 5912)
    Include:
    1. fee-for-service fees paid to consulting pathologists, radiologists, and other consulting physicians and/or nonphysician providers who are not included in the count of "Total physician" on line 82, FTE column, or the count of "Total nonphysician provider" on line 75, FTE column.

    Do not include:
    1. costs for purchased physician and/or nonphysician provider consultation services for capitation patients. Such cost is included in "Purchased services for capitation patients" on line 25.

Physicians
Lines 77, 78 and 79 request the FTE count for primary care physicians, nonsurgical specialty physicians and surgical specialty physicians. To compute the FTE numbers for the FTE column, add the number of full-time (1.0 FTE) physicians to the FTE count for the part-time physicians. A full-time physician works whatever number of hours the practice considers to be the minimum for a normal workweek, which could be 37.5, 40, 50 hours, or some other standard. To compute the FTE of a part-time physician, divide the total hours worked by the number of hours that your

Appendix F: Cost Survey: 2004 Guide to the Questionnaire Based on 2003 Data

practice considered to be a normal workweek. A physician working 30 hours compared to a normal workweek of 40 hours would be 0.75 FTE (30 hours divided by 40 hours). A physician working full-time for three months during a year would be 0.25 FTE (3 months divided by 12 months). A medical director devoting 50% effort to clinical activity would be 0.5 FTE. A physician cannot be counted as more than 1.0 FTE regardless of the number of hours worked.

Include:
1. practice physicians such as shareholders/ partners, salaried associates, employed and contracted physicians and locum tenens.
2. residents and fellows working at the practice.
3. only physicians involved in clinical care.

Do not include:
1. full-time physician administrators or the time that a physician devotes to medical director activities. The FTE and cost for such activities should be included as "General administrative" on line 34, FTE column and Cost column.

77. **Primary care physicians**
    Include:
    Family practice: general
    Family practice: sports medicine
    Family practice: urgent care
    Family practice: with obstetrics
    Family practice: without obstetrics
    Geriatrics
    Internal medicine: general
    Internal medicine: urgent care
    Pediatrics: adolescent medicine
    Pediatrics: general
    Pediatrics: sports medicine

78. **Nonsurgical specialty physicians**
    Include:
    Allergy/immunology
    Cardiology
    Cardiology: electrophysiology
    Cardiology: invasive
    Cardiology: invasive/interventional
    Cardiology: noninvasive
    Critical care: intensivist
    Dentistry
    Dermatology
    Emergency medicine
    Endocrinology/metabolism
    Gastroenterology

Gastroenterology: hepatology
Genetics
Hematology/oncology
Hospitalist
Infectious disease
Maternal and fetal medicine
Nephrology
Neurology
Nuclear medicine
Occupational medicine
Oncology (only)
Orthopedics: nonsurgical
Pathology: anatomic
Pathology: anatomic and clinical
Pathology: clinical
Pathology: general
Pediatrics: allergy and immunology
Pediatrics: cardiology
Pediatrics: child development
Pediatrics: clinical and lab immunology
Pediatrics: critical care intensivist
Pediatrics: emergency medicine
Pediatrics: endocrinology
Pediatrics: gastroenterology
Pediatrics: genetics
Pediatrics: hematology/oncology
Pediatrics: hospitalist
Pediatrics: infectious disease
Pediatrics: neonatal medicine
Pediatrics: nephrology
Pediatrics: neurology
Pediatrics: pulmonology
Pediatrics: rheumatology
Physical medicine and rehabilitation (physiatry)
Podiatry: general
Psychiatry: child and adolescent
Psychiatry: forensic
Psychiatry: general
Psychiatry: geriatric
Public health
Pulmonary medicine
Pulmonary medicine: critical care
Radiation oncology
Radiology: diagnostic-invasive
Radiology: diagnostic-noninvasive
Radiology: nuclear medicine
Reproductive endocrinology
Rheumatology

79. **Surgical specialty physicians**
    Include:
    Anesthesiology
    Anesthesiology: pain management

Appendix F: Cost Survey: 2004 Guide to the Questionnaire Based on 2003 Data

Anesthesiology: pediatric
Dermatology: MOHS surgery
Gynecology (only)
Gynecological oncology
Obstetrics
Obstetrics/gynecology
Ophthalmology
Ophthalmology: pediatric
Ophthalmology: retina
Otorhinolaryngology
Otorhinolaryngology: pediatric
Podiatry: surgical foot and ankle
Podiatry: surgical forefoot only
Surgery: cardiovascular
Surgery: cardiovascular pediatric
Surgery: colon and rectal
Surgery: general
Surgery: neurological
Surgery: oncology
Surgery: oral
Surgery: orthopedic
Surgery: orthopedic (foot and ankle)
Surgery: orthopedic (hand)
Surgery: orthopedic (hip and joint)
Surgery: orthopedic (oncology)
Surgery: orthopedic (pediatric)
Surgery: orthopedic (spine)
Surgery: orthopedic (sports medicine)
Surgery: orthopedic (trauma)
Surgery: pediatric
Surgery: plastic and reconstruction
Surgery: plastic and reconstruction, hand
Surgery: plastic and reconstruction, pediatric
Surgery: thoracic
Surgery: transplant
Surgery: trauma
Surgery: trauma, burn
Surgery: vascular
Urology
Urology: pediatric

80. **Total physician compensation** (8110-8160, 8180)
The total compensation paid to physicians who comprise "Total physician" on line 82, FTE column.
Include:
1. compensation for shareholders/partners, associates on salary, employed physicians, contract physicians, locum tenens, residents, fellows, etc.
2. compensation for full-time and part-time physicians.

3. salaries, bonuses, incentive payments, research contract revenue, honoraria and profit distributions.
4. voluntary employee salary deductions used as contributions to 401(k), 403(b), or Section 125 plans.
5. compensation attributable to activities related to revenue in "Nonmedical revenue" on line 84.
Do not include:
1. amounts included in "Provider consultant cost" on line 76, Cost column.
2. amounts included in "Total physician benefit cost" on line 81, Cost column.
3. expense reimbursements.

81. **Total physician benefit cost** (8210-8295)
The total benefits paid to physicians who comprise "Total physician" on line 82, FTE column.
Include:
1. employer's share of FICA (Federal Insurance Contributions Act), payroll and unemployment insurance taxes.
2. employer's share of health, disability, life and workers' compensation insurance.
3. employer payments to defined benefit and contribution, 401(k), 403(b) and nonqualified retirement plans.
4. deferred compensation paid or expensed during the year.
5. dues and memberships in professional organizations and state and local license fees, etc.
6. allowances for education, professional meetings, travel, automobile, etc.
7. entertainment, country/athletic club membership, travel for spouse, etc.
Do not include:
1. voluntary employee salary deductions used as contributions to 401(k) and 403(b) plans.
2. expense reimbursements.

82. **Total physician**
For "Total physician" FTE, add lines 77, 78 and 79, FTE column.
For "Total physician" cost, add lines 80 and 81, Cost column.

83. **Total provider**
For "Total provider" FTE, add lines 75 and 82 in the FTE column. For "Total provider" cost, add lines 75, 76 and 82 in the Cost column.

Appendix F: Cost Survey: 2004 Guide to the Questionnaire Based on 2003 Data

Nonmedical Revenue and Cost

84. Nonmedical revenue (9110-9160, 9300)
Include:
1. interest and investment revenue such as interest, dividends and/or capital gains earned on savings accounts, certificates of deposit, securities, stocks, bonds and other short-term or long-term investments.
2. gross rental revenue such as rent or lease income earned from practice-owned property not used in practice operations.
3. capital gains on the sale of practice real estate or equipment, etc.
4. interest paid by insurance companies for failure to pay claims on time.
5. bounced check charges paid by patients.
6. gross revenue from business ventures such as a billing service or parking lot. The direct costs of such ventures should be reported as "Nonmedical cost" on line 87.

Do not include:
1. cash received from loans, which is not reported anywhere on this survey.

85. Financial support for operating costs (4490, 9170)
Medical practices may receive operational support from a parent organization within a hospital or other integrated delivery system. If your response to "Net practice income or loss" on line 89 is a negative value, you may not have answered line 85 correctly. Please check your response.

Include:
1. operating subsidies received from a parent organization such as a hospital, health system, PPMC or MSO.

86. Goodwill amortization
When an IDS, hospital, PPMC, etc. purchases a medical practice, the purchase price can be thought of as having two components - the value of the tangible assets and the value of the goodwill. Goodwill is the premium paid in excess of the value of the tangible assets. Goodwill may be amortized over a period of time. The tangible assets are depreciated over a period of time. For this question, please report the annual amortization cost of goodwill on line 86.

Do not include:
1. depreciation of tangible assets such as the building or equipment. These depreciation costs are reported as a component of

"Information technology" cost on line 54, "Building and occupancy" cost on line 56, "Furniture and equipment" cost on line 57, "Clinical laboratory" cost on line 63, "Radiology and imaging" cost on line 64, and "Other ancillary services" cost on line 65.

87. Nonmedical cost (9200-9243, 9300)
Include:
1. income taxes based on net profit that is paid to federal, state, or local government. For cash basis accounting, income taxes equal the cash payment or refund for the 2002 tax year paid or received in 2003 plus periodic withholding paid for 2003 taxes during 2003. For accrual accounting, the income tax equals the total tax liability for 2003 regardless of when the tax was paid or refunds were received.
2. all costs required to maintain the productivity of income producing rental property and parking lots.
3. losses on the sale of real estate or equipment and losses from the sale of marketable securities.
4. other nonmedical cost.
5. all direct costs related to business ventures such as rental property, parking lots or billing services, for which gross revenue is reported as "Nonmedical revenue" on line 84, as long as these costs are not also included in "Total operating cost" on line 71.

88. Net nonmedical revenue
Add lines 84 and 85, then subtract lines 86 and 87.

Net Practice Income or Loss

89. Net practice income or loss
Subtract line 83, Cost column, from line 72, and add line 88.

To gain perspective on the income or loss amount, divide this amount by "Total physician (FTE)" on line 82, FTE column. The result is the income or loss per FTE physician. If the positive or negative amount is over $150,000 per physician, please check your totals for "Total medical revenue" on line 33, "Total support staff" on line 53, Cost column, "Total general operating cost" on line 70, "Total provider" on line 83, Cost column and "Net nonmedical revenue" on line 88.

Appendix F: Cost Survey: 2004 Guide to the Questionnaire Based on 2003 Data

If "Net practice income or loss" on line 89 is positive, this signifies that the practice retained earnings for the 12-month reporting period. Retained earnings can be used to make investments or to pay off the practice's debt. Retained earnings are not used to compensate the practice physicians.

If "Net practice income or loss" on line 89 is negative, this signifies that the practice experienced a reduction in the assets on its balance sheet due to the 12-month reporting period operations. You may not have answered "Financial support for operating costs" on line 85 correctly. Please read the definition for line 85 to make sure your response is in accordance with the definition.

Balance Sheet Data

90. **Current assets** (1110-1550)
    Cash and other assets expected to be converted to cash, sold or consumed in the normal course of operations within one year.

91. **Noncurrent and all other assets** (1600-1961)
    Include:
    1. investments and long term receivables such as long-term investments in securities, restricted cash, property not used for operations and receivables due beyond one year. Assets recorded in these accounts are not used to finance operations.
    2. noncurrent tangible assets such as long lived tangible assets used in practice operations. Assets recorded in these accounts generally have a useful life in excess of one year.
    3. intangible and other assets such as cost of property rights without physical substance that benefits future operations. Intangible assets are purchased from external sources, provide future benefit and are relatively long lived. Other assets include long term prepayments, deferred charges and assets not included in other categories.

92. **Total assets**
    Add lines 90 and 91.

93. **Current liabilities** (2100-2390)
    Include:
    1. payables such as liabilities that mature and require payment from current assets or through the creation of other liabilities within one year.

2. payroll liabilities such as amounts withheld from employees or otherwise accrued.
3. other current liabilities such as accrued nonpayroll liabilities, advances from settlements due to third-party agencies, patient deposits, estimated contract claims payable (incurred but not reported claims), deferred revenue, deferred income taxes.

94. **Noncurrent and all other liabilities** (2400-2480)
    Long-term liabilities that mature and require payment at some time beyond one year.

95. **Total liabilities**
    Add lines 93 and 94.

96. **Total net worth** (3000-3090)
    Subtract line 95 from line 92.

Accounts Receivable

97. **Current to 30 days**
    Amounts owed to the practice by patients, third-party payers, employer groups, unions, etc. for fee-for-service activities before adjustments for anticipated payment reductions, allowances for adjustments or bad debts. Amounts assigned to "Accounts receivable" are due to "Gross fee-for-service charges" on line 18. Assignment of a charge into "Accounts receivable" is initiated at the time an invoice is submitted to a payer or patient for payment. For example, if an obstetrics practice establishes an open account for accumulation of charges when a patient is accepted into a prenatal program and the account will not be invoiced until after delivery, then "Accounts receivable" will not reflect these charges until an invoice is created. Deletion of charges from "Accounts receivable" is done when the account is paid, turned over to a collection agency or written off as bad debt. "Accounts payable to patients and payers" are subtracted from "Accounts receivable" before reporting "Accounts receivable."
    Do not include:
    1. capitation payments owed to the practice by HMOs.

98-101. Use the same definition given for line 97.

102. **Total accounts receivable**
    Add lines 97 through 101.

Appendix F: Cost Survey: 2004 Guide to the Questionnaire Based on 2003 Data

103. Did your practice re-age accounts receivable when a balance was transferred to a secondary carrier or the patient's private account?
Answer "Yes" if accounts receivable were re-aged when a second insurance company or the patient was billed after the first insurance company refused to pay the entire billed amount.

Output Measures

When reporting procedure counts and gross charges for practice activities, it is necessary to identify whether the activity occurred inside or outside the practice's facilities. This inside/outside distinction enables the proper assignment of operating costs to develop cost per unit output statistics. The Centers for Medicare and Medicaid Services (CMS) "place of service" codes are used to make this inside/outside distinction. There is one "place of service" code, the "office" code (11), that indicates activity inside the practice's facilities. All other place of service codes (12-81) are for activities occurring outside the practice's facilities. Examples of "outside" locations are the patient's home, inpatient or outpatient hospital, psychiatric or rehabilitation facility, emergency room, freestanding ambulatory surgery center, birthing center, skilled nursing or custodial care facility, hospice, ambulance, independent laboratory or radiology and imaging center, ambulatory emergency center, etc.
Include:
1. procedures performed by all practice physicians, nonphysician providers and other health care professionals such as nurses, medical assistants and technicians.
2. purchased procedures from external providers and facilities on behalf of the practice's fee-for-service patients for which revenue is reported as a subset of "Net fee-for-service collections/revenue" on line 22 and for which costs are reported as a subset of "Clinical laboratory" on line 63, "Radiology and imaging" on line 64, "Other ancillary services" on line 65 and/or "Provider consultant cost" on line 76.
Do not include:
1. purchased procedures from external providers and facilities on behalf of the practice's capitation patients for which costs are reported as "Purchased services for capitation patients" on line 25.

If the observed medical practice uses Centers for Medicare and Medicaid Common Procedural Coding System (CMSCS) codes, please use your best judgment to assign the G, H, M, Q, S, and T code counts and gross charges to the appropriate categories.

The 5 digit numbers in the following lists are the Current Procedural Terminology (CPT) codes published in *Current Procedural Terminology CPT 2003* (American Medical Association, 2003).

104. Medical procedures conducted inside the practice's facilities
Include:
Evaluation and Management Services (given an appropriate location code)
1. 99201-99215, office or other outpatient services.
2. 99241-99245, office or other outpatient consultations.
3. 99271-99275, confirmatory consultations.
4. 99354-99360, prolonged and standby services.
5. 99361-99373, case management services.
6. 99374-99380, care plan oversight services.
7. 99381-99429, preventive medicine services.
8. 99431-99432, newborn care.
9. 99450-99499, special evaluation and management services.
Radiology Services (given an appropriate location code)
10. 77261-77799, radiation oncology.
11. 79000-79999, therapeutic nuclear medicine.
Medicine Services (given an appropriate location code)
12. 90281-99090.
13. 99170-99199.
Do not include:
1. 10021-69990, surgery procedures. These procedures are reported as "Surgery and anesthesia procedures" on line 106 or 107.
2. 70010-76499, diagnostic radiology. These procedures are reported as "Diagnostic radiology and imaging procedures" on line 109.
3. 76506-76999, diagnostic ultrasound. Report on line 109.

Appendix F: Cost Survey: 2004 Guide to the Questionnaire Based on 2003 Data

4. 78000-78999, diagnostic nuclear medicine. Report on line 109.
5. 80048-89399, clinical laboratory and pathology. These procedures are reported as "Clinical laboratory and pathology procedures," line 108.

105. Medical procedures conducted outside the practice's facilities
Include:
1. the 13 items listed under line 104, given an appropriate location code.
2. 99217-99220, hospital observation services.
3. 99221-99239, hospital inpatient services.
4. 99251-99255, initial inpatient consultations.
5. 99261-99263, follow-up inpatient consultations.
6. 99281-99290, emergency services.
7. 99291-99292, critical care services.
8. 99293-99294, pediatric critical care services.
9. 99295-99299, neonatal intensive care services.
10. 99301-99316, nursing facility services.
11. 99321-99333, custodial care services.
12. 99354-99360, prolonged services.
13. 99341-99350, home services.
14. 99431-99440, newborn care.
15. 99500-99600, home health services.

106. Surgery and anesthesia procedures conducted inside the practice's facilities
Include:
1. 00100-01999, anesthesia procedures.
2. 10021-69990, surgery procedures.
3. 99100-99142, anesthesia procedures.
4. surgery and anesthesia procedures performed in the practice's own ambulatory surgery unit.

107. Surgery and anesthesia procedures conducted outside the practice's facilities
The definition for line 106 is applicable to line 107 except that the location code for line 107 must be an outside code.
Include:
1. surgery and anesthesia procedures performed in an inpatient hospital or a free-standing ambulatory surgery center.

108. Clinical laboratory and pathology procedures
Include:
1. 80048-89399, a panel of tests represented by a single CPT code is considered to be one procedure.
2. HCPCS P codes.
3. all clinical laboratory and pathology procedures conducted by laboratories outside of the practice's facilities as long as the practice pays the outside laboratory directly for the procedures and the procedures are only for the practice's fee-for-service patients. The cost for these purchased laboratory services should be reported as a subset of "Clinical laboratory" on line 63.
4. all procedures done either at the practice (where the practice bills at a global rate for both the technical and professional components) or procedures done at an outside facility (where the practice bills at a professional rate only).

Do not include:
1. purchased laboratory services from external providers and facilities on behalf of the practice's capitation patients for which costs are reported as "Purchased services for capitation patients" on line 25.

109. Diagnostic radiology and imaging procedures
Include:
1. 70010-76499, diagnostic radiology.
2. 76506-76999, diagnostic ultrasound.
3. 78000-78999, diagnostic nuclear medicine.
4. all diagnostic radiology and imaging procedures conducted by laboratories outside of the practice's facilities as long as the practice pays the outside laboratory directly for the procedures and the procedures are only for the practice's fee-for-service patients.
5. all procedures done either at the practice (where the practice bills at a global rate for both the technical and professional components) or procedures done at an outside facility (where the practice bills at a professional rate only).

Do not include:
1. 77261-77799, radiation oncology.
2. 79000-79999, therapeutic nuclear medicine. Radiation oncology and therapeutic nuclear medicine activity is included in "Medical procedures" on line 104 or 105, depending on location code.

Appendix F: Cost Survey: 2004 Guide to the Questionnaire Based on 2003 Data

3. purchased radiology services from external providers and facilities on behalf of the practice's capitation patients for which costs are reported as "Purchased services for capitation patients" on line 25.

110. **Total procedures and procedural gross charges**
Add lines 104 through 109 in each column.

111. **Nonprocedural gross charges**
Other charges not reported on lines 104 through 109 in the Gross Charges column. Include:
1. facility fee charges for the operation of an ambulatory surgery unit.
2. facility fee charges in a hospital-affiliated practice that utilizes a split billing system where both facility fees and professional charges are billed.
3. charges for drugs and medications, administered inside the practice's facilities, such as chemotherapy drugs.
4. charges for HCPCS A, J, R, and V codes.
Do not include:
1. charges for the sale of medical goods and services. Such charges are not reported anywhere on this questionnaire. "Revenue from the sale of medical goods and services" is reported on line 28.

112. **Total gross charges**
Add lines 110 and 111, Gross Charges column.

113. **How many Resource Based Relative Value Scale (RBRVS) total and physician work relative value units (RVUs) and/or American Society of Anesthesiologists (ASA) units did your practice produce?**
An RVU is a nonmonetary standard unit of measure that indicates the value of services provided by physicians, nonphysician providers, and other health care professionals. It is very useful as an index of physician productivity and medical practice productivity. Compared to gross charges, which is a very common but problematic measure of medical practice productivity, the RVU has the advantage of being constant across all practices and physicians. For example, when a medical practice conducts a procedure, the price or gross charges that the Main Street Clinic charges might be very different from the price that the Oak Street

Clinic charges. Thus, gross charges, although very common, are not very useful when comparing the productivity of medical practices that utilize different fee schedules. For a given procedure, however, the RVUs for the Main Street Clinic will always be identical to the RVUs for the Oak Street Clinic. Thus, RVUs are a very effective method for comparing practice productivity.

The RVU system is explained in detail in the December 31, 2003 Federal Register, pages 80042 to 80166. Addendum B: Relative Value Units (RVUs) and Related Information presents a table of RVUs by CPT code. Your billing system vendor should be able to load these RVUs into your system if you are not yet using RVUs for management analysis.

The following description summarizes the Federal Register information so you can accurately respond to line 113.

The total RVUs for a given procedure consist of 3 components:
1. physician work RVUs.
2. practice expense (PE) RVUs.
3. malpractice RVUs.

Thus, total RVUs = physician work RVUs + practice expense RVUs + malpractice RVUs.

For 2003, there were 2 different types of practice expense RVUs:
1. Non-facility practice expense RVUs.
2. Facility practice expense RVUs.

"Non-facility" refers to RVUs associated with a medical practice that is not affiliated with a hospital and does not utilize a split billing system that itemizes facility (hospital) charges and professional charges. "Non-facility" also applies to services performed in settings other than a hospital, skilled nursing facility or ambulatory surgery center.
Include:
1. total RVUs on line 113 that are a function of "non-facility" practice expense RVUs.

"Facility" refers to RVUs associated with a hospital affiliated medical practice that utilizes a split billing fee schedule where facility (hospital) charges and professional charges are billed separately. "Facility" also

Appendix F: Cost Survey: 2004 Guide to the Questionnaire Based on 2003 Data

refers to services performed in a hospital, skilled nursing facility or ambulatory surgery center.

Do not include:
1. total RVUs on line 113 that are a function of "facility" practice expense RVUs.

If you are a hospital affiliated medical practice that utilizes a split billing fee schedule, you should report your total RVUs on line 113 as if you were a medical practice not affiliated with a hospital.

To summarize, there are 2 different types of total RVUs that you could potentially report on line 113:
1. Non-facility practice expense RVUs.
2. Facility practice expense RVUs.

The Federal Register Addendum B presents 7 columns of RVU data. The first column labeled "Physician Work RVUs" is what you should report when answering line 113b, "physician work RVUs." Non-facility total should be reported on line 113a.

Total RVUs, line 113a
Include:
1. RVUs for the "physician work RVUs," "malpractice RVUs" and "non-facility practive expense RVUs."
2. RVUs for all professional medical and surgical services performed by physicians, nonphysician providers and other physician extenders such as nurses and medical assistants.
3. RVUs for the professional component of laboratory, radiology, medical diagnostic and surgical procedures.
4. RVUs for the technical components (TC) of laboratory, radiology, medical diagnostic and surgical procedures.
5. RVUs for all procedures performed by the medical practice. For procedures with either no listed CPT code or with an RVU value of zero, RVUs can be estimated by dividing the total gross charges for the unlisted or unvalued procedures by the practice's known average charge per RVU for all procedures that are listed and valued.
6. RVUs for procedures for both fee-for-service and capitation patients.
7. RVUs for all payers, not just Medicare.

8. RVUs for purchased procedures from external providers on behalf of the practice's fee-for-service patients.

Do not include:
1. RVUs for other scales such as McGraw-Hill, California, etc.
2. RVUs for purchased procedures from external providers on behalf of the practice's capitation patients.
3. RVUs that have been weighted by a conversion factor. Do not weigh the RVUs by a conversion factor.
4. RVUs where the Geographic Practice Cost Index (GPCI) equals any value other than one. The GPCI must be set to 1.000 (neutral).

Physician Work RVUs, line 113b.
Include:
1. RVUs for the "physician work RVUs" only.
2. physician work RVUs for all professional medical and surgical services performed by physicians, nonphysician providers, and other physician extenders such as nurses and medical assistants.
3. physician work RVUs for the professional component of laboratory, radiology, medical diagnostic and surgical procedures.
4. physician work RVUs for all procedures performed by the medical practice. For procedures with either no listed CPT code or with an RVU value of zero, RVUs can be estimated by dividing the total gross charges for the unlisted or unvalued procedures by the practice's known average charge per RVU for all procedures that are listed and valued.
5. physician work RVUs for procedures for both fee-for-service and capitation patients.
6. physician work RVUs for all payers, not just Medicare.
7. physician work RVUs for purchased procedures from external providers on behalf of the practice's fee-for-service patients.

Do not include:
1. RVUs for "malpractice RVUs" or "non-facility practice expense RVUs."
2. RVUs for the technical components (TC) of laboratory, radiology, medical diagnostic and surgical procedures.
3. RVUs for other scales, such as McGraw-Hill, California, etc.

Appendix F: Cost Survey: 2004 Guide to the Questionnaire Based on 2003 Data

4. RVUs for purchased procedures from external providers on behalf of the practice's capitation patients.
5. RVUs that have been weighted by a conversion factor. Do not weigh the RVUs by a conversion factor.
6. RVUs where the Geographic Practice Cost Index (GPCI) equals any value other than one. The GPCI must be set to 1.000 (neutral).

ASA units, line 113c.
Include:
1. if your practice recorded ASA units, write the total number of ASA units based on the 2003 American Society of Anesthesiology Relative Guide Report, on line 113c.
Do not include:
1. duplicate services.

114. How many patients did your practice serve?
Individual Patients, line 114a.
The total number of individual patients that received services from the practice during the 12-month reporting period.
Include:
1. fee-for-service and capitation patients. A patient is simply a person who received at least one service from the practice during the 12-month reporting period, regardless of the number of encounters, procedures, etc. received by that person. If a person was a patient during 2002, but did not receive any services at all during 2003, that person would not be counted as a patient for 2003. A patient is not the same as a covered life. The number of capitated patients, for example, could be less than the number of capitated covered lives if a subset of the covered lives did not utilize any services during the 12-month reporting period.

Patient Encounters, line 114b.
The total number of patient encounters during the 12-month reporting period. A documented, face-to-face contact between a patient and a provider who exercises independent judgment in the provision of services to the individual. If the patient with the same diagnosis sees two different providers on the same day, it is one encounter. If patient sees two different providers on the same day for two different diagnoses, then it is considered two encounters. The total number of patient encounters should include only procedures

from the evaluation and management chapter (CPT codes 99201-99499) or the medicine chapter (CPT codes 90800-99199) of the Physicians' Current Procedural Terminology, Fourth Edition, copyrighted by the American Medical Association (AMA).
Include:
1. pre- and post-operative visits and other visits associated with a global charge.
2. for diagnostic radiologists, report the total number of procedures or reads.
3. for obstetric care, where a single CPT-4 code is used for a global service, count each ambulatory contact as a separate ambulatory encounter (e.g., each prenatal visit and postnatal visit is an ambulatory encounter). Count the delivery as a single surgical case.
4. administration of chemotherapy drugs.
5. administration of immunizations.
6. ambulatory encounters attributed to nonphysician providers.
7. visits where there is not an identifiable contact between a patient and a physician or nonphysician provider (i.e., patient comes into the practice solely for an injection, vein puncture, EKGs, EEGs, etc. administered by an RN or technician).
Do not include:
1. encounters for the physician specialties of pathology or diagnostic radiology. (see #2 under "Include" above)
2. encounters that include procedures from the surgery chapter (CPT codes 10040-69979) or anesthesia chapter (CPT codes 00100-01999).
3. number of procedures, since a single encounter can generate multiple procedures.

Breakout of Charges by Payer
Please estimate the percentage of your practice's "Total gross charges" (line 32) by type of payer. The sum of the percentages on lines 115 to 127 must add to 100%.

Managed care: Managed health care is a system in which the provider of care is incentivized to establish mechanisms to contain costs, control utilization, and deliver services in the most appropriate settings. There are three key factors: 1) controlling the utilization of medical services; 2) shifting financial risk to the provider; and 3) reducing the use of resources in rendering treatments to patients.

Appendix F: Cost Survey: 2004 Guide to the Questionnaire Based on 2003 Data

Capitation: Capitation is when a provider organization receives a fixed, previously negotiated periodic payment per member covered by the health plan in exchange for delivering specified health care services to the members for a specified length of time regardless of how many or how few services are actually required or rendered. Per member per month (PMPM) is the commonplace calculation unit for such capitation payments.

115. Medicare: fee-for-service
Fee-for-service gross charges, at the practice's established undiscounted rates, for all services provided to Medicare patients on a fee-for-service basis. If patients are covered by both Medicare and Medicaid or a similar state health care plan, all charges for such patients should be included as Medicare fee-for-service charges.

Do not include:
1. fee-for-service equivalent gross charges for services provided to Medicare/TEFRA (Tax Equity and Fiscal Responsibility Act) patients under capitated, prepaid or other "at-risk" arrangements.
2. charges for patients covered under discounted fee-for-service contract arrangements.

116. Medicare: managed care fee-for-service
Fee-for-service gross charges, at the practice's established undiscounted rates, for all services provided to Medicare patients through a managed care plan. If patients are covered by both Medicare and Medicaid or a similar state health care plan on a fee-for-service basis, all charges for such patients should be included as Medicare fee-for-service charges.

Include:
1. charges for patients covered under discounted fee-for-service contract arrangements.

Do not include:
1. fee-for-service equivalent gross charges for services provided to Medicare/TEFRA (Tax Equity and Fiscal Responsibility Act) patients under capitated, prepaid arrangements.

117. Medicare: capitation
Fee-for-service equivalent gross charges, at the practice's undiscounted rates, for all services provided to patients under a Medicare/TEFRA, received from a capitated contract.

Do not include:
1. charges for fee-for-service patients.
2. charges for patients covered under discounted fee-for-service contract arrangements.

118. Medicaid: fee-for-service
Fee-for-service gross charges, at the practice's established undiscounted rates, for all services provided to Medicaid or similar state health care program patients on a fee-for-service basis.

Do not include:
1. fee-for-service equivalent gross charges for services provided to Medicaid or other state health care program patients under capitated, prepaid or other "at-risk" arrangements.
2. charges for patients covered under discounted fee-for-service contract arrangements.

119. Medicaid: managed care fee-for-service
Fee-for-service gross charges, at the practice's established undiscounted rates, for all services provided to Medicaid or similar state health care program patients under a managed care plan. If patients are covered by both Medicare and Medicaid or a similar state health care plan on a fee-for-service basis, all charges for such patients should be included as Medicare fee-for-service charges.

Include:
1. charges for patients covered under discounted fee-for-service contract arrangements.

Do not include:
1. charges for fee-for-service patients.
2. fee-for-service equivalent gross charges for services provided to patients under capitated, prepaid arrangements.

120. Medicaid: capitation
Fee-for-service equivalent gross charges, at the practice's undiscounted rates, for all services provided to Medicaid or similar state health care program patients under a capitated contract.

Do not include:
1. charges for fee-for-service patients.
2. charges for patients covered under discounted fee-for-service contract arrangements.

Appendix F: Cost Survey: 2004 Guide to the Questionnaire Based on 2003 Data

121. **Commercial: fee-for-service**
Fee-for-service gross charges, at the practice's undiscounted rates, for all services provided to fee-for-service patients who were covered by commercial contracts that do not include a withhold but may or may not include a performance-based incentive. A commercial contract is any contract that is not Medicare, Medicaid, or workers' compensation.
Do not include:
1. charges for Medicare patients.
2. charges for Medicaid patients.
3. charges for capitation patients.
4. charges for patients covered by a managed care plan.
5. charges for workers' compensation patients.
6. charges for charity or professional courtesy patients.
7. charges for self-pay patients.

122. **Commercial: managed care fee-for-service**
Fee-for-service gross charges, at the practice's undiscounted rates, for all services provided to patients who were covered by managed care contracts that do include a withhold and may or may not include a performance based incentive. A commercial contract is any contract that is not Medicare, Medicaid, or workers' compensation.
Include:
1. charges for patients covered under discounted fee-for-service contract arrangements.
Do not include:
1. charges for Medicare patients.
2. charges for Medicaid patients.
3. charges for capitation patients.
4. charges for workers' compensation patients.
5. charges for charity or professional courtesy patients.
6. charges for self-pay patients.

123. **Commercial: capitation**
Fee-for-service equivalent gross charges, at the practice's undiscounted rates, for all services provided to patients under a commercial capitated contract.
Do not include:
1. charges for fee-for-service patients.
2. charges for patients covered under discounted fee-for-service contract arrangements.

124. **Workers' compensation**
Fee-for-service gross charges, at the practice's undiscounted rates, for all services provided to patients covered by workers' compensation insurance.
Do not include:
1. charges for Medicare patients.
2. charges for Medicaid patients.
3. charges for charity or professional courtesy patients.
4. charges for self-pay patients.

125. **Charity care and professional courtesy**
Fee-for-service gross charges, at the practice's undiscounted rates, for all services provided to charity patients. Charity patients are patients not covered by either commercial insurance or federal, state, or local governmental health care programs and who do not have the resources to pay for services. Charity patients must be identified at the time that service is provided so that a bill for service is not prepared. Professional courtesy charges are included in this category.

126. **Self-pay**
Fee-for-service gross charges, at the practice's undiscounted rates, for all services provided to patients who pay the medical practice directly. Note that these patients may or may not have insurance.
Include:
1. charges for patients who have no insurance but do have the resources to pay for their own care and do so.
2. charges for patients who have insurance but choose to pay for their own care and submit claims to their insurance company directly. Since the practice may or may not be aware of this situation, all charges paid directly by the patient should be considered as self-pay.

127. **Other federal government payers**
Fee-for-service gross charges, at the practice's undiscounted rates, for all services provided to patients who are covered by other federal government payers other than Medicare.
Include:
1. Charges for TRICARE patients.
Do not include:
1. Charges for Medicare and Medicaid patients.

Appendix F: Cost Survey: 2004 Guide to the Questionnaire Based on 2003 Data

Public Recognition Agreement

128. The *Performance and Practices of Successful Medical Groups: 2004 Report Based on 2003 Data* will be based upon observed medical practices that meet established "better performer" criteria. MGMA would like to publicly recognize the exceptional performance of the practices that have earned the "better performer" distinction. In the event your practice meets or exceeds the "better performer" criteria, does your practice agree to this public recognition? Answer "Yes" if you agree to have your practice publicly recognized in the event that it meets the criteria as a "better performer."

Questionnaire Contact

129 – 137. If we need to clarify any responses, it would be helpful to have the name of the person who is most familiar with the completed questionnaire. Please provide complete information.

138. **Please provide the Federal Tax ID# for the observed practice.**
Please provide the Federal Tax ID # for the observed practice reported in the questionnaire. This information will be used for internal tracking purposes only, and will not be released under any circumstances.

139. **Hours to complete**
Add together the total number of hours for each individual who worked on this questionnaire.

Questions 140 – 150
Participating organizations with at least one MGMA member will receive a copy of the *Cost Survey: 2004 Report Based on 2003 Data* and the *Cost Survey: 2004 Respondent Ranking Report Based on 2003 Data,* which is a customized benchmarking report that compares the performance of the responding medical practice to all responses in the same specialty as the responding medical practice.

Respondent Ranking Reports contain customized comparisons of an organization's self-reported data to median values compiled from the survey results. The individual identified on the questionnaire label will receive the Respondent Ranking Report and complimentary survey report for your organization. If this information is incorrect, please provide complete information on lines 140 through 150 for the appropriate recipient.

Parent Organization Information

Questions 151 – 154
The observed medical practice is the medical practice for which data has been reported. If you indicated in question 9 on page 3, ownership of the observed practice by a 'hospital/ integrated delivery system', 'MSO', 'PPMC', 'University' or 'Other' type of organization, please provide the name and location of the parent organization (owner) in the spaces provided.

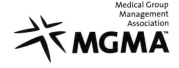

Medical Group
Management
Association

NOTES:

NOTES:

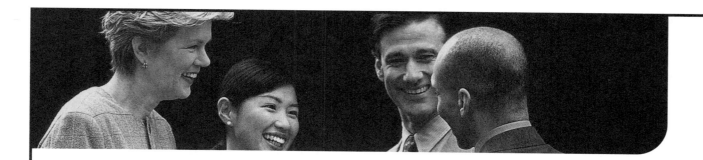

MGMA membership is great in theory.
It's *outstanding* in practice.

Vital resources. Valued results. That's why more than 19,000 of your peers and their practices depend on the benefits Medical Group Management Association (MGMA) membership provides. Whatever your professional needs, we're ready to help with:

INFORMATION. Fresh, relevant information gives you an advantage, whether you're making everyday decisions or planning long-term strategies. From industry-standard survey reports to the world-class MGMA Information Center, we keep you informed. The MGMA Health Care Consulting Group is also available to assist in improving finances, productivity and understanding benchmarking.

NETWORKING. Every professional knows the value of sharing ideas and advice with trusted colleagues. Online and in person, as an MGMA member you'll develop meaningful professional relationships that positively affect your career and your practice.

EDUCATION. We deliver varied opportunities to enhance your knowledge and skills. Online, in person, via audio and video — and special events — MGMA offers ongoing dynamic learning opportunities.

ADVOCACY. As the nation's principal voice for medical group practice, MGMA has been protecting your interests, keeping you abreast of crucial developments — and keeping you involved — for more than 75 years.

CERTIFICATION. If you want to be among the very best at the American College of Medical Practice Executives (ACMPE) can set you on the course toward respected professional board certification and Fellowship.

Want more information on membership?

Go to **www.mgma.com**, e-mail **membership@mgma.com** or call toll-free **877.275.6462**, ext. 889.

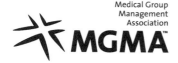

Medical Group
Management
Association

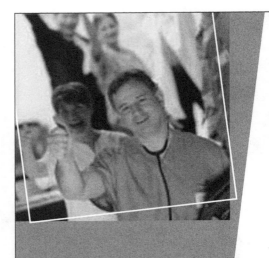

The MGMA Health Care Consulting Group

The key to practice improvement.

Your job is tough and you know you need to benchmark your practice's performance to move it to the next level of success. How do you start? How do you create more time?

The Medical Group Management Association (MGMA) health care consultants understand... first hand. We work with medical practices every day comparing their operations to the best performers in the nation. We deliver unique information and solutions.

How will you:
- Bolster low or stagnant revenue?
- Create equitable compensation plans?
- Improve inefficient operations?

If you're unsure of what to do or where to turn, the MGMA Health Care Consulting Group can help your practice set clear and measurable benchmarks. We have the expertise — with successful track records — as professional health care managers and administrators.

Contact us toll-free at 877.275.6462, ext. 877, or e-mail consulting@mgma.com.

Visit us online at www.mgma.com/consulting and pick up a few free self-assessment tools.

Toll-free *877.ASK.MGMA,* ext. *877*
consulting@mgma.com
www.mgma.com/consulting

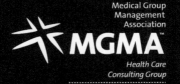

Medical Group
Management
Association

MGMA™

*Health Care
Consulting Group*

MGMA Survey Report Order Form

MGMA # _____

First name _____ MI _____ Last name _____

Title _____ Organization _____

Address _____ ☐ Work address ☐ Personal address

City _____ State _____ ZIP _____

Phone _____ Ext. _____ Fax _____ E-mail _____

☐ Male   Birth year _____   ☐ Please send me a **FREE** MGMA membership brochure. (MAA)

☐ Female Year started in medical practice management _____   ☐ Please send me a **FREE** ACMPE® board certification brochure. (AMD)

Item No.	Qty.	Description	Member	Affiliate	Other	Total Price
		Academic survey report				
PMM-6101		Academic Practice Compensation and Production Survey for Faculty & Management: 2004 Report Based on 2003 Data	$300	$350	$500	
		Cost survey reports				
PMM-6184		Cost Survey: 2004 Report Based on 2003 Data	$255	$305	$465	
PMM-6172		Cost Survey CD-ROM (Single user, additional licenses available)	$415	$465	$515	
PMM-6185		Cost Survey for Anesthesia Prac tices: 2004 Report Based on 2003 Data	$255	$305	$465	
PMM-6186		Cost Survey for Cardiovascular/Thoracic Surgery & Cardiology Practices: 2004 Report Based on 2003 Data	$255	$305	$465	
PMM-6189		Cost Survey for Integrated Delivery System Practices: 2004 Report Based on 2003 Data	$255	$305	$465	
PMM-6191		Cost Survey for Pediatric Practices: 2004 Report Based on 2003 Data	$255	$305	$465	
PMM-6193		Cost Survey for Orthopedic Practices: 2004 Report Based on 2003 Data	$255	$305	$465	
PMM-6194		Cost Survey for Urology Prac tic es: 2004 Report Based on 2003 Data	$255	$305	$465	
		Performance survey reports				
PMM-6220		Payer Performance Survey for Colorado: 2004 Report Based on 2004 Data	$ 95	$110	$160	
PMM-6198		Performance and Practices of Successful Medical Groups: 2004 Report Based on 2003 Data	$280	$330	$490	
PMM-6200		Ambulatory Surgery Center Performance Survey: 2004 Report Based on 2003 Data	$200	$270	$355	
PMM-6202		Freestanding Diagnostic Imaging Center Performance Survey: 2004 Report Based on 2003 Data	$255	$305	$465	
		Production and compensation reports				
PMM-6196		Physician Compensation and Production Survey: 2004 Report Based on 2003 Data	$270	$320	$480	
PMM-6178		Physician Compensation and Production Survey CD-ROM (Single user, additional licenses available)	$415	$465	$515	
PMM-6197		Management Compensation Survey: 2004 Report Based on 2003 Data	$130	$170	$200	
		Special offers				
PMM-6175		Cost Survey CD-ROM (single user) and report	$570	$670	$880	
PMM-6181		Physician Compensation and Production Survey CD-ROM (single user) and report	$585	$685	$895	
PMM-6205		Essentials in Benchmarking, set of four survey reports: Cost Survey; Physician Compensation and Production Survey; Management Compensation Survey; Performance and Practices of Successful Medical Groups	$805	$955	$1,435	

Online
The Store at
www.mgma.com
Search by the four-digit item number.

Phone
For credit card orders: Call toll-free
877.ASK.MGMA

Mail
Mail this form with your check payable to:
Medical Group Management Association
P.O. Box 17603
Denver, CO 80217-0603

Fax
Fax this form for credit card orders to:
303.643.4439

Shipping and handling

Orders are shipped via UPS. Federal Express is also available by request. International shipping is available. Call for pricing.

Special mail	Add
UPS Priority (next day air)	$15.50
UPS 2nd Day	$10.50

All orders must be prepaid

☐ Check enclosed

☐ Please charge my: ☐ VISA   ☐ MasterCard   ☐ AMEX

Card # _____   Exp. date _____

Card holder's name _____

Authorized signature _____

Today's date _____

Subtotal	
Shipping/Handling	$7.50
Sales tax*	
Special mail	
Total	

*Please add sales tax if a resident of:
Denver metro area 3.7%;
outside Denver metro area 2.9%;
Arapahoe County .25%;
District of Columbia 5.75%;
Texas 6.25%

Medical Group Management Association

✳MGMA®

Interactive (CD) Survey Report Order Form

Improve your bottom line with the Medical Group Management Association's (MGMA's) interactive (CD) survey reports. These interactive tools allow you to benchmark your practice performance, run customized data comparisons and identify opportunities for improvement.

Gain analytical and graphing capabilities with the CD. Use it as a complement to your reports.

We put it together. You put it to use.

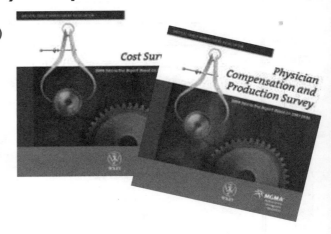

MGMA # _____

First name _____ MI _____ Last name _____

Title _____ Organization _____

Address _____ ❏ Work address ❏ Personal address

City _____ State _____ Zip _____

Phone _____ Ext. _____ Fax _____ E-mail _____

❏ Male Birth year _____ 　❏ Please send me a **FREE** MGMA membership brochure. (MAA)

❏ Female Year started in group practice management _____ 　❏ Please send me a **FREE** ACMPE® board certification brochure. (AMD)

Item No.	Qty.	Description	Member	Affiliate	Other	Total Price
Cost Survey Interactive (CD) Report						
PMM-6172		Single user, single computer system	$415	$465	$515	
PMM-6173		Network license, single site, single access	$725	$810	$895	
PMM-6174		Network license, single site, unlimited simultaneous access	$1,200	$1,350	$1,495	
Physician Compensation and Production Survey Interactive (CD) Report						
PMM-6178		Single user, single computer system	$415	$465	$515	
PMM-6179		Network license, single site, single access	$725	$810	$895	
PMM-6180		Network license, single site, unlimited simultaneous access	$1,200	$1,350	$1,495	

Subtotal	
Shipping/handling	**$7.50**
Sales tax*	
Special mail	
Total	

Online
The Store at
www.mgma.com
Search by the four-digit item number.

Phone
For credit card orders: Call toll-free
877.ASK.MGMA

Mail Mail this form with your check payable to:
Medical Group Management Association
P.O. Box 17603
Denver, CO 80217-0603

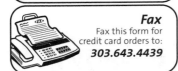

Fax
Fax this form for credit card orders to:
303.643.4439

Shipping and handling
Orders are shipped via UPS. Federal Express is also available by request. International shipping is available. Call for pricing.

Special mail	Add
UPS Priority (next day air)	$15.50
UPS 2nd day	$10.50

All orders must be prepaid

☐ Check enclosed

☐ VISA　☐ MasterCard　☐ AMEX

Card # _____ Exp. date _____

Cardholder's name _____

Authorized signature _____

Today's date _____

*Please add sales tax if a resident of:
Denver metro area 3.7%;
outside Denver metro area 2.9%;
Arapahoe County .25%;
District of Columbia, 5.75%;
Texas, 6.25%.

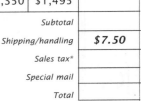

Medical Group
Management
Association

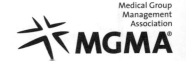